KT-448-103

ABERNATHY'S SURGICAL

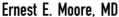

SECRETS

Sixth Edition

Alden H. Harken, MD
Professor and Chair
Department of Surgery
University of California, San Francisco–East Bay
Oakland, California
Chief of Surgery
Department of Surgery
Alameda County Medical Center
Oakland, California

Ernest E. Moore, MD
Professor and Vice Chairman
Department of Surgery
University of Colorado Health Sciences Center
Chief of Surgery and Trauma Services
Department of Surgery
Denver Health Medical Center
Denver, Colorado

MOSBY

ELSEVIER

ACQUISITION

1600 John F. Kennedy Blvd.
Ste 1800
Philadelphia, PA 19103–2899

ABERNATHY'S SURGICAL SECRETS, SIXTH EDITION   ISBN: 978-0-323-05711-0

Copyright © 2009, 2005, 2003, 2000, 1996, 1991, 1986 by Mosby, Inc., an affiliate of Elsevier Inc.

All rights reserved. No part of this publication may be reproduced or transmitted in any form or by any means, electronic or mechanical, including photocopying, recording, or any information storage and retrieval system, without permission in writing from the publisher. Permissions may be sought directly from Elsevier's Rights Department: phone: (+1) 215 239 3804 (US) or (+44) 1865 843830 (UK); fax: (+44) 1865 853333; e-mail: healthpermissions@elsevier.com. You may also complete your request on-line via the Elsevier website at http://www.elsevier.com/permissions.

NOTICE

Knowledge and best practice in this field are constantly changing. As new research and experience broaden our knowledge, changes in practice, treatment and drug therapy may become necessary or appropriate. Readers are advised to check the most current information provided (i) on procedures featured or (ii) by the manufacturer of each product to be administered, to verify the recommended dose or formula, the method and duration of administration, and contraindications. It is the responsibility of the practitioner, relying on their own experience and knowledge of the patient, to make diagnoses, to determine dosages and the best treatment for each individual patient, and to take all appropriate safety precautions. To the fullest extent of the law, neither the Publisher nor the Editor assumes any liability for any injury and/or damage to persons or property arising out of or related to any use of the material contained in this book.

The Publisher

Library of Congress Cataloging-in-Publication Data

Abernathy's surgical secrets. – 6th ed. / [edited by] Alden H. Harken, Ernest E. Moore.
   p. ; cm. – (The secrets series)
Includes bibliographical references and index.
ISBN 978-0-323-05711-0
1. Surgery–Examinations, questions, etc.   I. Abernathy, Charles.   II.
Harken, Alden H. III. Moore, Ernest Eugene. IV. Title: Surgical secrets.
V. Series.
[DNLM: 1.   Surgical Procedures, Operative–Examination Questions. WO 18.2 A146
2009]
RD37.2.S975 2009
617.0076–dc22   2008031054

Acquisitions Editor: Jim Merritt
Developmental Editor: Christine Abshire
Project Manager: Mary Stermel
Marketing Manager: Alyson Sherby

Printed in China

Last digit is the print number: 9   8   7   6   5   4   3   2   1

Working together to grow
libraries in developing countries

www.elsevier.com | www.bookaid.org | www.sabre.org

ELSEVIER   BOOK AID International   Sabre Foundation

DEDICATION

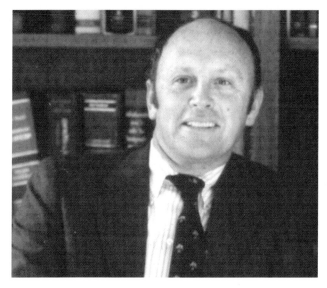

Charles M. Abernathy, M.D.
1941–1994

CONTENTS

III. ABDOMINAL SURGERY

IV. ENDOCRINE SURGERY

V. BREAST SURGERY

VI. OTHER CANCERS

IX. PEDIATRIC SURGERY

X. TRANSPLANTATION

XI. UROLOGY

XII. HEALTH CARE

CONTRIBUTORS

Brett B. Abernathy, MD
Clinical Instructor, Division of Urology, Department of Surgery, University of Colorado Health Sciences Center, Denver, Colorado; The Urology Center of Colorado, Denver, Colorado

Jason Q. Alexander, MD
Chief, Vascular Surgery, Kaiser Oakland Medical Center, Oakland, California; General Surgery Residency Site Director, Division of Vascular and Endovascular Therapy, University of California, San Francisco–East Bay, Oakland, California

David Altman, MD, MBA
Chief Medical Officer, Alameda County Medical Center, Oakland, California

Nancy C. Andersen, MD
Resident, Department of General Surgery, University of North Carolina Hospitals, Chapel Hill, North Carolina

Benjamin O. Anderson, MD
Director, Breast Health Center, Professor, Department of Surgery, University of Washington School of Medicine, Seattle, Washington

Ashok N. Babu, MD
General Surgery Resident, Department of Surgery, University of Colorado, Denver, Colorado

Thomas E. Bak, MD
Department of Transplant Surgery, University of Colorado Denver, Aurora, Colorado; University of Colorado Hospital, Denver, Colorado

Carlton C. Barnett, Jr., MD
Assistant Professor, Department of Surgery, University of Texas Southwestern Medical Center, Dallas, Texas

Joel Baumgartner, MD
Surgery Resident, Department of Surgery, University of Colorado, Denver, Colorado

Bernard Timothy Baxter, MD
Professor, Department of Surgery, University of Nebraska Medical Center, Omaha, Nebraska; Staff Surgeon, Department of Surgery, Methodist Hospital, Omaha, Nebraska

Kathryn Beauchamp, MD
Assistant Professor, Department of Neurosurgery, University of Colorado at Denver, Denver, Colorado; Neurosurgeon, Department of Neurosurgery, Denver Health Medical Center, Denver, Colorado

Allen T. Belshaw, MD
Assistant Clinical Professor, Department of Surgery, University of Colorado Health Sciences Center, Denver, Colorado; General Surgeon, Yampa Valley Medical Center, Steamboat Springs, Colorado

Denis D. Bensard, MD
Professor of Surgery, Department of Pediatric Surgery, University of Cincinnati and The Cincinnati Children's Hospital Medical Center, Cincinnati, Ohio; Director, Department of Pediatric Surgery, The Peyton Manning Children's Hospital at St. Vincent, Indianapolis, Indiana

Walter L. Biffl, MD, FACS
Assistant Professor of Surgery, Department of Surgery, University of Colorado Denver School of Medicine, Denver, Colorado; Acute Care Surgeon, Assistant Director of Patient Quality and Safety, Department of Surgery, Denver Health Medical Center, Denver, Colorado

Natasha D. Bir, MD, MHS
Resident, Department of Surgery, University of California, San Francisco–East Bay, Oakland, California

Elizabeth C. Brew, MD
Department of Surgery, Foothills Surgical Associates, Wheat Ridge, Colorado

Laurence H. Brinckerhoff, MD
Chief, General Thoracic Surgery, Assistant Professor, Department of Surgery, Tufts Medical Center, Boston, Massachusetts

Jamie M. Brown, MD
Associate Professor of Surgery, Department of Surgery, University of Maryland, Baltimore, Maryland; Associate Professor of Surgery, Department of Surgery, University of Maryland Medical Center, Baltimore, Maryland

Mark P. Cain, MD
Professor, Department of Urology, Indiana University, Indianapolis, Indiana; Riley Hospital for Children, Indianapolis, Indiana

Kristine E. Calhoun, MD
Assistant Professor, Department of Surgery, University of Washington School of Medicine, Seattle, Washington

Brian P. Callahan, MD
Chief Resident, Department of Neurosurgery, University of Colorado Health Sciences Center, Denver, Colorado

Jeffrey Campsen, MD
Surgical Transplant Fellow, Department of Transplantation, University of Colorado Health Sciences Center, Aurora, Colorado

Anne Cannon, RN, BSN
Ventricular Assist Device Coordinator, Department of Cardiothoracic Surgery, University of Colorado Hospital, Aurora, Colorado

Mario F. Chammas, Jr., MD
Urologist, Department of Urology, University of Colorado Denver, Aurora, Colorado; Urologist, Department of Urology, Denver Health Medical Center, Denver, Colorado

David J. Ciesla, MD, MS
Associate Professor, Department of Surgery, University of South Florida, Tampa, Florida; Director of Trauma and Surgical Critical Care, Department of Surgery, Tampa General Hospital, Tampa, Florida

Joseph C. Cleveland, Jr., MD
Associate Professor of Surgery, Surgical Director, Cardiac Transplant and MCS, Department of Surgery, University of Colorado at Denver, Aurora, Colorado; Associate Professor, Department of Surgery, University of Colorado Hospital, Aurora, Colorado; Chief, CT Surgery, Department of Surgery, Denver Veterans Affairs Medical Center, Denver, Colorado

C. Clay Cothren, MD
Assistant Professor, Department of Surgery, University of Colorado School of Medicine, Denver, Colorado; Program Director, Surgical Critical Care & TACS Fellowships, Department of Surgery, Denver Health Medical Center, Denver, Colorado

Paul R. Crisostomo, MD
Research Fellow, Department of Surgery, Indiana University, Indianapolis, Indiana; Resident in Surgery, Department of Surgery, Indiana University, Indianapolis, Indiana

Elizabeth L. Cureton, MD
Resident in General Surgery, Department of Surgery, University of California, San Francisco–East Bay, Alameda County Medical Center, Oakland, California

Laura DiMatteo, MD
Orthopaedic Surgery Resident, Department of Orthopaedics, University of Colorado Health Sciences Center, Denver, Colorado

Alexander Q. Ereso, MD
Chief Resident, Department of Surgery, University of California, San Francisco–East Bay, Alameda County Medical Center, Oakland, California

Michael E. Fenoglio, MD
General Surgeon, Department of General Surgery, Presbyterian St. Luke's Hospital, Denver, Colorado; General Surgeon, Department of General Surgery, St. Joseph's Hospital, Denver, Colorado; General Surgeon, Department of General Surgery, University of Colorado Health Sciences Center, Denver, Colorado

Christina A. Finlayson, MD
Associate Professor, Department of Surgery, University of Colorado Denver, Aurora, Colorado; Director, Diane O'Connor Thompson Breast Center, University of Colorado Hospital, Aurora, Colorado

David A. Fullerton, MD
Professor and Division Head, Department of Cardiothoracic Surgery, University of Colorado Denver, Aurora, Colorado; Faculty Surgeon, Department of Surgery, Division of Cardiothoracic Surgery, University Hospital, Aurora, Colorado; Faculty Surgeon, Department of Cardiothoracic Surgery, The Children's Hospital, Aurora, Colorado; Faculty Surgeon, Department of Cardiothoracic Surgery, Veterans Administration Medical Center, Denver, Colorado

Glenn W. Geelhoed, MD, MPH, MA, DTMH, ScD (Hon), MA, MPhil, EdD, FACS
Professor of Surgery, International Medical Education, Microbiology, Immunology, and Tropical Medicine, Departments of Surgery and Microbiology, Immunology, and Tropical Medicine, Office of the Dean, George Washington University Medical Center, Washington, DC; Distinguished Global Professor of International Medicine, Center for Creative Learning, University of Toledo Medical Sciences Center, Toledo, Ohio; Distinguished Professor of Obstetrics and Gynecology, Department of Obstetrics and Gynecology and Maternal Fetal Medicine, State University of New York Upstate, Syracuse, New York

Ricardo J. Gonzalez, MD
Assistant Professor of Surgery, Department of Surgery, University of Colorado, Aurora, Colorado

Raffi Gurunluoglu, MD, PhD
Associate Professor, Department of Plastic Surgery, University of Colorado Health Sciences Center, Denver, Colorado; Chief and Associate Professor, Department of Plastic Surgery, Denver Health Medical Center, Denver, Colorado

Richard-Tien V. Ha, MD
Surgery Resident, Department of Surgery, University of California, San Francisco–East Bay, Oakland, California

James B. Haenel, RRT
Surgical Critical Care Specialist, Department of Surgery, Denver Health Medical Center, Denver, Colorado

Alden H. Harken, MD
Professor and Chair, Department of Surgery, University of California, San Francisco–East Bay, Oakland, California; Chief of Surgery, Department of Surgery, Alameda County Medical Center, Oakland, California

Tabetha R. Harken, MD, MPH
Fellow in Obstetrics and Gynecology, University of California at San Francisco, San Francisco, California

Richard J. Hendrickson, MD
Pediatric Surgeon, Indianapolis, Indiana

Laurel R. Imhoff, MD, MPH
Surgical Resident, Department of Surgery, University of California, San Francisco–East Bay, Alameda County Medical Center, Oakland, California

Ramin Jamshidi, MD
Resident, Department of Surgery, University of California, San Francisco, San Francisco, California

Jeffrey L. Johnson, MD
Director, SICU, Department of Surgery, Denver Health Medical Center, Denver, Colorado; Assistant Professor of Surgery, University of Colorado Denver School of Medicine, Aurora, Colorado

Darrell N. Jones, PhD
Administrator, Vascular Surgery, Department of Surgery, University of Colorado Denver, Aurora, Colorado; Director, Department of Vascular Diagnostics, University of Colorado Hospital, Aurora, Colorado

Janeen R. Jordan, MD
Resident, Department of Surgery, University of Colorado Denver Health Sciences Program, Denver, Colorado; Resident, Department of Surgery, Denver Health Medical Center, Denver, Colorado; Department of Surgery, University of Colorado Hospital, Denver, Colorado

Sarah Judkins, MD
General Surgery Resident, Department of Surgery, University of Colorado Health Sciences Center, Denver, Colorado

Frederick M. Karrer, MD
Professor of Surgery and Pediatrics, University of Colorado Denver School of Medicine; Professor, Department of Surgery, The Children's Hospital, Denver, Colorado

Jeffry L. Kashuk, MD, FACS
Assistant Professor of Surgery, Department of Surgery Trauma, Denver Health Rocky Mountain Trauma Center, Denver, Colorado; Assistant Professor, Department of Surgery, University of Colorado Health Sciences Center, Denver, Colorado

Jarrod N. Keith, MD
General Surgery Resident, Department of Surgery, University of Colorado Health Sciences Center, Denver, Colorado

Fernando J. Kim, MD, FACS
Associate Professor, Director of Minimally Invasive Urological Oncology, University of Colorado Health Sciences Center, Tony Grampsas Cancer Center, Denver, Colorado; Chief of Urology, Department of Surgery, Denver Medical Center, Denver, Colorado

G. Edward Kimm, Jr., MD
Assistant Clinical Professor, Department of Surgery, University of Colorado Health Sciences Center, Denver, Colorado; Attending Surgeon, Department of Surgery, Denver Health Medical Center, Denver, Colorado

Ann Marie Kulungowski, MD
General Surgery Resident, Department of General Surgery, University of Colorado Hospital, Aurora, Colorado

Adam H. Lackey, MD
Resident, Department of Surgery, University of Colorado Health Sciences Center, Denver, Colorado

Michael L. Lepore, MD, FACS
Professor, Department of Otolaryngology–Head and Neck Surgery, University of Colorado School of Medicine, Denver, Colorado; Director of Otolaryngology–Head and Neck Surgery, Department of Surgery, Denver Health Medical

Center, Denver, Colorado; Professor, Department of Surgery, Department of Veterans Affairs, Denver, Colorado; Professor, Department of Otolaryngology–Head and Neck Surgery, University Hospital, Denver, Colorado

Kathleen R. Liscum, MD
Associate Professor, Department of Surgery, Baylor College of Medicine, Houston, Texas; Chief of General Surgery, Department of Surgery, Ben Taub General Hospital, Houston, Texas

Andrew E. Luckey, MD
Private Practice, General and Laparoscopic Surgery, Los Angeles, California

Joyce A. Majure, MD
Department of Surgery, St. Joseph Regional Medical Center, Lewiston, Idaho

Martin D. McCarter, MD
Associate Professor, Division of GI Tumor and Endocrine Surgery, University of Colorado Denver School of Medicine, Denver, Colorado; University of Colorado Hospital, Aurora, Colorado

Robert C. McIntyre, Jr., MD
Associate Professor, Department of Surgery, University of Colorado Denver School of Medicine, Aurora, Colorado

Nadia McMillan
Student, Johns Hopkins University, Baltimore, Maryland

Margaret M. McQuiggan, MS, RD, CNSD
Clinical Research Specialist, Department of Surgery, The Methodist Hospital Research Institute, Houston, Texas

Randall B. Meacham, MD
Professor, Division Head, Residency Program Director, Division of Urology, University of Colorado Denver School of Medicine, Aurora, Colorado; Practice Director, Department of Urology, University of Colorado Hospital, Aurora, Colorado; Staff, Department of Surgery/Urology, Veterans Administration Medical Center, Denver, Colorado; Staff, Department of Urology, Denver Medical Center, Denver, Colorado

Daniel R. Meldrum, MD, FACS
Director of Research, Associate Professor, Department of Cardiothoracic Surgery, Indiana University, Indianapolis, Indiana; Staff Cardiothoracic Surgeon, Department of Cardiothoracic Surgery, VA Medical Center, Indianapolis, Indiana; Staff Cardiothoracic Surgeon, Department of Cardiothoracic Surgery, Indiana University Medical Center, Indianapolis, Indiana

Kirstan K. Meldrum, MD
Assistant Professor, Department of Pediatric Urology, Indiana University School of Medicine, Indianapolis, Indiana

Ryan P. Merkow, MD
Department of Surgery, University of Colorado Denver Medical School, Denver, Colorado; Department of Surgery, University of Colorado Hospital, Denver, Colorado

Ernest E. Moore, MD
Professor and Vice Chairman, Department of Surgery, University of Colorado Health Sciences Center, Denver, Colorado; Chief of Surgery and Trauma Services, Department of Surgery, Denver Health Medical Center, Denver, Colorado

Frederick A. Moore, MD, FACS
Professor, Department of Surgery, Weill Cornell Medical College, New York, New York; Head, Division of Surgical Critical Care and Acute Care Surgery, Department of Surgery, The Methodist Hospital, Houston, Texas

Steven J. Morgan, MD, FACS
Associate Professor, Department of Orthopaedics, University of Colorado School of Medicine, Denver, Colorado; Associate Director, Department of Orthopaedics, Denver Health Medical Center, Denver, Colorado

Mark R. Nehler, MD
Program Director, Department of Surgery, University of Colorado Health Sciences Center, Denver, Colorado; Associate Professor of Surgery, Department of Surgery, Denver VA Medical Center, Denver, Colorado

Tony T. Nguyen, DO
Chief Surgery Resident, Department of Surgery, University of California, San Francisco–East Bay Surgical Residency Program, Oakland, California

Lawrence W. Norton, MD
Emeritus Professor, Department of Surgery, University of Colorado School of Medicine, Aurora, Colorado

Trevor L. Nydam, MD
Resident, Department of Surgery, University of Colorado Denver School of Medicine, Aurora, Colorado

Kagan Ozer, MD
Associate Professor, Department of Orthopedic Surgery, University of Colorado, Denver, Colorado; Chief of Hand Surgery, Department of Orthopedic Surgery, Denver Health Medical Center, Denver, Colorado

Cyrus J. Parsa, MD
Chief Resident, Department of Thoracic Surgery, Duke University, Durham, North Carolina

David A. Partrick, MD
Associate Professor, Department of Pediatric Surgery, University of Colorado, Denver, Colorado; Chief of Pediatric Surgery, Denver Health Medical Center, Denver, Colorado; Associate Professor, Pediatrics, The Children's Hospital, Denver, Colorado

Nathan W. Pearlman, MD
Professor, Department of Surgery, University of Colorado Health Science Center, Denver, Colorado; Attending Surgeon, Department of Surgery, Denver VA Medical Center, Denver, Colorado

Erik D. Peltz, DO
Surgical Resident, Department of Surgery, University of Colorado at Denver, Denver, Colorado; Surgical Resident, Surgical Research Fellow, Department of Surgery/Trauma Research Center, Denver Health Medical Center, Denver, Colorado

Steven L. Peterson, DVM, MD
Associate Professor, Department of Surgery, Oregon Health Sciences University, Portland, Oregon; Hand & Plastic Surgery Service, Division of Plastic Surgery, Department of Surgery, Portland Veterans Administration, Portland, Oregon

Marvin Pomerantz, MD
Professor of Surgery and Director of the Center for the Surgical Treatment of Lung Infections, Department of Surgery, Division of Cardiothoracic Surgery, University of Colorado Denver, Aurora, Colorado; Professor of Surgery, Department of Surgery, University of Colorado Hospital, Aurora, Colorado

Craig H. Rabb, MD
Associate Professor, Department of Neurosurgery, University of Colorado School of Medicine, Denver, Colorado; Chief, Neurosurgery, Department of Neurosurgery, Denver Health Medical Center, Denver, Colorado

Christopher D. Raeburn, MD
Assistant Professor, Department of Surgery, University of Colorado Denver School of Medicine, Aurora, Colorado

T. Brett Reece, MD
Resident, PGY IX, Division of Cardiothoracic Surgery, University of Colorado Denver, Aurora, Colorado; Resident, PGY IX, Department of Surgery, Division of Cardiothoracic Surgery, University Hospital, Aurora, Colorado

Thomas F. Rehring, MD, FACS
Associate Clinical Professor of Surgery, Vascular Surgery Section, University of Colorado Denver Health Sciences Center, Denver, Colorado; Director, Department of Vascular Therapy, Chief, Vascular and Endovascular Surgery, Colorado Permanente Medical Group, Denver, Colorado

John A. Ridge, MD, PhD
Chief, Head and Neck Surgery Section, Department of Surgical Oncology, Fox Chase Cancer Center, Philadelphia, Pennsylvania

Jonathan P. Roach, MD
Resident, Department of Surgery, University of Colorado Denver, Denver, Colorado

Thomas N. Robinson, MD
Assistant Professor, Department of Surgery, University of Colorado at Denver Health Sciences Center, Aurora, Colorado; Department of Surgery, University of Colorado Hospital, Aurora, Colorado

Christina L. Roland, MD
Research Fellow, Department of Surgery, University of Texas Southwestern Medical Center, Dallas, Texas

Carlos A. Rueda, MD
General Surgery Resident, Department of Surgery, University of Colorado Denver, Denver, Colorado; General Surgery Resident, Department of Surgery, University of Colorado Denver Hospital, Denver, Colorado; General Surgery Resident, Department of Surgery, Denver Health Medical Center, Denver, Colorado

Craig H. Selzman, MD
Associate Professor, Department of Surgery, Division of Cardiothoracic Surgery, University of Utah School of Medicine, Salt Lake City, Utah

Amandeep Singh, MD
Assistant Clinical Professor of Medicine, Division of Emergency Medicine, Department of Medicine, University of California, San Francisco, San Francisco, California; Attending Physician, Department of Emergency Medicine, Alameda County Medical Center–Highland General Hospital, Oakland, California

Wade R. Smith, MD
Professor, Department of Orthopaedics, University of Colorado School of Medicine, Aurora, Colorado; Director, Department of Orthopaedics, Denver Health Medical Center, Denver, Colorado; Department of Orthopaedics, Veterans Affairs Medical Center, Denver, Colorado

David E. Stein, MD
Assistant Professor, Department of Surgery, Drexel University College of Medicine, Philadelphia, Pennsylvania; Chief, Division of Colorectal Surgery; Department of Surgery, Hahnemann University Hospital, Philadelphia, Pennsylvania

Gregory V. Stiegmann, MD
Professor of Surgery, Department of Surgery, University of Colorado Denver School of Medicine, Denver, Colorado; Vice President Clinical Affairs, University of Colorado Hospital, Aurora, Colorado; Staff Surgeon, Department of Surgery, Denver Veterans Affairs Hospital, Denver, Colorado

Karyn Stitzenberg, MD, MPH
Surgical Oncology, Fox Chase Cancer Center, Philadelphia, Pennsylvania

U. Mini B. Swift, MD
Physician Advisor, Alameda County Medical Center, Oakland, California

Alex J. Vanni, MD
Resident, Department of Urology, Lahey Clinic, Burlington, Massachusetts

Gregory P. Victorino, MD
Associate Professor, Department of Surgery, University of California, San Francisco–East Bay, Alameda County Medical Center, Oakland, California; Chief, Division of Trauma, Department of Surgery, Alameda County Medical Center, Oakland, California

Thomas A. Whitehill, MD
Associate Professor, Department of Surgery, University of Colorado, Denver, Colorado; Chief of Surgical Services, VA Medical Center, Denver, Colorado

Jennifer M. Worth, MD
General Surgery Resident, Department of General Surgery, University of Nebraska Medical Center, Omaha, Nebraska

Franklin L. Wright, MD
Resident, Department of Surgery, University of Colorado Denver, Denver, Colorado

Michael Zimmerman, MD
Assistant Professor, Division of Transplant Surgery, University of Colorado Health Sciences Center, Aurora, Colorado

PREFACE

When we refer to a work of art, music, or literature as a "classic", one of the observations that we make is that the work has stimulated a wide variety of treatments and interpretations. Imitation is, of course, the most visible and credible form of flattery. When Charlie Abernathy initially assaulted our surgical clinical comfort zone with a barrage of questions neither he, nor we, predicted that his irritating efforts would spawn a whole "Secrets Series" of challenging Abernathyisms in almost all medical disciplines.

But, characteristically, Charlie had his fingers capably placed on the pulse of progress. Casey Stengel famously noted: "In baseball, more games are lost than won." If you are not investigating, learning, or questioning, you are losing. In medicine, and certainly surgery, you cannot stand still. Alfred North Whitehead, the U.S. philosopher, observed: "No man of science could subscribe without qualification . . . to all of his own scientific beliefs of ten years ago." We must be flexible, to evolve, to question. Happily, surgeons are almost unique in our ability to be self-critical. We must never march, like a legion of lemmings, into a sea of intellectual acceptance.

This sixth edition of *Surgical Secrets* is again dedicated to Abernathy's irritatingly penetrating series of questions. Charlie never took much stock in the ponderously traditional answer. Intellectually active surgeons should never get too comfortable. Challenging dogma is good; comfort is bad. Dinosaurs were inflexible and are extinct. Surgeons will never be either.

Alden H. Harken, MD
Ernest E. Moore, MD
April, 2008

TOP 100 SECRETS

Andrew E. Luckey, MD, and Cyrus J. Parsa, MD

These secrets are 100 of the top board alerts. They summarize the concepts, principles, and most salient details of surgical practice.

1. Primary goal in treating cardiac dysrhythmias is to achieve a ventricular rate between 60 and 100 beats per minute; secondary goal is to maintain sinus rhythm.

2. Clinical determinants of brain death are the loss of the papillary, corneal, oculovestibular, oculocephalic, oropharyngeal, and respiratory reflexes for >6 hours. The patient should also undergo an apnea test, in which the P_{CO_2} is allowed to rise to at least 60 mm Hg without coexistent hypoxia. The patient should be observed for the absence of spontaneous breathing.

3. The estimated risks of hepatitis B virus (HBV), hepatitis C virus (HCV), and human immunodeficiency virus (HIV) transmission by blood transfusion in the United States are 1 in 205,000 for HBV; 1 in 1,935,000 for HCV; and 1 in 2,135,000 for HIV.

4. The most common location of an undescended testicle is the inguinal canal.

5. The most common solid renal mass in infancy is a congenital mesoblastic nephroma, and in childhood, it is a Wilms' tumor.

6. Ogilvie's syndrome is an acute massive dilatation of the cecum and the ascending and transverse colon without organic obstruction.

7. The best screening method for prostate cancer is digital rectal examination combined with serum prostate-specific antigen (PSA).

8. The most common histologic type of bladder cancer is transitional cell carcinoma.

9. Carcinoma in situ of the bladder is treated with immunotherapy with intravesical bacillus Calmette-Guérin.

10. The most common cause of male infertility is varicocele.

11. The most common nonbacterial cause of pneumonia in transplant patients is cytomegalovirus (CMV).

12. Chimerism is leukocyte sharing between the graft and the recipient so that the graft becomes a genetic composite of both the donor and the recipient.

13. OKT3 is a mouse monoclonal antibody that binds to and blocks the T-cell CD3 receptor.

14. The most common disease requiring liver transplant is hepatitis C.

15. Cystic hygroma is a congenital malformation with a predilection for the neck. It is a benign lesion that usually presents as a soft mass in the lateral neck.

16. In neuroblastomas, age at presentation is the major prognostic factor. Children younger than 1 year have an overall survival rate >70%, whereas the survival rate for children older than 1 year is <35%.

17. The most feared complication of diaphragmatic hernia is persistent fetal circulation.

18. The three most common variants of tracheoesophageal fistula are (1) proximal esophageal atresia with distal tracheoesophageal fistula, (2) isolated esophageal atresia, and (3) tracheoesophageal fistula with esophageal atresia.

19. Atresia can occur anywhere in the gastrointestinal (GI) tract: duodenal (50%), jejunoileal (45%), or colonic (5%). Duodenal atresia arises from failure of recanalization during the eighth to tenth week of gestation; jejunoileal and colonic atresia are caused by an in utero mesenteric vascular accident.

20. The two types of aortic dissection are ascending (type A) dissection, which begins in the ascending aorta and may continue into the descending aorta, and descending dissection (type B), which involves only the descending aorta.

21. The likelihood that a solitary lung nodule is cancer is the same as the age of the patient; thus, a 60-year-old patient's nodule is 60% likely to be cancer.

22. Mediastinal staging (mediastinoscopy) is indicated if: (1) the lung nodule is >2 cm; (2) the mediastinum is "full" as seen on a computerized tomography (CT) scan; and (3) the nodule is "kissing" up against the mediastinum. A lung resection is contraindicated if: (1) "high" ipsilateral paratracheal nodes are positive; (2) contralateral nodes are positive; or (3) undifferentiated ("oatcell") histology is identified.

23. The most common causes of aortic stenosis are now congenital anomalies and calcific (degenerative) disease.

24. In mitral regurgitation, the left ventricle ejects blood via two routes: (1) antegrade through the aortic valve, or (2) retrograde through the mitral valve. The amount of each stroke volume ejected retrograde into the left atrium is the regurgitant fraction. To compensate for the regurgitant fraction, the left ventricle must increase its total stroke volume. This ultimately produces volume overload of the left ventricle and leads to ventricular dysfunction.

25. The indications for coronary artery bypass graft (CABG) are (1) left main coronary artery stenosis; (2) three-vessel coronary artery disease (70% stenosis) with depressed left ventricular (LV) function or two-vessel coronary artery disease (CAD) with proximal left anterior descending (LAD) involvement; and (3) angina despite aggressive medical therapy.

26. Hibernating myocardium is improved by CABG. Myocardial hibernation refers to the reversible myocardial contractile function associated with a decrease in coronary flow in the setting of preserved myocardial viability. Some patients with global systolic dysfunction exhibit dramatic improvement in myocardial contractility after CABG.

27. The surgical treatment of ulcerative colitis is total colectomy with ileoanal pouch anastomosis.

28. Dieulafoy's ulcer is a gastric vascular malformation with an exposed submucosal artery, usually within 2 to 5 cm of the gastroesophageal junction. It presents with painless, often massive, hematemesis.

29. The role of blind subtotal colectomy in the management of massive lower GI bleeding is limited to a small group of patients in whom a specific bleeding source cannot be identified. The procedure is associated with a 16% mortality rate.

30. Colorectal polyps <2 cm have a 2% risk of containing cancer; 2-cm polyps have a 10% risk; and polyps >2 cm have a cancer risk of 40%. Sixty percent of villous polyps are >2 cm, and 77% of tubular polyps are <1 cm at the time of discovery.

31. Patients with colorectal cancer with lymph node involvement (Dukes' classification) should receive chemotherapy postoperatively to treat micrometastases.

32. Goodsall's rule states the location of the internal opening of an anorectal fistula is based on the position of the external opening. An external opening posterior to a line drawn transversely across the perineum originates from an internal opening in the posterior midline. An external opening anterior to this line originates from the nearest anal crypt in a radial direction.

33. Incarcerated inguinal hernia: structures in the hernia sac still have a good blood supply but are stuck in the sac because of adhesions or a narrow neck of the hernia sac. Strangulated inguinal hernia occurs when hernia structures have a compromised blood supply because of anatomic constriction at the neck of the hernia.

34. Chvostek's sign is spasm of the facial muscles caused by tapping the facial nerve trunk. Trousseau's sign is carpal spasm elicited by occlusion of the brachial artery for 3 minutes with a blood pressure cuff. Both signs indicate hypocalcemia.

35. The two surgical options for Graves' disease are subtotal thyroidectomy or near-total thyroidectomy.

36. The only biochemical test that is routinely needed to identify patients with unsuspected hyperthyroidism is serum thyroid-stimulating hormone (TSH) concentration.

37. The surgically correctable causes of hypertension are renovascular hypertension, pheochromocytoma, Cushing's syndrome, primary hyperaldosteronism, coarctation of the aorta, and unilateral renal parenchymal disease.

38. The "triple negative test" or "diagnostic triad" for diagnosing a palpable breast mass includes physical examination, breast imaging, and biopsy.

39. Chest wall radiation is indicated after mastectomy in patients with greater than 5 cm primary cancers, positive mastectomy margins, or more than four positive lymph nodes, all of which are associated with heightened locoregional recurrence rates.

40. Sentinel lymph nodes are the first stop for tumor cells metastasizing through lymphatics from the primary tumor.

41. The most common site of origin of subungual melanomas is the great toe. Amputation at or proximal to the metatarsal phalangeal joint and regional sentinel lymph node biopsy are advised.

42. Ramus marginalis mandibularis, the lowest branch of the nerve that innervates the depressor muscles of the lower lip, is the most commonly injured facial nerve branch during parotidectomy.

43. Waldeyer's ring is the mucosa of the posterior oropharynx covering a bed of lymphatic tissue that aggregates to form the palatine, lingual, pharyngeal, and tubal tonsils. These structures form a ring around the pharyngeal wall. This may be the site of primary or metastatic tumor.

44. A patient in whom the head and neck examination is completely normal but fine needle aspiration (FNA) of a cervical node reveals squamous cancer should have examination of the mouth, pharynx, larynx, esophagus, and tracheobronchial tree under anesthesia (triple endoscopy). If nothing is seen, blind biopsy of the nasopharynx, tonsils, base of tongue, and pyriform sinuses should be done at the same sitting.

45. The microorganisms implicated in atherosclerosis include *Chlamydia pneumoniae*, *Helicobacter pylori*, streptococci, and *Bacillus typhosus*.

46. The cumulative 10-year amputation rate for claudication is 10%. Vascular disease is systemic, therefore, many of these patients die before amputation.

47. The absolute reduction in risk of stroke is 6% over a 5-year period in asymptomatic patients with >60% stenosis who undergo carotid endarterectomy (CEA) plus aspirin versus patients treated with aspirin alone (5.1%; surgery versus 11% medical Rx). This is from the Asymptomatic Carotid Atherosclerosis Study (ACAS) study (see Required Reading Chapter 1).

48. The average expansion rate of an abdominal aortic aneurysm is 0.4 cm/year.

49. Heparin binds to antithrombin III, rendering it more active.

50. The patient with suspected intermittent claudication should initially be evaluated by obtaining ankle brachial index (ABI) or segmental limb pressures at rest. Typically, ABI of 0.6 reflects claudication and ABI of <0.3 reflects limb threat.

51. Shock is suboptimal consumption of oxygen (O_2) and excretion of carbon dioxide (CO_2) at the cellular level.

52. Nitric oxide is synthesized in vascular endothelial cells by constitutive nitric oxide synthase (NOS) and inducible NOS, using arginine as the substrate.

53. Saliva has the highest potassium concentration (20 mEq), followed by gastric secretions (10 mEq), and then pancreatic and duodenal secretions (5 mEq).

54. Basal caloric expenditure equal to 25 kilocalories per kilogram a day with a requirement of approximately 1 g of protein per kilogram per day.

55. Six and one-fourth grams of protein contain 1 g of nitrogen.

56. Dextrose has 3.4 kcal/g; protein has 4 kcal/g; and fat 9 kcal/g (20% lipid solution delivers 2 kcal/ml).

57. Maximal glucose infusion rates in parenteral formulas should not exceed 5 milligrams per kilogram per minute.

58. Refeeding syndrome occurs in moderately to severely malnourished patients (e.g., chronic alcoholism or anorexia nervosa) who, with a large nutrient load, develop clinically significant decreases in serum phosphorus, potassium, calcium, and magnesium levels. Hyperglycemia is common secondary to blunted insulin secretion. Adenosine triphosphate (ATP) production is mitigated, and the respiratory failure is common.

59. Glutamine is the most common amino acid found in muscle and plasma. Levels decrease after surgery and physiologic stress. Glutamine serves as a substrate for rapidly replicating cells (interestingly, it is also the number one metabolic substrate for neoplastic cells), maintains the integrity and function of the intestinal barrier, and protects against free radical damage by maintaining glutathione (GSH) levels. Glutamine is unstable in intravenous (IV) form unless linked as a dipeptide.

60. Fever is caused by activated macrophages that release interleukin-1, tumor necrosis factor (TNF), and interferon in response to bacteria and endotoxin. The result is a resetting of the hypothalamic thermoregulatory center.

61. Cardiac output (CO) is equal to heart rate multiplied by stroke volume; normal CO is 5 to 6 L/min and cardiac index is 2.4 to 3.0 liters per minute per square meter.

62. Systemic vascular resistance (SVR) is equal to mean arterial pressure (MAP) minus central venous pressure (CVP) divided by CO multiplied by 80; and it is written as: SVR = to $[(MAP - CVP)/CO] \times 80$. Normal SVR is 800 to 1200 dyne·sec/cm^{-5}.

63. The signs of hypovolemic shock are low CVP and pulmonary capillary wedge pressure (PCWP), low CO and mixed venous oxygen saturation (SVO$_2$), and high SVR.

64. The signs of cardiogenic shock are high CVP and PCWP, low CO and SVO$_2$, and variable SVR.

65. The signs of septic shock are low or normal CVP and PCWP, high CO initially, high SVO$_2$, and low SVR.

66. Kehr's sign is concurrent left upper quadrant (LUQ) and left shoulder pain, indicating diaphragmatic irritation from a ruptured spleen or subdiaphragmatic abscess. Anatomically, the diaphragm and the back of the left shoulder enjoy parallel innervation.

67. Rebound tenderness (rubbing the peritoneal surfaces against each other) implies peritoneal inflammation (peritonitis).

68. The five Ws of postoperative fever are **w**ound (infection), **w**ater (urinary tract infection; UTI), **w**ind (atelectasis, pneumonia), **w**alking (thrombophlebitis), and **w**onder drugs (drug fevers).

69. Cricothyroidotomy should not be performed in patients <12 years old or any patient with suspected direct laryngeal trauma or tracheal disruption.

70. The palpable radial (wrist) pulse reflects systolic blood pressure (SBP) >80 mm Hg; palpable femoral (groin) pulse reflects SBP >70 mm Hg; and palpable carotid (neck) pulse reflects SBP >60 mm Hg.

71. A general rule for crystalloid infusion to replace blood loss is a 3:1 ratio of isotonic crystalloid to blood.

72. Raccoon eyes (periorbital ecchymosis) and Battle's sign (mastoid ecchymosis) are clinical indicators of basilar skull fracture.

73. Cerebral perfusion pressure (CPP) is equal to MAP minus intracranial pressure (ICP); and it is written as CPP = MAP − ICP. Some debate exists on the minimum allowable CPP, but consensus indicates that a CPP of 50 to 70 mm Hg is necessary.

74. Violation of the platysma defines a penetrating neck wound.

75. Tension pneumothorax is air accumulation in the pleural space eliciting increased intrathoracic pressure and resulting in a decrease in venous return to heart.

76. The most common site of thoracic aortic injury in blunt trauma is just distal to the take-off of the left subclavian artery.

77. The most common manifestation of blunt myocardial injury is arrhythmia.

78. Indications for thoracotomy in a stable patient with hemothorax include an immediate tube thoracostomy output of >1500 ml and ongoing bleeding of 250 ml/h for 4 consecutive hours.

79. Beck's triad is hypotension, distended neck veins, and muffled heart sounds (think of pericardial tamponade).

80. The hepatic artery supplies approximately 30% of blood flow to the liver, and the portal vein supplies the remaining 70%. The oxygen delivery, however, is similar for both at 50%.

81. Pringle's maneuver, which is used to reduce liver hemorrhage, is a manual occlusion of the hepatoduodenal ligament to interrupt blood flow to the liver.

82. Splenectomy significantly decreases immunoglobulin M (IgM) levels.

83. Ninety percent of trauma fatalities resulting from pelvic fractures are the result of venous bleeding and bone oozing; only 10% of fatal pelvic bleeding from blunt trauma is arterial (most common site is superior gluteal artery).

84. The protocol for intraperitoneal bladder rupture from blunt trauma is operative management, whereas the protocol for extraperitoneal rupture is observant management.

85. Pseudoaneurysm is a disruption of the arterial wall leading to a pulsatile hematoma contained by vascular adventitia and fibrous connective tissue (but not all three arterial wall layers, which is what defines a true aneurysm).

86. The earliest sign of lower extremity compartment syndrome is neurologic in the distribution of the peroneal nerve with numbness in the first dorsal webspace and weak dorsiflexion.

87. Posterior knee dislocations are associated with popliteal artery injuries and are an indication for angiography.

88. Management of suspected navicular fracture despite negative radiography is short-arm cast and repeat x-ray in 2 weeks; these fractures are also at high risk for avascular necrosis.

89. The Parkland formula is lactated Ringer's at 4 ml/kg × percentage of total body surface area (TBSA) burned (second- and third-degree only). Infuse 50% of volume in first 8 hours and the remaining 50% over the subsequent 16 hours.

90. The metabolic rate peaks at 2.5 times the basal metabolic rate in severe burns >50% TBSA.

91. Gallstones and alcohol abuse are the two main causes of acute pancreatitis.

92. Alcohol abuse accounts for 75% of cases of chronic pancreatitis.

93. Isolated gastric varices with hypersplenism indicate splenic vein thrombosis and are an indication for splenectomy.

94. The treatment for gallstone pancreatitis is cholecystectomy and intraoperative cholangiogram during the same hospital stay once the pancreatitis has subsided.

95. Proton pump inhibitors (PPIs) irreversibly inhibit the parietal cell hydrogen ion pump.

96. Definitive treatment of alkaline reflux gastritis after a Billroth II includes a Roux-en-Y gastro-jejunostomy from a 40-cm efferent jejunal limb.

97. Cushing's ulcer is a stress ulcer found in critically ill patients with central nervous system (CNS) injury. It is typically single and deep with a tendency to perforate.

98. Curling's ulcer is a stress ulcer found in critically ill patients with burn injuries.

99. Marginal ulcer is an ulcer found near the margin of gastroenteric anastomosis, usually on the small bowel side.

100. The most common cause of small bowel obstructions is adhesive disease; the second most common cause is a hernia.

I. GENERAL TOPICS

ARE YOU READY FOR YOUR SURGICAL ROTATION?

Tabetha R. Harken, MD, MPH, U. Mini B. Swift, MD, Alden H. Harken, MD

CHAPTER 1

Surgery is a participatory, team, and contact sport. Present yourself to patients, residents, and attendings with enthusiasm (which covers a multitude of sins), punctuality (type A people do not like to wait), and cleanliness (you must look, act, and smell like a doctor).

1. **Why should you introduce yourself to each patient and ask about his or her chief complaint?**
   Symptoms are perception, and perception is more important than reality. To a patient, the chief complaint is not simply a matter of life and death; it is much more important. Patients routinely are placed into compromising, uncomfortable, embarrassing, and undignified predicaments. Patients are people, however, and they have interests, concerns, anxieties, and a story. As a student, you have an opportunity to place your patient's chief complaint into the context of the rest of his or her life. This skill is important, and the patient will always be grateful. You can serve a real purpose as a listener and translator for the patient and his or her family.
   Patients want to trust and love you. This trust in surgical therapy is a formidable tool. The more a patient understands about his or her disease, the more the patient can participate in getting better. Recovery is faster if the patient helps.
   Similarly, the more the patient understands about his or her therapy (including its side effects and potential complications), the more effective the therapy is (this principle is not in the textbooks). You can be your patient's interpreter. This is the fun of surgery (and medicine).

2. **What is the correct answer to almost all questions?**
   Thank you. Gratitude is an invaluable tool on the wards.

3. **Are there any simple rules from the trenches?**
   1. **Getting along with the nurses.** The nurses do know more than the rest of us about the codes, routines, and rituals of making the wards run smoothly. They may not know as much about pheochromocytomas and intermediate filaments, but about the stuff that matters, they know a lot. Acknowledge that, and they will take you under their wings and teach you a ton!
   2. **Helping out.** If your residents look busy, they probably are. So, if you ask how you can help and they are too busy even to answer, asking again probably would not yield much.
      Always leap at the opportunity to shag x-rays, track down lab results, and retrieve a bag of blood from the bank. The team will recognize your enthusiasm and reward your contributions.
   3. **Getting scuted.** We all would like a secretary, but one is not going to be provided on this rotation. Your residents do a lot of their own scut work without you even knowing about it. So if you feel like scut work is beneath you, perhaps you should think about another profession.
   4. **Working hard.** This rotation is an apprenticeship. If you work hard, you will get a realistic idea of what it means to be a resident (and even a practicing doctor) in this specialty. (This has big advantages when you are selecting a type of internship.)
   5. **Staying in the loop.** In the beginning, you may feel like you are not a real part of the team. If you are persistent and reliable, however, soon your residents will trust you with more important jobs.

6. **Educating yourself, and then educating your patients.** Here is one of the rewarding places (as indicated in question 1) where you can soar to the top of the team. Talk to your patients about everything (including their disease and therapy), and they will love you for it.

7. **Maintaining a positive attitude.** As a medical student, you may feel that you are not a crucial part of the team. Even if you are incredibly smart, you are unlikely to be making the crucial management decisions. So what does that leave: attitude. If you are enthusiastic and interested, your residents will enjoy having you around, and they will work to keep you involved and satisfied. A dazzlingly intelligent but morose complainer is better suited for a rotation in the morgue. Remember, your resident is likely following 15 sick patients, gets paid less than $2 an hour, and hasn't slept more than 5 hours in the last 3 days. Simple things such as smiling and saying thank you (when someone teaches you) go an incredibly long way and are rewarded on all clinical rotations with experience and good grades.

8. **Having fun!** This is the most exciting, gratifying, rewarding, and fun profession and is light years better than whatever is second best (this is not just our opinion).

4. **What is the best approach to surgical notes?**

Surgical notes should be succinct. Most surgeons still move their lips when they read. See Table 1-1.

TABLE 1-1. BEST APPROACH TO SURGICAL NOTES

Admission Orders

Admit to 5 West (attending's name)

Condition:	Stable
Diagnosis:	Abdominal pain; r/o appendicitis
Vital signs:	q 4 h
Parameters:	Please call HO for:
T >38° C	
160 < BP < 90	
120 < HR < 60	
Diet:	NPO
Fluids:	1000 LR w 20 mEq KCl @ 100 ml/h
Med[ication]s:	ASA 650 mg PR prn for T >38.5° C

Thank you.

Sign your name/leave space for resident's signature (your beeper number)

History and Physical Examination (H & P)

Mrs. O'Flaherty is a 55 y/o w ♀[white woman] admitted with a cc [chief complaint]: "my stomach hurts." Pt [patient] was in usual state of excellent health until 2 days PTA [prior to admission] when she noted gradual onset of crampy midepigastric pain. Pain is now severe (7/10; 7 on a scale of 10) and recurring q 5 minutes. Pt described + vomiting (+ bile, −blood) [with bile, without blood].

PMH [past medical history]

Hosp[italizations]:	Pneumonia (1991)
	Childbirth (1970, 1972)

TABLE 1-1. BEST APPROACH TO SURGICAL NOTES—CONT'D

Surg[ery]:	splenectomy for trauma (1967)
Allergies:	Codeine, shellfish
Social:	ETOH [alcohol]
Tobacco:	1 ppd [pack per day] x 25 years
ROS [review of systems]	
Resp[iratory]:	productive cough
Cardiac:	ō chest pain [o = not observed, noncontributory, or not here]
	ō MI [myocardial infarction]
Renal:	ō dysuria
	ō frequency
Neuro[logic]:	WNL [within normal limits]
Physical Examination (PE)	
BP:	140/90
HR:	100 (regular)
RR [respiratory rate]:	16 breaths/min
Temp:	38.2° C
WD [well-developed], WN [well-nourished], mildly obese, 55 y/o ♀ in moderate abdominal distress	
HEENT [head, eyes, ears, nose, and throat]: WNL	
Resp:	Clear lungs bilat[erally]
	ō wheeze
Heart:	ō m [murmur]
	RSR [regular sinus rhythm]
Abdomen:	Mildly distended
	High-pitched rushes that coincide with crampy pain
	Tender to palpation (you do not need to hurt the patient to find this out)
	ō Rebound
Rectal:	(Always do; never defer the rectal exam on your surgical rotation)
Hematest—negative for blood	
No masses, no tenderness	
Pelvic:	No masses
	No adnexal tenderness
	No cervical motion tenderness or chandelier sign; if quick motion of cervix makes your patient hit the chandelier → non specific peritoneal sign, possibly pelvic inflammatory disease (PID; gonorrhea)

(Continued)

TABLE 1-1. BEST APPROACH TO SURGICAL NOTES—CONT'D

Extremities:	Full ROM [range of motion]
	ō edema
	Bounding (3+) pulses
Imp[ression]:	Abdominal pain
	r/o SB [small bowel] obstruction 2° [secondary] to adhesions
Rx:	NG [nasogastric] tube
	IV fluids
	Op[erative] consent
	Type and hold

[Signature]

Notes on the surgical H&P

- A surgical H&P should be succinct and focused on the patient's problem.
- Begin with the chief complaint (in the patient's words).
- Is the problem new or chronic?
- PMH: always include prior hospitalizations and medications.
- ROS: restrict review to organ systems (lung, heart, kidneys, and nervous system) that may affect this admission.
- PE: always begin with vital signs (including respiration and temperature); that is why these signs are vital.
- Rebound means inflammatory peritoneal irritation or peritonitis.

Preop[erative] note

The preoperative note is a checklist confirming that you and the patient are ready for the planned surgical procedure. Place this note in the Progress Notes:

Preop dx [diagnosis]:	SB obstruction 2° to adhesions
CXR [chest x-ray]:	Clear
ECG [electrocardiogram]:	NSR w/ST-T wave changes
Blood:	Type and cross-match x 2 u
Consent:	In chart

Operative note

The operative note should provide anyone who encounters the patient after surgery with all the needed information:

Preop dx:	SB obstruction
Postop dx:	Same, all bowel viable
Procedure:	Exp[loratory] Lap[arotomy] with lysis of adhesions
Surgeon:	Name him or her
Assistants:	List them
Anesthesia:	GEA [general endotracheal anesthesia]

TABLE 1-1. BEST APPROACH TO SURGICAL NOTES—CONT'D	
I&O [intake and output]:	In: 1200 ml Ringer's lactate (R/L)
	Out: 400 ml urine
EBL [estimated blood loss]:	50 ml
Specimen:	None
Drains:	None
[Sign your name]	

ASA, aspirin; *BP*, systolic blood pressure; *BRP*, bathroom privileges; *h*, hour; *HO*, house officer; *HR*, heart rate; *NPO*, nothing by mouth (this includes water and pills); *OOB*, out of bed; *PR*, per rectum; *PRN*, as needed; *q*, every; *r/o*, rule out; *T*, temperature.
Note: You cannot be too polite or too grateful to patients or nurses.

HOSPITAL DISCHARGE

5. What is a care transition?
It is a fancy word for any change in a clinical care setting. Examples include: from hospital to home, from home to emergency department (ED), and from nursing home to home.

6. What is one of the most dangerous things that you can do to your patient?
Discharge them from the hospital.

7. Why is a hospital discharge a dangerous procedure?
Hospitals are designed for maximal support. Procedures are managed; diet is controlled; and even the increasingly obligate poly-pharmacy is orchestrated such that each pill is swallowed with metronomic precision. Then, much like, a baby eaglet, the patient is unceremoniously "pushed out" of this federally regulated inpatient nest. And again, like the baby iglet, we expect that patient to take flight at home.

8. What would improve safety at discharge?
Follow through on the "last sign out." Sign out to your patient, their family members, and the next doctor who is going to take care of them in the nursing home or clinic.

9. What are the most important elements of the final sign out (discharge summary)?
Discharge summaries should include:
  Primary and other diagnoses
  Pertinent medical history and physical findings
  Dates that they were hospitalized and brief hospital course (assume that the doctor on the outside knows how to treat hyperkalemia)
  Results of procedures
  Abnormal lab tests
  Recommendations of the specialists that you consulted
  Information that you gave to the patient and family
Discharge Medications:
  Details of follow-up arrangements
  To do list of appointments, pending tests or procedures to be scheduled or checked
  Name and contact information of the inpatient doctor

The idea that a hospital discharge is a risky business, but the risk can be reduced by a conscientious physician or medical student comes from:

Kripalani S, LeFevre F, Phillips CO et al.: Deficits in communication and information transfer between hospital-based and primary care physicians, JAMA 297:831-841, 2007.

APPENDIX: REQUIRED READING

Kristin Kanka, DO, and Terrence H. Liu, MD

Unlike medical rounds, where to keep up you need to "one up" by quoting a current (preferably yesterday's) journal article, in surgery, you can flourish by knowing the following references, but you need to know them cold.

1. **Mangano DT, Goldman L: Pre-operative assessment of patients with known or suspected coronary disease, N Engl J Med 333:1750-1756, 1995.**

   This is an update of Goldman's original (N Engl J Med, 1977) article in which he pioneered the concept of "risk adjusted surgical outcome." You should copy Table 2, Three Commonly Used Indexes of Cardiac Risk, and always carry it with you. Intuitively, a triathlete will weather a surgical stress better than a Supreme Court judge, but this article provides a point system with which you can calculate objective perioperative risk.

2. **Veronesi U, Cascinelli N, Mariani L et al.: Twenty-year follow-up of a randomized study comparing breast conserving surgery with radical mastectomy for early breast cancer, N Engl J Med 347:1227-1232, 2002.**

   Seven hundred women with <2-cm breast cancer were randomized to radical mastectomy or quadrantectomy and radiation therapy. After 1976, patients with positive axillary nodes also received adjuvant cyclophosphamide, methotrexate, and 5-fluorouracil (CMF). After 20 years, 30 women in the conservative treatment group and 8 women in the radical mastectomy group suffered local recurrence ($p = 0.01$). Conversely, the incidence of deaths from all causes at 20 years was identical at 41%. The authors conclude that breast conservation therapy is the "treatment of choice" for women with "relatively small breast cancers."

3. **Fisher B, Anderson S, Bryant J et al.: Twenty-year follow-up of a randomized trial comparing total mastectomy, lumpectomy and lumpectomy plus irradiation for the treatment of invasive breast cancer, N Engl J Med 347:1223-1241, 2002.**

   Clinical investigation is hard to do. The National Surgical Adjuvant Breast and Bowel Project (NSABP) Trials, initiated 25 years ago, continue to serve as the benchmark for superb prospective, randomized investigations. In this study, 1851 women were randomized after the breast tumor was excised and the nodal status was documented. The authors conclude that lumpectomy followed by breast irradiation is appropriate therapy. To appreciate the huge problems in interpreting clinical trials, you must read this article carefully. Radiation did decrease death from breast cancer, but this reduction was partially offset by an increase in deaths from other causes.

4. **Barnett HJ, Taylor DW, Eliasziw M et al.: Benefit of carotid endarterectomy in patients with symptomatic moderate or severe stenosis, N Engl J Med 339:1415-1425, 1998.**

   This is the North American Symptomatic Carotid Endarterectomy Trial (NASCET) initiated in 1987. NASCET randomized patients with severe carotid stenosis (70% to 99%) and moderate stenosis (<70%) into standard medical therapy or carotid endarterectomy (CEA). By 1991, the clear advantage of surgery in symptomatic patients with severe stenosis was so clear that the study was stopped for this group. This manuscript reports a 5-year reduction in ipsilateral stroke from 22.2% (medical) to 15.7% (surgical) ($p = 0.045$) in patients with moderate (50% to 69%) stenosis. Once a patient with carotid disease becomes symptomatic, that is ominous. As you witness various diseases, you subconsciously compile a list of diseases you do not want. A big burn and a big stroke are on the top of everyone's list.

5. **Endarterectomy for asymptomatic carotid artery stenosis. Executive Committee for the Asymptomatic Carotid Atherosclerosis Study, JAMA 273:1421-1428, 1995.**

   The Asymptomatic Carotid Atherosclerosis Study (ACAS) randomized 1662 asymptomatic patients with >60% carotid artery stenosis to medical prescription (one aspirin a day plus risk factor modification) or CEA. After only 2.7 years, the projected 5-year risk of ipsilateral stroke and death was 5.1% in the surgical group and 11% in the medical group. This is an aggregate (including perioperative trouble) risk reduction of 53%. This article concludes that an asymptomatic patient with a 60% or greater carotid artery lesion, who is an acceptable risk (atherosclerosis is a systemic disease) for elective surgery will enjoy a reduction in 5-year risk of ipsilateral stroke if the surgery can be accomplished with less than a 3% aggregate morbidity or mortality.

6. **Selzman CH, Miller SA, Zimmerman MA et al.: The case for beta-adrenergic blockade as prophylaxis against perioperative cardiovascular morbidity and mortality, Arch Surg 136:286-290, 2001.**

When patients suffer perioperative morbidity and mortality, the cardiovascular system is typically the culprit. Patients with coronary artery disease (CAD) cannot increase coronary blood flow to meet the enhanced oxygen demand associated with surgical stress. Beta-adrenergic blockade decreases myocardial oxygen consumption, and cardioselective beta-blockers do not exacerbate bronchospasm in patients with chronic obstructive pulmonary disorder (COPD). These authors argue that all patients over 40 years old will benefit from beta-adrenergic blockade initiated 2 weeks before elective surgery.

7. **Van den Berghe G, Wouters P, Weekers F et al.: Intensive insulin therapy in critically ill patients, N Engl J Med 345:1359-1367, 2001.**

Both hyperglycemia and insulin resistance are characteristic of critically ill patients. These authors randomized 1548 surgical intensive care unit (SICU) patients to either aggressive blood glucose control (maintained at 80 to 110 mg/100 dl) or conventional therapy (give insulin only if blood glucose exceeds 215 mg/100 dl). Aggressive glucose control decreased intensive care unit (ICU) mortality from 8% to 4.6% ($p = 0.04$) with the largest impact in patients with multiple organ failure from a septic focus.

In surgery, attention to detail counts big:

- Keep blood sugar between 80 and 110 mg/100 dl.
- Give prophylactic antibiotics 0 to 2 hours preoperatively so the patient will have a good antibiotic blood level at the time of the incision.
- Keep your patient warm (37° C).
- Hyperoxia reduces infection.

8. **Van De Vijver MJ, He YD, van't Veer LJ et al.: A gene expression signature as a predictor of survival in breast cancer, N Engl J Med 347:1999-2009, 2002.**

The authors postulate that 70 of our 35,000 genes dictate the character of breast cancer. So cancer, unlike cystic fibrosis and sickle cell disease, requires a constellation of genetic mutations, not just one. They followed 295 patients for 12 years and report that this "70 gene signature" predicts survival better than the classical indicators of patient age, tumor size, tumor histology, pathologic grade, hormone receptor status, and even lymph node disease. The latter is the shocker. The authors observe that distant metastasis kills you, positive lymph nodes do not. In patients with either positive or negative lymph nodes, gene profile determines survival. Each cancer does not acquire an ability to metastasize as it grows, that capability is programmed into the first neoplastic cell that establishes residence in your patient.

9. **Sandham JD, Hull RD, Brant RF et al.: A randomized controlled trial of the use of pulmonary artery catheters in high risk surgical patients, N Engl J Med 348:5-14, 2003.**

This is a superb study in which 1994 surgical ICU patients were randomized to goal-directed therapy guided by a pulmonary artery (PA) catheter or standard care without a PA catheter. The patients were sick and, to be included for randomization, had to be over 60 years old, have estimated ASA class III or IV risk (major disease), and scheduled for elective or urgent surgery. Hospital mortality and survival at 6 and 12 months were essentially identical. Following years of impassioned debate, the utility of a PA catheter, even in sick surgical patients, can no longer be justified. Conversely, if, after you have given fluid and low-dose cardiotonic agents, your patient is not improving or still presents a confusing picture, place a PA catheter and get more information. When your patient improves, pull it out.

10. **Harken AH: Enough is enough, Arch Surg 134:1061-1063, 1999.**

This article explores the surgeon's responsibility to assess surgical risk, to relate risk to anticipated physiologic and psychological benefit, and to develop common sense strategies to appreciate individual patient happiness. When benefits exceed anticipated operative risks—this is easy—proceed with surgery. When risks exceed benefits, this can be uncomfortable, but sensitive recognition of this relatively common problem by the surgeon can limit extension of the patient's and family's grief, prevent the squandering of limited resources, and appropriately divert decision-making guilt from the family to the surgeon.

11. **Eatock FC, Chong, P, Menezes N et al.: A randomized study of early nasogastric versus nasojejunal feeding in severe acute pancreatitis, Am J Gastroenterol 100:432-439, 2005.**

Early feeding in some patients with acute pancreatitis (AP) causes pain and is traditionally believed to be the result of worsening disease produced by premature stimulation of the pancreas. Recent scientific evidence suggests that over-stimulation of pancreatic acinar cells may not be the underlying cause of AP, therefore leading physicians to question the benefits of resting the pancreas. The delivery of nutrients into distal small bowel has been shown beneficial during severe AP. This study is the first randomized prospective study in which 50 adult patients with severe AP were randomized to receive early feeding by either nasogastric tubes or nasojejunal tubes. Measured endpoints included disease severity measured by how sick the patient is (APACHE II scores), the magnitude of systemic inflammation (C-reactive protein [CRP] levels), clinical progression, and pain. Overall 24.5% mortality was observed, with no difference in mortality between the groups. No difference in complication rates, CRP changes, APACHE II changes, or pain level changes were observed. This study is significant in that it scientifically challenges the surgical bias that resting the pancreas helps patients with AP recover faster.

12. **McFalls EO, Ward HB, Moritz TE et al.: Coronary-artery revascularization before elective major vascular surgery, N Engl J Med 351:2795-2804, 2004.**

This is a Veterans Administration prospective randomized trial that was conducted to assess the benefits of preoperative coronary revascularization in patients undergoing major vascular surgery. Five hundred ten patients were randomized to coronary revascularization by coronary artery bypass graft (CABG), percutaneous approach, or standard medical therapy. Patient characteristics were similar in both groups; $\approx$40% were diabetics, 45% were smokers, 40% with history of myocardial infarction (MI), $\approx$30% with three-vessel coronary disease, and 20% with history of cerebrovascular accident (CVA) or transient ischemic attack (TIA). Patient outcome was assessed during hospitalization and in long-term follow up. The results showed no difference in postoperative complications or in-hospital mortality rates between the treated groups. At 2.7 years after randomization, no difference in mortality was observed between the groups. Significant delays in treatment occurred in the preoperative revascularization patients (54 days versus 18 days). These results demonstrated that unless patients exhibit acute coronary syndrome (ACS), there are no clear short-term or long-term benefits in routine coronary revascularization before major vascular surgical procedures.

13. **Andre T, Boni C, Mounedji-Boudiaf L et al.: Oxaliplatin, fluorouracil, and leucovorin as adjuvant treatment for colon cancer, N Engl J Med 2343-2351, 2004.**

Roughly one half of the patients undergoing curative surgery for colorectal cancer relapses and dies of metastatic disease. The presence or absence of lymph node metastases is one of the most important prognosticators for survival. Previous studies have shown that patient with stage III (node-positive) colon cancer had improved survival with adjuvant 5-FU and leucovorin (FL) therapy in comparison to surgery alone. This randomized control trial compared FL to FL plus oxaliplatin therapy for 6 months in patients with stage II and stage III colon cancer. Primary endpoint was disease-free survival. Over 1100 patients were randomized to each arm of the study, and after a median follow up of 40 months, a highly statistically significant difference in survival was seen between the groups (26.1% versus 21.1%; $p = 0.002$). Disease-free survival for the groups was significantly different at 78.2% versus 72.9%. Treatment-related complications, including GI symptoms, sensory neuropathy, and fevers occurred more commonly in the FL + oxaliplatin patients. Subgroup analyses showed the greatest benefit among Stage III patients. This study is called the MOSAIC trial and is responsible for the current chemotherapy treatment standards for patients with stage III colon cancer.

14. **Fitzgibbons RJ Jr, Giobbie-Hurder A, Gibbs JO et al.: Watchful waiting vs repair of inguinal hernia in minimally symptomatic men: a randomized clinical trial, JAMA 295:285-292, 2006.**

Deciding if and when to operate is one of the most important decisions you will make as a surgeon. This trial put that decision to the test as it pertains to men with minimally symptomatic inguinal hernias. Fitzgibbons is a nationally recognized expert in the field of hernia surgery and presented the results of this prospective, randomized, multicenter study in the Society of American Gastrointestinal and Endoscopic Surgeons (SAGES) Grand Round Master Series (to view the video go to: www.medscape.com/viewarticle/553466). In this trial, 720 men with mildly symptomatic inguinal hernias were randomized into two groups: watchful waiting versus tension-free repair. They were followed for 2 to 4.5 years. No significant difference between the two groups was found based on the main outcomes of the trial, pain and discomfort interfering with activity, and changes from baseline in the physical component score (PCS) of the Short Form-36 health-related quality-of-life survey. Therefore watchful waiting in this subset of patients is permissible because the risk of incarceration is rare (1.8/1000 patient-years).

15. **Neumayer L, Giobbie-Hurder A, Jonasson O et al.: Open mesh vs laparoscopic mesh repair of inguinal hernia, N Engl J Med 350:1819-1827, 2004.**

With the development of minimally invasive surgery in the late 1980s, many operations, including inguinal hernia repair, were adapted to the laparoscopic approach. The advantages of laparoscopic repair include significantly less postoperative pain and speedier return to usual activities. However, laparoscopy does carry risk. The best approach to repair of inguinal hernias has been controversial, multifactorial, and inconclusive. Laparoscopic operations must be performed under general anesthesia, and there is increased potential for serious complications, including but not limited to bowel perforation and major vessel injury. Many studies have proven an overall advantage of laparoscopic over open tension-free techniques, but most of these studies were done at specialized centers. This large multicenter, prospective, randomized trial, conducted at the Veterans Administration, is the notable exception and may be more representative of the general population. Two thousand one hundred sixty-four patients were randomized to laparoscopic versus Lichtenstein or open tension-free repair of inguinal hernias. Though patients in laparoscopic group had less pain and returned to work sooner, recurrence was significantly more common (10.1% versus 4.9%). Based on recurrence and safety, open tension-free repair was found to be superior to laparoscopic repair. This study, and the subsequent editorial by Dr. Jacobs, raises many questions regarding the learning curves for laparoscopic procedures, surgeon skill, and future resident training.

16. **Poldermans D, Boersma E, Bax J et al.: The effect of bisoprolol on perioperative mortality and myocardial infarction in high-risk patients undergoing vascular surgery, N Engl J Med 341:1789-1794, 1999.**

    This study is a nice follow-up to the study by Mangano and colleagues that evaluated the cardioprotective effects of beta blockade in patients undergoing major surgery (N Eng J Med 335:1713-1720, 1996.) The patient population in Mangano's study either had or was at-risk for CAD and underwent various surgical procedures. On 2-year follow-up, they found beta blockade did not significantly reduce the incidence of perioperative MI or death from cardiac causes during hospitalization. The patient population studied was not at high risk for perioperative cardiac complications, and therefore they were unable to significantly show a benefit to perioperative beta blockade. To prove the advantage of perioperative beta blockade, Poldermans and colleagues selected patients who were high risk for cardiac complications based on preoperative testing including positive dobutamine echocardiography. They also chose patients who were specifically undergoing vascular procedures. In this high-risk population, beta blockade did in fact significantly reduce perioperative mortality from cardiac causes and nonfatal MI by 34%. This is a great example of the importance in risk-stratifying patients accurately. In the future all surgeons' "report cards" will be public knowledge. It is critical for us to accurately risk-stratify our patients.

    The recommendations for the use of perioperative beta-blockade in high-risk surgical patients are:

    - Beta blockade should be started 1 to 2 weeks preoperatively
    - Preoperative target heart rate less than 70 beats per minute
    - Immediate postoperative heart rate less than 80 beats per minute

17. **Giger UF, Michel JM, Opitz I et al.: Risk factors for perioperative complications in patients undergoing laparoscopic cholecystectomy: analysis of 22,953 consecutive cases from the Swiss Association of Laparoscopic and Thoracoscopic Surgery Database, J Am Coll Surg 203:723-728, 2006.**

    Using the Swiss database, the authors identified a number of risk factors for local and systemic complications in patients undergoing laparoscopic cholecystectomy (LC). There are no surprises reported during this investigation; however, the findings seem to be useful for all of us to recognize so that we can adjust and control surgeon related variables, including skill levels of trainee and supervisor involved in the complex cases and timing of surgery for the complex patients.

18. **Hebert P, Wells G, Blajchman M et al.: A multicenter, randomized, controlled clinical trial of transfusion requirements in critical care, N Eng J Med 340:409-417, 1999.**

    Red cells are responsible for the delivery of oxygen to tissues, and the augmentation of oxygen delivery is generally presumed to be beneficial in critically ill patients; therefore a transfusion threshold of (hemoglobin) 10.0 g had often been deemed acceptable in the critical care setting. Both the risks and benefits of blood transfusions can be significant. Given that blood transfusions are associated with excess volume infusion, immunosuppression, and infection transmission, the benefits of a liberal transfusion strategy had not been clearly established and potentially exposed many patients who did not necessarily need a transfusion to avoidable risks. This multicenter, randomized, controlled trial randomized 838 euvolemic, intensive care patients to either a "restrictive" or "liberal" transfusion strategy. In the restrictive group, patients were given red blood cells when their hemoglobin dropped below 7 g/dl. In the liberal group, patients were transfused at hemoglobin of 10 g/dl. Patients who were less acutely ill and were younger than 55, had a much lower 30-day mortality in the restrictive arm of the study than those in the liberal group (8.7% to 16.1% and 5.7% to 13%, respectively). Patients in the restrictive group also received fewer transfusions (mean of 2.6 units versus 5.6 units) and experienced lower in-hospital mortality (22.2% versus 28.1%; $p = 0.05$). Cardiac events including pulmonary edema and MI occurred more frequently among the liberal transfusion patients during their ICU stay. These findings suggest that a restrictive transfusion strategy with hemoglobin values of 7.0 to 9.0 may be safely applied for most critically ill patients, with the exception of patients with ACS. By shining a light on traditional transfusion triggers, this trial encourages physicians to justify the use and assess the risks and the benefits of blood transfusions.

19. **The Clinical Outcomes of Surgical Therapy Study Group. A comparison of laparoscopic assisted and open colectomy for colon cancer, N Engl J Med 350:2050-2059, 2004.**

Studies comparing laparoscopic and open abdominal operations have generally demonstrated shorter hospitalization and recovery for patients treated laparoscopically; however, as a result of concerns with inadequate oncologic resections and a potential compromise in patient survival, laparoscopic colectomy had not been widely accepted for the management of colon cancer. This randomized control trial was designed to evaluate outcomes in patients undergoing laparoscopic colectomy for colon cancer. A total of 872 patients were randomized to open colectomy or laparoscopic colectomy, with similar patient demographics and distributions of tumor locations in both treatment arms. The findings of the study indicated no difference in complication rates, 30-day mortality, and surgical margin status between the treatment arms. However, perioperative recovery was faster among the patients treated laparoscopically with significant shorter hospital stay and reduced duration of narcotic analgesic usage reported. At 3-year follow up, there was no difference in recurrence rates, overall survival, and disease-free survival. These results along with similar findings reported from a European trial (Lancet Oncol 6:477-484, 2005) have clearly established laparoscopic colectomy as an acceptable surgical treatment for colon cancer. To view a laparoscopic colectomy for cancer, go to www.websurg.com.

20. **Lee T, Marcantonio E, Mangione C et al.: Derivation and prospective validation of a simple index for prediction of cardiac risk of major noncardiac surgery, Circulation 100:1043-1049, 1999.**

During the preoperative evaluation the risks and benefits of the operation should be established and discussed with the patient. The cardiovascular system is challenged during the perioperative period and cardiac complications carry significant morbidity. Therefore, risk stratification for cardiac complications is essential for each patient. Historically, guidelines including Goldman's criteria and the Cardiac Risk Index were devised to determine cardiac risk. The use of these systems has been limited by their complexity. This study proposed a much simpler Revised Cardiac Risk Index (RCRI) to predict the risk of cardiac complications in major elective noncardiac procedures. The study was performed at a highly reputable academic hospital and included 4315 patients. The main outcome measures were cardiac complications. Six independent, equal predictors of complications were identified including: high-risk type of surgery, history of ischemic heart disease, history of congestive heart failure (CHF), history of cerebrovascular disease, preoperative treatment with insulin, and a preoperative serum creatinine >2.0 mg/dl. The RCRI can be calculated quickly and is a valuable tool currently used to accurately risk-stratify patients for cardiac complications in major elective noncardiac procedures.

21. **Gurm HS, Yadav JS, Fayad P et al., for the SAPPHIRE Investigators: Long-term results of carotid stenting versus endarterectomy in high-risk patients, N Engl J Med 358:1572-1579, 2008.**

The authors note that there is a direct relationship between the degree of carotid stenosis and ipsilateral stroke. In the hands of experienced vascular surgeons and interventionalists, this disease can be managed and patients can anticipate extraordinarily good results. The morbidity and mortality of a surgical CEA, even in debilitated patients, is quite low. When an angioplasty catheter is inflated in the cerebral circulation, there is a risk that a tiny bit of crumbled plaque floats north, causing memory loss. So, a fishing net that is placed distal to the deployment of the angioplasty balloon and stent was developed (the first two authors acknowledge that they are the inventors and hold patents on the emboli protection device). In a prospective randomized trial of 260 patients, the authors conclude that carotid artery stenting with protection by the emboli protection device is "not inferior" to CEA at 1 month, 1 year, and 3 years.

CHAPTER 2

CARDIOPULMONARY RESUSCITATION

Amandeep Singh, MD

1. What is cardiac arrest and sudden cardiac death?
Cardiac arrest is the sudden cessation of effective cardiac pumping function as a result of either ventricular asystole (electrical or mechanical) or pulseless ventricular tachycardia or ventricular fibrillation. Sudden cardiac death is the unexpected natural death from a cardiac cause within 1 hour of onset of symptoms; in a person without a previous condition, that would appear fatal.

2. What is the most common dysrhythmia encountered during sudden cardiac death?
Ventricular fibrillation (VF) is the predominate rhythm encountered in the first 3 to 5 minutes after sudden cardiac arrest. VF is characterized by chaotic rapid depolarizations and repolarizations that cause the heart to quiver so that it is unable to pump blood effectively.

3. What is the initial treatment for a patient found to be in ventricular fibrillation?
Immediate therapy with defibrillation is the only effective treatment for VF and is most effective if performed within 5 minutes of collapse. Initiation of cardiopulmonary resuscitation (CPR) with chest compressions and ventilation provides a small but critical amount of blood to the heart and brain while waiting for a defibrillator to arrive.

4. Is endotracheal intubation mandatory during cardiopulmonary resuscitation?
No. Adequate ventilation may be achieved with proper airway positioning, an oropharyngeal or nasopharyngeal airway, and a bag-valve mask attached to an oxygen source. Insertion of an endotracheal tube may be deferred until the patient fails to respond to initial CPR and defibrillation.

5. How is the airway positioned during a resuscitation attempt?
In an unconscious patient, the most common airway obstruction is the patient's tongue, which falls back into the throat when the muscles of the throat and tongue relax. Opening the airway to relieve the tongue from obstruction can be done using the head tilt-chin lift maneuver, or in the patient with suspected cervical spine injury, the jaw-thrust maneuver. If available, an oral airway or nasal trumpet should be inserted.

6. Describe the head tilt-chin lift and jaw-thrust maneuvers
The head tilt-chin lift maneuver consists of two separate maneuvers. First, one hand is placed on the forehead and is used to rotate the head into a "sniffing" position (i.e., neck fully extended and head tilted backwards). Second, the other hand is used to lift the chin forward and up. In the jaw-thrust maneuver, the rescuer places both hands at the sides of the victim's face, grasps the mandible at its angle, and lifts the mandible forward.

7. What is the proper method of chest compressions in children and adults?
The proper position for your hands during chest compressions in children and adults (about 1 year of age and older) is in the center of the chest at the nipple line. Using the heel of both

hands, the rescuer should compress the chest approximately 1½ to 2 inches for adults. The same method is used for children, however one hand is often adequate to compress the chest and the depth of compression should be one third to one half the depth of the chest. Rescuers should push hard, push fast (rate of 100 compressions per minute), allow for complete chest recoil between compressions, and minimize interruptions in compressions for all victims.

8. **What is the interposed abdominal compression cardiopulmonary resuscitation technique?**
   The interposed abdominal compression CPR technique uses a dedicated rescuer to provide manual compression of the abdomen (midway between the xiphoid and the umbilicus) during the relaxation phase of chest compression. This technique is thought to enhance venous return during CPR and has been shown to increase return of spontaneous circulation and short-term survival for in-hospital resuscitations.

9. **What respiratory rate should be achieved during a resuscitation attempt?**
   Rescuers should deliver 8 to 10 breaths per minute during CPR, with each breath delivered over 1 second at a tidal volume sufficient to produce chest rise (approximately 6 to 7 ml/kg or 500 to 600 ml). A number of commercially available devices can be added in-line with a bag-valve mask device to assist in delivering the proper number of breaths per minute. Hyperventilation should be avoided.

10. **What are the advantages to central line insertion during cardiac resuscitation?**
    Advantages to central line insertion
    - Delivery of large fluid volumes can be facilitated with a large-bore central catheter.
    - Peak drug concentrations are higher and circulation times are shorter with central catheters.
    - Supraclavicular insertion into the subclavian vein requires minimal interruption in chest compressions.
    - May be quicker to obtain central access with ultrasound guidance compared to peripheral access in a patient who is severely hypotensive.

    Although certain advantages exist with central line insertion, there is no data to suggest improved outcome with central line placement. In most cases a large-bore peripheral intravenous (IV) or intraosseous (IO) cannulation is adequate for cardiac resuscitation.

11. **Which advanced cardiac life support medications have demonstrated improved survival of neurologically intact patients at hospital discharge?**
    There are no advanced cardiac life support (ACLS) medications that have proven useful in this regard. To date no placebo-controlled trials have shown that administration of any vasopressor agent at any stage of pulseless ventricular tachycardia (VT), VF, pulseless electrical activity (PEA), or asystole increases the rate of neurologically intact survival to hospital discharge.

12. **What is the sequence for treatment of ventricular fibrillation or pulseless ventricular tachycardia?**
    As soon as possible, 120 to 200 J of electricity should be delivered through a biphasic defibrillator (or 360 J through a monophasic defibrillator). A period of CPR should precede defibrillation if the arrest was not witnessed. Immediately following defibrillation, CPR is continued for 2 minutes at which point a brief pulse and rhythm check is done as the defibrillator is recharged. In patients with persistent VF/VT, CPR should be resumed until the charge is complete, and only withheld as the shock is delivered. This sequence of CPR-SHOCK-CPR-RHYTHM CHECK should be continued as long as the patient remains in VF/VT. When IV or IO

access is available, 1 mg of epinephrine IV or IO should be repeated every 3 to 5 minutes or a single dose of 40 U of vasopressin IV or IO should be given. Consider amiodarone 300 mg IV or IO (with an additional 150 mg IV or IO given for patients with refractory VF or VT). Chest compression should not be interrupted for the administration of medications.

13. **What is the sequence for treatment of asystole/pulseless electrical activity?**
CPR should be initiated immediately and continued for 2 minutes before a brief pulse and rhythm check. CPR is continued following the pulse and rhythm check. This sequence of CPR-RHYTHM CHECK should be continued as long as the patient remains in asystole/PEA. When IV or IO access is available, 1 mg of epinephrine IV or IO repeated every 3 to 5 minutes or a single dose of 40 U of vasopressin IV or IO should be given; 1 mg of atropine IV repeated every 3 to 5 minutes (to a maximum of three doses) is given for asystole or slow PEA rate. Chest compression should not be interrupted for the administration of medications.

14. **What are the common treatable contributing factors for cardiac arrest?**
Hypovolemia
Hypoxia
Hydrogen ion (acidosis)
Hypokalemia or Hyperkalemia
Hypoglycemia
Hypothermia
Toxins
Tamponade, cardiac
Tension pneumothorax
Thrombosis, coronary
Thrombosis, pulmonary
Trauma
An easy way to remember the etiology for treatable cardiac arrest is to remember that there are six "H" causes and six "T" causes.

15. **Is there a role for routine fibrinolysis in patients with pulseless electrical activity cardiac arrest?**
No. The results from a recent large clinical trial failed to show any significant treatment effect when a fibrinolytic agent (tPA) was given to out-of-hospital patients with undifferentiated cardiac arrest unresponsive to initial interventions. Individual patients in cardiac arrest in whom a strong suspicion for PEA exists (e.g., immobilized patient, peripartum, deep venous thrombosis [DVT] by history or suggested by physical examination) may benefit from the use of fibrinolytics as a last-ditch, life-saving intervention.

16. **What are the initial objectives of postresuscitation support?**
Optimize cardiopulmonary function and systemic perfusion, especially perfusion to the brain. Try to identify the precipitating cause of the arrest and institute measures to prevent recurrence. Institute measures that may improve long-term, neurologically intact survival.

17. **What is postresuscitation therapeutic hypothermia?**
Postresuscitation induction of hypothermia (cooled to 32°C to 34°C for 12 to 24 hours) for comatose patients with return of spontaneous circulation has been shown to lead to improved neurologic outcome in patients with cardiac arrest. Although most clinical studies of cooling have used external cooling techniques (e.g., cooling blankets and frequent application of ice bags), more recent studies suggest that internal cooling techniques (e.g., cold saline, endovascular cooling catheter) can also be used to induce hypothermia.

18. **What is the role of end-tidal CO_2 monitoring?**

End-tidal carbon dioxide (CO_2) monitoring is a safe and effective noninvasive indicator of cardiac output (CO) during CPR. During cardiac arrest, CO_2 continues to be generated throughout the body. The major determinant of CO_2 excretion is its rate of delivery from the peripheral production sites to the lungs. In the low-flow state during CPR, ventilation is relatively high compared to blood flow, so that end-tidal CO_2 concentration is low. If ventilation is reasonably constant, then changes in end-tidal CO_2 concentrations reflect changes in CO.

19. **What electrolyte abnormalities can lead to cardiac arrest?**

Malignant ventricular dysrhythmias may result from significantly elevated or depleted potassium levels and from hypomagnesemia. Cardiorespiratory arrest can result from severe hypermagnesemia.

20. **What advanced cardiac life support modifications are required in patients with severe electrolyte abnormalities?**

Hyperkalemic cardiac arrest can be seen in patients with renal failure, metabolic acidosis, hemolysis, tumor lysis from chemotherapy, and rhabdomyolysis. It is also seen in patients who receive multiple blood transfusions and in those taking certain medications. Sudden cardiac death in patients with documented or suspected severe hyperkalemia (>7 mEq/L with toxic electrocardiogram [ECG] changes) mandates immediate treatment with IV doses of 1000 mg of calcium chloride, 50 mEq of sodium bicarbonate, 25 g of glucose, and 10 units of regular insulin.

Hypokalemic cardiac arrest is seen in patients with severe hypokalemia (<2.5 mEq/L). Hypokalemia is suspected in patients with alcoholism, diuretic use, severe diarrhea, and diabetes mellitus (DM). Immediate treatment with 10 mEq of IV potassium given over 5 minutes is indicated for patients with malignant ventricular dysrhythmia. Concurrent hypomagnesemia is common in patients with hypokalemia.

Hypomagnesemia is seen in patients with alcoholism, diuretic use, severe diarrhea, diabetic ketoacidosis (DKA), and severe burns. Cardiac arrest resulting from severe hypomagnesemia is often preceded by torsades de pointes on a cardiac monitor. These patients require 2 g MgSO4 IV push over 5 minutes.

Cardiorespiratory arrest from hypermagnesemia is treated with 1000 mg of calcium chloride IV over 2 minutes, along with aggressive volume and respiratory support.

21. **What are the common causes for cardiac arrest resulting from anaphylaxis?**

Life-threatening anaphylaxis is seen with reactions to antibiotics (especially parenteral penicillins and other b-lactams), aspirin and nonsteroidal antiinflammatory drugs, and IV contrast agents. Certain foods, including nuts, seafood, and wheat are associated with life-threatening anaphylaxis from bronchospasm and asphyxia.

22. **What advanced cardiac life support modifications are required in patients with cardiac arrest resulting from anaphylaxis?**

Cardiac arrest from anaphylaxis is as a result of acute airway obstruction coupled with profound venous vasodilation leading to cardiovascular collapse. Early endotracheal intubation, prolonged CPR, aggressive volume administration (typically between 4 and 8 L of isotonic crystalloid), and adrenergic drugs are the cornerstones of therapy. Patients with full cardiac arrest may receive high-dose epinephrine (i.e., escalating from 1 mg to 3 mg to 5 mg over 5 minutes). Surgical or needle cricothyrotomy is indicated if airway edema precludes endotracheal intubation.

23. **What advanced cardiac life support modifications are required in patients with cardiac arrest associated with trauma?**
Basic and advanced life support for the trauma patient is fundamentally the same as that for the patient with a primary cardiac arrest. Hypovolemia, tension pneumothorax, and pericardial tamponade must be quickly evaluated and addressed during resuscitation.

24. **Should all patients in cardiac arrest receive cardiopulmonary resuscitation?**
No. Legitimate reasons to withhold CPR include:
The patient has a valid do not resuscitate (DNR) order.
The patient has signs of irreversible death (e.g., rigor mortis, decapitation, decompensation, or dependent lividity).
No physiologic benefit can be expected because vital functions have deteriorated despite maximal therapy (e.g., progressive septic or cardiogenic shock).

25. **When should resuscitative efforts be terminated?**
The decision to terminate resuscitative efforts rests with the treating physician in the hospital and is based on consideration of many factors, including time to CPR, time to defibrillation, comorbid disease, pre-arrest state, and initial arrest rhythm. None of these factors alone or in combination is clearly predictive of outcome. Reports indicated that prolonged CPR could be effective in cardiac arrest resulting from hypothermia, drug overdose, and anaphylaxis.

26. **When should a "slow-code" be initiated?**
Never. The practice of knowingly providing ineffective resuscitation compromises the ethical integrity of healthcare providers and undermines the physician-patient or nurse-patient relationship.

27. **Can family members be present during resuscitation of a loved one?**
Yes. Not only do the majority of family members surveyed prior to a resuscitation state that they would like to be present during a resuscitation attempt, many family members say that it is comforting to be at the side of their loved one and eases the grief associated with a sudden or expected loss.

28. **What are the most common causes of perioperative cardiac arrest in children?**
About 50% of cases are related to anesthesia, 25% are a result of failure to wean from cardiopulmonary bypass, and 20% related to uncontrolled surgical hemorrhage. Among the cases related to anesthesia, cardiovascular causes were the most common (41% of all arrests), with hypovolemia from blood loss and hyperkalemia from transfusion of stored blood the most common identifiable cardiovascular causes. Among respiratory causes of arrest (27% of all arrests), airway obstruction from laryngospasm was the most common cause. Medication-related cardiac arrest accounted for 18% of all arrests. Vascular injury incurred during placement of central venous catheters was the most common equipment-related cause of arrest.

29. **What is the revised cardiac risk index?**
The revised cardiac risk index (RCRI) accurately predicts major cardiac events (e.g., myocardial infarction [MI], pulmonary embolus [PE], VF, heart block, or cardiac arrest) in adults undergoing major noncardiac surgery. Each risk factor is assigned a single point: high-risk surgical procedure, history of ischemic heart disease, history of congestive heart failure (CHF), history of cerebrovascular disease, preoperative treatment with insulin, preoperative serum creatinine >2.0 mg/dl. The risk of a major cardiac event is <1% if there is none or one risk factor present. A 6.6% risk of major cardiac event occurs if two risk factors are present, and increases to 11% if three or more risk factors are present.

BIBLIOGRAPHY

1. Ali B, Zafari AM: Narrative review: cardiopulmonary resuscitation and emergency cardiovascular care: review of the current guidelines, Ann Intern Med 147:171-179, 2007.

2. American Heart Association: American Heart Association guidelines for cardiopulmonary resuscitation and emergency cardiovascular care, Circulation 112 (suppl), 2005.

3. Bhananker SM, Ramamoorthy C, Geiduschek JM et al.: Anesthesia-related cardiac arrest in children: update from the pediatric perioperative cardiac arrest registry, Anesth Analg 105:344-350, 2007.

4. Ibrahim WH: Recent advances and controversies in adult cardiopulmonary resuscitation, Postgrad Med J 83:649-654, 2007.

5. Lee TH, Marcantonio ER, Mangione CM et al.: Derivation and prospective validation of a simple index for prediction of cardiac risk of major noncardiac surgery, Circulation 100:1043-1049, 1999.

6. Greene RS, Howes D: Hypothermic modulation of anoxic brain injury in adult survivors of cardiac arrest: A review of the literature and an algorithm for emergency physicians, Can J Emerg Med 7:42-47, 2005.

CHAPTER 3

EVALUATION AND TREATMENT OF CARDIAC DYSRHYTHMIAS

Laurel R. Imhoff, MD, MPH, and Alden H. Harken, MD

1. Are cardiac dysrhythmias and cardiac arrhythmias the same?

Yes. Some purists will tell you that an arrhythmia can be only the absence of a cardiac rhythm. But these are the same purists who use the word iatrogenic to mean "caused by a physician," when, of course, the only thing that can truly be "iatrogenic" is a physician's parents.

2. Are all cardiac dysrhythmias clinically important?

Most are not. Many of us have isolated premature ventricular contractions (PVCs) or premature ventricular depolarizations (PVDs) all the time. Superbly conditioned athletes frequently exhibit resting heart rates in the 30s. A clinically important cardiac dysrhythmia is a rhythm that bothers the patient. As a rule, if the patient's ventricular rate is 60 to 100 beats per minute (regardless of mechanism), cardiac rhythm is not a problem.

3. State the goals in the treatment of cardiac dysrhythmias.

The primary goal is to control ventricular rate between 60 and 100 beats per minute, and the secondary goal is to maintain sinus rhythm.

4. How important is sinus rhythm?

It depends on the patient's ventricular function. Induction of atrial fibrillation in a medical student volunteer causes no measurable hemodynamic effect. Your ventricular compliance is so good that you do not need an atrial "kick" to fill the ventricle completely.
Conversely, the worse (the stiffer) the patient's heart, the more you should try to maintain sinus rhythm. We observed a patient with a 7% left ventricular (LV) ejection fraction (EF) whose cardiac output (CO) decreased by 40% when he spontaneously developed atrial fibrillation.

5. Do you need to be ankle-deep in electrocardiogram paper and personally acquainted with Drs. Mobitz, Lown, and Ganong to treat cardiac dysrhythmias in the intensive care unit (ICU)?

No.

6. When you are called by the ICU nurse to see a patient with an arrhythmia, what questions do you ask yourself?

1. *Does the patient really exhibit an arrhythmia?* What is the patient doing? Is the stuff that looks like ventricular fibrillation (VF) really just the patient brushing his or her teeth? Or is the rhythm strip that looks like asystole really just a loose lead? If the patient does exhibit an arrhythmia, ask yourself the following questions.

2. *Does the arrhythmia require intervention?* Isolated PVCs usually can be ignored safely. Similarly a resting bradycardia in a triathlete is normal. This is the occasion to launch into your "2-second physical exam." Is the patient sweaty and confused or alert and happy?

3. *What is a 2-second physical exam?* You look into the patient's eyes, hoping to determine whether he or she is perfusing his or her brain. If the patient looks back at you, you have some time. If the patient requires therapy, ask yourself the following questions.

4. *How soon is therapy required?* At this point, the patient becomes (paradoxically) irrelevant. The most robust indicator dictating velocity of intervention is not how sick the patient is, but how frightened you are. You must determine rapidly whether delay in therapy is likely to put the patient at risk. If the cardiac arrhythmia is likely to inflict psychopathologic (hypoxemic) consequences not only on the patient, but also, by extension, on his or her extended (societal) family, you should be frightened. If you are frightened, you must ask yourself:

5. *What is the safest and most effective therapy?*

7. If the patient requires antiarrhythmic therapy, what is the safest and most effective strategy?

Therapy for cardiac arrhythmias is simple and comprises three comprehensible concepts:

1. If the patient is hemodynamically unstable (the sole determinant of instability is whether you are frightened), cardiovert with 360 J. (For lower energy, see Chapter 2.)

2. If the patient has a wide-complex tachycardia, cardiovert with 360 J.

3. If the patient has a narrow-complex tachycardia, infuse an atrioventricular (AV) nodal blocker intravenously (IV). If at any time the patient becomes unstable, proceed with cardioversion.

8. In assessing a cardiac impulse, how do you distinguish supraventricular from ventricular origin?

Supraventricular origin: When an impulse originates above the AV node (supraventricular), it can access the ventricles only through the AV node. The AV node connects with the endocardial Purkinje system, which conducts impulses rapidly (2 to 3 m/sec). A supraventricular impulse activates the ventricles rapidly (<0.08 sec, 80 msec, or two little boxes on the electrocardiogram [ECG] paper), producing a narrow-complex beat.

Ventricular origin: When an impulse originates directly from an ectopic site on the ventricle, it takes longer to access the high-speed Purkinje system. A ventricular impulse activates the entire ventricular mass slowly (<0.08 sec, 80 msec, or two little boxes on the ECG paper), producing a wide-complex beat (See Fig. 3-1).

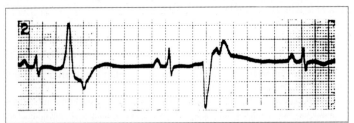

Figure 3-1. Wide-complex beats are of ventricular origin. Narrow-complex beats are of supraventricular origin.

9. **Extra credit: Correlate the ECG with cardiomyocyte membrane ion flux.**
   See Fig. 3-2.

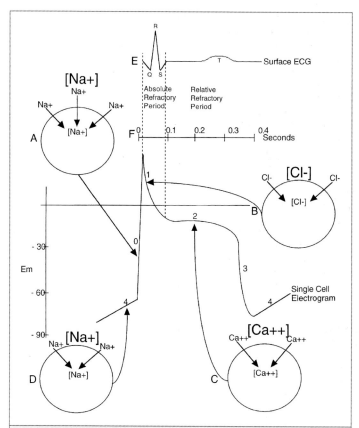

Figure 3-2. Typical action potential of a cardiac myocyte, the ionic shifts responsible for each phase, and correlation with the surface ECG. **A,** Phase 0 = rapid depolarization, characterized by rapid influx of sodium (Na+) through the voltage-gated Na+ channels. **B,** Phase 1 = brief repolarization, characterized by transient influx of chloride (Cl-). **C,** Phase 2 = plateau phase, characterized by a rapid rise in calcium (Ca2+) permeability through L-type Ca2+ channels. Phase 3 = repolarization with potassium (K+) exiting the cell. **D,** Slow depolarization of pacemaker cells caused by slow influx of Na+. (From Meldrum DR, Cleveland JC, Sheridan BC et al.: Cardiac surgical implications of calcium dyshomeostasis in the heart, Ann Thorac Surg 61:1273-1280, 1996, with permission.)

10. **Do all wide-complex beats derive from the ventricles?**
    No, but most do. An impulse of supraventricular origin that is conducted with aberrancy through the ventricle can take enough time to make it a wide-complex beat. In one study, 89% of 100 patients presenting to an emergency department (ED) with a wide-complex tachycardia eventually proved to exhibit ventricular tachycardia, whereas 11% were diagnosed with supraventricular tachycardia with aberrancy.

11. **What do you do if you cannot tell whether a ventricular complex is wide or narrow?**
    Acutely and transiently (for 5 seconds) block the AV node by giving 6 mg of adenosine IV; if the ventricular complex persists, it is ventricular. If the ventricular complex stops, it was supraventricular.

12. **To prevent lots of supraventricular impulses from getting to the ventricles, how do you block the atrioventricular node pharmacologically?**
    In *seconds,* give 6 mg adenosine IV push.
    In *minutes,* draw up 20 mg Diltiazem (calcium channel blocker), infuse as IV over 2 minutes. If necessary start continuous IV infusion of 5-10 mg/hr to be started immediately following IV bolus. (For IV infusion do not exceed 15 mg/hr and the drug should not be infused for more than 24 hours.)
    In *hours,* put 0.5 mg digoxin in 100 ml of Ringer's lactate and infuse by IV drip over 30 minutes.

KEY POINTS: CHARACTERIZATION OF CARDIAC DYSRHYTHMIAS

1. Supraventricular origin: when an impulse originates above the AV node, it can access the ventricles only through the AV node to reach the Purkinje system, which conducts and activates the ventricles rapidly, producing a narrow-complex beat (<2 small boxes on ECG).

2. Ventricular origin: when an impulse originates from an ectopic site on the ventricle, it takes longer to access the high-speed Purkinje system. A ventricular impulse activates the entire mass, slowly producing a wide-complex beat (>2 small boxes on ECG).

3. Not all wide-complex beats are ventricular in origin.

4. To distinguish ventricular from supraventricular tachycardia, transiently block AV node with adenosine intravenous push. If ventricular complex persists, it is ventricular tachycardia; if the complex stops, it is supraventricular tachycardia.

13. **Why give digoxin?**
    Digoxin is an effective AV nodal blocker, but it makes cardiomyocytes more excitable. By giving digoxin, you make supraventricular impulses more likely; but by blocking the AV node, you render these impulses less dangerous.

14. **Why infuse digoxin over 30 to 60 minutes intravenously?**
    Studies indicate that a big pulse of digoxin (IV push) concentrates in the myocardium, making the myocytes hyperexcitable. Digoxin infused more slowly avoids this problem.

15. **List the steps in calling a dysrhythmia by name.**
    Bradycardia: <60 beats per minute
    Tachycardia: 100 to 250 beats per minute
    Flutter: atrial or ventricular rate 250 to 400 beats per minute
    Fibrillation: atrial or ventricular rate >400 beats per minute

WEBSITES

www.blaufuss.org/

www.americanheart.org/presenter.jhtml?identifier=10000056#P

BIBLIOGRAPHY

1. Echahidi N, Pibarot P, O'Hara G et al.: Mechanisms, prevention, and treatment of atrial fibrillation after cardiac surgery, J Am Coll Cardiol 51:793-801, 2008.
2. Harken AH: Cardiac dysrhythmias. In Wilmore DW, Cheung L, Harken AH et al., editors: Scientific American surgery, New York, 1999, Scientific American.
3. Meldrum DR, Cleveland JC, Sheridan BC et al.: Cardiac surgical implications of calcium dyshomeostasis in the heart, Ann Thorac Surg 61:1273-1280, 1996.
4. Vukanovic-Criley JM, Criley S, Warde CM et al.: Competency in cardiac examination skills in medical students, trainees, physicians, and faculty: a multicenter study, Arch Intern Med 166:610-616, 2006.
5. Walsh SR, Tang T, Wijewardena C et al.: Postoperative arrhythmias in general surgical patients, Ann R Coll Surg Engl 89:91, 2007.

CHAPTER 4

HOW TO THINK ABOUT SHOCK

Laurel R. Imhoff, MD, MPH, and Alden H. Harken, MD

1. **Define shock.**
   Shock is:
   - Not just low blood pressure.
   - Not just decreased peripheral perfusion.
   - Not just limited systemic oxygen delivery.

   Ultimately, shock is decreased tissue respiration. Shock is suboptimal consumption of oxygen and excretion of carbon dioxide (CO_2) at the cellular level.

2. **Is shock related to cardiac output?**
   Yes. A healthy medical student can redistribute blood flow preferentially to vital organs. After a 3- to 4-unit bleed, your typical young gunslinger can still think and can tell you: "four dudes jumped me." From this history you have no idea what happened to him, but you do know that he is still perfusing his brain.

3. **Is organ perfusion democratic?**
   No. Limited blood flow always is redirected toward the carotid and coronary arteries. Peripheral vasoconstriction steals blood initially from the mesentery, then skeletal muscle, and then kidneys and liver.

4. **Is this vascular autoregulatory capacity uniform in all patients?**
   No. With age and atherosclerosis, patients lose their ability to redistribute limited blood flow. A 20% decrease in cardiac output (CO), or a fall in blood pressure to 90 mm Hg, can be life-threatening to a Supreme Court justice, whereas it may be undetectable in a triathlete.

5. **For diagnostic and practical therapeutic purposes, can shock be classified?**
   Yes.
   1. **Hypovolemic shock** mandates volume resuscitation.
   2. **Cardiogenic shock** mandates cardiac stimulation (pharmacologic and eventually mechanical).
   3. **Peripheral vascular collapse shock** mandates pharmacologic manipulation of the peripheral vascular tone (and direct attention to the cause of the vasodilation—typically sepsis).

6. **Is it advisable to treat all shock in the same sequential fashion?**
   Ultimately, yes. Whether a cigar-chomping banker presents with a big gastrointestinal (GI) bleed (hypovolemic shock) or crushing substernal chest pain (cardiogenic shock), the surgeon should take the following steps in order:
   1. **Optimize volume status;** give volume until further increase in right-sided (central venous pressure [CVP]) and left-sided (pulmonary capillary wedge pressure [PCWP]) preload confers no additional benefit for CO or blood pressure (BP). (This step is Starling's law; place the patient's heart at the top of the Starling curve.)

2. If CO, BP, and tissue perfusion remain inadequate despite adequate preload, the patient has a pump (cardiogenic shock) problem. **Infuse cardiac inotropic drugs** (β-agonist) to the point of toxicity (typically cardiac ectopy), which will have lots of frightening premature ventricular contractions. For pharmacologically refractory cardiogenic shock, insert an intraaortic balloon pump (IABP).

3. If the patient exhibits a surprisingly high CO and a paradoxically low BP (such unusual loss of vascular autoregulatory control is associated typically, but not always, with sepsis), **infuse a peripheral vasoconstrictor drug** (α-agonist).

7. What is the preferred access route for volume infusion?

Flow depends on catheter length and radius. Volume may be infused at twice the rate through a 5-cm, 14-gauge peripheral catheter as through a 20-cm, 16-gauge central line. Assessment of CVP (and left-sided filling pressure) is necessary if the patient fails to respond to initial volume resuscitation.

8. Should one infuse crystalloid, colloid, or blood?

If the goal is only to improve preload and to repair CO and BP, crystalloid solution should be sufficient. It is controversial whether infused colloid remains in the vascular compartment. If the goal is to augment systemic oxygen delivery, red blood cells bind much more oxygen than plasma (see Chapter 7). Crystalloid should enhance flow, and blood should augment oxygen delivery.

9. When cardiac preload is adequate, which inotropic agents are useful?

Dobutamine, epinephrine, and norepinephrine are the chocolate, vanilla, and strawberry of the 32 flavors of cardiogenic drugs. These three drugs are all that the surgeon really needs.

10. Is dopamine the same as dobutamine?

No. Dopamine stimulates renal dopaminergic receptors and may be useful in low doses (2 milligrams per kilogram per minute) to counteract the renal arteriolar vasoconstriction that accompanies shock. Dopamine has no place as a primary cardiac inotropic agent.

11. Discuss the use of dobutamine, epinephrine, and norepinephrine.

See Table 4-1.

TABLE 4-1. USE OF DOBUTAMINE, EPINEPHRINE, AND NOREPINEPHRINE

Dobutamine is a β_1-agonist (cardiac inotrope), but it also has some β_2 effects (peripheral vasodilation).

Start at: 5 micrograms per kilogram per minute and increase to point of toxicity (cardiac ectopy).

Note: Infuse to desired effect (do not stick rigidly to a preconceived dose). Because dobutamine has some vasodilating effects, it may be frightening to infuse into typically hypotensive patients in shock.

Epinephrine is a combined β- and α-adrenergic agonist, with the β effects predominating at lower doses and progressive vasoconstriction accompanying increased doses.

Start at: 0.05 micrograms per kilogram per minute and increase to point of toxicity (cardiac ectopy).

Note: As with dobutamine, infuse to desired effect.

(Continued)

TABLE 4-1.   USE OF DOBUTAMINE, EPINEPHRINE, AND NOREPINEPHRINE—CONT'D
Norepinephrine is a combined α- and β-adrenergic agonist, with the α effects predominating at all doses.
Start at: 0.05 milligrams per kilogram per minute and increase to point of toxicity (cardiac ectopy).
Note: Relatively pure peripheral vasoconstriction rarely is indicated and should be used only to modulate the peripheral vascular tone in peripheral vascular collapse shock.

12. When is an intraaortic balloon pump indicated?

Mechanical circulatory support is indicated when the preload to both ventricles (CVP and PCWP) has been optimized and further cardiac stimulatory drugs are limited by frightening runs of premature ventricular contractions. Do not be afraid to resort to mechanical support.

KEY POINTS: SUMMARY OF ADRENERGIC AGENTS

1. Dobutamine: β_1 agonist (cardiac inotrope) with mild-to-moderate β_2 effects (peripheral vasodilation).

2. Epinephrine: combined β- and α-adrenergic agent, with the β effects predominating at lower doses and progressive vasoconstriction accompanying increased doses.

3. Norepinephrine: combined β- and α-adrenergic agonist, with the α effects predominating at all doses.

13. What does an intraaortic balloon pump do?

It provides diastolic augmentation and systolic unloading.

14. What is diastolic augmentation?

A soft 40-ml balloon is inserted percutaneously through the common femoral artery into the descending thoracic aorta. The balloon is not occlusive (it should not touch the aortic walls). When it is inflated, it displaces 40 ml of blood and is exactly like acutely transfusing 40 ml of blood into the aorta, augmenting each LV stroke volume by 40 ml. Balloon infusion is triggered off the QRS complex from a surface ECG (any lead). The balloon is always inflated during diastole to increase diastolic blood pressure (DBP) and augment coronary blood flow (CBF). Eighty percent of CBF occurs during diastole.

KEY POINTS: INTRAAORTIC BALLOON PUMP

1. Indicated for cardiogenic shock refractory to pharmacologic manipulation.

2. Triggered by QRS complex of surface ECG; inflates during diastole (T wave) and deflates on systole (R wave or at dicrotic notch on aortic pressure curve).

3. Eighty percent of CBF occurs during diastole.

4. Mechanistically results in diastolic augmentation and systolic unloading (afterload reduction).

15. **What is systolic unloading?**
Balloon deflation is an active (not a passive) process. Helium abruptly is sucked out of the balloon, leaving a 40-ml empty space in the aorta. The left ventricle can eject the first 40 ml of its stroke volume into this empty space at dramatically reduced workload. An intraaortic balloon increases CBF during diastole, while decreasing cardiac oxygen consumption just presystole.

16. **Name the contraindications to intraaortic balloon pump.**
The two main contraindications to an IABP are aortic insufficiency and atrial fibrillation.
Aortic insufficiency is when diastolic augmentation distends and injures the left ventricle.
Atrial fibrillation is when balloon inflation and deflation cannot be appropriately timed.

WEBSITES

www.aic.cuhk.edu.hk/web8/IABP.htm

www.ccmtutorials.com/index.htm

www.acid-base.com/

BIBLIOGRAPHY

1. Harken AH: Cardiac dysrhythmias. In Wilmore DW, Cheung L, Harken AH et al., editors: Scientific American surgery, New York, 1999, Scientific American.

2. Hirshberg A, Hoyt DB, Mattox KL: From "leaky buckets" to vascular injuries: understanding models of uncontrolled hemorrhage. J Am Coll Surg 204:665-672, 2007.

3. Holcroft JW: Shock. In Wilmore DW, Cheung L, Harken AH et al., editors: American college of surgeons surgery, New York, 2002, WebMD Corporation.

4. Peters MJ, Brierley J: Back to basics in septic shock. Intensive Care Med 34(6):991-993. Epub 2008.

5. Vincent JL, Weil MH: Fluid challenge revisited. Crit Care Med 34:1333-1337, 2006.

CHAPTER 5

WHAT IS PULMONARY INSUFFICIENCY?

Alden H. Harken, MD

1. **What is pulmonary insufficiency?**
   The alveolar-capillary surface of the lung is the size of a singles tennis court. The purpose of the lung is to match alveolar ventilation (V) to blood flow (Q). V/Q mismatching leads to pulmonary insufficiency.

2. **How is alveolar ventilation and blood flow mismatching characterized?**
   Shunt: decreased ventilation relative to regional blood flow; pulmonary arterial (unoxygenated) blood "shunts" by hypoventilated alveoli.
   Dead space: decreased pulmonary regional blood flow relative to ventilation.
   So, both shunt (less ventilation than flow) and dead space (ventilated zones that are not perfused) qualify as V/Q mismatch.

3. **How much energy is expended in the work of breathing?**
   A healthy medical student expends about 3% of total oxygen consumption (energy use) on work of breathing. After injury, particularly a big burn, patients may increase fractional energy expenditure of breathing to 20% of their total energy use.

4. **Which surgical incisions most significantly compromise a patient's vital capacity?**
   Intuitively an extremity incision or injury influences vital capacity least, followed sequentially by a lower abdominal incision, median sternotomy, thoracotomy, and upper abdominal incision. An upper abdominal incision is worse than a thoracotomy!

5. **Is a chest radiograph helpful in assessing respiratory failure?**
   Yes, but the radiograph must be interpreted carefully. It can be difficult to standardize x-ray technique, especially in an intensive care unit (ICU).

6. **What should you look for on the chest radiograph of a patient with impending respiratory failure?**
   1. Are both lungs fully expanded?
   2. Are there localized areas of infiltrate, atelectasis, or consolidation?
   3. Are there generalized areas of infiltrate, atelectasis, or consolidation?
   4. Are the endotracheal and other tubes in proper position?
   5. Why is the local versus generalized distinction important in assessing respiratory failure?
   A local process may be produced by tumor or aspiration, and both are diagnosed and treated by bronchoscopy. Generalized multilobar infiltrates are more likely to represent a diffuse alveolar-capillary leak syndrome, such as adult respiratory distress syndrome (ARDS).

7. **What is adult respiratory distress syndrome?**
   ARDS is a diffuse, multilobar capillary transudation of fluid into the pulmonary interstitium that dissociates the normal concordance of V with Q.

8. **What governs fluid flux across pulmonary capillaries into the interstitium of the lung?**
Starling initially described the balance between intravascular hydrostatic pressure (Pc), which tends to push fluid out of the capillaries, and colloid oncotic pressure (COP), which sucks fluid back in across the capillary endothelial barrier (K):

$$\text{Fluid flux} = 5 \, K(Pc - COP)$$

9. **What causes ARDS?**
Anything that increases lung dysfunction by promoting wet lung:
   1. **Heart failure** backs up pulmonary intravascular Pc, forcing fluid into the pulmonary interstitium.
   2. **Malnutrition and liver failure** decrease plasma protein and therefore COP. Fluid is not sucked back out of the lung (if the total protein and albumin are low).
   3. **Sepsis** may break down the capillary endothelial barrier (K), permitting water and protein to leak into the lung.

KEY POINTS: CLINICAL FEATURES OF ACUTE RESPIRATORY DISTRESS SYNDROME

1. Severe hypoxemia refractory to increased inspired oxygen concentration
2. Diffuse pulmonary infiltrates
3. Low lung compliance
4. Large ventilation/perfusion (V/Q) mismatch

10. **Explain high-pressure versus low-pressure ARDS.**
Purists appropriately note that lung congestion resulting from high intravascular Pc hydrostatic pressure secondary to heart failure is really not primary respiratory distress syndrome. If the pulmonary capillary wedge pressure (PCWP) is >18 mm Hg, the diagnosis is high-pressure pulmonary edema (not ARDS). A patient with pure mitral stenosis may have (high-pressure) lung congestion, whereas a malnourished patient may develop (low-pressure) lung congestion; neither of these is, strictly speaking, ARDS, although patients with ARDS frequently have components of both.

11. **What is a normal colloid oncotic pressure (COP)?**
It is 22 mm Hg.

12. **How is COP calculated?**
Of COP, 75% normally is created by serum albumin along with globulins and fibrinogen:

$$COP = 2.1 \, (\text{total protein})$$

If an osmotically active molecule such as hetastarch is infused, this calculation is fouled up.

13. **Define low-pressure ARDS.**

   Low-pressure ARDS is a redundant term. To make the diagnosis of ARDS, the PCWP must be <18 mm Hg. Pure ARDS exists only if the PCWP is >4 mm Hg less than the COP.

14. **How can the pulmonary capillaries leak if the COP exceeds the PCWP?**

   The current concept involves a septic expression of neutrophil CD11 and CD18 adhesion receptors, which stick to pulmonary vascular endothelial intercellular adhesion molecules. Septic stimuli provoke the adherent neutrophils to release intravascular proteases and oxygen radicals. Resultant endovascular damage breaks down the K, permitting the lung leak-even at low Pc.

15. **What is a Lasix sandwich?**

   Many surgeons, when their backs are against the wall, give 25 g of albumin followed in 20 minutes by 20 mg of furosemide (Lasix) intravenously (IV). They reason that the albumin pulls fluid out of the water-logged lung and the Lasix promotes diuresis to rid the patient of extra water. This therapeutic concept probably works only in patients who are not very sick. The sicker the patient, the faster the infused albumin leaks and equilibrates across the damaged endovascular endothelial barrier. Little water is sucked out of the sick lung in preparation for diuresis.

16. **List the goals of therapy for ARDS.**

   1. Reduce lung edema (typically with a diuretic).
   2. Reduce oxygen toxicity (inspired oxygen concentration <60% is safe).
   3. Limit lung barotrauma (avoid peak inspiratory pressure in >40 cm H_2O).
   4. Promote matching of V and Q; frequently positive end-expiratory pressure (PEEP) is useful.
   5. Maintain systemic oxygen delivery (arterial oxygen content × cardiac output [CO]).

17. **What governs the distribution of lung perfusion?**

   It is governed mostly by gravity. The dependent portions of the lung always are better perfused.

18. **Discuss hypoxic pulmonary vasoconstriction (HPV).**

   Most students believe that after dedicating the entire second year of medical school to pheochromocytoma and hypoxic pulmonary vasoconstriction (HPV), both entities may be safely forgotten. At least in the case of HPV, this is not true. A patient who has just undergone carotid endarterectomy (CEA) illustrates the relevance of HPV. As the patient awakens from anesthesia, the blood pressure (BP) is 220/120 mm Hg and arterial partial pressure of oxygen (PO_2) with 100% oxygen is 500 mm Hg. So that the patient will not blow the carotid anastomosis, the surgeon urgently infuses nitroprusside. In 20 minutes, the blood pressure is 120/80 mm Hg, but PO_2 (still with 100% oxygen) has dropped to 125 mm Hg!

   Did the lab technician screw up the blood gas analysis? No; this is an example of the clinical significance of HPV, which directs pulmonary arteriolar delivery of deoxygenated blood toward ventilated alveoli and away from poorly ventilated lung regions. The patient was using HPV to attain a PO_2 of 500 mm Hg. All antihypertensive agents (e.g., nitroprusside) and most general anesthetics block HPV. The PO_2 increment from 125 to 500 mm Hg is as a result of HPV. HPV steered perfusion toward ventilated areas of the lung.

19. **What governs the distribution of ventilation in lung?**

   A large pleural pressure gradient (more negative at the top of the lung by 20 cm H_2O) squeezes gas primarily out of the dependent lung during each exhaled breath. The regional compliance of dependent lung is much better than that of lung apex, which still is distended with gas at the end of exhalation. The usual approach is to perfuse and ventilate dependent lung preferentially.

KEY POINTS: THERAPEUTIC GOALS IN ACUTE RESPIRATORY DISTRESS SYNDROME

1. Reduce lung edema
2. Reduce oxygen toxicity (FiO_2 <60%)
3. Minimize barotraumas (keep peak inspiratory pressure <40 cm H_2O)
4. PEEP to promote V/Q matching
5. Maintain systemic oxygen delivery (arterial oxygen content × CO)

---

20. **How does ARDS compromise lung function?**
    The trachea is held open with cartilaginous rings, but terminal bronchioles are not. Wet lung collapses the terminal bronchioles, trapping distal alveolar gas. Persistent perfusion of these poorly ventilated regions is a shunt that results in hypoxia.

21. **How long does it take for pulmonary arterial (deoxygenated) blood to equilibrate completely with trapped (poorly oxygenated) alveolar gas?**
    It takes about three fourths of a second. After that, no more oxygen is added, and no more carbon dioxide (CO_2) is eliminated from the perfusing blood. Terminal bronchiolar closure producing trapped alveolar gas is bad.

22. **What is the therapy for terminal airways closure and resultant shunt secondary to the wet lung of ARDS?**
    PEEP should hold open terminal bronchioles, promoting ventilation of previously trapped alveoli and minimizing the shunt.

23. **When may the patient come off mechanical ventilation and be extubated safely?**
    The patient should be sufficiently alert to protect his or her airway, require an inspired oxygen concentration (FiO_2) no greater than 0.4, and be comfortable breathing on a T-piece (without mechanical ventilation) for 60 minutes at a respiratory rate <20 and a minute ventilation <10 L/min. The patient should be able to generate a negative inspiratory force >−20 cm H_2O. Finally, after 1 hour on the T-piece, oxygenation should provide a hemoglobin saturation >85% without respiratory acidosis (see Chapter 7).

24. **What is nitric oxide?**
    Nitric oxide (NO) is synthesized in vascular endothelial cells by constitutive nitric oxide synthase (cNOS) and inducible NOS (iNOS). Intuitively, inhaled NO should diffuse across ventilated alveoli to increase regional perfusion and improve matching of V and Q.

25. **Does inhaled NO work in ARDS?**
    Almost 24 randomized controlled clinical trials have assessed the therapeutic efficacy of inhaled NO. Although systemic oxygenation and pulmonary hypertension improve transiently, ventilator time and ultimate survival are not influenced.

WEBSITES

www.ardsnet.org

www.nlm.nih.gov/medlineplus/ency/article/000103.htm

BIBLIOGRAPHY

1. Bartlett R: Pulmonary insufficiency, New York, 2006, American College of Surgeons, Surgery WebMd Corporation.

2. Chetta A, Tzani P, Marangio E et al.: Respiratory effects of surgery and pulmonary function testing in the preoperative evaluation. Acta Biomed 77:69-74, 2006.

3. Davidson TA, Caldwell ES, Curtis JR et al.: Reduced quality of life in survivors of acute respiratory distress syndrome compared with critically ill control patients. JAMA 281:354-360, 1999.

4. Gust R, McCarthy TJ, Kozlowski J et al.: Response to inhaled nitric oxide in acute lung injury depends on distribution of pulmonary blood flow prior to its administration. Am J Respir Crit Care Med 159:563-570, 1999.

5. Pesenti A, Fumagalli R: PEEP: blood gas cosmetics or a therapy for ARDS? Crit Care Med 27:253-254, 1999.

6. Wang T, Tagayun A, Bogardus A et al.: How accurately can we predict forced expiratory volume in one second after major pulmonary resection? Am Surg 73:1047-1051, 2007.

7. Westwood K, Griffin M, Roberts K et al.: Incentive spirometry decreases respiratory complications following major abdominal surgery. Surgeon 5:339-342, 2007.

CHAPTER 6

MECHANICAL VENTILATION

Jeffrey L. Johnson, MD, and James B. Haenel, RRT

1. **Why do patients need mechanical ventilation?**

   There are three basic categories of need when it comes to mechanical ventilation (MV): (1) inadequate respiratory drive; (2) inability to maintain adequate alveolar ventilation; and (3) hypoxia. The decision to provide MV should be based on clinical examination and assessment of gas exchange by arterial blood gas (ABG) analysis as needed. It is an individualized decision because arbitrary cutoff values for the partial pressure of oxygen (PO_2), partial pressure of carbon dioxide (pCO_2), or acid-base balance (pH) may not be germane to all patients. Common derangements necessitating the need for MV include primary parenchymal disorders, such as pneumonia, pulmonary edema, or pulmonary contusion, and systemic disease that indirectly compromises pulmonary function, such as sepsis or central nervous system (CNS) dysfunction.

2. **Does mechanical ventilation make the lung better?**

   Not really. In the setting of respiratory failure, the aim is to support gas exchange while the underlying disease process is reversed. Certain techniques can be used to recruit more airspace for gas exchange, but overall it is much easier to hurt the lung with a ventilator (i.e., ventilator induced lung injury [VILI]) than to fix it.

3. **How many modes of ventilation can you name?**

   Common modes include controlled mechanical ventilation (CMV), assist-control ventilation (ACV), intermittent mandatory ventilation (IMV), synchronized IMV (SIMV), pressure-controlled ventilation (PCV), pressure-support ventilation (PSV), inverse ratio ventilation (IRV), airway pressure-release ventilation (APRV), mandatory minute ventilation (MMV), high-frequency ventilation (HFV), and dual control modes, such as pressure regulated volume control (PRVC). The most basic difference between these modes of ventilation is based on whether they deliver *mandatory breaths* (whether inspiration is machine triggered or machine cycled) versus *spontaneous breaths* (whether inspiration is patient triggered and patient cycled).

4. **What three elements can characterize all of the aforementioned mechanical ventilation modes?**

   Each mode can be described by how a breath is *triggered* (by the patient or by the machine), how it is *cycled* (switches from inhalation to exhalation), and how it is *limited* (for example by time, by pressure, or by flow).

5. **What are the most commonly used modes of positive-pressure ventilation?**

   ACV, IMV, SIMV, and PSV, which all differ primarily in how the breaths are triggered and cycled.

6. **How does assist-control ventilation work?**

   The ACV mode delivers a set minimum number of machine triggered breaths and also allows the patient to trigger a breath. Every breath (mandatory or patient triggered spontaneous) is *cycled* when a preset volume has been delivered at a preset flow rate. Because the patient receives a full tidal volume with every breath, even when tachypneic, ACV may result in respiratory alkalosis more often and may promote auto-positive end-expiratory pressure (PEEP).

7. **How does intermittent mechanical ventilation differ from assist-control ventilation?**

Like ACV, the ventilator provides a preset number of machine triggered breaths at a preset tidal volume and flow rate in the IMV mode. Unlike ACV, however, the patient-triggered breaths are not cycled at a preset volume. Rather, spontaneous breaths are cycled based on the patient's own respiratory efforts (usually by sensing the end of patient effort as the flow rate falls). IMV may allow a decreased mean airway pressure (Paw) and possibly less barotrauma, because not every breath is a full positive-pressure breath.

8. **Compare intermittent mechanical ventilation with synchronized intermittent mechanical ventilation**

SIMV prevents "stacking" of breaths by deferring a machine-triggered breath if it would occur in the middle of a spontaneous breath. It is therefore easier to synchronize the patient's effort with the ventilator in the SIMV mode. In practice, most IMV is delivered as SIMV. Both modes involve additional work of breathing on the patient's part. Pressure support can be added during the spontaneous breaths to alleviate this work. It may be advantageous to relieve as much work of breathing as possible in the early part of respiratory failure.

9. **What are the pressure-limited types of ventilation?**

PSV, PRVC, HFV, and PCV. PSV is a mode of ventilation used in spontaneously breathing patients to decrease the imposed work of breathing from the endotracheal tube and to overcome resistance in the breathing circuit. It is often used to "wean" or determine the readiness of a patient to discontinue MV. PSV is a pure assisted form of ventilation. The patient must always trigger the breath (not the machine). This causes the ventilator to deliver a clinician-determined preset pressure, augmenting the tidal volume (V_T). PEEP or continuous positive airway pressure (CPAP) may be added. PCV is a machine-triggered mode (based on time) in which a set pressure (limit) is applied. It is cycled based on a preset amount of *time*, regardless of the size of the breath that was delivered during that time.

10. **Summarize the advantages and limitation of pressure-controlled ventilation.**

Advantages include (1) limiting of peak pressure and theoretical prevention of overdistention and (2) better matching of patient flow requirement than with a set flow rate. Potential limitations include variation in delivered volumes as a result of increased airway resistance, decreased pulmonary compliance, and decreased patient effort.

11. **What are phase variables?**

There are four basic phase variables: pressure, volume, flow, and time. These are the same variables incorporated by the ventilator to detect the end of the inspiratory flow phase of a breath, (i.e., pressure cycled, volume cycled, flow cycled, and time cycled). Phase variables may be controlled either by the patient or by the ventilator.

12. **What are trigger variables?**

Trigger variables describe how a ventilator initiates inspiration. One or more of the phase variables may be used: time, pressure, flow, or volume. For example, in the CMV mode, time is the only trigger option available; no matter what the patient does, they cannot trigger a breath. In the ACV or SIMV mode, the patient may receive a breath based on time; however, a patient-generated decrease in baseline pressure (pressure-triggered) or patient-generated gas flow (flow-triggered) can also initiate a breath.

13. **What are limit variables?**

The limit variables (pressure, volume, and flow) are parameters that cannot be exceeded during inspiration. During an inspiration the pressure, flow, and volume will rise, and if they do not exceed a preset value, a breath is said to be limited by the primary variable.

14. **What are the goals of mechanical ventilation in patients with acute respiratory failure?**

In patients with acute respiratory failure (ARF), the goals are to preserve or improve arterial oxygenation and ventilation, to optimize lung mechanics, and to promote patient comfort while preventing ventilator-induced lung inquiry. Complications may arise from elevated alveolar pressures or persistently high inspired concentrations of oxygen (FiO_2).

15. **What are the initial ventilator settings in acute respiratory failure?**

There are lots of possibilities and styles, but generally a mode that provides full support is desired. Evidence from the ARDS-Net trial is centered on ACV, which ensures delivery of a preset volume; this mode is simply most well studied. Pressure-cycled modes are acceptable but probably offer only theoretical advantage. In any mode, the FiO_2 begins at 1.0 and is titrated downward as tolerated. High FiO_2 in the face of acute lung injury results in worsening of intrapulmonary shunt, possibly as a result of absorption atelectasis. Tidal volume is based on ideal body weight (IBW) and the pathophysiology of lung injury. Volumes of 8 to 10 ml/kg of IBW are probably acceptable if the plateau pressure is within a safe range. However, in the setting of acute respiratory distress syndrome (ARDS) or acute lung injury (ALI), large pressures or volumes may exacerbate the underlying lung injury. Therefore, smaller volumes ($\leq$6 ml/kg IBW) are delivered at a higher frequency.

16. **Which ventilator variables control the inspiratory/expiratory (I/E) ratio?**

The inspiratory/expiratory (I/E) ratio is the net effect of four ventilator settings: the respiratory rate (RR), Vt, peak flow, and the waveform setting. The peak flow rate is the maximal flow rate delivered by the ventilator during the inspiratory part of the respiratory cycle. An initial flow rate of 50 to 80 L/min is usually satisfactory. In a volume-cycled mode (e.g., ACV), then, a higher flow rate means a shorter inspiratory time, and a lower I/E ratio. An I/E ration of 1:2 to 1:3 is reasonable in most situations. Patients with chronic obstructive pulmonary disease (COPD) may require longer expiratory times to allow adequate exhalation. This can be accomplished by increasing flow, thus decreasing the I/E ratio. High flow rates may increase airway pressures and worsen gas distribution in some cases; slower flow rates may reduce airway pressures and improve gas distribution by increasing the I/E ratio. The ventilator waveform (e.g., square versus decelerating) will also effect the I/E ratio. Without changing the peak flow setting the square waveform results in a higher peak airway pressure and longer E time than the selection of a decelerating waveform.

17. **What is positive end-expiratory pressure?**

PEEP is an elevation of the baseline pressure above atmospheric pressure at end exhalation.

18. **What does positive end-expiratory pressure do?**

PEEP prevents alveolar collapse, recruits atelectatic alveoli, increases functional residual capacity, and reverses hypoxemia. In all patients early in the course of their respiratory failure PEEP probably needs to be manipulated in response to periods of desaturation (after common causes for hypoxemia have been ruled out, such as mucous plugging and barotrauma) to assess for recruitment potential.

19. **What is intrinsic or auto-positive end-expiratory pressure?**

Intrinsic PEEP (PEEPi) is the development of positive pressure and continued flow within the alveoli at end expiration without application of extrinsic PEEP (PEEPe). Patients with high minute ventilation requirements or patients receiving high I/E ratios are at risk for PEEPi. In healthy lungs during MV, if the respiratory rate is too rapid or the expiratory time is too short, there is insufficient time for full exhalation, resulting in stacking of breaths and generation of positive airway pressure at end exhalation. Small-diameter endotracheal tubes may also limit exhalation and contribute to PEEPi. Patients with increased airway resistance and decreased pulmonary compliance are at high risk for PEEPi. Such patients have difficulty in exhaling gas because of small airway obstruction or collapse and are prone to development of PEEPi during spontaneous ventilation and MV. PEEPi has the same side effects as PEEPe, but detecting it requires more vigilance.

Failure to recognize the presence of auto-PEEP can lead to inappropriate ventilator changes. The only way to detect and measure PEEPi is to occlude the expiratory port at end expiration while monitoring airway pressure. Decreasing rate or increasing inspiratory flow (to decrease I/E ratio) may allow time for full exhalation. Consider administering bronchodilator therapy in the setting of bronchospasm.

20. **What are the side effects of positive end-expiratory pressure?**
    a. Barotrauma may result from overdistention of alveoli.
    b. Cardiac output (CO) may be decreased as a result of intrathoracic pressure, producing an increase in transmural right atrial pressure and a decrease in venous return. PEEP also increases pulmonary artery pressure, potentially decreasing right ventricular output. Dilation of the right ventricle may cause bowing of the interventricular septum into the left ventricle, thus impairing filing of the left ventricle, decreasing CO, especially if the patient is hypovolemic.
    c. Incorrect interpretation of cardiac filing pressures: Pressure transmitted from the alveolus to the pulmonary vasculature may falsely elevate the readings. A rule of thumb is to subtract one half of the PEEP applied over five from the pulmonary artery occlusion pressure.
    d. Overdistention of alveoli from excessive PEEP decreases blood flow to these areas, increasing dead space volume (V_D; V_D/V_T).
    e. Work of breathing may be increased with PEEP because the patient is required to generate a larger negative pressure to trigger flow from the ventilator.
    f. Increase in intracranial pressure (ICP) and fluid retention.
    g. Increase in lung water.

21. **What is a ventilator bundle?**
    The term *ventilator bundle* encompasses several preventative measures that virtually all ventilated patients should receive. Use of such bundles can minimize the incidence of ventilator associated pneumonia (VAP) and other complications. Simple bedside techniques such as oral care and elevating the head of bed, for example, have been shown to decrease VAP. The need for prolonged MV also places the patient at risk for gastrointestinal (GI) bleeding and deep venous thrombosis (DVT) and therefore prophylaxis from stress ulceration and DVTs should be initiated as part of the ventilator bundle.

22. **What is controlled hypoventilation with permissive hypercapnia?**
    Controlled hypoventilation (or permissive hypercapnia) is a pressure- or volume-limiting, lung-protective strategy whereby pCO_2 is allowed to rise, placing more importance on protecting the lung than on maintaining eucapnia. The set V_T is lowered to a range of approximately 4 to 6 ml/kg of IBW in an attempt to keep the alveolar pressure (static pressure) less than 30 cm H_2O. Several studies in ARDS and status asthmaticus have shown a decrease in barotrauma, intensive care days, and mortality using this approach. The pCO_2 is allowed to rise slowly to a level up to 80 to 100 mm Hg. If cardiovascular instability results as the pH falls, then the addition of intravenous sodium bicarbonate may be necessary. Alternatively one may wait for the normal kidney to retain bicarbonate in response to the hypercapnia. Permissive hypercapnia is usually well tolerated. Potential adverse effects include cerebral vasodilatation leading to increased ICP and intracranial hypertension is the only absolute contraindication to permissive hypercapnia. Increased sympathetic activity, pulmonary vasoconstriction, and cardiac arrhythmias may occur but are rarely significant. Depression of cardiac contractility may be a problem in patients with underlying ventricular dysfunctions. In cases of ARF, worsening of acid-base may preclude or limit aggressive permissive hypercapnia.

23. What is compliance? How is it determined?

Compliance is a measure of distensibility and is expressed as the change in volume for a given change in pressure. Determination of compliance involves the interrelationship between pressure, volume, and resistance to airflow. The two relevant pressures that must be monitored during MV are peak and static pressures.

24. How is peak pressure measured?

Peak pressure is measured during the delivery of airflow at the end of inspiration. It is influenced by the inflation volume, airway resistance, and elastic recoil of the lungs and chest wall and reflects the dynamic compliance of the total respiratory system.

25. How is static pressure measured?

Static or plateau pressure is measured during an end-inspiratory pause, during a no-flow condition, and reflects the static compliance of the respiratory system, including the lung parenchyma, chest wall, and abdomen.

26. How is compliance calculated?

Both dynamic and static compliance should be calculated as a routine part of ventilator monitoring. Dynamic compliance is calculated as V_T (Paw − total PEEP), and plateau or static compliance is V_T (plateau pressure − total PEEP). Normal values for both dynamic and static compliance are 60 to 100 ml/cm H_2O. A decrease in dynamic compliance without a change in the static compliance suggests an acute increase in airway resistance and can be assessed further by comparing peak pressure and plateau pressure. The normal gradient is approximately 10 cm H_2O. A gradient >10 cm H_2O may be secondary to endotracheal tube obstruction, mucous plugging, or bronchospasm. If volume is constant, acute changes in both dynamic and static compliance suggest a decrease in respiratory system compliance that may be caused by worsening pneumonia, ARDS, atelectasis, or increasing abdominal pressures.

Compliance is a global value and does not describe what is happening regionally in the lungs with ARDS, in which diseased regions are interspersed with relatively healthy regions. Compliance values of 20 to 40 cm H_2O are common in advanced ARDS. Decreased lung compliance reflects the compliance of the lung that is participating in gas exchange, not the collapsed or fluid-filled alveoli. As a general rule when static compliance is <25 ml/cm H_2O ventilator weaning may be difficult secondary to tachypnea during spontaneous breathing trials.

27. Is ventilation in the prone position an option for patients who are difficult to oxygenate?

Absolutely! PaO_2 improves significantly in approximately two thirds of patients with ARDS when they are placed prone. The mechanisms include (1) recruitment of collapsed dorsal lung fields by redistribution of lung edema to ventral regions; (2) increased diaphragm motion enhancing ventilation; (3) elimination of the compressive effects of the heart on the inferior lower lung fields, thus improving regional ventilation; (4) maintenance of dorsal lung perfusion in the face of improved dorsal ventilation, which leads to improved ventilation/perfusion (V/Q) matching; and (5) a change in the pleural pressure gradient from the ventral to dorsal regions of the lung.

28. What are the indications for prone ventilation?

Indications for prone ventilation are not clearly established. We initiate a prone trial in any patient who remains hypoxemic or requires high FiO_2 concentrations after the performance or recruitment/PEEP maneuvers. The best predictor of improved outcome during prone ventilation may be a decrease in the $PaCO_2$ and not improved oxygenation.

29. Junior O'Flaherty is "fighting the ventilator." What do I do?

Initially, the potential causes are separated into ventilator (machine, circuit, and airway) problems and patient-related problems. Patient-related causes include hypoxemia, secretions or mucous plugging, pneumothorax, bronchospasm, infection (pneumonia or sepsis), pulmonary embolus, myocardial ischemia, GI bleeding, worsening PEEPi, and anxiety. The ventilator-related issues include system leak or disconnection; inadequate ventilator support or delivered FiO_2; airway-related problems, such as extubation, obstructed endotracheal tube, cuff herniation, or rupture; and improper triggering sensitivity or flows. Until the problem is identified, the patient should be ventilated manually with 100% O_2. Breath sounds and vital signs should be immediately checked. ABG analysis and portable chest radiograph are valuable, but if a tension pneumothorax is suspected, immediate decompression precedes the chest radiograph.

30. Should neuromuscular blockage be used to facilitate mechanical ventilation?
Neuromuscular blocking agents (NMBAs) are commonly used to facilitate MV during ARDS, but despite wide acceptance, there are few data and as yet no consensus available for when these agents should be used. Gainnier and colleagues (2004) were the first to report the effects of a 48-hour NMBA infusion on gas exchange in patients with early ARDS. All patients were ventilated according to the ARDSNet protocol. Significant improvements in oxygenation and ability to lower PEEP occurred in the NMBA group and were sustained beyond the 48-hour infusion period. Although it remains to be elucidated why muscle paralysis improves oxygenation, NMBAs are thought to decrease oxygen consumption, promote patient-ventilator interface, and increase chest wall compliance.

Muscle paralysis may also be of benefit in specific situations, such as intracranial hypertension or unconventional modes of ventilation (e.g., IRV or extracorporeal techniques). Drawbacks to the use of these drugs include loss of neurologic examination, abolished cough, potential for prolonged paralysis, diaphragmatic atrophy, and death associated with inadvertent ventilator disconnects. Use of NMBAs must not be taken lightly. Adequate sedation should be attempted first; if deemed absolutely necessary, use of NMBAs should be limited to 24 to 48 hours to prevent potential complications.

KEY POINTS

1. Inadequate alveolar ventilation, hypoxia, and impaired respiratory drive are the three reasons patients may need MV.

2. All modes of ventilation can be described based on how a breath is triggered, cycled, and limited.

3. Initial ventilator settings for ARF should provide full support. ACV mode is the most studied.

4. Hypoventilation and letting pCO_2 rise is permissible—and beneficial—if it allows the physician to limit alveolar pressure and stretch (permissive hypercapnia).

5. When a patient appears to be "fighting" the ventilator, the first step is to remove the ventilator and manually ("bag") ventilate the patient. This allows you to eliminate ventilator variables as a cause and assess patient variables that may need urgent treatment (e.g., tension pneumothorax).

BIBLIOGRAPHY

1. Abroug F, Ouanes-Besbes L, Elatrous S et al.: The effect of prone positioning in acute respiratory distress syndrome or acute lung injury: a meta-analysis. Areas of uncertainty and recommendations for research. Int Care Med, in press 2008.

2. Burger CD, Resar RK: "Ventilator bundle" approach to prevention of ventilator-associated pneumonia. Mayo Clin Proc 81(6):849-850, 2006.

3. Campbell RS, Davis BR: Pressure-controlled versus volume-controlled ventilation: does it matter? Respir Care 47(4):416-424, 2002.

4. Gainnier M, Roch A, Forel JM et al.: Effect of neuromuscular blocking agents on gas exchange in patients presenting with acute respiratory distress syndrome. Crit Care Med 32:113-119, 2004.

5. Levine S, Nguyen T, Taylor N et al.: Rapid disuse atrophy of diaphragm fibers in mechanically ventilated humans. N Engl J Med 358(13):1327-1335, 2008.

6. Meade MO, Cook DJ, Guyatt GH et al.: Ventilation strategy using low tidal volumes, recruitment maneuvers, and high positive end-expiratory pressures for acute lung injury and acute respiratory distress syndrome: a randomized controlled trial. JAMA 299(6):637-645, 2008.

7. Mercat A, Richard JM, Vielle, B et al.: Positive end-expiratory pressure setting in adults with acute lung injury and acute respiratory distress syndrome. JAMA 299(6):646-655, 2008.

8. Pierson, DJ: Indications for mechanical ventilation in adults with acute respiratory failure. Respir Care 47(3):249-262, 2002.

CHAPTER 7

WHY GET ARTERIAL BLOOD GASES?

Alden H. Harken, MD

1. **Is breathing really overrated?**
   It may be. A Japanese yoga master survived just fine breathing once per minute for 1 hour (see reference 3).

2. **Mr. O'Flaherty has just undergone an inguinal herniorrhaphy under local anesthesia. The recovery room nurse asks permission to sedate him. She says that he is confused and unruly and keeps trying to get out of bed. Is it safe to sedate Mr. O'Flaherty?**
   No. A confused, agitated patient in the recovery room or surgical intensive care unit (SICU) must be recognized as acutely hypoxemic until proved otherwise.

3. **Mr. O'Flaherty is moved to the SICU, and at 2:00 AM the SICU nurse calls to report that he has a partial pressure of oxygen (PO_2) of 148 mm Hg on facemask oxygen. Is it okay to roll over and go back to sleep?**
   No. More information is needed.

4. **You glance at the abandoned cup of coffee sitting on your well-worn copy of *Surgical Secrets*. What is the PO_2 of that cup of coffee?**
   It is 148 mm Hg.

5. **How can Mr. O'Flaherty and the coffee have the same PO_2?**
   The abandoned coffee presumably has had time to equilibrate completely with atmospheric gas. At sea level, the barometric pressure is 760 mm Hg. To obtain the partial pressure of oxygen (PO_2) in the coffee, subtract water vapor pressure (47 mm Hg) and multiply by the concentration of oxygen (20.8%) in the atmosphere:

$$PO_2 = (760 - 47) \times 20.8\% = 148 \text{ mm Hg}$$

6. **What is the difference between Mr. O'Flaherty's and the coffee's PO_2?**
   Nothing. Both represent the partial pressure of oxygen in fluid. A complete set of blood gases is necessary.

7. **What constitutes a complete set of blood gases?**
   PO_2
   pCO_2
   pH
   Hemoglobin saturation
   Hemoglobin concentration

8. **If Mr. O'Flaherty and the coffee have the same PO_2, how would Mr. O'Flaherty do if he were exchange-transfused with coffee?**
   Badly.

9. **Why?**
   Although the oxygen tensions are the same, the *amount* of oxygen in blood is vastly greater.

10. **How does one quantify the amount of oxygen in blood?**
    Arterial oxygen content (CaO_2) is quantified as ml of oxygen/100 ml of blood. (*Watch out:* Almost all other concentrations traditionally are provided per ml or per L and *not* per 100 ml.) Because ml of oxygen is a volume in 100 ml of blood, these units frequently are abbreviated as vol %.

11. **Why is blood thicker than coffee (or wine)?**
    Because hemoglobin binds a huge amount of oxygen. A total of 10 g of fully saturated hemoglobin (hematocrit about 30%) binds 13.4 ml of oxygen, whereas 100 ml of plasma at a PO_2 of 100 mm Hg contains only 0.3 ml of oxygen.

12. **Does the position of the oxyhemoglobin dissociation curve make any difference?**
    - An increase in pCO_2
    - An increase in hydrogen ion concentrations **(not pH)**
    - An increase in temperature

    All shift the oxyhemoglobin curve to the right; that is, oxygen is released more easily in the tissues. Within physiologic limits, however, Mae West probably said it best: "There is less to this than meets the eye."

KEY POINTS: MEDIATORS OF OXYHEMOGLOBIN DISSOCIATION CURVE

Right Shift	Left Shift
1. Increase in pCO_2	1. Decrease in $[H+^+]$, higher pH
2. Increase in $[H+^+]$, lower pH	2. Higher altitudes/elevation
3. Increase in temperature	3. Decrease in 2,3-DPG (e.g., at 4 weeks storage, blood maintains *no* 2,3-DPG)
4. Increase in 2,3-DPG	

---

13. **If arterial oxygen content (CaO_2) or ultimately systemic oxygen delivery (cardiac output $\times$ CaO_2) is what the surgeon really wants to know, why does the nurse report Mr. O'Flaherty's PO_2 instead of his CaO_2 at 2:00 AM?**
    No one knows.

14. **What is the fastest and most practical method of increasing Mr. O'Flaherty's CaO_2?**
    Transfusion of red blood cells. The patient's CaO_2 is increased by 25% with transfusion from a hemoglobin concentration of 8 to 10 g/dl. The patient's CaO_2 is affected negligibly by an increase in arterial PO_2 from 100 to 200 mm Hg (hemoglobin is fully saturated in both instances).

15. **What is a transfusion trigger?**
    The hematocrit at which a patient is automatically transfused. This is *not* a useful concept. The NIH Consensus Conference, drawing data from Jehovah's Witnesses, patients with renal failure, and monkeys concluded that it is not necessary to transfuse a patient until the

hematocrit is 21%. Traditional surgical dogma mandates a hematocrit >30%. When the patient is in trouble, however, authorities in surgical critical care encourage transfusion to a hematocrit of 45% to optimize systemic oxygen delivery.

16. **What governs respiratory drive?**

pCO_2 and pH are inextricably intertwined by the Henderson-Hasselbalch equation. By juggling this equation in the cerebrospinal fluid (CSF) of goats, it is clear that CSF hydrogen ion concentration (not pCO_2) controls respiratory drive. This distinction is not clinically important, however. What is important is that if a person becomes acidotic either with diabetic ketoacidosis (DKA) or by running up a flight of stairs, minute ventilation (V_E) is increased.

17. **How tight is respiratory control? Or, if you hold your breath for 1 minute, how much do you want to breathe?**

A lot (unless you are a yoga master approaching nirvana).

18. **After 60 seconds of apnea, what happens to $PaCO_2$?**

It increases only from 40 to 47 mm Hg. Tiny changes in pCO_2 (and pH) translate into a huge respiratory stimulus. Normally, respiratory compensation for metabolic acidosis is tight.

19. **Define base excess.**

Base excess is a poor man's indicator of the metabolic component of acid-base disorders. After correcting the pCO_2 to 40 mm Hg, the base excess or base deficit is touted as an indirect measure of serum lactate. Although many parameters directing volume resuscitation in shock are more practical and direct (see Chapter 4), base deficit has been advertised as helpful. The base excess or deficit is calculated from the Sigaard-Anderson nomogram in the blood gas laboratory. Normally, there is no base excess or deficit. Acid-base status is "just right."

BIBLIOGRAPHY

1. Catheline JM, Bihan H, Le Quang T et al.: Preoperative cardiac and pulmonary assessment in bariatric surgery. Obes Surg 18:271-277, 2008.

2. Dekerle J, Baron B, Dupont L et al.: Maximal lactate steady state, respiratory compensation threshold, and critical power. Eur J Appl Physiol 89:280-288, 2003.

3. Miyamura M, Nishimura K, Ishida K et al.: Is a man able to breathe once a minute for an hour? The effect of yoga exercises on blood gases. Jpn J Physiol 52:313, 2002.

4. Tada T, Hashimoto F, Matsushita Y et al.: Study of life satisfaction and quality of life of patients receiving home oxygen therapy. J Med Invest 50:55-63, 2003.

CHAPTER 8

FLUIDS, ELECTROLYTES, GATORADE, AND SWEAT

Alden H. Harken, MD

1. **What is hypertonic saline?**

   Normal saline is 0.9% sodium chloride. Hypertonic saline is 7.5% sodium chloride (8 times as concentrated as normal saline).

KEY POINTS: ION CONCENTRATIONS IN CRYSTALLOID SOLUTIONS

1. One half normal saline or 0.45% NaCl: 77 mEq of Na+, 77 mEq of Cl−

2. Normal saline or 0.9% NaCl: 154 mEq of Na+, 154 mEq of Cl−

3. Hypertonic normal saline or 7.5% NaCl: 1283 mEq of Na+, 1283 mEq of Cl−

4. Lactated Ringer's: 130 mEq of Na+, 110 mEq of Cl−, 38 mEq of lactate, 4 mEq of K+, and 3 mEq Ca+

2. **What is hypertonic saline good for?**

   Resuscitation. The initial hypothesis was that a little hypertonic saline would pull extravascular water into the intravascular compartment, rapidly restoring volume. It now appears that an osmotic jolt (even a transient jump from 140 to 180 mOsm) would pacify circulating neutrophils so that they do not stick to the endovasculature and provoke posttraumatic inflammation.

3. **Is hypertonic saline good for anything else?**

   Pacification of "primed" neutrophils should decrease the risk of posttraumatic multiple organ failure.

4. **How do you convert 1 g of sodium into milliequivalents (mEq)?**

   Divide by the atomic weight of sodium:

   $$1 \, g \, (1000 \, mg) \text{ of sodium} \div 23 = 43.5 \, mEq$$

5. **How many mEq of sodium are in 1 teaspoon of salt?**

   104 mEq (or 2400 mg).

6. **How many mEq of sodium are in an 8-oz bottle of Gatorade?**

   5 mEq.

7. **How much does a 40-lb block of salt cost?**

   $3.40 at the feed store.

8. **What is the electrolyte content of intravenous fluids?**
   See Table 8-1.

TABLE 8-1. ELECTROLYTE CONTENT OF INTRAVENOUS FLUIDS

Solution (mEq/L)	Sodium	Potassium	Chloride	Bicarbonate/Lactate
Normal saline (0.9% NaCl)	154	—	154	—
Ringer's lactate solution	130	4	109	28*
5% dextrose ½ normal saline	77	—	77	—

*Lactate is converted immediately to bicarbonate.

9. **How do these concentrations relate to body fluid and electrolyte compartments?**
   See Table 8-2.

TABLE 8-2. ELECTROLYTE CONCENTRATIONS IN BODY FLUIDS

Compartment (mEq/L)	Sodium	Potassium	Chloride	Bicarbonate/Lactate
Plasma	142	4	103	27
Interstitial fluid	144	4	114	30
Intracellular fluid	10	150	—	10

10. **What are the daily volumes (mL/24 h) and electrolyte contents (mEq/L) of body secretions for a 70-kg medical student?**
    See Table 8-3.

TABLE 8-3. DAILY VOLUMES AND ELECTROLYTE CONTENTS OF BODY SECRETIONS

	ml/24 h	Sodium	Potassium	Chloride	Bicarbonate
Saliva	+1500	10	25	10	30
Stomach	+1500	50	10	130	—
Duodenum	+1000	140	5	80	—
Ileum	+3000	140	5	104	30
Colon	−6000	60	30	40	—
Pancreas	+500	140	5	75	100
Biliary	+500	140	5	100	30
Sweat*	+1000	50	—	—	—
Gatorade	—	21	—	21	—

*See question 6.

11. **Are sweat glands responsive to aldosterone? Can they be trained?**
Yes and yes. Archie Bunker's sweat contains 100 mEq/L sodium, whereas an Olympic marathon runner retains sodium (sweat sodium may be as low as 25 mEq/L).

12. **Is Gatorade really just flavored athlete's sweat?**
Yes.

13. **What are the daily maintenance fluid and electrolyte requirements for a 70-kg medical student?**

Total fluid volume	2500 ml
Sodium	70 mEq (1 mEq/kg)
Potassium	35 mEq (0.5 mEq/kg)

14. **Does the routine postoperative patient require intravenous sodium or potassium supplementation? Routine serum electrolyte testing?**
No and no.

15. **Can a patient with a good heart and kidneys overcome all but the most woefully incompetent fluid and electrolyte management?**
Yes.

16. **Can one throw a healthy medical student into congestive heart failure by intravenous infusion of 100 ml of 5% dextrose in saline solution per kilogram per hour?**
No. One will simply be ankle-deep in urine.

17. **What is subtraction alkalosis?**
Vigorous nasogastric suction of a patient with a lot of gastric acid eliminates hydrochloric acid, leaving the patient alkalotic.

18. **Which electrolyte is most useful in repairing a hypokalemic metabolic alkalosis?**
Chloride.

19. **List the best indicators of a patient's volume status.**
Heart rate
Blood pressure
Urine output
Big-toe temperature

20. **Does a warm big toe indicate a hemodynamically stable patient?**
Most likely. The vascular autoregulatory ability of a young healthy patient is huge. The carotid and coronary circulations are maintained until the bitter end. Conversely, if the patient's big toe is warm and perfused, the patient is stable.

21. **What is the minimal adequate postoperative urine output?**
It is 0.5 milliliters per kilogram per hour.

22. **What is a typical postoperative urine sodium?**
It is <20 mEq/L.

23. Why?

Surgical stress prompts mineralocorticoid (aldosterone) secretion so that the normal kidney retains sodium.

24. Explain paradoxical aciduria.

Postoperative patients, by virtue of nasogastric suction (loss of gastric acid), blood transfusions (the citrate in blood is converted to bicarbonate), and hyperventilation (decreased pco_2), are typically alkalotic. Patients also are stressed, and their kidneys retain sodium and water. The renal tubules must exchange some other cations for the retained sodium. The kidney chooses to exchange potassium and hydrogen ions. Even in the face of systemic alkalosis, the postoperative kidney absorbs sodium and excretes hydrogen ions, producing a paradoxical aciduria.

25. What is third spacing?

Hypotension and infection prime neutrophils (CD11 and CD18 receptor complexes), promoting adherence to vascular endothelial cells. Subsequent activation of adherent neutrophils spews out proteases and toxic superoxide radicals, blowing big holes in the vascular lining. Water and plasma albumin leak through the holes. The volume pulled out of the vascular space into the third space of the interstitial and hollow viscus (gut) creates relative hypovolemia and requires additional fluid replacement.

26. What is a Lasix sandwich?

It is 25 gms albumin followed by 20 mg of furosemide (Lasix) intravenously (IV). If the patient is edematous, the intravenous albumin theoretically sucks water osmotically out of the interstitial third space. As the excessive water enters the vascular compartment, Lasix produces a healthy diuresis. In most patients in the intensive care unit (ICU), however, the infused albumin rapidly equilibrates across the damaged vascular endothelium. No additional water is pulled into the blood volume. Although surgeons often order Lasix sandwiches, they probably work only in healthy patients who do not need them.

BIBLIOGRAPHY

1. Brown MD: Evidence-based emergency medicine: hypertonic versus isotonic crystalloid for fluid resuscitation in critically ill patients. Ann Emerg Med 40:113-114, 2002.

2. Bunn F, Roberts I, Tasker R et al.: Hypertonic versus isotonic crystalloid for fluid resuscitation in critically ill patients. Cochrane Database Syst Rev (1):CD002045, 2002.

3. Dellinger RP, Levy MM, Carlet JM et al.: Surviving Sepsis Campaign: international guidelines for management of severe sepsis and septic shock: 2008. Crit Care Med 36:296-327, 2008.

4. Greaves I, Porter KM, Revell MP: Fluid resuscitation in pre-hospital trauma care: a consensus view. J R Coll Surg Edinb 47:451-457, 2002.

5. Perel P, Roberts I: Colloids versus crystalloids for fluid resuscitation in critically ill patients. Cochrane Database Syst Rev (4):CD000567, 2004.

6. Traber DL: Fluid resuscitation after hypovolemia. Crit Care Med 30:1922, 2002.

CHAPTER 9

NUTRITIONAL ASSESSMENT, PARENTERAL, AND ENTERAL NUTRITION

Margaret M. McQuiggan, MS, RD, CNSD, and Frederick A. Moore, MD, FACS

NUTRITIONAL ASSESSMENT

1. What does a nutritional assessment include?

The **medical and surgical history** determine pre-existing conditions, metabolic stress, and alterations in organ function that influence nutritional support. The **physical exam** evaluates muscle mass, adipose stores, skin integrity, and hydrational state. **Laboratory data** include serum sodium (Na), potassium (K), carbon dioxide (CO_2), chloride (Cl), blood urea nitrogen (BUN), creatinine, glucose, ionized calcium (Ca), serum phosphate (PO_4), magnesium (Mg), and complete blood count (CBC) with differential. Arterial blood gases (ABGs) to assess acid-base status and CO_2 retention, albumin, transferrin, prealbumin and urinary nitrogen are useful. Glycosylated hemoglobin (HgbA1C), lipid profile, C-reactive protein (CRP), 25-OH vitamin D, trace elements and liver function tests (LFTs) may also be valuable. The **drug profile** reveals agents that affect the metabolism of nutrients (insulin, levothyroxine, corticosteroids), alter energy expenditure (β-blockers, Diprivan), or affect gastrointestinal (GI) function (prokinetic agents, antibiotics). **Anthropometric data** include height, weight, waist and hip circumference. Skinfold testing with calipers is useful once edema has resolved, but is rarely used in the fat-free acute care setting. **Bioelectrical impedance analysis (BIA)** quantifies adipose reserve, intracellular and extracellular water, and third space fluid in stable surgical patients. Dual energy x-ray absorptiometry (DEXA) is effective for tracking bone mineral density that may be compromised with age, hormonal status, drug therapy, and chronic disease. The **nutrition history** reveals information on the nutritional practices of the individual. The **social history** explores economic data, social support network, or substance abuse behaviors and may predict the likelihood of adequate home care and treatment compliance for the patient, once discharged.

2. What are primary malnutrition and secondary malnutrition?

Primary malnutrition results when the individual consumes inadequate kilocalories, protein, vitamins, or minerals. It may occur as a result of poor food choices, anorexia, poverty, alcoholism, suboptimal support regimens, or after bariatric surgery. **Secondary malnutrition** occurs even when adequate food is infused or consumed. It may result from organ dysfunction (hypoalbuminemia with cirrhosis), malabsorption (Crohn's disease), immobility (muscle wasting), drug therapy (insulin resistance with corticosteroids), or the inflammatory state (acute phase response).

3. What is the significance of serum proteins in nutritional assessment?

The most commonly cited and readily available proteins for nutritional assessment are albumin, transferrin, and prealbumin, which are produced in the liver (see Table 9-1). All three constitutive proteins plummet shortly after injury or surgery because the liver reprioritizes the production of acute phase proteins. Then, as the stress response resolves, the liver resumes

TABLE 9-1. SERUM PROTEINS

Protein	Synthetic Site	Clinical Significance	Half-Life	Limitations	Interpretation
Albumin	Liver	Relates to outcomes; relates to edema	20–21 days	Best case scenario for hepatic production—12–25 g/24 hours; dilutional effects; long half-life; used alone, sensitivity poor	Normal <3.5 g/dl Mild depletion 2.8–3.5 g/dl Moderate 2.2–2.8 g/dl Severe <2.2 g/dl
Prealbumin	Liver	Indicates nutritional deficits before albumin	2–4 days	Short half life	Normal >18 mg/dl Mild depletion 10–18 mg/dl Moderate 5–10 mg/dl Severe <5 mg/dl
Transferrin	Liver	More sensitive than albumin; relatively useful parameter in liver disease compared with albumin; can calculate from TIBC	8–10 days	Poor marker of early repletion; sensitive to changes in body iron	Mild depletion 150–200 mg/dl Moderate 100–150 mg/dl Severe <100 mg/dl
C-Reactive Protein (CRP)	Liver	Increases abruptly after injury. Early and reliable indicator of disease or injury severity.	48–72 hours	May be increased with obesity and other chronic inflammatory states	Baseline normal <3 mg/dl Bacterial infection 30–35 mg/dl Viral infection <20 mg/dl Peaks 48–72 hours post-trauma up to 35 mg/dl

TIBC, total iron-binding capacity.

production of constitutive proteins. Adequate kilocalories and protein facilitate this process. As a result of shorter half-lives, prealbumin and transferrin are most useful in the intensive care unit (ICU) and should be limited to patients with creatinine clearance >50 ml/min. Prealbumin travels in the circulation bound to retinol binding protein (RBP) and vitamin A. Levels of prealbumin may be elevated in renal failure despite nutritional compromise resulting from decreased catabolism and excretion of RBP. Transferrin is elevated with iron depletion, independent of the effects of nutrition.

4. **How are protein requirements determined?**
   Protein need is determined based on patient weight, current stress factors, extraordinary skin losses, and organ function. Although the recommended daily intake (RDI) for protein for healthy individuals is only 0.8 g of protein/kg of body weight, the following guidelines may be used in the surgical patient:

Injury Level	Protein Requirement
Mild stress/injury	1.2 to 1.4 g of protein/kg
Moderate stress/injury	1.5 to 1.7 g of protein/kg
Severe stress/injury	1.8 to 2.5 g of protein/kg

5. **What is the significance of urinary nitrogen in nutritional assessment?**
   Total urinary nitrogen (TUN) is the most reliable indicator of nitrogen use and excretion in the patient who is in the surgical intensive care unit (SICU). However, urinary urea nitrogen (UUN) is more readily available in most hospital laboratories. Although TUN and UUN are nearly equal in healthy ambulatory patients with normal renal and hepatic function, critically ill patients have a poor correlation between the two. A 12-hour urine collection compares well with a 24-hour collection (Graves). Optimal nutrition support promotes a +3 to +5 nitrogen balance. Estimate the protein needs of the patient by adding:

   [24h UUN (g) + 2 g N insensible losses + 3] × 6.25 = required amount of protein (g)

   Remember that 6.25 g of protein yields 1 g of nitrogen. Insensible losses are increased with burns, decubiti, wound vacuums, and large wounds. UUN is not useful as a guide for nutritional prescription in hepatic failure, renal dysfunction (<50 ml/min creatinine clearance), or recent spinal cord injury.

6. **Should protein be severely restricted in the surgical patient with hepatic failure or renal failure?**
   Limit protein to 0.6 to 0.8 g/kg in the patient with hepatic encephalopathy, if the encephalopathy produces significant clinical consequences. However, only about 10% of chronic liver disease patients are protein sensitive; thus, other causes of encephalopathy, such as infection, constipation, and electrolyte disturbance, should be explored. Otherwise, give a more typical postsurgical protein load (1.3 to 1.5 g/kg).
   In injured and acutely ill patients with **renal failure,** balance the need for increased protein with the need for increased dialysis. Giving adequate protein may require more frequent dialysis. Amino acid losses and requirements increase with more intensive hemodialysis (HD) (10 to 12 g of amino acids removed with each HD, or 5 to 12 g of amino acids daily with continuous venovenous hemodialysis [CVVHD]).

7. **How are kilocalorie needs determined?**
   There are numerous methods for setting kilocalorie targets in the surgical patient: (a) prediction equations, (b) kcal/kg estimations or, (c) indirect calorimetry. One common **prediction equation,** the Harris Benedict (HBE), was developed in 1919 for use on ambulatory, fasted, healthy people but is of limited usefulness in hospitalized patients.
   A number of prediction equations have been developed but most physicians employ a total **kcal/kg goal** as shown in Table 9-2.

TABLE 9-2. KILOCALORIE GOALS IN SURGICAL PATIENT

Patient	Feeding Level (kcal/kg)	Level by Indirect Calorimetry
Normal weight patients	25–30	REE* × 1.0
Underweight patients	30–35	REE × 1.2
Obese patients	20–25†	REE × 0.85
Morbidly obese	10–20†	REE × 0.75

*Basal energy expenditure (BEE) is the number of kilocalories expended at rest, in a fasted state. Resting energy expenditure (REE) is measured in a fed state and is 5% to 10% higher than BEE.
†Adjusted weight = [(Actual weight− Ideal weight) × 0.25] + Ideal weight

8. **What is indirect calorimetry, and when is it useful?**
Indirect calorimetry is a respiratory test that measures the patient's production of CO_2 and consumption of oxygen for approximately 30 minutes, until steady state is achieved. Results are worked into the modified Weir equation:

$$REE = [(3.796 \times VO_2) + (1.214 \times VCO_2)] \times 1440 \text{ min/day}$$

Where:
REE = resting energy expenditure (kcal/day)
VO_2 = oxygen consumption (L/min)
VCO_2 = CO_2 exhaled (L/min)
The report indicates the number of kilocalories the patient consumes in 24 hours and the respiratory quotient (RQ). $RQ = VCO_2/VO_2$ and provides information on the type of substrate being used. The RQ for the metabolism of fat, protein, and carbohydrate are 0.7, 0.83, and 1.0, respectively. Overfeeding will result in an RQ >1.0, as a result of increased CO_2 production associated with lipogenesis.
The test is useful in the patient on mechanical ventilation (MV) once a patient is relatively stable, with a fractional concentration of oxygen in inspired gas (FiO_2) <60% and peak end-expiratory pressure (PEEP) <10. Studies are helpful:
a. When overfeeding (diabetes mellitus, chronic obstructive pulmonary disease, obesity) is undesirable
b. When underfeeding (renal failure, large wounds) is detrimental.
c. In patients whose physical or clinical factors promote alterations in energy expenditure (spinal cord injury).
d. When drugs are used that significantly alter energy expenditure (paralytic agents, β-blockers).
e. In patients who do not respond as expected to calculated regimens.

ENTERAL NUTRITION

9. **When should enteral nutrition be considered?**
Always, but especially when a patient is unlikely to meet >70% of nutritional needs by mouth. Patients who have sustained major head injury (Glasgow Coma Scale <8), major torso trauma, major trauma to the pelvis and long bones, or major chest trauma benefit from enteral nutrition. Approximately 85% of patients (even those undergoing GI surgery) tolerate early enteral feeding within 24 hours postoperatively.

10. **How do you access the gastrointestinal tract for feeding?**
Pursue access by blind placement of a nasogastric (NG) tube or a nasoduodenal tube. Place a nasojejunal tube (NJ) blindly, endoscopically or fluoroscopically. Achieve gastric decompression with concurrent nasojejunal feeds with an endoscopic percutaneous gastrostomy/jejunostomy (PEG/PEJ). Alternatively, place a gastrostomy or feeding jejunostomy intraoperatively.

11. **What types of enteral formulas are available?**
Polymeric enteral feedings are soy-based, lactose-free products containing intact protein, carbohydrate, and fat. Most offer 1 kcal/ml and 37 to 62 g of protein per liter. Special modifications of the standard formulas include dietary fiber or "**immune-enhancing**" agents, such as fish oil, arginine, glutamine, and nucleotides. "**Elemental**" formulas contain amino acids, di-, tri-, and quatra-peptides, dextrose, and minimal fat. Several **concentrated** formulas (2 kcal/ml) are available for use in patients with congestive heart failure (CHF), renal failure, and hepatic failure. In general, products that are "**disease-specific**" or contain nutrients in elemental form are more expensive than standard products.

12. **Are specialized formulas necessary for the patient with diabetes mellitus who is critically ill?**
No. Formulas with reduced carbohydrate and increased fat loads are marketed as being superior in maintaining glycemic control. These products have not shown superior, clinically significant outcome in hospitalized patients in randomized controlled trials. The use of standard high protein formulas in an isocaloric or hypocaloric load, combined with appropriate insulin therapy, is the most effective treatment for hyperglycemia in the stressed patient with type 2 DM. The level of glycemic control associated with enhanced outcome is best achieved with insulin, as opposed to carbohydrate restriction. Furthermore, gastric feedings with high fat formulas in the diabetic patient with gastroparesis may delay gastric emptying and increase risk of aspiration.

13. **Should specialized "pulmonary" formulas be used on all patients on ventilators?**
No. Specialized, high omega-6 fat formulas have been marketed to reduce CO_2 production in COPD patients who retain CO_2. In theory, these formulas minimize CO_2 production and facilitate weaning. However, avoiding overfeeding is more important for reducing CO_2 production than providing high fat formula. Gastric feeding with these products increases the risk of aspiration.

14. **What complications are related to enteral support?**
Enteral feeding may produce electrolyte abnormalities, hyperglycemia, GI intolerance, pulmonary aspiration, and nasopharyngeal erosions. Surgical complications of enteral access include leaks, tube dislodgement, volvulus, soft tissue infection, and bowel necrosis.

15. **Should one wait for bowel sounds or flatus before beginning enteral feedings?**
No.

16. **Should one delay nutrition support longer in obese patients assuming they have increased reserves?**
No. Obese patients have more fat, but during stress all patients become hypermetabolic and break down endogenous protein stores to mobilize amino acids for gluconeogenesis, protein production, and adenosine triphosphate. As with patients who are of normal weight, patients who are obese require high protein nutritional supplementation to meet increased nitrogen demands.

17. Should enteral formulas be diluted for initial presentation?

No. Dilution delays the attainment of feeding goals and increases the likelihood of bacterial contamination. Solution osmolarity is a relatively minor culprit in producing diarrhea.

18. How should enteral feeding-related diarrhea be managed?

Mild diarrhea usually requires no treatment. With moderate to severe diarrhea, consider feeding reduction, antidiarrheal agents, and stool studies for *clostridium difficile*. Evaluate the medication profile for sorbitol-containing elixirs, laxatives, stool softeners, and prokinetic agents. Monitor sanitation issues related to formula handling. Some success has been reported with soluble fiber or lactobacillus (yogurt) in antibiotic-associated diarrhea.

19. During gastric feeding, at what level of gastric residual volume (GRV) should one hold feedings?

Always use measurements of gastric residual volume (GRV) in tandem with clinical assessment. Increase vigilance at 200 to 500 ml of GRV and start prokinetic agents. Hold feedings if GRV >500 ml.

20. Do enteral feedings contain enough water to meet all fluid needs?

Most 1 kcal/ml formulas (standard) contain 85% water by volume, whereas 2 kcal/ml formulas contain 70% water. Water is generally not an issue in the patient in ICU receiving multiple intravenous (IV) fluids and drugs. However, post-ICU, or in patients bound for home or extended care facilities, it is essential to write a water prescription with the tube feeding order. General guidelines for the total water needs are shown in Table 9-3.

For example, if the total calculated need for fluid is 2400 ml for a 60-kg patient and 2400 cc of the tube feeding provides approximately 2000 ml of free water, write an order to give 200 ml of water to the patient twice daily.

TABLE 9-3. DAILY WATER NEEDS IN RELATION TO AGE		
Patient	**Age**	**Daily Water Needs**
Average adult	25–55 years	35 ml/kg
Young, active adult years	16–35	40 ml/kg
Adult	>55–65 years	30 ml/kg
Elderly	>65 years	25 ml/kg

21. How is enteral nutrition infused?

Enteral nutrition is infused continuously, in bolus form or cyclically. Continuous infusion is best in the patient who is critically ill requiring postpyloric feedings. Bolus feedings are used in more stable patients with gastric feedings. Cyclic feedings or nocturnal feedings are useful for the patient who is on concurrent oral intake and in transition to full oral support, or for those requiring feeding-free periods for physical therapy or activities of daily living.

22. Is enteral nutrition better than total parenteral nutrition?

Yes. Substrates delivered enterally are better tolerated, are associated with fewer metabolic and hepatic complications, and help preserve normal mucosal integrity. Eighty percent of the body's immune tissue is in the gut and needs local and systemic nutrition. A review of 13 studies describing a total of 856 patients who were critically ill, contrasting total parenteral nutrition (TPN) with enteral nutrition, concluded that enteral nutrition reduces infectious complications and is typically more cost-effective than parenteral nutrition.

23. **Should you discontinue enteral feeding at midnight on all patients undergoing elective surgery with general anesthesia?**

    No. The American Society of Anesthesiologists recommends that healthy adults cease intake of solids for at least 6 hours and liquids for 2 hours before undergoing elective procedures. The guidelines may need to be modified for patients with coexisiting diseases that may affect gastric emptying-pregnancy, obesity, DM, hiatal hernia, gastroesophageal reflux disease (GERD), ileus or bowel obstruction, emergency care, or enteral tube feeding. Recent clinical investigation shows enhanced immunologic and functional recovery of the GI tract with decreased perioperative fasting periods.

24. **Is the clear liquid diet mandatory after surgery?**

    No. Clinical outcomes are similar when patients are fasted or given clear liquids until the appearance of flatus or BM as opposed to receiving a regular diet beginning one day postoperatively.

25. **Does preoperative nutrition with immune-enhancing diets improve surgical outcome?**

    Yes. Perioperative immune-enhancing diets (IEDs) can reduce postoperative complications and infections and enhance postoperative immunocompetence in properly selected patients. The consensus recommendations from the U.S. Summit on Immune-Enhancing Enteral Therapy (2001) advise giving IEDs to severely malnourished patients undergoing lower GI surgery 5 to 7 days before surgery. Emerging data suggest a benefit for patients who are not clinically malnourished.

26. **Should actual, ideal, or adjusted body weight be used in nutrition calculations for the patient with obesity?**

    Studies using an obesity-adjusted weight in kilocalorie calculations [ideal body weight (IBW) + .25 (actual-IBW)] correlate better with measured energy expenditure than when using actual weight.

ENTERAL CONTROVERSIES

27. **What are probiotics, and when are they useful?**

    Probiotics are live microbes that benefit the host. Clinical studies show therapeutic or preventive use of varied probiotic strains for antibiotic-associated diarrhea, rotavirus-associated diarrhea and pouchitis. Results are promising for irritable bowel syndrome, ulcerative colitis, and for side-effect reduction in antibiotic therapy for *helicobacter pylori*.

28. **Which is more important: nitrogen or caloric balance?**

    Ultimately, maintaining positive nitrogen balance may be more important than achieving positive kilocalorie balance.

29. **Are postpyloric feedings superior to gastric feedings?**

    Following major surgery or injury, gastric emptying is impaired for several days. Early enteral feeding, with its known benefits, may not easily occur through a gastric feeding in the early stages of injury. Postpyloric feedings deliver more kilocalories, more timely return to anabolism, and promote a lower rate of infectious complications than continuous gastric feeding.

30. **When should immune-enhancing formulas be used?**

    Rarely. Patients in randomized controlled trials have demonstrated that IEDs improve outcome and reduce septic morbidity in patients prone to intraabdominal sepsis after major torso trauma and after major operative resection of upper GI cancers. The use of IEDs should be restricted to these patients, and duration should be limited because of the increased expense. The IEDs have not been adequately tested in other types of patients, and, when tested in a variety of patients in the ICU, there is some evidence to suggest that they could be harmful. There is concern that administering arginine in patients with sepsis, who have upregulated expression of inducible nitrous oxide synthase (iNos), will result in excessive nitrous oxide production and resultant exaggerated vasodilation and oxidant stress.

31. **Should formula with increased fish-oil formula be used in patients who are going into acute respiratory distress syndrome?**
Two industry-funded, randomized controlled trials demonstrate superior outcome in patients with acute respiratory distress syndrome (ARDS) when provided a high omega-3 fatty acid enteral product as opposed to a high omega-6 "pulmonary" formula. Unfortunately, the control diet, a high omega-6 fatty acid formula, is not the standard of care and may worsen ARDS. High omega-6 fatty acids increase inflammation and produce lipid mediators that worsen ventilation/perfusion (V/Q) mismatch in the lung and worsen oxygenation in ARDS. A randomized controlled trial comparing standard, moderate-fat polymeric formula and a high omega-3 formula is needed.

PARENTERAL NUTRITION

32. **What is parenteral nutrition?**
Parenteral nutrition is the provision of protein as amino acids (4 kcal/g), dextrose (3.4 kcal/g), and fat (lipid 20% solution delivers 2 kcal/ml), vitamins, minerals, trace elements, fluid, and sometimes insulin through an IV infusion.

33. **What are the indications for parenteral nutrition?**
Use parenteral nutrition when the GI tract is totally nonfunctional, e.g., major bowel resection, "short gut," peritonitis, intestinal hemorrhage, paralytic ileus, high volume enterocutaneous fistulae, ileus, and severe intractable diarrhea (>1 liter/day).

34. **What types of access are available for the delivery of parenteral nutrition?**
Central parenteral solutions have osmolarities up to 3000 mOsm/L. These require delivery into a large lumen vein (e.g., subclavian, or less commonly, a femoral vein). If a multiple-port catheter is used, a "virgin port" should be reserved exclusively for nutrient infusion. When prolonged parenteral nutrition infusion is necessary in the postacute setting, consider a long-term access device such as a Hickman or Broviac catheter. This may not be necessary, however, when the central venous catheter is placed under sterile conditions and the patient and caretakers deliver meticulous care.

35. **Should patients with pancreatitis be exclusively fed parenterally?**
Although patients with pancreatitis have traditionally been given "gut rest" and TPN, studies demonstrate improved outcome with enteral feeding past the ligament of Treitz. Enteral feedings delivered into the jejunum promote decreased infectious morbidity, shorter hospital length of stay, fewer complications, a faster resolution of systemic inflammatory response syndrome (SIRS) and a shorter disease course than parenteral nutrition. If enteral nutrition is not tolerated, parenteral nutrition should be considered no sooner than 5 days into the hospitalization.

36. **Are intravenous lipids contraindicated in pancreatitis?**
In extremely rare instances of pancreatitis caused by congenital hyperlipidemia, lipids should be withheld. However, in most cases of severe pancreatitis where enteral nutrition is not tolerated, it is best to avoid IV lipid emulsions until the inflammatory response has subsided.

37. **What complications are associated with parenteral nutrition?**
Fluid and electrolyte imbalance, altered glucose metabolism, increased LFTs, hepatic steatosis, systemic candidiasis, site infections, and gut atrophy are associated with TPN. Hemothorax or pneumothorax may occur during central line placement. Although rare, air emboli or extravascular placement of central lines occur.

38. **Why do parenterally fed patients often develop hyperglycemia?**
Patients who are fed parenterally may develop hyperglycemia as a result of increased stress and the inflammatory response, limited mobility, concurrent steroid therapy, and excessive kilocalorie intake.

39. **How should hyperglycemia be managed?**
Evaluate information on the home glucose control regimen from the medication history. A continuous insulin infusion is often necessary during critical illness to achieve adequate glycemic control. When insulin requirements are predictable and the patient becomes more stable metabolically and moves outside of the ICU, insulin is added to the TPN. NPH insulin is geared toward patients consuming meals at regular intervals and thus, is not appropriate with continuous IV feedings. Glucose infusion rates should not exceed 5 milligrams per kilogram per minute.

40. **Why are intravenous fat emulsions used, and when are they contraindicated?**
Theoretically, fat emulsions are employed to prevent essential fatty acid deficiency. In reality, this condition is rare, takes several weeks to develop, and requires only 3% to 4% of kilocalories as linoleic acid (or 10% of kilocalories as a standard fat emulsion). Fat emulsions are also used to provide additional kilocalories once glucose delivery exceeds 5 kilocalories per kilogram per minute. When delivered in total-nutrient-admixtures (3-in-1 solutions) lipid emulsions are stable for 24 hours. When infused as a sole nutrient, limit hang times to <12 hours to prevent bacterial growth. Avoid fat emulsions with hyperlipidemia-induced pancreatitis, and when serum triglycerides are significantly elevated (e.g., >500 mg/dl). Because they are associated with increased mortality early after trauma, and increased infections in critical illness, IV fat emulsion risk outweighs benefit during the early acute-phase response.

41. **What is refeeding syndrome, and how is it managed or prevented?**
Refeeding syndrome occurs when a patient is moderately to severely malnourished and has limited substrate reserves, usually as a result of chronic alcoholism, anorexia nervosa, post-bariatric surgery, or chronic starvation. When presented with a large nutrient load, the patient rapidly develops a clinically significant decline in serum K, phosphorus (P), Ca, and Mg because of compartment shifts or increased utilization of these ions. Hyperglycemia is common as a result of blunted basal insulin secretion (see Kraft). Provide ample quantities of K, P, Ca, and Mg with the initial parenteral mixture, within the solubility limits of the solution. Reduce the initial kilocalorie load by 25% of goal by limiting dextrose kilocalories. Monitor blood glucose 4 times daily, and, serum K, P, Ca, and Mg daily for 5 days after initiating feeding, while advancing kilocalories to goal levels.

42. **How should parenteral nutrition be monitored?**
Parenteral nutrition should be monitored daily with serum chemistries (Na, K, Cl, CO_2, glucose, Mg, P, and Ca) during the initial days of therapy in the critical care setting. Check blood glucose every 6 hours. With acceptable fluid and electrolyte balance, reduce frequency to 1 to 2 times weekly. The adequacy of the nutrition regimen may be assessed by evidence of proper wound healing, maintenance of hydrational status, preservation of body cell mass, and a timely repletion of constitutive protein levels. Overfeeding may present as insulin resistance, hypertriglyceridemia, increased LFTs, and hypercapnia.

43. What infusion schedules are used for TPN?

TPN is usually infused continuously. In more ambulatory patients, and those on home therapy, a cyclic or nighttime infusion schedule (12- to 18-hour cycle) increases patient freedom.

44. How should TPN be discontinued?

To discontinue TPN, reduce the infusion rate by half for 2 hours, halved again for 2 hours, and then turn it off. This "ramp down" prevents reactive hypoglycemia.

45. What is the cost of parenteral nutrition?

Parenteral solution costs vary widely depending on the constituents. The cost of TPN solution components, preparation, access devices, and laboratory monitoring costs up to 10 times that of a standard enteral feeding. Many third-party payers do not provide more reimbursement for parenteral therapy than enteral in the hospital setting.

46. How much gut is necessary to avoid TPN dependence after small bowel resection?

The normal adult small bowel is 300 to 800 cm in length. Loss of more than two thirds is considered short-bowel syndrome. The condition of the remnant small bowel is important.

PARENTERAL CONTROVERSIES

47. Should TPN solutions contain the same percentage of fat kilocalories that are recommended in the diet of healthy Americans (i.e., 30% of total kilocalories)?

The American Heart Association (AHA) recommendations for 30% of total kilocalories as fat are geared toward cardiovascular disease prevention in healthy people and were never intended for IV feeding in individuals who are critically ill. Furthermore, AHA suggests that those kilocalories be distributed among saturated, monounsaturated and polyunsaturated fat, including omega-3 series fatty acids. Current lipid formulations available in the United States are made from either soybean oil or a mixture of soybean and safflower oil; thus, they are predominately polyunsaturated (omega-6) fat. Glucose kilocalories are the most cost-effective kilocalories, followed by standard amino acid kilocalories, then lipid calories. Lipid infusions exceeding 1 g/kg of body weight are associated with decreased immunocompetence and impaired oxygenation in patients who are critically ill.

48. Does supplemental glutamine enhance outcome in surgical patients?

Glutamine, the amino acid found in greatest concentration in muscle and plasma, decreases after surgery, injury, or stress. Thus, it is a conditionally essential amino acid. It plays a role as a metabolic substrate for rapidly replicating cells, maintains the integrity and function of the intestinal barrier, and protects the enterocyte from free radical damage. Glutamine is not included in standard amino acid solutions because of limited solubility and stability. Supplementation may reduce infectious complication rates and decrease hospital stay in surgical patients.

49. Should recombinant growth hormone, glutamine, and a modified diet be used routinely to maximize gut adaptation after intestinal resection?

Five clinical trials have appeared in the past decade. Three showed negative results, whereas two showed positive results. Positive results are short-lived. Until further research occurs, this expensive therapy should not be routine, and intensive nutrition and pharmacologic management should remain the mainstay of care.

BIBLIOGRAPHY

1. Brady M, Kinn S, Stuart P: Preoperative fasting for adults to prevent perioperative complications, Cochrane Database Syst Rev CD004423, 2003.

2. Heyland DK, Dhaliwal R, Day A et al.: Canadian Critical Care Clinical Practice Guidelines Committee. Canadian clinical practice guidelines for nutrition support in mechanically ventilated, critically ill adult patients, JPEN 27:355-373, 2003.

3. Frankenfield D, Hise M, Malone A et al.: Prediction of resting metabolic rate in critically ill adult patients: results of a systematic review of the evidence. J Am Diet Assoc 107:1552-1561, 2007.

4. Gadek JE, DeMichele SJ, Karlstad MD et al.: Effect of enteral feeding with eicopentaenoic acid, gamma-linolenic acid, and antioxidants in patients with acute respiratory distress syndrome. Crit Care Med 27:1409-1420, 1999.

5. Graves C, Saffle J, Morris S: Comparison of urine urea nitrogen collection times in critically ill patients. Nutr Clin Pract 20:271-275, 2005.

6. Haugen HA, Chan LN, Li F: Indirect calorimetry: a practical guide for clinicians. Nutr Clin Pract 22:377-388, 2007.

7. KDOQI clinical practice guidelines for nutrition in chronic renal failure. Am J Kidney Dis 35(6 Suppl 2); S1-S140, 2000.

8. Konstantinides FN, Konstantinides NN, Li JC et al.: Urinary urea nitrogen: too sensitive for calculating nitrogen balance studies in surgical clinical nutrition. JPEN 15:189-193, 1991.

9. Kozar R, McQuiggan M, Moore F: Nutritional support of trauma patients. In Shikora S, Martindale RG, Schwaitzburg S, editors: Nutritional considerations in the intensive care unit. Silver Springs, MD, 2002, ASPEN Publishers.

10. Kraft MD, Btaiche IF, Sacks GS: Review of the refeeding syndrome. Nutr Clin Pract 20:625-633, 2005.

11. Matarese LE, O'Keefe SJ, Kandil HM et al.: Short-bowel syndrome: clinical guidelines for nutrition management. Nutr Clin Pract 20:493-502, 2005.

12. McClave SA: Nutrition support in acute pancreatitis. Gastroenterol Clin North Am 36:65-74, 2007.

13. Novak F, Heyland DK, Avenell A et al.: Glutamine supplementation in serious illness: a systematic review of the evidence. Crit Care Med 30:2022-2029, 2002.

14. Pontes-Arruda A, Aragão AM, Albuquerque JD: Effects of enteral feeding with eicosapentaenoic acid, gamma-linolenic acid, and antioxidants in mechanically ventilated patients with severe sepsis and septic shock. Crit Care Med 34: 2325-2333, 2006.

15. Van den Berghe G, Wouters P, Weekers F et al.: Intensive insulin therapy in critically ill patients. N Engl J Med 345:1359-1367, 2001.

CHAPTER 10

WHAT DOES POSTOPERATIVE FEVER MEAN?

Alden H. Harken, MD

1. **What is a fever?**

   Normal core temperature varies between 36° C and 38° C. Because humans hibernate a little at night, we are cool (36° C) just before rising in the morning; after revving our engines all day, we are hot at night (38° C). A fever is a pathologic state reflecting a systemic inflammatory process. The core temperature is >38° C but rarely >40° C.

2. **What is malignant hyperthermia?**

   A rare, life-threatening response to inhaled anesthetics or some muscle relaxants. Core temperature rises >40° C. Abnormal calcium metabolism in skeletal muscle produces heat, acidosis, hypokalemia, muscle rigidity, coagulopathy, and circulatory collapse.

3. **How is malignant hyperthermia treated?**
   - Stop the anesthetic.
   - Give sodium bicarbonate (2 mEq/kg intravenously [IV]).
   - Give dantrolene (calcium channel blocker at 2.5 mg/kg IV).
   - Continue dantrolene (1 mg/kg every 6 hours for 48 hours).
   - Cool patient with alcohol sponges and ice.

KEY POINTS: MALIGNANT HYPERTHERMIA

1. Rare, familial (autosomal dominant with variable penetrance) catastrophic response to inhaled anesthetics or muscle relaxants.

2. Mechanism: abnormal calcium metabolism in skeletal muscle.

3. Clinical manifestations: core temperature >40° C, trismus, hypercapnia, tachycardia, tachypnea, hypertension, cardiac dysrhythmias, metabolic acidosis, hypoxemia, myoglobinuria, or coagulopathy.

4. Management: halt anesthetic; administer dantrolene over 48 hours, supplemental sodium bicarbonate; actively cool patient.

4. **What causes fever?**

   Macrophages are activated by bacteria and endotoxin. Activated macrophages release interleukin-1, tumor necrosis factor (TNF), and interferon, which reset the hypothalamic thermoregulatory center.

5. **Can fever be treated?**
   Yes. Aspirin, acetaminophen, and ibuprofen are cyclooxygenase inhibitors that block the formation of prostaglandin E_2 in the hypothalamus and effectively control fever.

6. **Should fever be treated?**
   This is controversial. No evidence suggests that suppression of fever improves patient outcome. Patients are more comfortable, however, and the surgeon receives fewer calls from the nurses.

7. **Should fever be investigated?**
   Yes. Fever indicates that something (frequently treatable) is going on. The threshold for inquiry depends on the patient. A transplant patient with a temperature of 38° C requires scrutiny, whereas a healthy medical student with an identical temperature of 38° C 24 hours after an appendectomy can be ignored.

8. **Summarize a fever work-up.**
   - Order blood cultures, urine Gram stain and culture, and sputum Gram stain and culture.
   - Look at the surgical incisions.
   - Look at old and current intravenous sites for evidence of septic thrombophlebitis.
   - If breath sounds are worrisome, obtain a chest x-ray.

9. **What is the most common cause of fever during the early postoperative period (1 to 3 days)?**
   The traditional answer is atelectasis. A total pneumothorax does not cause fever, however. Why does a little atelectasis cause fever, whereas a lot of atelectasis (pneumothorax) does not? The most likely explanation is that sterile atelectasis (and early postoperative lung collapse typically is not infected) has nothing to do with fever.

10. **Do surgical incisions compromise spontaneous breathing patterns?**
    Yes. Vital capacity was measured in a large group of patients 24 hours after various surgical procedures. An upper abdominal incision was the worst, followed by lower abdominal incision, then (counterintuitively) thoracotomy, median sternotomy, and extremity incision.

11. **Should atelectasis be treated with incentive spirometry?**
    Yes, but not to avoid fever.

12. **Define a wound infection.**
    A wound infection contains $>10^5$ organisms per gram of tissue. An infected incision appears erythematous (red), edematous (swollen), and tender.

13. **Are certain wounds prone to infection?**
    Each milliliter of human saliva contains 10^8 aerobic and anaerobic, gram-positive and gram-negative bacteria. All human bite wounds must be considered as contaminated. Animal bite wounds typically are less contaminated. (It is safer to kiss your dog than your fiancé[e].)

14. **Do incisions become infected early after surgery?**
    The incision must be examined in a patient with a fever (39° C) <12 hours after surgery. Look for a foul-smelling, serous discharge in a particularly painful wound (all incisions hurt) with or without crepitus. Gram stain of the serous discharge for gram-positive rods confirms or excludes the diagnosis of clostridial infection.

15. **Summarize the therapy for clostridial gas gangrene.**
    - The wound should be opened immediately, with fluid resuscitation of the patient. The mainstay of therapy is aggressive surgical debridement of necrotic tissue (skin, muscle, and fascia). Make a big hole, and do not worry about closing it.
    - Give penicillin, 12 million U/day IV for 1 week.
    - Hyperbaric oxygen is not helpful.

16. **Are nonclostridial necrotizing wound infections a cause of concern?**
    Hemolytic streptococcal gangrene, idiopathic scrotal gangrene, and gram-negative synergistic necrotizing cellulitis are distinct entities but have been lumped into the single category of necrotizing fasciitis. All require the same initial approach:
    1. Fluid and electrolyte resuscitation.
    2. Broad-spectrum antibiotics ("triples").
    3. Aggressive surgical debridement of all necrotic tissue.

17. **What are triple antibiotics?**
    A shotgun approach to potentially life-threatening infections when the patient is seriously ill and the surgeon is seriously concerned:
    1. Gram-positive coverage (e.g., ampicillin)
    2. Gram-negative coverage (e.g., gentamicin)
    3. Anaerobic coverage (e.g., metronidazole [Flagyl])
    To avoid overgrowth of yeast and resistant bacteria, focus on the culprit bacteria as soon as the cultures define it.

KEY POINTS: CLOSTRIDIAL VERSUS NONCLOSTRIDIAL ✓ NECROTIZING WOUND INFECTIONS

1. Clostridial infection involves underlying muscle resulting in myonecrosis or gas gangrene.

2. Nonclostridial infection involves subcutaneous fascia (also known as necrotizing fasciitis).

3. Similar management: fluid and electrolyte resuscitation, antibiotics (high-dose penicillin for clostridial infection, broad-spectrum triples for necrotizing fasciitis), and aggressive surgical debridement of necrotic tissue.

18. **Give the doses for triple antibiotics.**
    Ampicillin 1 g every 6 hours IV in adults
    40 mg/kg every 6 hours IV in children
    Gentamicin 7 mg/kg IV every 24 hours (this single daily dose is less nephrotoxic than 2 mg/kg IV every 8 hours)
    Metronidazole 500 mg IV every 6 hours in adults
    7.5 mg/kg IV every 6 hours in children

19. **Which surgical procedures are predisposed to wound infections?**
    Gastrointestinal (GI) procedures, especially when the colon is opened.

20. **When do wound infections typically occur?**
    They occur between 12 hours and 7 days postoperatively.

21. **How is a wound infection treated?**
    The wound should be opened and completely drained.

22. **Is it necessary to irrigate an infected wound?**
Tap water irrigation decreases the bacterial load and promotes healing. Alcohol is toxic to tissues. Sodium hydrochlorite (Dakin solution) and hydrogen peroxide kill fibroblasts and slow epithelialization. As a rule of thumb, put nothing into a wound that you would not put in your eye.

23. **When do urinary tract infections occur?**
The longer the urethral (Foley) catheter is in place, the more likely the urinary tract infection (UTI). Urologic instrumentation at the time of surgery may accelerate the process considerably. Germs crawl up the outside of the urethral catheter, and by 5 to 7 days after surgery, most patients harbor infected urine.

24. **How is a urinary tract infection diagnosed?**
A UTI has a urine culture with $>10^5$ bacteria/ml. White blood cells on urinalysis are highly suspicious.

25. **Name the most common late causes of postoperative fever.**
Septic thrombophlebitis (from an intravenous line) and occult (usually intraabdominal) abscesses tend to present about 2 weeks after surgery.

WEBSITES

www.mhacanada.org

www.anes.ucla.edu/dept/mh.html

BIBLIOGRAPHY

1. Bansal BC, Wiebe RA, Perkins SD et al.: Tap water for irrigation of lacerations. Am J Emerg Med 20:469-472, 2002.
2. da Luz Moreira A, Vogel JD, Kalady MF et al.: Fever evaluations after colorectal surgery: identification of risk factors that increase yield and decrease cost. Dis Colon Rectum 51: 1202-1207, 2008.
3. Helmer KS, Robinson EK, Lally KP et al.: Standardized patient care guidelines reduce infectious morbidity in appendectomy patients. Am J Surg 183:608-613, 2002.
4. Lewis RT: Oral versus systemic antibiotic prophylaxis in elective colon surgery: a randomized study and meta-analysis send a message from the 1990s. Can J Surg 45:173-180, 2002.
5. Singer AJ, Quinn JV, Thode HC Jr et al.: Determinants of poor outcome after laceration and surgical incision repair. Plast Reconstr Surg 110:429-435, 2002.

CHAPTER 11

SURGICAL WOUND INFECTION

Steven L. Peterson, DVM, MD

1. Why should we worry about surgical wound infection?

Approximately 30 million patients undergo surgery each year in the United States, and 20% of these patients acquire at least one nosocomial infection in the postoperative period. Infections at surgical sites are the third most common form of these infections and complicate 1% to 12% of all operations. The risk of death is 4 times higher in patients who develop wound infections, and each infection costs $12,000 to $30,000 to treat.

Commonly reported rates for specific operations are:

Cholecystectomy	3%	Inguinal herniorrhaphy	2%
Appendectomy	5%	Thoracotomy	6%
Colectomy	12%		

2. What comprises a surgical wound infection?

Surgical wound infections more appropriately are called surgical site infections (SSIs) and must occur within 30 days of surgery unless a foreign body is left in situ. In the case of implanted foreign material, 1 year must elapse before surgery can be excluded as causative. SSIs are subdivided based on depth of tissue involvement into three clinically relevant categories.

1. Superficial incisional SSIs involve only the skin and subcutaneous tissue.
2. Deep incisional SSIs involve deep soft tissue layers, such as fascial or muscle layers of the incision.
3. Organ space SSIs involve any anatomic structure opened or manipulated during the operative procedure.

3. List the classic signs of superficial incisional, deep incisional, and organ space surgical site infections.

Superficial and deep incisional SSIs:

- Calor (heat)
- Rubor (redness)
- Tumor (swelling)
- Dolor (pain)
- Purulent drainage

Organ space SSIs should be suspected in the presence of systemic signs and symptoms:

- Fever
- Ileus
- Shock

Definitive diagnosis of organ space SSIs may require imaging studies.

4. Why do these infections occur?

Many factors contribute, however, the fundamental principle is that traumatic and surgical wounds violate the normal protective layer of skin. The importance of an intact integument has been shown experimentally in which it was determined that an inoculum of 8 million bacteria is required for infection of intact skin, 1 million are required for violated skin, and only 100 are required when foreign material is present.

5. **Surgery always violates the skin, and we often leave foreign material. How can we avoid SSIs?**
   Although it is true that the basic act of surgery compromises the patients' defenses, we can take steps to prevent wound infection. These steps involve the surgeon and the patient.

6. **What can the surgeon do to decrease SSIs?**
   The first step the surgeon can take is appropriate hand washing. The classic surgical scrub consists of 3 minutes of brushing with povidone-iodine or chlorhexidine gluconate. This protocol has been shown to have a high rate of noncompliance, which may contribute to SSIs. Data indicate improved compliance with comparable SSI rates using a much simpler protocol consisting of a 1-minute hand wash with nonantiseptic soap followed by hand-rubbing with a liquid aqueous alcoholic solution. Whether such simpler scrub protocols also can be applied in the future to the preparation of the patient is unknown.

7. **What else can the surgeon do to control SSIs?**
   The surgeon may limit the duration of surgery and follow good surgical principles by eliminating dead space, controlling hemorrhage, minimizing placement of foreign material (including excessive suture), and exhibiting gentle tissue handling. The surgeon should ensure that the patient remains warm during the perioperative period. This simple act of warming was shown in two prospective studies to decrease significantly the incidence of SSIs.

8. **Can't the surgeon predict who is going to get infected and just give them lots of antibiotics to stop infection from happening?**
   To a degree, SSIs can be anticipated. Factors that have been shown to have some predictive value to the surgeon are the physical status of the patient as classified by the American Society of Anesthesiologists, results of intraoperative cultures, and duration of preoperative hospital stay. Adequacy of regional blood supply also is important, as evidenced by the low infection rate in facial wounds. The classic description of wounds based on degree of gross contamination also may be of value. This scheme places wounds into one of four categories:
   1. **Clean wounds** are atraumatic wounds in which no inflammation is encountered, no breaks in sterile technique occur, and no hollow viscus is entered.
   2. **Clean-contaminated wounds** are identical except that a hollow viscus is entered.
   3. **Contaminated wounds** are caused by trauma from a clean source or by minor spillage of infected materials.
   4. **Dirty-infected wounds** are caused by trauma from a contaminated source or gross spillage of infected material into an incision.

   Reported infection rates for each category are 2.1%, 3.3%, 6.4%, and 7.1%, respectively. Antibiotics can help but only when used appropriately.

9. **How do I use antibiotics correctly to prevent SSIs?**
   First by knowing what organism you are targeting, then choosing an appropriate antibiotic and delivering it at the appropriate time via the appropriate route. Because you usually will not have a preoperative culture to guide therapy, you need to base your choice of antibiotic on predicted organisms. Staphylococci are the most common skin organism and the most common etiologic agent in SSIs. Cefazolin, a first-generation cephalosporin, is usually the recommended antibiotic for prophylaxis in clean surgical procedures. In circumstances in which known contamination has occurred, initial antibiotics should be tailored based on the violated organ's common flora. If the gut was entered, enterobacteriaceae and anaerobes are common; biliary tract and esophageal incisions yield these organisms plus enterococci. The urinary tract or vagina may contain group D streptococci, *Pseudomonas,* and *Proteus* species.

10. **If antibiotics are used, how and when should they be administered?**
Maximal benefit is obtained when tissue concentrations are therapeutic at the time of contamination. Efficacy is enhanced when prophylactic antibiotics are administered intravenously (IV) less than 1 hour before surgical incision; late administration is similar to no administration. Multiple-dose regimens have no proven benefit over single-dose regimens. Indiscriminate antibiotic selection outside recommended hospital protocols may increase the incidence of SSIs. In special circumstances, administration routes other than IV may be indicated.

KEY POINTS: WOUND CLASSIFICATION AND INFECTION RATE

1. Clean wound is atraumatic, with no breaks in sterile technique, no entry into respiratory, alimentary, or genitourinary tract. Incidence is 2.1%.

2. Clean-contaminated wound is same as clean wound except entry into respiratory, alimentary, or genitourinary tract. Incidence is 3.3%.

3. Contaminated wound has trauma from a clean source or minor spillage of infected materials. Incidence is 6.4%.

4. Dirty wound is trauma from a contaminated source or spillage of infected materials. Incidence is 7.1%.

11. **Name other routes that you would use for prophylactic antibiotic administration.**
In patients with nasal carriage of *Staphylococcus aureus*, intranasal administration of mupirocin ointment may have some efficacy in decreasing nosocomial and SSIs. In elective colon surgery, a meta-analysis of published studies indicated that orally administered antibiotics combined with intravenous antibiotics are superior to intravenous antibiotics alone in preventing surgical site infections.

12. **Does all that pulsatile lavage the surgeon uses in the operating room really do any good?**
Yes. High-pressure pulsatile lavage has been evaluated extensively in soft tissue contamination and shown to be 7 times more effective in reducing bacterial load than bulb syringe lavage. The inherent elastic recoil of the soft tissues allows particulate matter to escape between pulses of fluid. The optimal pressure and pulse frequency seems to be 50 to 70 lb/in.^{2} and 800 pulses/min. Adding antibiotics to lavage solutions, although commonly practiced, has not been shown definitively to improve outcome.

13. **What can the patient do to help decrease SSIs?**
Stop smoking. Although obesity, poor nutritional status, advanced age, and diabetes are risk factors for SSIs, cigarette smoking is probably the leading preventable patient factor for SSIs just like it is the leading preventable cause of death and disability in the United States. Half of all people who smoke eventually die from a smoking-related illness. Smoking not only kills, but also more than triples that risk of incisional wound breakdown. In one study, smoking increased the incidence of SSIs in clean operative procedures sixfold, from 0.6% to 3.6%. Tobacco use results in decreased blood flow and decreased oxygen delivery to the wound. Toxic tobacco by-products also directly impede all stages of wound healing. Despite this knowledge, surgeons continue to operate electively on smokers, and most smokers continue to smoke up until the day of surgery.

14. **When prevention fails, what do you do for SSIs?**

The first line of therapy in SSIs is drainage. This is established by reopening the wound or, in the case of deep space infections, using techniques that are guided by computed tomography (CT) or ultrasound for drain placement or presurgical planning. Antibiotic therapy is used to control associated cellulitis and generalized sepsis.

15. **What may happen with untreated superficial or deep incisional SSIs?**

Locally the wound breaks down, and infection dissects through the tissue planes and continues to advance. If the infection progresses rapidly, necrotizing fasciitis may develop. Finally, the strength layers of the wound closure break open (dehisce).

16. **Define wound dehiscence.**

The partial or total disruption of any or all layers of the operative wound.

17. **Define evisceration.**

Rupture of the abdominal wall and extrusion of the abdominal viscera.

18. **What factors predispose to dehiscence?**

Age >60 years, obesity, increased intraabdominal pressure, malnutrition, renal or hepatic insufficiency, diabetes mellitus (DM), use of corticosteroids or cytotoxic drugs, and radiation have been implicated in wound dehiscence. Infection also plays an important role; an infective agent is identified in more than half of wounds that undergo dehiscence. Despite these excuses, the most important factor in wound dehiscence is the adequacy of closure. Fascial edges should not be devitalized. Ideally the linea alba sutures should be placed neither too laterally nor too medially. Excessive lateral placement may incorporate the variable blood supply of the rectus abdominis muscle and compromise fascial circulation. Excessive medial placement misses the point of maximal strength at the transition zone between the linea alba and rectus abdominis sheath. In addition, sutures should be tied correctly without excessive tension, and suture material of adequate tensile strength should be chosen.

19. **When does wound dehiscence occur?**

It may occur at any time after surgery; however, it is most common between the fifth and tenth postoperative days, when wound strength is at a minimum.

20. **What are the signs and symptoms of wound dehiscence?**

Normally a ridge of palpable thickening (healing ridge) extends about 0.5 cm on each side of the incision within 1 week. Absence of this ridge may be a strong predictor of impending wound breakdown. More commonly, leakage of serosanguineous fluid from the wound is the first sign. In some instances, sudden evisceration may be the first indication of abdominal wound dehiscence. The patient also may describe a sensation of tearing or popping associated with coughing or retching.

21. **Describe the proper management of wound dehiscence.**

If the dehiscence is not associated with infection, elective reclosure may be the appropriate therapeutic course. If the condition of the patient or wound makes reclosure unacceptable, however, the wound should be allowed to heal by second intention. An unstable scar or incisional hernia may be dealt with at a later, safer time. Dehiscense of a laparotomy wound with evisceration is a surgical emergency with a reported mortality of 10% to 20%. Initial treatment in this instance consists of appropriate resuscitation while protecting the eviscerated organs with moist towels; the next step is prompt surgical closure. Exposed bowel or omentum should be lavaged thoroughly and returned to the abdomen; the abdominal wall should be closed; and the skin wound should be packed open. Vacuum-assisted wound closure may be valuable in select cases.

WEBSITE

www.acssurgery.com/abstracts/acs/acs0102.htm

BIBLIOGRAPHY

1. Barie PS: Modern surgical antibiotic prophylaxis and therapy: less is more. Surg Infect 1:23-29, 2000.
2. Garner GB, Ware DN, Cocanour CS et al.: Vacuum-assisted wound closure provides early fascial reapproximation in trauma patients with open abdomens. Am J Surg 182:630-638, 2001.
3. Harbarth S, Fankhauser C, Schrenzel J et al.: Universal screening for methicillin-resistant *Staphylococcus aureus* at hospital admission and nosocomial infection in surgical patients. JAMA 299:1149-1157, 2008.
4. Kluytmans J, Voss A: Prevention of postsurgical infections: some like it hot. Curr Opin Infect Dis 15:427-432, 2002.
5. Krueger JK, Rohrich RJ: Clearing the smoke: the scientific rationale for tobacco abstention with plastic surgery. Plast Reconstr Surg 108:1063-1073, 2001.
6. Morange-Saussier V, Giraudeau B, van der Mee N et al.: Nasal carriage of methicillin-resistant *Staphylococcus aureus* in vascular surgery. Ann Vasc Surg 20:767-772, 2006.
7. Myles PS, Iacono GA, Hunt JO et al.: Risk of respiratory complications and wound infection in patients undergoing ambulatory service. Anesthesiology 97:842-847, 2002.
8. Parienti JJ, Thibon P, Heller R et al.: Hand-rubbing with an aqueous alcoholic solution vs traditional surgical hand scrubbing and 30-day surgical site infection rates: a randomized equivalence study. JAMA 288:722-727, 2002.
9. Perl TM, Cullen JJ, Wenzel RP et al.: Intranasal mupirocin to prevent postoperative *Staphylococcus aureus* infections. N Engl J Med 346:1871-1877, 2002.
10. Seltzer J, McGraw K, Horsman A et al.: Awareness of surgical site infections for advanced practice nurses. ACCN Clin Iss 13:398-409, 2002.

CHAPTER 12

PRIORITIES IN EVALUATION OF THE ACUTE ABDOMEN

Alden H. Harken, MD

1. **What is the surgeon's responsibility when confronted by a patient with an acute abdomen?**
   1. To identify how sick the patient is (treat the patient first and *then* the disease).
   2. To determine whether the patient (a) needs to go directly to the operating room, (b) should be admitted for resuscitation or observation, or (c) can be sent safely home.

2. **Which is the most dangerous course in a patient with an acute abdomen?**
   To send the patient home.

3. **Is it important to make the diagnosis in the emergency department?**
   No. Frequently time spent confirming a diagnosis in the emergency department (ED) is lost to in-hospital resuscitation or treatment in the operating room. The only patient who needs a relatively firm diagnosis is a patient who is to be sent home.

4. **If the essential goal is not to make the diagnosis, what should the surgeon do?**
   1. Resuscitate the patient. Most patients do not eat or drink when they are getting sick. Most patients are depleted of at least several liters of fluid. Fluid depletion is worse in patients with diarrhea or vomiting.
   2. Start a big intravenous (IV) line.
   3. Replace lost electrolytes (see Chapter 8).
   4. Insert a Foley catheter.
   5. Examine the patient (frequently).

5. **Are symptoms and signs uniquely misleading in any groups of patients?**
   Yes. Watch out for the following groups:
   - The very young, who cannot talk.
   - Diabetics because of visceral neuropathy.
   - The very old, in whom, much as in diabetics, abdominal innervation is dulled.
   - Patients taking steroids, which depress inflammation and mask everything.
   - Patients with immunosuppression (a heart or kidney transplant patient may act cheerful even with dead or gangrenous bowel).

6. **Summarize the history needed.**
   1. **The patient's age.** Neonates present with intussusception; young women present with ectopic pregnancy, pelvic inflammatory disease, and appendicitis; the elderly present with colon cancer, diverticulitis, and appendicitis.
   2. **Associated problems.** Previous hospitalizations, prior abdominal surgery, medications, heart and lung disease? An extensive gynecologic history is valuable; however, it is probably safer to assume that all women between 12 and 40 years old are pregnant.

3. **Location of abdominal pain.** *Right upper quadrant:* gallbladder or biliary disease, duodenal ulcer. *Right flank:* pyelonephritis, hepatitis. *Midepigastrium:* duodenal or gastric ulcer, pancreatitis, gastritis. *Left upper quadrant:* ruptured spleen, subdiaphragmatic abscess. *Right lower quadrant:* appendicitis (see Chapter 37), ectopic pregnancy, incarcerated hernia, rectus hematoma. *Left lower quadrant:* diverticulitis, incarcerated hernia, rectus hematoma. ***Note:*** Cancer, unless it obstructs (colon cancer), and bleeding (diverticulosis) typically do not hurt.

4. **Duration of pain.** The pain of a perforated duodenal ulcer or perforated sigmoid diverticulum is sudden, whereas the pain of pyelonephritis is gradual and persistent. The pain of intestinal obstruction is intermittent and crampy. *Note:* Although the surgeon is rotating through a gastrointestinal (GI) service, the patient may not know this and may present with urologic, gynecologic, or vascular pathology.

PHYSICAL EXAMINATION

7. **Are vital signs important?**
Yes. They are vital. If heart rate (HR) and blood pressure (BP) are on the wrong side of 100 (heart rate >100 beats/min, systolic blood pressure <100 mm Hg), watch out! Tachypnea (respiratory rate >16) reflects either pain or systemic acidosis. Fever may develop late, particularly in the immunosuppressed patient who may be afebrile in the face of florid peritonitis.

8. **What is rebound?**
The peritoneum is well innervated and exquisitely sensitive. It is not necessary to hurt the patient to elicit peritoneal signs. Depress the abdomen gently and release. If the patient winces, the peritoneum is inflamed **(rebound tenderness)**.

9. **What is mittelschmerz?**
Mittelschmerz is pain in the middle of the menstrual cycle. Ovulation frequently is associated with intraperitoneal bleeding. Blood irritates the sensitive peritoneum and hurts.

10. **What do bowel sounds mean?**
If something hurts (e.g., a sprained ankle), the patient tends not to use it. Inflamed bowel is quiet. Bowel contents squeezed through a partial obstruction produce high-pitched tinkles. Bowel sounds are notoriously unreliable, however.

11. **Explain the significance of abdominal distention.**
Distention may derive from either intraenteric or extraenteric gas or fluid (worst of all, blood). Abdominal distention is always significant and bad.

12. **Is abdominal palpation important?**
Yes. Remember, the patient is (or should be) the surgeon's friend. There is no need to cause pain. Palpation guides the surgeon to the anatomic zone of most tenderness (usually the diseased area). It is best to start palpation in an area that does not hurt. Rectal (test stool for blood) and pelvic examinations localize pathology further.

13. **What is Kehr's sign?**
The diaphragm and the back of the left shoulder enjoy parallel innervation. Concurrent left upper quadrant and left shoulder pain indicate diaphragmatic irritation from a ruptured spleen or subdiaphragmatic abscess.

14. **What is a psoas sign?**
Irritation of the retroperitoneal psoas muscle by an inflamed retrocecal appendix causes pain on flexion of the right hip or extension of the thigh.

LABORATORY STUDIES

15. How is a complete blood count helpful?
1. **Hematocrit.** If the hematocrit is high (>45%), the patient is most likely dry or may have chronic obstructive pulmonary disease (COPD). If it is low (<30%), the patient probably has a more chronic disease (associated with blood loss; always do a rectal and test the stool for blood).
2. **White blood cell count.** It takes hours for inflammation to release cytokines and elevate the white blood cell count. A normal white blood cell count is entirely consistent with significant abdominal trouble.

16. Is urinalysis necessary?
Yes. White blood cells in the urine may redirect attention to the diagnosis of pyelonephritis or cystitis. Hematuria points to renal or ureteral stones. Because an inflamed appendix may lie directly on the right ureter, red and white blood cells may be found in the urine of patients with appendicitis.

17. What is a "three-way of the abdomen"?
1. **Upright chest radiograph:** Look for free air under the diaphragm (perforated viscus) and pneumonia or pneumothorax.
2. **Upright abdomen:** Look for free air under the diaphragm and air-fluid levels (intestinal obstruction). Remember to look for sigmoid or rectal air (partial obstruction).
3. **Supine abdomen:** This radiograph tells nothing.
Most ureteral stones can be visualized. Only 10% of gallstones are radiopaque, and appendiceal fecaliths are rarely noted.
Honors: Air in the biliary system indicates a biliary-enteric fistula; this in association with intestinal air-fluid levels makes the diagnosis of gallstone ileus.

KEY POINTS: RADIOGRAPHIC EVALUATION FOR THE ACUTE ABDOMEN

1. May assist in diagnostic evaluation but should not supplant physical examination in evaluation of an acute abdomen.
2. Three-way of the abdomen: look for free air under the diaphragm, intrathoracic pathology, air-fluid levels, dilated alimentary canal, and distal air in rectum.
3. Ultrasound: useful for biliary, ob-gyn, and vascular assessments; may note intraperitoneal or retroperitoneal fluid collections.
4. CT: increasing use in clinical arena, with excellent visualization of abdominal structures. Drawbacks: cost, radiation exposure.

18. What is a sentinel loop?
Except in children (who swallow everything, including air), small bowel gas is always pathologic. A single loop of small bowel gas adjacent to an inflamed organ (e.g., the pancreas) may point to the diseased organ.

19. Is ultrasound valuable?
Yes, if the working diagnosis is cholecystitis, gallstones, ectopic pregnancy, ovarian cyst, abdominal aortic aneurysm, or intraperitoneal/retroperitoneal fluid.

20. Is abdominal computed tomography valuable?
Yes, if the working diagnosis is an intraabdominal abscess (sigmoid diverticulitis), pancreatitis, retroperitoneal bleeding (leaking abdominal aortic aneurysm; this patient should have gone straight to the operating room), or intrahepatic or splenic pathology.

21. What is a double-contrast computed tomography scan?
The bowel is delineated with barium or Gastrografin. The blood vessels are delineated with an iodinated vascular dye. The CT scan precisely displays the abdominal contents relative to vascular and intestinal landmarks. Contrast CT of pancreatitis is valuable to assess zones of perfusion or necrosis.

SURGICAL TREATMENT

22. If the patient is sick (and not getting better), what should be done?
After fluid resuscitation, the patient's abdomen should be explored. An exploratory laparotomy has been touted as the logical conclusion of a complete physical examination.

23. Is a negative laparotomy harmful?
Yes, but patients can uncomfortably survive a negative laparotomy, whereas missed bowel infarction (or appendicitis) can be life-threatening.

24. Name the most challenging problem in all of medicine?
An acute abdomen.

WEBSITE

www.acssurgery.com/abstracts/acs/acs0301.htm

BIBLIOGRAPHY

1. D'Agostino J: Common abdominal emergencies in children. Emerg Med Clin N Am 20:139-153, 2002.
2. Dhillon S, Halligan S, Goh V et al.: The therapeutic impact of abdominal ultrasound in patients with acute abdominal symptoms. Clin Radiol 57:268-271, 2002.
3. Forster MJ, Akoh JA: Perforated appendicitis masquerading as acute pancreatitis in a morbidly obese patient. World J Gastroenterol 14:1795-1796, 2008.
4. Gajic O, Urrutia LE, Sewani H et al.: Acute abdomen in the medical intensive care unit. Crit Care Med 30:1187-1190, 2002.
5. Rozycki GS, Tremblay L, Feliciano DV et al.: Three hundred consecutive emergent celiotomies in general surgery patients: influence of advanced diagnostic imaging techniques and procedures on diagnosis, Ann Surg 235:681-689, 2002.

CHAPTER 13

SURGICAL INFECTIOUS DISEASE

Glenn W. Geelhoed, MD, MPH, MA, DTMH, ScD (Hon), MA, MPhil, EdD, FACS

1. **Have modern antibiotic developments controlled many, if not most, of the problems of surgical infection?**
   No. In seriously ill surgical patients in intensive care unit (ICU) settings, the problems of sepsis have increased and remain among the principal causes of death in ICU patients, especially those with multiple organ failure (MOF) and impairments of host defense. Antibiotic treatment may change the biographical sketch of the flora associated with patients' deaths but cannot overcome the multiple causes of failing host resistance to infection that accompany barrier breeches to microbial invasion and the inflammatory and immunologic responses to the "usual suspects."

2. **What kinds of barrier breech allow microbial invasion that may set up surgical site infection?**
   The skin and mucosal linings of the body maintain a barrier between the multifloral outside world and the sterile interior milieu of the tissues and organs (even when the outside world is a tube of heavily populated flora through the middle of usually sterile body cavities, such as the gastrointestinal [GI] tract). It is easy to see the barrier breech when a knife penetrates the skin, carrying exterior flora beneath the skin, or when that knife perforates and spills the contaminated contents of the gut into the abdomen. It is less obvious when the breech is caused by a low-flow state or when inadequate nutrition or toxins impair mucosal immunoglobulins, making the "bug-body barrier" permeable. These polymicrobial communities of organisms may begin to invade through the breech in such barriers, particularly if there are further failures in the third line of defense in humoral and cellular resistance.

3. **What is the difference between contamination and infection?**
   The presence of microorganisms does not an infection make!
   Resident communities of flora on body surfaces do little harm, and gut flora are even beneficial when contained in the gut. It is even possible for bacteria to be transiently present outside their usual commensal residences without constituting an infection in the normally intact host. For example, in vigorously brushing one's teeth, gram-negative bacteria of various kinds that are resident in the oral cavity are introduced into the bloodstream but probably quickly were eliminated by normal defense mechanisms, unless they met lowered host resistance or seeded a prosthetic heart valve.

4. **How can the enormous load of bacteria in the lower gastrointestinal tract be beneficial?**
   Bugs can be beautiful. These are the same bacteria that have lived with and in humans symbiotically for millennia. They synthesize vitamin K—something we literally cannot do without—or crowd out pathogenic organisms by their overwhelming numbers. They also help to metabolize bile salts and play a role in detoxifying some environmental hazards, similar to septic systems.

5. **Whenever intraabdominal bowel spillage is encountered, is it mandatory to culture the fecal contamination and obtain sensitivities of all identified organisms?**

No. There is a difference between contamination and infection. Therefore, cultures of fecal spillage into the peritoneum will not provide useful information. The contaminant, just because of its change in position with reference to the bowel wall, is not likely to be sterile. When would you like the laboratory to quit? Will you be content to hear a report of *Escherichia coli* and bacteroides, two of the more than 800 species that even the most compulsive laboratory can hardly be competent to identify, given the exposure to air and time lapse until processing on different media? How will information from a sampling error of mixed, community-acquired contaminants change your therapy? If, for instance, no anaerobes are identified from the fecal specimen, will you be so confident that they are not present as to exclude these species from coverage?

The lesson to be learned is that culture of community-acquired **contaminants** is expensive, incomplete, and unedifying; the culture of invading microbes in **infections,** particularly hospital-acquired microbes that persist after treatment, may give critical information and is a more appropriate use of microbiologic resources.

6. **What are preps (e.g., bowel preps)?**

Preps are decontamination procedures, designed to reduce resident flora before an elective invasive procedure. Preps may take the form of a simple process such as an alcohol swab smeared over the skin before a quick prick of the subcutaneous injection or may involve preparation of a larger area of the skin surface for the surgical field of incision (see question 7).

A bowel prep is similarly designed to reduce the resident flora in the gut through (1) mechanical catharsis (i.e., purge); (2) osmotic or volume dilution with large volumes of saline, other electrolyte solutions, or mannitol; or (3) oral administration of nonabsorbed antibiotics. Of these methods, the most important is clearly mechanical catharsis because it purges huge amounts of flora, which may account for up to two thirds the dry weight of colon contents. One of the most cogent reasons for the choice of certain oral antibiotics in bowel preps (see question 9) is their vigorous cathartic action.

7. **How is the skin or mucosal cavities of a patient sterilized to prepare a sterile field for operative incision?**

There is one way, hardly recommended, by which patients can be "sterilized"; similar to instruments and drapes, they can be placed in an autoclave. But short of this absurd example, the skin is never sterile. Decontamination processes are never perfect, particularly in so complex a tissue with crevices and accessory skin structures in which bacteria reside. Resting gloved hands on a "sterile field" does not include the skin or mucosal surfaces.

At best, we simply reduce the flora to the low-level inoculum that can be handled by most intact host defense systems—as in the example of brushing your teeth—but living tissue surfaces are never sterile. A method that kills all microbial organisms from such surfaces would also devitalize mammalian cells and render them more susceptible to lower-level microbial inocula.

8. **What means can be used to reduce surface resident flora without further injuring the skin or mucosa?**
   - **Volume lavage** (for mnemonic value only: dilution is the solution to pollution)
   - **Defatting,** which solubilizes the sebaceous oils that may trap flora
   - **Microbicidal killing** with a bacteriostatic agent

To an amazing extent, one cheap, simple fluid that may serve as a diluent, fat solvent, and antimicrobial is alcohol. Alcohol is nearly ideal as prepping solution, with the minor disadvantages that it is dehydrating and minimally flammable. Because it vaporizes and disappears, flora may spread from interstices, outside the field, or even via aerosolized fallout onto the field, thus requiring the addition of extended-duration bacteriostasis to the alcohol prep.

Iodine also kills bacteria but with a greater hazard to sensitive mammalian cells (it oxidizes the cell walls of small plants). A lower initial concentration of iodine and a longer duration of action can be achieved by incorporation of an iodophor, a substance in nearly universal use in preps. The application of moisture- and vapor-permeable "incise drapes" or desiccation-preventing "ring drapes" may further retard repopulation of flora over the prepped (but still not sterile) field.

9. **What are "pipe cleaner" antibiotics?**
Pipe cleaners are orally administered antibiotic regimens that reduce the flora in the GI tract, from which they are not well absorbed. They are an almost ideal component of bowel preps because they are potent cathartic agents and accomplish the vast majority of their "pipe cleaning" by mechanical purgative action. The most popular pipe cleaners include a neomycin or erythromycin base.

10. **What is selective gut decontamination? How does it work?**
It does not work. This method used pipe cleaners in patients at high risk for the development of sepsis from MOF with the theoretic aim of reducing the risk involved in barrier breech of the GI tract and inoculation with gut flora. Good experimental evidence indicated that this method should reduce the high mortality rate in seriously ill patients at high risk of surgical sepsis. After prolonged clinical trials, however, it failed to demonstrate a benefit in patient survival. The likely reason is that whereas the laboratory studies were done in intact animal models with functioning host defense systems, failures of defense beyond the barrier breech may explain why selective gut decontamination failed to benefit seriously ill patients. Furthermore, resident hospital flora repopulated the purged gut over time, but with virulent forms of microbes selected by their resistance to the broad-spectrum antibiotics. The method still has some use in patients undergoing procedures such as high-dose chemotherapy or bone marrow transplantation and in some patients isolated in "life islands" (e.g., patients with immunodeficiency diseases or burns).

ANTIBIOTICS

11. **Are antibiotics the classic wonder drugs?**
Only because you wonder if they are going to work, if they are going to cause more harm than good, and if the next generation will be unaffordable or toxic.

Skepticism is healthy with regard to any procedure or agent in heath care but especially with regard to antibiotics, which are embraced almost universally as agents that both prevent and cure infections. The primacy of the host defense in this vital process and the potential interference by the very drugs given credit for infection control are overlooked. We must look critically at the limited role that antibiotics should play in health care and restrain their overuse, which generates even more harm than unnecessary expense.

12. **What is meant by generations of antibiotics, as in third-generation cephalosporins?**
The earliest antibiotics were bacteriostatic, largely through interference in protein synthesis, so that they might keep a microorganism from reproducing even if they did not kill it. The difference between **infestation** (presence of living microbes in the host) and **infection**

(replication and spread of microorganisms in the host) may be useful in understanding how previous drugs possibly controlled infection but were less capable of eliminating organisms in any brief period of therapy.

Penicillin changed all that. It may be the first antibiotic with a legitimate claim to the title "wonder drug" because it has the microbicidal capability of eradicating sensitive organisms. Penicillin was the first generation of the beta-lactam antibiotics, joined by the congener first-generation cephalosporins (e.g., cefazolin). They shared beta-lactam structure and had good gram-positive coverage with less range in any effect over gram-negative microbes.

The second-generation beta-lactam antibiotics (e.g., cefoxitin) covered new classes of microbes beyond gram-positive aerobes, such as many of the *Bacteroides* species, but had little effect on gram-negative aerobic microbes. Because the third-generation cephalosporins covered some of the latter microbes, they were touted as single-agent therapy for all principal-risk floras.

As with penicillin, the original wonder drug, the wonderment waned with failures of the new agents because of rapidly induced antimicrobial resistance. The most easily measured and calculated difference in the generations is cost: wholesale values are about $2.00/g for the first generation, $5.00/g for the second, and $30.00/g for the third. Despite this bracket creep in cost, the higher generations lose some of their potency against the original gram-positive organisms for which the first-generation agents were truly wonderful. Therefore, it takes 2 g of moxalactam to be half as good as 1 g of cefazolin for gram-positive coverage. It does not take a pharmacoeconomist to ask, "What have I got in return for this sixtyfold surcharge?"

13. What is the role of third-generation cephalosporins in surgical prophylaxis?
None (no more wondering here!). If the principal-risk flora are gram-positive, the first generation is better; if the anaerobic risk is sizable, the second generation is better. And either class is cheaper by far and seems to have generated less resistance than the third-generation cephalosporins, which are unconscionably expensive for use in prophylaxis and rarely as effective as other single-agent therapy for established surgical site infection (SSI). Specific indications, such as pediatric meningitis, hospital-acquired pneumonia, or other specific infections outside the indications of surgical predominance, might use or exclude these agents.

14. How do enzyme inhibitors combined with antibiotics enhance their antimicrobial spectrum?
Microorganisms have defense mechanisms of their own, and the strains that have the capacity to make antibiotic-degrading enzymes achieve an unnatural selection advantage with the widespread use of antibiotics. This is what happened to penicillin: penicillinases emerged. But clever pharmaceutical manufacturers closed that loophole for bacterial ingenuity in degrading penicillin by strategic placement of a methyl group to ruin the survival fitness of penicillinase producers. Methicillin was the result, but the persistence of the microbes means that we now have a plague of methicillin-resistant *Staphylococcus aureus* (MRSA). Besides, microbes outnumber pharmaceutical manufacturers and have a shorter turnaround time than the approval process of the Food and Drug Administration (FDA). Microbes will always be ahead of us in ingenuity if only because of their numbers.

Newer strategies by the bacteria included the production of beta-lactamases. The response of the pharmaceutical industry was a group of inhibitors of beta-lactamase, such as clavulanic acid or sulbactam. The combination of a beta-lactamase inhibitor with a modified penicillin such as ampicillin should have enhanced activity against bacteria that produce beta-lactamase, provided that they were ampicillin sensitive in the first place. Higher doses of the original agent for a shorter time may accomplish the same effect, often at lower cost, because the combined drugs were developed much more recently and are under patent protection.

15. **What are the most expensive kinds of antibiotic therapy?**
    - Drugs that are given when they are not needed.
    - Drugs that are badly needed but do not work.
    - Drugs that cause more harm than good because of host toxicity, whatever their antibiotic potential.

16. **Can oral antibiotics be given in place of intravenous antibiotics in seriously ill surgical patients?**
    Yes, if only they could take them! These patients almost invariably can take nothing by mouth (NPO), are often unconscious, and are as likely as not to be on a ventilator. In addition, the gut has been put out of commission by nasogastric (NG) suction tubes, laparotomy, and ileus, and primary intraabdominal problems often associated with the need for the antibiotics, such as intraabdominal sepsis and pancreatitis. Usually such patients are on complete gut rest and are likely to be on parenteral nutrition as well.

    The attempt to use some form of gut-delivered antibiotic is based on the favorable pharmacokinetics and spectrum of quinolones, which can be started intravenously and switched as soon as possible to the oral form when feeding has resumed. Nearly all such patients begin on some form of intravenous (IV) antibiotic program and the start-up of the antibiotic regimen is more important than the form to which patients are tapered before treatment is discontinued.

PROPHYLAXIS

17. **Should systemic antibiotic prophylaxis be used in elective colon resection?**
    Yes, beyond any statistical shadow of a doubt. At least two dozen clinical trials have been carried out using placebo controls against a variety of antibiotics, principally those active against at least the anaerobic-predominant flora, and nearly all have shown a reduction in infectious complications in the antibiotic group. Never again should this point need repeating, and no patient should be placed at risk when systemic antibiotic prophylaxis has been established as the standard of care. No new clinical trials against placebo in this group of patients with known risk can be performed ethically given the confirmed risk reduction.

    Other risk groups (e.g., cesarean section after membrane rupture) besides patients undergoing colon resection have been standardized by trials in large patient populations and have shown similar risk reduction. The benefit of prophylaxis has been demonstrated. In other groups of patients that cannot be standardized because of unusual contamination factors or unique factors of host resistance impairment, guidelines for rational prophylaxis should follow similar principles.

18. **Are two prophylactic doses better than one in preventing infection? Are three doses better still?**
    Only one dose (the dose in systemic circulation at the time of the inoculum) of prophylactic antibiotic can be proved, beyond statistical or clinical doubt, to be efficacious. Whether the dose needs to be repeated one or more times during the 24 hours after the inoculum depends on the blood levels of the drug, which are largely a function of protein binding and clearance rate. We also know for sure that 10 days of the same prophylactic drug that is efficacious if given immediately before the inoculum results in a higher risk of infection than no antibiotic at all.

KEY POINTS: PREOPERATIVE ANTIBIOTIC PROPHYLAXIS

1. Timing of administration is the most important factor.

2. Dose 30 minutes before incision so that antibiotic is circulating before the inoculum.

3. No evidence supports continuation of prophylaxis beyond 24 hours.

19. **What factors determine the timing of antibiotic administration under the criteria of prophylaxis?**

The most important element in timing of prophylaxis is that the drug be circulating before the inoculum. When should it stop? When the reduction in infection risk is no longer provable and before continued use will defeat the prophylactic purpose (as explained previously). To summarize with an arbitrary rule of thumb: *There is no justification for prophylactic antibiotic 24 hours after the inoculum of an invasive procedure.*

What does this rule imply? Should we not continue prophylaxis for weeks to cover the presence of a prosthetic hip joint? Presumably, the prosthetic hip will be in the patient for many years; but surely you do not argue that the antibiotic should continue on a daily basis as long as the hip is in place! What is "prophylaxed" is not the prosthetic hip but the procedure of implantation. And it is not only implantation that poses a risk to the patient with a prosthesis, so does the hemorrhoidectomy done years later, for which prophylaxis is made mandatory by the presence of the hip prosthesis.

The prosthetic or rheumatic heart valve is a risk, but the indication for the use of prophylactic antibiotics is an invasive procedure; a root canal is an example in which an inoculum is unavoidable. *Operations* are covered by prophylactic antibiotics; the conditions that are risk factors during the operation are not.

20. **To be safe, why not administer prophylactic antibiotics to all patients undergoing any kind of operation?**

Can you give me the indication for a prophylactic antibiotic in a patient undergoing a clean elective surgical procedure that implants no prosthesis, such as hernia repair?

"Sure," one of my brighter students once responded, "the patient who has a serious impairment in host response, such as acute granulocytic leukemia in blast crisis."

I responded, "Why on earth are you fixing his hernia? That is a clean error (hopefully not a clean kill) in surgical judgment that has nothing to do with antibiotics at all. A patient with that degree of host impairment does not undergo an elective surgical procedure."

Rule of thumb: If you can provide the indication for a prophylactic antibiotic to cover a clean elective nonprosthetic operation for a patient, you have provided the contraindication for the operation.

MANAGEMENT OF SURGICAL SITE INFECTIONS

21. **What is the drug of choice for the treatment of an abscess?**

A knife. Surgically drain the abscess. Abscesses have no circulation of blood within them to deliver an antibiotic. The antibiotic, even if injected directly into the abscess, would be worthless because the abscess contains a soup of dead microorganisms and white blood cells (WBCs). Even if the organisms were barely alive, they would not be reproducing and incorporating the antibiotic. The drug most likely would not work at all at the acid-base balance (pH) and pKa conditions of the abscess environment.

If there is an indication for an antibiotic, it would be in the circulation around the compressed inflammatory edge of the abscess and the cellulitis (at the vascularized "peel of the orange") and uncontaminated tissue planes through which the necessary drainage must be carried out. A *focal* infection is managed by a *local* treatment, which is both *necessary* in all abscesses and *sufficient* treatment in many. Adjunctive systemic antibiotics are occasionally indicated for protection of the tissues through which drainage is carried out. If it helps to make this fundamental surgical principle clear, here is the rule of thumb for management of abscesses: *Where there is pus, let there be steel.* Perhaps one of the most gratifying procedures in all of medicine is the drainage of pus with immediate relief of local and systemic symptoms (e.g., a perirectal abscess).

22. Which abscess treatment is the important one in determining the outcome of a patient with intraabdominal sepsis?

It is the drainage of the *last* abscess that counts. There should be little applause for drainage of a pelvic abscess in the patient who retains a subphrenic abscess. The patient responds dramatically when the *last* pus is drained.

This has been an area of significant advance in managing surgical infections because noninvasive scanning capability has facilitated the finding of multiple pockets of pus. Furthermore, such modalities as the computed tomography (CT) scan not only *find* but also percutaneously *direct the fixing* of the last abscess. What might have been an indication for an exploratory return trip to the operating room only a decade before (i.e., a failing patient on appropriate therapy should trigger the first response, "Where's the pus?") is now a good indication for a CT scan to find and drain the focal infection.

23. Which is preferred for draining an intraabdominal abscess, a needle or a knife?

Which can be done most expeditiously? The patient with intraabdominal sepsis is quite ill, and the earliest, safe drainage is the procedure of choice. There may be advantages to the less invasive CT scanning, which can be repeated and has less morbidity if the results are negative. Surgery, on the other hand, can fix associated conditions that may have caused the abscess, such as the devitalized loop of bowel or the leak in the anastomosis that can be exteriorized. Each method is likely to find multiple collections, and each can leave external drains for lavage and continuing drainage. Whether by needle or by knife, the urgency and adequacy of local treatment of focal infection determine which methods takes precedence.

24. What is the role of gallium scintiscanning in early finding of abscesses in the abdomen?

There is none. Ordering a gallium scan is a temporizing means of self-deception that some progress is being made in finding out what is wrong with the patient. In fact, it merely postpones decisions about intervention in critical illness for several days, often to a point beyond salvage. Gallium scanning involves bowel prepping, a vigorous WBC response from an active bone marrow, and false-positive test results at the sites of tubes and incisions. It is a time-consuming and unreliable test that is the obverse of the principles of *early* and *definitive* management. Do not order a gallium scan to satisfy a consultant that "something is being done for this patient."

EXTRA CREDIT QUESTIONS

25. Should all patients undergoing elective laparotomy receive prophylactic antibiotic coverage?

No. Doing so would contribute to driving up the cost of antibiotics and their complication rate and devaluing formerly good drugs by rendering them useless against common flora against which they were once highly potent. Operating room nurses have always classified the kind of operation by its status with respect to microbial exposure: clean, contaminated, or septic. These categories are approximation of the microbial risk exposure, and if additionally are superimposed categories of patient resistance (higher risk associated with aging, obesity or other malnutrition, concomitant drugs, or viral or mycobacterial or neoplastic disease immune compromise), these same strata are called class I, II, and III.

26. Which abscess is the most important one to be drained?

It is the *last* abscess that counts in drainage because the patient's dramatic response is often only achieved when the last pus is drained. Draining a pelvic abscess, for example, but leaving behind a subphrenic abscess, would not result in the quenching of the inflammatory mediators of the sepsis syndrome.

27. Is postoperative fever the earliest and most frequent sign of an incisional infection?

Postoperative fevers are much more frequent than are wound infections, and the typical wound infection presents far later. The principal sources of postoperative fever are:

Wind (atelectasis or pneumonia)
Water (urinary tract infection)
Walk (get your patient up and around; thrombophlebitis)
Wound

28. Should you begin amphotericin at the first isolation of *Candida* species drawn from any intravenous catheter line?

No. Again, remember the distinction between colonization and infection, and the source from which the specimen is taken. The IV lines through which hyperalimentation solutions are infused make colonization possible. The presence of a fungus such as *Candida* species is frequent in patients who do not have an invasive fungal infection or a true candidemia. The latter might be distinguished from catheter colonization by a blood culture drawn from another source, such as a venopuncture. If evidence of any invasive fungal infection is also present (e.g., as endoscopic biopsy of inflammatory mucositis), a choice of antifungal therapies is now indicated.

Topical fungal solutions (e.g., mycostatin mouthwashes or lavage) may control the local fungal infection and may sometimes be instituted as prophylaxis in high-risk patients (e.g., patients on antirejection therapy for bone marrow or solid organ transplantation).

Systemic antifungal agents include fluconazole, caspifungin, and amphotericin.

29. Are antibiotic drug combinations always superior to a single antibiotic agent?

Monotherapy is superior to combination antibiotic treatment regimens, but this is provable probably only in the highest-risk patients. With the carbapenem class antibiotic agents, a large multicenter clinical trial proved imipenem therapy superior to aminoglycoside and a macrolide antibiotic, with survival demonstrably superior only in the patients with the highest acute physiology and chronic health evaluation (APACHE) scores. Ertapenem monotherapy was the equivalent of ceftriaxone and metronidazole in a smaller, more recent trial.

More is not always better, and the *R* and *S* on culture reports do not translate directly to the *M* and *M* (morbidity and mortality) at the Death and Complications Conference reports. It is not just important that the effective antibiotic regimen kills the bacteria; also important are *how* this microbicidal effect is carried out, and what effect it may have on the patient in quenching or prolonging the systemic inflammatory response.

30. Is antibody treatment of circulating endotoxin a clinically important tool?

Not yet. The neutralization of circulating endotoxin might give a theoretic benefit to patients with sepsis, and animal studies looked promising. But antigen/antibody complexes initiate complement cascade and release of activate leukocyte products such as leukotrienes that may further augment the inflammatory process. The complexes are also filtered in the kidney where they may further impair renal function. To date, no clinical therapeutic benefit has been demonstrated for such monoclonal antibody therapy.

31. **What is the role of human recombinant activated protein C in patients with sepsis?**
Of the multiple clinical trials of mediator neutralization or receptor blockade, the evidence to date seems marginally favorable only for a few, and the major response to treatment comes from early and complete control of the focus of sepsis (not the cytokine sequelae).

WEBSITES

www.acssurgery.com/abstracts/acs/acs0102.htm

www.medscape.com

Search: preoperative antibiotics

BIBLIOGRAPHY

1. Bartlett JG: Intra-abdominal sepsis. Med Clin North Am 79:599-617, 1995.

2. Bernard GR, Vincent JL, Laterre PF et al.: Efficacy and safety of recombinant human activated protein C for severe sepsis. N Engl J Med 344:699, 2001.

3. Bilik R, Burnweit C, Shandling B: Is abdominal cavity culture of any value in appendicitis? Am J Surg 175:267-270, 1998.

4. Castaldo ET, Yang EY: Severe sepsis attributable to community-associated methicillin-resistant *Staphylococcus aureus*: an emerging fatal problem. Am Surg 73:684-687; discussion 687-688, 2007.

5. Christou NV, Turgeon P, Wassef R et al.: Management of intra-abdominal infections. The case for intraoperative cultures and comprehensive broad-spectrum antibiotic coverage. The Canadian Intra-abdominal Infection Study Group. Arch Surg 131:1193-1201, 1996.

6. Ciftci AO, Tanyei FC, Buyukpamukcu N et al.: Comparative trial of four antibiotic combinations for perforated appendicitis in children. Eur J Surg 163:591-596, 1997.

7. Falagas ME, Barefoot L, Griffith J et al.: Risk factors leading to clinical failure in the treatment of intra-abdominal or skin/soft tissue infections. Eur J Clin Microbiol Infect Dis 15:913-921, 1996.

8. Geelhoed GW: Preoperative skin preparation: evaluation of efficacy, timing, convenience, and cost. Infect Surg 85:648-669, 1985.

CHAPTER 14

RISKS OF BLOOD-BORNE DISEASE

Natasha D. Bir, MD, MHS

1. **What infectious diseases are transmissible via blood transfusion?**

   Viruses, parasites, and bacteria and the diseases they transmit have all been found in donated blood. Donor screening and testing have dramatically decreased the risk of transfusion-related infections in the developed world; however, infection remains a significant risk in less-developed countries, where over 10 million units of blood are not screened for HIV or the hepatitides. The most common transmitted diseases in developed nations include hepatitis B virus (HBV) and hepatitis C virus (HCV); human immunodeficiency virus (HIV) and cytomegalovirus (CMV) transmission are far less common. Parasites such as malaria *(Plasmodium)*, Chagas' disease *(Trypanosoma cruzii)*, toxoplasmosis *(Toxoplasma gondii)*, and babesiosis *(Babseium)*, are only a problem where these diseases are endemic. Lymphomas and leukemias can be caused by human T-cell lymphotropic virus (HTLV-1), and infectious mononucleosis by Epstein-Barr virus (EBV). Bacterial contamination of blood products occurs most often in platelets, which are stored at room temperature. Bacterial contamination can result in sepsis or a toxic shocklike syndrome.

2. **What are the estimated risks of HBV, HCV, and HIV transmission by blood transfusion in the United States?**

   Rates of viral disease transmission are lower than ever, particularly after nucleic acid testing for HIV, HBV, and HCV began in 1999. At present time, mathematical models are employed to estimate risks of viral transmission.

Disease	Frequency per Million Units of Blood	Risk of Disease per Actual Unit Transfused
HBV	17	1/60,000 to 1/200,000
HCV	1	1/800,000 to 1/1,600,000
HIV	1	1/1,400,000 to 1/2,400,000
Bacterial transmission; packed red blood cells	2	1/500,000
Bacterial transmission; platelets	500	1/2,000

3. **Which blood-borne pathogens pose a risk to surgeons?**

   More than 8 million healthcare workers are exposed to blood or other body fluids annually. Eighty-two percent are exposed through percutaneous injury such as needlesticks, and another 14% through contact with the mucosal membranes of the eyes, mouth, or nose. HIV, HBV, and HCV are diseases of concern to surgeons because of the morbidity and mortality associated with these diseases. As of 2003 (the most recent data available in 2008) only 57 confirmed cases of healthcare-worker HIV infection by patients have been reported, including six physicians (all non-surgeons). In all cases, the inciting injury involved significant cuts or penetration with large-bore hollow needles. Solid needlesticks have never resulted in HIV transmission. HIV transmission between patient and surgeon in the operating room has never been documented in the United States.

HBV infection of surgeons has declined with the widespread use of the HBV vaccine (see below). A hollow needlestick can result in HBV transmission in as many as 30% of cases.

The risk of HCV in the operating room remains significant because there is no available vaccine and the number of chronically infected patients numbers more than 4 million. After exposure, the rate of seroconversion to HCV is approximately 10%. Fifty to eighty percent of seroconverters develop a persistent chronic HCV infection, and 20% of these advance to hepatic cirrhosis. Given the lack of cure and potentially devastating consequences of this disease, HCV infection is the greatest threat to surgeons.

4. What is the risk to healthcare workers of exposure to hepatitis B virus?
In the United States, there are 2 million people with HBV—approximately 100,000 new cases each year. The highest prevalence is in individuals aged 20 to 49 years. Thirty percent of acute HBV cases are clinically occult, and 10% remain chronic carriers for life. About 25 percent of people with chronic HBV eventually die of hepatic disease. Among healthcare workers, vaccination and the adoption of universal precautions led to a sharp decline in new HBV infections–from 12,000 cases in 1985 to approximately 1,000 in 1994. However, two-hundred fifty healthcare workers die from chronic HBV every year.

5. What is the risk to healthcare workers of exposure to hepatitis C virus (HCV)?
HCV is transmitted via blood, and patients at higher risk include injection drug users, patients who received a blood transfusion before 1999, hemophiliacs, patients on hemodialysis, and healthcare workers. Acute HCV infection is asymptomatic in 70% of cases. Sixty percent of acute HCV infections result in chronic, persistent infection. Although these data are still controversial, 50% of patients infected with HCV will develop cirrhosis, and half of them will go on to develop a hepatoma. Approximately 10% of needlesticks result in acute HCV infection.

6. What is the risk to healthcare workers of exposure to HIV?
Among healthcare workers only 57 confirmed cases and 139 "possible" cases (unconfirmed as a result of poor documentation) of HIV transmission have occurred since 1983. The majority of confirmed cases were nurses (n=24), while six were physicians. None were surgeons. Eighty-four percent of the cases suffered percutaneous routes of transmission—that is, cuts or punctures. The risk of seroconversion to HIV after a percutaneous exposure is 0.3%. There have been no documented cases of transmission from a patient who is HIV positive to a surgeon.

7. How well does hepatitis B vaccination protect against the disease?
Ninety percent of individuals who complete the three-dose immunization series for HBV develop anti-HBV surface antibody (anti-HBs) titres of $\geq$ 10 mIU/ml. An additional 8% display appropriate titre levels after additional doses. An anti-HBs level of 10 or more mIU/ml confers a protective efficacy of nearly 100%. While about half of successfully vaccinated adults demonstrate a decreased or non-detectable titre level within 10 years, a lifelong "immune memory" to the viral antigen persists and people do not require booster doses.

A bivalent vaccine immunizing against both hepatitis A and B was approved in 2001 by the U.S. Food and Drug Administration (FDA) for individuals 18 years of age and older, and it is as successful as the monovalent vaccine in conferring protection against HBV infection with the added benefit of protecting against hepatitis A viral infection. There are also two brands of monovalent recombinant DNA vaccines available.

8. **Are patients at risk of infection from surgeons who are infected with HBV?**

   Some cases of surgeon-to-patient transmission of HBV have been documented. Those
   with the highest chance of transmitting disease to patients are positive for the e-antigen
   of hepatitis B, a degradation product of the viral nucleocapsid that represents active
   replication in the liver. E-antigen positive people generally exhibit a high viral load.
   However, transmission of disease has been documented even when a surgeon was negative
   for e-antigen.

9. **What is the proper response after percutaneous exposure to a patient with
   known hepatitis B?**

   For practitioners who have been immunized and ever demonstrated positive titres, no additional
   response is necessary. Some people's titre levels may decline with time so titre levels at the time
   of exposure is not indicated. People who were immunized or who had a weak or incomplete
   response to vaccine should receive a dose of hepatitis B immunoglobulin and then begin the
   vaccination series anew.

10. **What are the recommendations for hepatitis B immunization?**

    Vaccination against hepatitis B is required for surgical trainees and strongly encouraged for all
    healthcare workers. The recommendations of the United States Public Health Service are
    that all healthcare workers who perform tasks the may involve exposure to blood or body
    fluids should receive a 3-dose series of hepatitis B vaccine at 0-, 1- and 6-month intervals.
    They should then be tested for hepatitis B surface antibody (anti-BHs) 1 to 2 after vaccination,
    to document immunity. If the anti-BHs is at least 10 mIU/ml then the patient is immune.
    If less than 10 mIU/ml, the patient remains unprotected; another 3-dose series of vaccination
    should be given and titres should be rechecked 1 to 2 months. If titres are adequate, the
    patient is immune. If still less than 10 mIU/ml, the patient is deemed a non-responder.
    They should be considered susceptible to HBV and should maintain strict precautions and
    obtain hepatitis B immunoglobulin for any known or probable exposure.

11. **What are the recommendations for hepatitis C immunization?**

    There are none.

    The only effective protection against HCV is the rigorous use of universal precautions to
    prevent exposure to infected body fluids. There is no effective vaccine, and immunoglobulin
    does not confer protection.

12. **Does laparoscopic surgery minimize the risk of HIV contamination?**

    Laparoscopic technique reduces exposure to blood and sharp instruments. However, discharge
    of pneumoperitoneum can release aerosolized blood and peritoneal fluid into the operating
    room if not evacuated into a closed system.

13. **Is double gloving an effective method of protection?**

    Yes, the contact rates between blood and skin decrease by 70% with the addition of a
    second pair of gloves. The nondominant index finger is the most common target.

14. **Are non-percutaneous exposures (eye splash) a major threat to surgeons?**

    According to the Centers for Disease Control and Prevention (CDC), the risk of seroconversion
    after mucocutaneous exposure (eyes, nose, or mouth) is 0.1%, or about 1 in 1000.
    Mucocutaneous contact is responsible for 13% of documented HIV transmissions. Among
    surgeons, eye splash injuries are often overlooked as a major risk for disease transmission. One
    study of surgical procedures examined the eye shields of 160 surgeons and assistants. All
    operations were 30 minutes or greater. Although the surgeons were aware of spray in only 8%
    of cases, blood splashes were macroscopically visible in 16% of cases, and microscopically
    positive in 44% of cases. Eye protection is important.

15. What is the surgeons' rate of exposure to blood and body fluids?

Exposure is widely underreported but percutaneous exposure occurs in an estimated 1% to 6% of operative procedures and mucocutaneous exposure in up to 50% of surgical cases. No healthcare worker has even been infected by exposure through intact skin.

16. Again, what are the seroconversion rates for HIV, HBV, and HCV exposure?

Seroconversion rates from a hollow needlestick are 0.3% for HIV, 10% for HCV, and range between 6% and 30% for HBV.

17. Are there effective methods to reduce the risk of transmission of blood-borne diseases to surgeons?

Obviously, the most effective way to reduce disease transmission is to limit exposure to infected blood or body fluid (universal barrier precautions). For HBV, postexposure immunoglobulin administration reduces infection. A highly effective vaccine exists and is required for most healthcare workers. Surprisingly, most surgeons over 50 have not been vaccinated.

18. What is the risk to surgeons in training?

A recent multicenter survey of surgeons in training noted that needlesticks are frequent and often go unreported. Number of needlesticks increased with each year in training (postgraduate year (PGY)-2, 3.7; PGY-3, 4.1; PGY-4, 5.3; and PGY-5, 7.7), and by their final year of training, 99% of residents had at least one needlestick. About half of residents had been exposed to blood from high-risk patients (patients with a history of HIV, HBV, HCV, or injection drug use). The most common reason for not reporting a needlestick was "lack of time."

BIBLIOGRAPHY

1. Barrie PS, Patchen Dellinger E, Dougherty SH et al.: Assessment of hepatitis B virus immunization status among North American surgeons. Arch Surg 129:27-32, 1994.

2. Bell DM: Occupational risk of human immunodeficiency virus infection in healthcare workers: an overview. Am J Med 102(suppl 5B):81S-85S, 1997.

3. Dodd RY, Notari EP, Stramer SL: Current prevalence and incidence of infectious disease markers and estimated window-period risk in the American Red Cross blood donor population. Transfusion 42:975-979, 2002.

4. Eubanks S, Newman L, Lucas G: Reduction of HIV transmission during laparoscopic procedures. Surg Laparosc Endosc 3:2-5, 1993.

5. Fry DE: Occupational blood-borne diseases in surgery. Am J Surg 190(2):249-254, 2005.

6. Gershon RR, Sherman M, Mitchell C et al.: Prevalence and risk factors for bloodborne exposure and infection in correctional healthcare workers. Infect Control Hosp Epidemiol 28(1):24-30, 2007.

7. Goodnough, LT: Risks of blood transfusion, Anes Clin N Am 23:241-252, 2005.

8. Jaffray CE, Flint LM: Blood-borne viral diseases and the surgeon. Curr Probl Surg 40(4):195-251, 2003.

9. Klein HG, Spahn DR, Carson JL: Red blood cell transfusion in clinical practice. Lancet 370(9585):415-426, 2007.

10. Koff RS: Hepatitis A, hepatitis B, and combination hepatitis vaccines for immunoprophylaxis: an update. Digest Dis Sci 47:1183-1194, 2002.

11. Makary MA, Al-Attar A, Holzmueller CG et al.: Needlestick injuries among surgeons in training. N Engl J Med 356(26):2693-2699, 2007.

12. Marasco S, Woods S: The risk of eye splash injuries in surgery. Aust N Z J Surg 68:785-787, 1998.

13. Mast EE, Weinbaum CM, Fiore AE et al.: A comprehensive immunization strategy to eliminate transmission of hepatitis B virus infection in the United States: recommendations of the Advisory Committee on Immunization Practices (ACIP) Part II: immunization of adults. MMWR Recomm Rep 55(RR-16):1-33, 2006.

14. Weiss ES, Makary MA, Wang T et al.: Prevalence of blood-borne pathogens in an urban, university-based general surgical practice. Ann Surg 241(5):803-807; discussion 807-809, 2005.

INITIAL ASSESSMENT

Jeffry L. Kashuk, MD, FACS

CHAPTER 15

1. **What is the "golden hour"?**
   This first hour of injury provides a unique opportunity to initiate life-saving interventions. More than half of trauma deaths occur during this time period as a result of brain injury or exsanguinating hemorrhage, therefore, rapid transport, appropriate triage, and organized systems of assessment (advanced trauma life support [ATLS]) are important standardized procedures that can save lives.

2. **Name the major components of the initial assessment of the trauma patient.**
   Primary survey, resuscitation, secondary survey, reevaluation, and definitive care.

3. **What is the purpose of the primary survey?**
   To identify life threatening injuries via a reproducible prioritized system and time frame.

4. **Define the ABCDE mnemonic of the primary survey that reinforces the fact that life-threatening injuries kill in a predicable order.**
   Airway control with cervical spine protection
   Breathing with oxygenation and ventilation
   Circulation with hemorrhage control
   Disability or neurologic status
   Exposure of patient with temperature control

5. **What are the adjuncts to the primary survey?**
   All trauma patients should initially receive high-flow supplemental oxygen by nasal cannula or face mask. Continuous monitoring should include pulse oximetry, cardiac electrocardiogram (ECG) monitor, and a cycled blood pressure (BP) cuff. Two large-bore intravenous (IV) lines are placed as blood is drawn for screening tests, including blood type and cross-match. Nasogastric (NG) or orogastric tubes are placed for gastric decompression and to prevent aspiration. A Foley catheter is inserted to assess urine flow and character of urine. Radiographs should include the "big three" for major trauma "mechanism": cervical spine, chest x-ray, and pelvic x-ray. Cervical spine x-ray may be deferred if the patient is going to computed tomography (CT) scan.

6. **Identify the one concept that can prevent unexpected acute deterioration of the trauma patient during initial assessment.**
   Reevaluation: If deterioration occurs, proceed back to the ABCs in sequential order.

7. **Name the two major causes of death during the first 24 hours after injury.**
   Exsanguination secondary to bleeding from traumatic wounds, and central nervous system (CNS) injury.

8. How is the airway assessed?

Ask the patient a question. A response in a normal voice suggests that the airway is not in immediate danger. A horse, weak, or stridorous response may imply airway compromise. An agitated or combative response indicates hypoxia, until proven otherwise. No response indicates the need for a "definitive airway" (ideally, a cuffed tube in the trachea).

9. What are the causes of upper airway obstruction in the trauma patient?

The tongue, followed by blood, loose teeth or dentures, vomit, and soft tissue edema.

10. What are the initial maneuvers used to restore an open airway?

The chin lift and jaw thrust physically displace the mandible and the tongue anteriorly to open the airway, which will facilitate manual clearance of debris and suctioning of the oropharynx to optimize patency. Oropharyngeal and nasopharyngeal airways (trumpets) are useful adjuncts in maintaining an open airway in an obtunded patient. One should always assume the presence of a cervical spine injury until proven otherwise, performing in-line stabilization while evaluating the airway.

11. What are the indications for a definitive airway?

Apnea, inability to maintain or protect the airway (compromised consciousness), inability to maintain oxygenation, hemodynamic instability, need for muscle relaxation or sedation, and need for hyperventilation.

12. List the types of definitive airway that are available in their order of priority.

- Orotracheal intubation.
- Nasotracheal intubation.
- Surgical airway (cricothyroidotomy or tracheostomy).

13. What are the indications for a surgical airway?

Extensive maxillofacial and trauma, high-risk anterior neck trauma, or any situation in which airway intubation cannot be accomplished safely.

Contraindications include: direct laryngeal trauma, suspected tracheal disruption, and children, who have a greatly increased risk of stenosis in this region after the procedure. Preferred options in this group are tracheostomy and transtracheal ventilation.

14. How does one "clear the C-spine"?

Injury must be excluded before moving the head or neck of a trauma patient. Alert patients without other significant "distracting injuries" may be cleared if they are asymptomatic and have no tenderness on exam by direct palpation. Other patients require radiologic evaluation. Most bony injuries may be found with definitive CT scan of the neck, reserving magnetic resonance imaging (MRI) evaluation for suspected soft tissue ligamentous injury that can cause instability. In the absence of CT scan capability, a three-view cervical spine series (anteroposterior [AP], lateral, and odontoid) are required, with visualization to the level of C7-T1. This level is frequently difficult to view, requiring a "swimmers view" to accentuate the visualization of this anatomic region.

15. What are the five non-airway conditions that pose an immediate threat to breathing in the trauma patient?

Tension pneumothorax: air in the pleural space under pressure that obstructs the venous outflow by kinking the vena cava, treated with urgent decompression with needle or tube thoracostomy.

Open pneumothorax: an open wound of the chest wall casing free communication of the pleural space with the air interfering with the thoracic bellows mechanism treated with tube thoracostomy.

Flail chest: multiple rib fractures with a free-floating segment and potential underlying pulmonary contusion, treated with tube thoracostomy and frequently endotracheal intubation.

Massive hemothorax: a large collection of blood in the pleural space that limits lung ventilation and oxygenation treated with tube thoracostomy and possible thoracotomy.

Pericardial tamponade: inhibition of diastolic filling and associated cardiac output (CO)—the major cause of cardiogenic shock in trauma—requires evacuation of the tamponade initially by aspiration if possible, and subsequent emergency thoracotomy with correction of the underlying injury.

16. **What are the preferred sites of emergent intravenous access?**

Peripheral venous access in the upper extremities with large bore (14- to 16-gauge) catheter. Other options include ankle or groin saphenous vein. Central venous access (subclavian or jugular routes) is indicated for measurement of central venous pressure (CVP) after the initial fluid boluses to assess hemodynamic instability. In children <6 years, the interosseous route at the distal femur or proximal tibia is an effective alternative.

17. **What are common, simple measures of assessing hemodynamic stability in a trauma patient?**

Mental status (**a**lert, **v**erbal, **p**ain, or **u**nresponsive).

Skin perfusion (pink/warm versus pale/cool).

Hemodynamic parameters (BP, heart rate [HR], and respiratory rate [RR]).

Gross estimates of systolic blood pressures: radial pulse: >80 mm Hg; femoral: >70 mm Hg; carotid: >60 mm Hg. Urine flow of >½ milliliters per kilogram per hour suggests good end organ perfusion.

18. **What is the Glasgow Coma Scale and what does it measure?**

The Glasgow Coma Scale (GCS) is an assessment of mental status, papillary status, and best motor activity.

Best eye-opening response, scored 1 to 4

Best verbal response, scored 1 to 5

Best motor response, scored 1 to 6

Points are added up. An overall score of 13 to 15 indicates a mild head injury, 9 to 12 indicates moderate injury, and <8 indicates a severe injury and mandates endotracheal intubation.

19. **What fluids should be used for initial resuscitation?**

Lactated Ringer's or normal saline are the mainstay of fluid resuscitation via rapid infusion. Early blood and plasma should be administered to optimize oxygen carrying capacity and prevent progressive coagulopathy in patients who present with signs of acidosis (pH <7.25), hypothermia (temperature <34° C), coagulopathy (international normalized ratio [INR] >1.5) in the face of severe shock (systolic BP <70 mm Hg).

Colloid infusions are more expensive and have no proven advantage in the trauma setting.

20. **What does FAST mean, and how does it help in trauma evaluation?**

FAST stands for focused abdominal sonography in trauma. The four areas examined by ultrasound include the pericardial area, right upper quadrant, left upper quadrant, and the pelvis. The test is reported as positive (blood) or negative.

21. **What is DPL, and does it have a role in trauma evaluation?**

DPL stands for diagnostic peritoneal lavage, in which a small catheter is inserted into the patient to assess for intraperitoneal bleeding. Its chief usefulness in the era of FAST and CT scan is in the hemodynamically unstable patient whose initial FAST is negative to better rule out the abdomen as a source of hemorrhage.

22. How can I learn proficiency at initial assessment?

Take the ATLS course of the American College of Surgeons, which emphasizes the skills necessary to initially treat the trauma patient.

KEY POINTS OF INITIAL ASSESSMENT

1. Follow the ABCDEs of the ATLS system when evaluating a trauma patient, and return to the same sequential order when reevaluating the patient.

2. Assume every trauma patient has a cervical spine injury until proven otherwise, and carefully assess methods to evaluate or clear the cervical spine.

3. Establish a secure airway based on the injury pattern present, or the neurological status of the patient (GCS).

4. Evaluate for presence of shock and initiate fluid, blood, or plasma resuscitation based on the level of shock and associated signs of coagulopathy, hypothermia, and acidosis via large-bore peripheral IV infusions.

5. Establish central venous catheterization to help assess homodynamic stability.

6. Use FAST, DPL, and CT scan to evaluate the extent of injuries and triage the patient appropriately.

BIBLIOGRAPHY

1. American College of Surgeons Committee on Trauma: Advanced Trauma Life Support Course 7th ed., Chicago, 2004, American College of Surgeons.
2. Cha J, Kashuk JL, Moore EE: Diagnostic peritoneal lavage remains a valuable adjunct to modern imaging techniques. J Trauma, in press.
3. Cothren CC, Moore EE: Emergency department thoracotomy In: Trauma, 6th ed., New York, 2008, McGraw Hill.
4. Fisher A, Young WF: Is the lateral cervical spine x-ray obsolete during the initial evaluation of patients with acute trauma? Surg Neurol 70(1):25-28, 2008.
5. Kashuk JL, Moore EE, Johnson JL et al.: Post-surgery life threatening coagulopathy: is 1:1 FFP: RBC the answer? J Trauma 66:xx, 2008.
6. Kaufmann CR: Initial assessment and management. In Trauma, 6th ed., New York, 2008, McGraw-Hill.
7. Rabb CH, Johnson JL, VanSickle D et al.: Are upright lateral cervical radiographs in the obtunded trauma patient useful? A retrospective study, World J Emerg Surg 2:4, 2007.
8. Sanchez B, Waxman K, Jones T et al.: Cervical spine clearance in blunt trauma: evaluation of a computed tomography-based protocol. J Trauma 59:179, 2005.

CHAPTER 16

POSTTRAUMATIC HEMORRHAGIC SHOCK

Ryan P. Merkow, MD, and Ernest E. Moore, MD

1. Are hemorrhagic shock and hypovolemic shock the same?
Yes.

2. What is hemorrhagic shock?
Shock exists when the cardiovascular system is no longer able to meet the body's metabolic and oxygen needs resulting in cellular injury. In other words, the tissues are not adequately perfused to meet their oxygen and nutrient requirements.

3. What is the initial management of hemorrhagic or hypovolemic shock?
Prompt and aggressive fluid resuscitation in attempt to restore circulating blood volume. Hemorrhage is the most common cause of shock in the injured patient. Depletion of the blood volume results in a decreased driving pressure returning blood to the heart, a decreased end-diastolic ventricular volume, and a decreased stroke volume; resulting in a decreased cardiac output (CO).

4. Describe the cellular manifestations of hemorrhagic shock.
The inadequate tissue perfusion results in decreased cellular oxygen tension and disruption of normal oxidative phosphorylation with a decrease in the generation of adenosine triphosphate (ATP). The Na+ K+ ATPase slows, and the cell can no longer maintain membrane polarization integrity impairing a number of important cellular processes. Anaerobic metabolism ensues resulting in the production of lactic acid, creating a "gap" metabolic acidosis. The first evidence of this dysfunction is swelling of the endoplasmic reticulum, followed by mitochondrial damage, lysozyme rupture, and entry of interstitial water into the cell as intracellular sodium (Na+) accumulates. This loss of extracellular water exacerbates the intravascular volume deficit.

5. List the clinical manifestations of hemorrhagic shock.
- Heart rate (HR) >100 beats per minute and blood pressure (BP) <90 mm Hg.
- Altered mental status with lethargy and confusion.
- Decrease in urine output <0.5 milliliters per kilogram per hour and low central venous pressure (CVP).

6. How can blood volume be estimated in adults and children?
In adults and children, the average blood volume represents 7% and 9% of ideal body weight, respectively. Therefore, in adults multiply the ideal weight in kg × 7% (70 ml/kg). In children, multiply ideal weight in kg × 9% (90 ml/kg).

7. State the first physiologic response to hypovolemia.
The patient tries to compensate for the decrease in stroke volume by increasing HR (tachycardia).

8. What are the skin manifestations?
The skin becomes cool, clammy, and pale. The subcutaneous veins collapse (making it hard to start an intravenous [IV] line). Capillary refill is delayed 2 to 3 seconds. This results from the body's attempt to redistribute oxygen delivery to vital organs.

9. **Can the neck veins tell you anything?**

Lack of pulsations or collapsed external jugular veins indicate low right-sided heart filling pressure (i.e., hypovolemia); conversely, distended veins indicate heart failure or cardiogenic shock, including pericardial tamponade.

10. **Is the hematocrit a reliable guide for estimating acute blood loss?**

No. A decrease in the hematocrit occurs with refill of the intravascular space from the interstitial space or during administration of exogenous crystalloid resuscitation fluid. However, this process is not immediate, and serial hematocrits are more helpful to assess blood loss.

11. **What is the appropriate choice for intravenous solution during resuscitation?**

Lactated Ringer's or normal saline. Isotonic crystalloid fluid requirements in hemorrhagic shock are estimated at 3 times the blood loss (3:1 rule). The initial volume replacement should be directed by the response to therapy rather than relying on estimated blood loss. Do *not* add dextrose to the initial fluids; this exacerbates the physiologic hyperglycemia and provokes an osmotic diuresis. Dextrose 5% is added to IV solutions after initial resuscitation for its protein-sparing effect in the fasting trauma patient.

12. **What is base deficit, and how is it useful during resuscitation?**

The base deficit reflects the degree of metabolic acidosis in blood and is used in hemorrhagic shock as a surrogate marker of tissue hypoxia. The worse the base deficit (the more positive it is), the worse (less adequate) the patients peripheral perfusion. Base deficit depends on the hematocrit, acid-base balance (pH), and partial pressure of carbon dioxide (pCO_2); if you correct the pCO_2 back to 40 mm Hg, the pH should be 7.40. If your patient is still acidotic, they have a base deficit.

13. **What are the clinical classifications of shock and the associated clinical manifestations?**

See Table 16-1. These are estimates and not nearly as accurate or valuable as determining your patient's response to therapy or resuscitation.

TABLE 16-1. CLINICAL CLASSIFICATIONS OF SHOCK		
Class	**Description**	**Clinical Manifestations**
Class 1	Blood volume loss = 15% Can compare this with a blood donor	Mild tachycardia, headache, and postural dizziness
Class 2	Blood volume loss = 30%	Moderate tachycardia, tachypnea, and decreased pulse pressure
Class 3	Blood volume loss = 40%	Marked tachycardia, tachypnea, decreased mental status, hypotension, and decreased urine output
Class 4	Blood volume loss >40%	Marked tachycardia, marked tachypnea, decreased systolic blood pressure, obtundation to unconscious mental status, and no urine output

14. **What are the other types of shock, and how do they differ from hemorrhagic shock?**

In addition to **hemorrhagic** or **hypovolemic shock,** there are neurogenic, cardiogenic, and septic types of shock. **Neurogenic shock** (this is uncommon) is caused by sudden loss of autonomic vascular tone, resulting in vasodilation. The systolic BP is low, the pulse pressure is low, but the skin remains warm. **Cardiogenic shock** results from pump failure secondary to intrinsic heart muscle damage (myocardial infarction [MI]) or mechanical compression (cardiac tamponade). In this setting, CO is low, however intravascular volume is adequate reflected by increased CVP. **Septic shock** (more common in surgical intensive care unit [SICU] patients) is characterized by hypotension and low systemic vascular resistance (SVR). It is important to remember these categories of shock do not always exist in isolation. For example, a trauma patient may have cardiac tamponade and also be hemorrhaging into his pelvis.

15. **When should fluid resuscitation be initiated on the patient with multiple traumas?**

Immediately! Begin therapy (fluid through large-bore IV lines) while you are doing the primary survey directed at life-threatening injuries. It is inappropriate to wait until the trauma patient fits a precise physiologic classification of shock before starting aggressive volume restoration.

16. **What are the potential sources of occult blood loss when trying to ascertain a patient's hemodynamic status?**

The pleural spaces, abdominal cavity, retroperitoneal or pelvic space (pelvic fractures), major long bone fractures, and at the scene externally ("on the sidewalk"). Femur fractures can hide >1 L of blood, whereas each rib fracture can account for 150 ml.

17. **What is the patient called who becomes unstable after the initial resuscitation, and why is it important to recognize this phenomenon?**

This patient is a "transient responder." This indicates ongoing blood loss! Mismanagement in this setting can be fatal.

18. **When is blood transfusion indicated during initial resuscitation?**

If the patient arrives who is not responding to aggressive ("wide open") crystalloid infusion, the patient should receive uncrossed, O-negative packed red blood cells. Do not wait for type-specific blood if immediate infusion is required; the blood bank is not generally using the same clock (they are not as frightened because they cannot see the patient).

19. **How does hemorrhagic shock lead to multiple organ failure?**

Multiple organ failure (MOF) is a syndrome that represents a complicated and dynamic pathophysiologic pathway leading to organ functional derangement and eventual death. Severe hemorrhagic shock begins an inflammatory cascade that cannot be reversed in some patients despite adequate resuscitation. This pathway is thought to begin within hours of injury. During the Vietnam War, the patients in hemorrhagic shock were treated rapidly, but later died as a result of pulmonary failure or adult respiratory distress syndrome (ARDS). Patients with ARDS can be mechanically ventilated but later die from a combination of liver, cardiac, and bone marrow failure or MOF. MOF is the leading cause of late postinjury mortality in 85% of these deaths. In addition to the cellular derangement in ATP synthesis; shock causes the release of platelet-activating factor, interleukin-8, and arachidonic acid metabolites that prime neutrophils to adhere to endothelial cells and release cytotoxic mediators, which produce defects in the endovasculature, flooding the interstitial space and causing organ damage. The mesenteric circulation is a hotbed of proinflammatory mediator synthesis (the gut is the "motor for MOF") and appears to release agents (probably arachidonate and other toxic lipids) into the mesenteric lymph that causes systemic neutrophil priming and ultimately acute lung injury.

KEY POINTS: CLASSIFICATIONS OF SHOCK

1. Hemorrhagic: most common cause of posttraumatic shock; low filling pressures and CO, low mixed venous oxygen saturation (SVO_2), high SVR.

2. Neurogenic: uncommon; low SVR with bradycardia; skin remains warm.

3. Cardiogenic: pump failure secondary to intrinsic myocardial damage (MI) or mechanical compression (tamponade); high filling pressures, low CO, low SVO_2.

4. Septic: more common in surgical intensive care unit than in trauma bay; initially high CO, low SVR, high SVO_2.

BIBLIOGRAPHY

1. Ciesla DJ, Moore EE, Johnson JL et al.: A 12-year prospective study of postinjury multiple organ failure: has anything changed? Arch Surg 140(5):432-438; discussion 438-440, 2005.

2. Durham RM, Moran JJ, Mazuski JE et al.: Multiple organ failure in trauma patients. J Trauma 55(4):608-616, 2003.

3. Feliciano DV, Mattox KL, Moore EE: Trauma, 6th ed., New York, 2008, McGraw-Hill.

4. Gonzalez EA, Moore FA, Holcomb JB et al.: Fresh frozen plasma should be given earlier to patients requiring massive transfusion. J Trauma 62(1):112-119, 2007.

5. Gutierrez G, Reines HD, Wulf-Gutierrez ME: Clinical review: hemorrhagic shock. Crit Care 8(5):373-381, 2004.

6. Moore FA, Moore EE, American College of Surgeons: ACS surgery: principles and practice 2006. Section 7 Initial Management of Life-Threatening Trauma. New York: 2006, WebMD Professional Pub.

7. Moore FA, McKinley BA, Moore EE: The next generation in shock resuscitation. Lancet 363(9425):1988-1996, 2004.

CHAPTER 17

TRAUMATIC BRAIN INJURY

Brian P. Callahan, MD, and Craig H. Rabb, MD

1. **Is traumatic brain injury (TBI) a common problem?**
   Yes. In the United States, 1 in 12 deaths are due to injury. About 40% of traumatic deaths are associated with TBI. Of deaths resulting from motor vehicle accidents, 60% are a result of brain injury. Even more common is minor TBI, which accounts for 75% of admissions for head trauma. There are over 200,000 patients hospitalized with TBI in the United States per year and over 1.7 million mild TBIs that require a physician's attention. It is estimated that 2 to 6 million people in the United States are living with TBI-associated disabilities.

2. **What is a concussion?**
   The definition of concussion or mild TBI per the Centers for Disease Control and Prevention (CDC) is a complex pathophysiologic process secondary to trauma that results in a constellation of physical, cognitive, emotional, or sleep-related symptoms that may or may not involve loss of consciousness (LOC). The symptoms include headache, dizziness, amnesia, and vomiting. There are about 128/100,000 population concussions in the United States per year. In pediatric patients, sports is the most common cause, whereas falls and motor vehicle accidents are the most common cause in adults. The Glasgow Coma Scale (GCS) score is used to categorize brain injuries as follows: mild, 13 to 14; moderate, 9 to 12; and severe, 8.

3. **How is the GCS score derived?**
   The GCS is a means of identifying change in neurologic status. Its principal strengths are ease of use and reproducibility among observers. It is a 15-point scale; 15 is the best score, and 3 is the worst. The score is derived from the addition of the three individual components: best eye-opening response (1 to 4 points), best verbal response (1 to 5 points), and best motor response (1 to 6 points). The GCS is insensitive to pupillary response and focality.

4. **When should a neurosurgeon be consulted?**
   For patients with LOC and subsequent neurologic abnormality or abnormality on computed tomography (CT) scan. These patients often have a GCS score equal to 13.

5. **How do you initially assess the patient with a brain injury?**
   Just like any trauma patient. The first steps are assessment of the ABCs (airway, breathing, and circulation) and rapid physiologic resuscitation. The neurologic examination is crucial. The initial examination includes (1) GCS assessment; (2) assessment of cranial nerve reflexes, including pupil size and reactivity, oculocephalic reflex (doll's eyes), corneal reflex, and gag reflex; (3) and motor examination. Repetition of the neurologic examination is also crucial. Finally, evaluate for concurrent cervical spine injury.

6. **What takes priority in a patient who is hypotensive also with a traumatic brain injury?**
   Hypotension in patients with head injury frequently accompanies other injuries. Do not assume that hypotension is a result of the brain injury alone. A single episode of hypotension doubles the mortality rate. Also, hypoxemia, as defined as a PaO_2 less than 60 or O_2 saturation less than 90%, significantly increases mortality in TBI.

7. **What is the significance of anisocoria in a patient with a decreased level of consciousness?**

Anisocoria (unequal pupils) is a true neurologic emergency. Commonly a mass lesion (e.g., subdural or epidural hematoma, contusion, or diffuse swelling of one hemisphere) leads to uncal herniation and stretching of the ipsilateral third nerve. Time is crucial. Give mannitol, get a CT scan, and proceed with surgical decompression (if possible).

8. **What if the larger pupil is reactive?**

If the larger pupil is reactive, the third cranial nerve is functioning. Think of Horner's syndrome (miosis, ptosis, and anhydrosis) on the other side. This syndrome may be a result of injury to the sympathetic nerves traveling with the carotid artery in the neck. Consider evaluation (angiography) for a carotid dissection.

9. **Is the term "*semicomatose*" inaccurate?**

Yes. Patients are either **alert, lethargic** (arousal is maintained by verbal interaction), **obtunded** (constant mechanical stimulation to maintain arousal), or **comatose** (neither verbal nor mechanical stimulation elicits arousal). Change in level of consciousness is often the first sign of increasing intracranial pressure (ICP); it is also the most poorly documented part of the neurologic examination. Document all findings!

10. **How is motor response tested?**

Ascertain the ability to follow commands by asking the patient to hold up fingers and move his or her arms and legs. If the patient does not follow commands, test response to painful central stimulus. Localization of painful stimulus is confirmed by the patient's hand reaching toward a sternal rub. The patient may be in more danger if in response to pain he or she exhibits flexor posturing (decorticate), extensor posturing (decerebrate), or no response. Flexor posturing indicates a high brainstem injury, and extensor posturing is associated with low brainstem dysfunction.

11. **What is the significance of periorbital ecchymosis (raccoon eyes) and ecchymosis over the mastoid (Battle's sign)?**

In the absence of direct trauma to the eyes or mastoid regions, periorbital ecchymosis and ecchymosis over the mastoid are reliable signs of basilar skull fractures. Of patients with basilar skull fractures, 10% have cerebrospinal fluid (CSF) leaks, including rhinorrhea or otorrhea. Persistent CSF leaks are associated with meningitis; however, prophylactic antibiotics do not decrease the risk of meningitis.

12. **Should scalp lacerations be explored in the emergency department?**

Usually not. A CT scan should be performed first to look for intracranial pathology or skull fracture. If surgical pathology is seen on the CT, the laceration will be closed in the operating room (OR). If not, the laceration can be washed and closed in the emergency department (ED). If bleeding cannot be controlled before CT, then the laceration should be closed with staples to stop the blood loss.

13. **Which patients need CT scans of the head?**

The CT scan is used partly as a triage tool with minor brain injuries and can be cost effective compared with admission to the intensive care unit (ICU) for observation. Conversely, patients with focality on examination do not proceed to the OR without a CT scan. Patients who definitely need a CT scan after mild TBI are those less than age 16 or greater than 65, who are intoxicated, not dependable, on anticoagulants, have persistent amnesia or other neurological symptoms, signs of a basilar skull fracture, or abnormal neurological exam.

14. **What are the common traumatic surgical lesions?**

If the ventricles are large (ventriculomegaly), a ventriculostomy can drain excessive CSF if ICP is elevated. Epidural hematomas (from arterial bleeding), subdural hematomas (from venous bleeding), and intraparenchymal hematomas with significant mass effect should be surgically evacuated. A depressed skull fracture or foreign body (e.g., a bullet) may require a trip to the operating room in certain clinical situations.

15. **When is intracranial pressure monitoring indicated?**

ICP should be monitored in all salvageable patients with a severe TBI (GCS 3 to 8 after resuscitation) *and* an abnormal CT (defined as hematomas, contusions, swelling, herniation, or compressed cisterns). ICP monitoring is also indicated in patients with severe TBI and *normal* CT if 2 or more of the following are noted: age >40, posturing, or systolic blood pressure (SBP) <90 mm Hg.

16. **Describe the initial treatment of patients with a suspected increase in ICP.**

The brain, similar to every other organ, must have adequate blood flow and oxygen delivery. The ABCs come first. Airway should be established, and the patient should be intubated if necessary. Keep the systolic blood pressure >100 mm Hg and avoid hypoxia. The head of the bed should be elevated, and cervical spine precautions followed. Mannitol should be given if patient has signs of impending herniation, such as anisocoria, or focal neurological signs on examination such as posturing.

17. **Should all patients with elevated ICP be hyperventilated?**

Decreasing the partial pressure of carbon dioxide (pCO_2) is the most rapidly effective treatment for elevated ICP. The goal is usually a pCO_2 of 30 to 35 mm Hg. Any patient with a depressed level of consciousness and inability to protect the airway should be intubated. Before a CT scan is obtained, patients thought to have a mass lesion by neurologic examination should be hyperventilated until definitive treatment is achieved. Avoid chronic hyperventilation, which can cause ischemic brain injury as a result of vasoconstriction of cerebral blood vessels and decrease of cerebral blood flow (CBF). Because of this effect on CBF, hyperventilation should only be used as a temporizing measure.

18. **In hemodynamically stable patients, how do you decrease ICP?**

Mannitol, 1 g/kg, as an intravenous (IV) bolus. More recent evidence also suggests that hypertonic saline may decrease ICP and maintain hemodynamic stability. Hypertonic saline may be given as a continuous infusion with a goal serum sodium or as bolus injections for bumps in ICP. The bolus dose varies from 100 ml of 3% normal saline to 10 ml of 23.4% normal saline. Also be sure the cervical collar is not obstructing venous outflow through the jugular system.

19. **What is the end point of treatment with diuretics?**

Serum sodium of 150 mEq/L and serum osmolality of 320 mOsm are usually the upper limits of diuresis. Anticipate intravascular hypovolemia and treat accordingly. The recent SAFE (Saline vs Albumin Fluid Evaluation) trial comparing albumin versus saline in resuscitation of patients with TBI has shown that resuscitating with albumin increases mortality and is more expensive than crystalloids. Thus, crystalloids should be used to replace the lost volume secondary to diuresis in TBI.

20. **What is the significance of cerebral perfusion pressure (CPP)?**

CPP is the difference between mean arterial pressure (MAP) and ICP:

$$CPP = MAP - ICP$$

CPP is important. Neurologic outcome is best in patients with CPPs in the 60s, and CPP<50 should be avoided. Some patients require treatment with pressors and fluids to maintain the CPP, however, aggressively maintaining CPP >70 should be avoided because of the increased risk of adult respiratory distress syndrome (ARDS).

21. **Why should all children with TBI be undressed and examined thoroughly?**
Half of children suffering nonaccidental trauma (child abuse) have TBI. A thorough examination may reveal additional injuries.

22. **Should posttraumatic seizures be treated prophylactically?**
Patients with brain parenchymal abnormalities on CT scan after head injury may benefit from 1 week of antiseizure prophylaxis. Early seizures can increase the metabolic demand of the injured brain and adversely affect ICP. Of patients who have seizures within the first 7 days of injury, 10% also have late seizures. Prevention of early seizures does not reduce the incidence of late seizures, however. Patients at increased risk of seizures are those with GCS <10, contusions, depressed skull fractures, brain hematomas, or penetrating injuries.

23. **Which coagulopathy is associated with severe brain injury?**
Disseminated intravascular coagulation. The presumed mechanism is massive release of thromboplastin from the injured brain into the circulation. The serum levels of fibrin degradation products roughly correlate with the extent of brain parenchymal injury. All patients who are severely brain injured should be evaluated with prothrombin time, partial thromboplastin time, platelet counts, and fibrinogen levels.

24. **What other medical complications may result from severe head injury?**
Diabetes insipidus (DI) secondary to the inadequate secretion of antidiuretic hormone is caused by injury to the pituitary or hypothalamic tracts. The kidney is unable to decrease free water loss. Usually the urine output is >200 ml/hr, and the urine specific gravity is <1.003. The serum sodium may rise precipitously if DI is not treated promptly. The treatment of choice in trauma is IV infusion of synthetic vasopressin (Pitressin), which has a 20-minute half-life and can be titrated to produce the appropriate urine output. Because most trauma-induced DI is self-limited, long-term 1-deamino-8-D-arginine vasopressin (DDAVP), which has a 12-hour half-life, is usually not necessary.

25. **If a patient is awake with significant neurologic symptoms but no abnormality on CT scan, what are the likely explanations?**
A spinal cord injury or carotid or vertebral artery dissection.

26. **Are gunshot wounds that cross the midline of the brain uniformly fatal?**
No. The tract that the bullet takes is important, but so is the energy that it imparts to the brain.

27. **What is the significance of concussion?**
In most studies of minor TBI, >50% of patients have complaints of headache, fatigue, dizziness, irritability, and alterations of cognition and short-term memory. This constellation of symptoms has been called the postconcussive syndrome. It is important to alert the patient to the likelihood of developing these symptoms. The neurobehavioral problems significantly affect patients' lives. The symptoms usually resolve within 3 to 6 months after injury.

28. **Can patients with minor TBIs be discharged from the emergency department?**
Patients whose examination (including short-term memory) returns to normal and who have a normal head CT scan can be discharged to home if they are accompanied by a responsible person and given written instructions to return to the hospital if headache continues to worsen, increasing vomiting, weakness, drowsiness, or CSF leak appears.

29. **Is brain injury permanent? Is the outcome always poor?**
No and no. Brain injury occurs in two phases. The primary injury occurs at the moment of impact. Secondary injury is preventable and treatable. Examples include hypoxia, hypotension, elevated ICP, and decreased perfusion to the brain secondary to ischemia, brain swelling,

and expanding mass lesions. Rapid surgical management and avoidance of secondary injury improve outcome. Although previously it was believed that the brain was not capable of repair, it is now clear that neuronal repair and reorganization occur after injury.

30. What is the threshold for treating increased ICP?
Most studies agree that the threshold for treating ICP should be 20 to 25 mm Hg.

31. Should high dose steroids be given to TBI patients to treat increased ICP?
No. There is evidence (CRASH [Corticosteroid Randomization After Significant Head Injury] study) that shows that high dose steroids in TBI are associated with increased morbidity and mortality.

32. Are patients with traumatic brain injury at risk for deep venous thrombosis and pulmonary embolus?
Yes. The risk of deep venous thrombosis (DVT) and pulmonary embolus (PE) in patients with TBIs can be as high as 30%. SCDs have been shown to reduce the rate of DVT/PE and should be used in all patients with TBIs unless a lower extremity injury prevents their use. Low-molecular weight heparin (LMWH) has also been shown to decrease the risk, but can also increase the risk of brain hemorrhage.

KEY POINTS

1. Hypotension and hypoxia must be avoided in TBI.

2. Think of carotid or vertebral artery dissection in trauma patients with neurologic symptoms but a normal CT scan.

3. CPP = MAP − ICP. Try to maintain CPP between 50 and 60 mm Hg in severe TBI, especially in patients with ongoing ICP problems. Do not overtreat (CPP >70), as this increases the risk of ARDS.

4. Do not use high dose steroids in TBI.

WEBSITES

www.acssurgery.com/abstracts/acs/acs0501.htm

www.surgery.ucsf.edu/eastbaytrauma/Protocols/ER%20protocol%20pages/closedheadinjury.htm

www.emedicine.com/pmr/topic212.htm

www.cdc.gov/ncipc/tbi/mtbi/report.htm

BIBLIOGRAPHY

1. Brain Trauma Foundation; American Association of Neurological Surgeons; Congress of Neurological Surgeons; Joint Section on Neurotrauma and Critical Care, AANS/CNS: Guidelines for the management of severe traumatic brain injury. J Neurotrauma 24 Suppl 1: S1-S106, 2007.

2. Brain Trauma Foundation: Management and prognosis of severe traumatic brain injury, New York, 2000, Brain Trauma Foundation. Available at www.braintrauma.org.

3. Carson J, Tator C, Johnston K et al.: New guidelines for concussion management. Can Fam Physician 52:756-757, 2006.

4. Marion DW: Evidenced-based guidelines for traumatic brain injuries. Prog Neurol Surg 19:171-196, 2006.

5. Mazzola CA, Adelman PD: Critical care management of head trauma in children. Crit Care Med 30:S393-S401, 2002.

6. Narayan RK, Michel ME, Ansell B et al.: Clinical trials in head injury. J Neurotrauma 19:503-557, 2002.

7. Ogden AT, Mayer SA, Connolly ES Jr: Hyperosmolar agents in neurosurgical practice: the evolving role of hypertonic saline. Neurosurgery 57(2):207-215, 2005.

8. Ropper AH, Gorson KC: Clinical practice. Concussion. N Engl J Med 356(2):166-172, 2007.

9. SAFE Study Investigators; Australian and New Zealand Intensive Care Society Clinical Trials Group; Australian Red Cross Blood Service et al.: Saline or albumin for fluid resuscitation in patients with traumatic brain injury. N Engl J Med 357(9):874-884, 2007.

10. Shaw NA: The neurophysiology of concussion. Prog Neurobiol 67:281-344, 2002.

CHAPTER 18

SPINAL CORD INJURIES

Brian P. Callahan, MD, and Craig H. Rabb, MD

1. What is the difference between a spinal injury and a spinal cord injury?

Spinal injuries include damage to the bone, disc, or ligaments. These injuries sometimes result in spinal instability. They also may be associated with spinal cord injury (SCI), which is damage to the neural tissue, often with clinical deficit. It is crucial to determine whether there is (1) a spinal injury, (2) an SCI, or (3) spinal instability.

2. Describe the evaluation of a patient with a suspected spine injury.

First, be sure that the patient is adequately immobilized, and everyone knows to maintain spinal precautions. Second, inspect and palpate the spine for external trauma and step-off. Finally, do a complete neurologic examination including all four extremities. Assess strength, sensation (light touch/proprioception and pain/temperature), muscle tone, reflexes, and rectal tone. Carefully document your results.

3. How do you minimize the risk of additional spine injury in hospital?

Trauma patients should be protected with a rigid cervical collar. The thoracic and lumbar spine are protected using initial spine board immobilization. The patient should be logrolled during initial evaluation, then removed from the board and transferred to an appropriate hospital bed to prevent decubitus ulcers. Spine precautions should be maintained until the spine is "cleared," meaning there is no spinal instability or the instability has been identified.

4. How is the level of the spinal cord injury defined?

The level does not refer to the level of the injury to the spinal column (vertebrae, discs, and ligaments) but to the most caudal level in the cord with intact function. If a patient has normal function of the deltoids (C5) and little or no function of the biceps (C6) or below, the patient has a C5 motor level injury. Right and left sides should be documented separately.

5. Which type of injury is commonly associated with cervical spine injury?

Head injury. Forces associated with significant head and brain injury may be transmitted through to the cervical spine. Of patients with spinal cord injuries, 50% have associated head injuries. Approximately 15% of patients with one spine injury have a second injury elsewhere in the spine.

6. How can the spinal cord be evaluated in patients with associated head injury?

All patients should have a rectal examination to evaluate tone. A patulous anus is a good indication of spinal cord or cauda equina injury. Flaccid motor tone and absent reflexes should raise suspicion of SCI. These findings are extremely unusual with isolated brain injury. Priapism is common with SCI but not caused by head injury. Radiographic imaging should be used liberally when an SCI is suspected.

7. Which other significant injury may mimic, at presentation, a high thoracic cord injury?

Thoracic aortic dissection may present as a T4 region cord injury. T4 is a watershed zone in the cord between the vertebral arterial distribution and the aortic radicular arteries.

8. **What is spinal shock?**

   Absence of all spinal cord function below the level of the lesion results in flaccid motor tone and areflexia. Neurogenic shock, by contrast, refers to the hypotension that may result from cervical or upper thoracic complete spinal cord lesions. The hypotension is the result of the lack of sympathetic vasomotor innervation below the lesion and is characterized by bradycardia from unbalanced vagal input to the heart. Fluid resuscitation and pressors should be used to keep the systolic blood pressure (SBP) >90 mm Hg. Atropine may be necessary to treat the bradycardia.

9. **Describe an adequate radiologic evaluation.**

   Awake, alert, and reliable patients with no neck pain or tenderness do not require imagining. A three-view cervical spine series (anteroposterior [AP], lateral, and odontoid views) is recommended for radiographic evaluation of the cervical spine in patients who are symptomatic after traumatic injury. The relationship between C7 and the top of T1 must be visualized. This should be supplemented with computed tomography (CT) to further define areas that are suspicious or not well visualized on the plain cervical x-rays. Cervical spine immobilization in awake patients with neck pain or tenderness and normal cervical spine x-rays (including supplemental CT as necessary) may be discontinued after either (a) normal and adequate (with at least 30-degree excursion in each direction) dynamic flexion/extension radiographs, or (b) a normal magnetic resonance imaging (MRI) study is obtained within 48 hours of injury or (c) at the discretion of the treating spine attending physician. Obtunded patients with normal cervical spine x-rays should undergo high-quality CT imaging with coronal and sagittal reconstructed images. This may be supplemented with MRI.

   For the thoracic and lumbosacral spine, anteroposterior and lateral views are obtained. Patients with evidence of possible fractures on plain films should have CT scans to define the injury in greater detail. MRI is also useful to look for herniated discs and ligamentous injury. Currently, these areas can be satisfactorily imaged by images reconstructed from body imaging done during the trauma workup (CT chest, abdomen, and pelvis).

10. **Describe the proper way to read a lateral cervical spine film.**

    Make a habit of doing a thorough systematic review in the same way with every film. First look at the prevertebral soft tissue space, which may be the only radiographic abnormality in 40% of C1 and C2 fractures. The space anterior to C3 should not exceed one third of the body of C3. At the C6 level, the entire body of C6 generally fits into the prevertebral soft tissue space. Check the alignment of the anterior, then posterior edges of the vertebral bodies. Be sure that the intervertebral disc spaces are of relatively equal height. Assess each facet joint. Check the spinous processes for alignment and abnormal splaying. Finally, evaluate each vertebra for fracture.

11. **What about the anteroposterior film?**

    Carefully inspect the alignment of the midline spinous processes. Abrupt angulations suggest unilateral facet dislocation. More subtle changes may indicate facet instability or fracture. Body fractures may be more obvious in the AP view.

12. **Can a patient have a spinal cord injury and normal plain radiographs?**

    Spinal cord injury without radiographic abnormality (SCIWORA) is defined as neurologic signs and symptoms consistent with traumatic myelopathy despite normal x-rays. SCIWORA is rare and is most common in children, where most series quote about 15% of SCI. This rate can be as high as 40% in children <9 years old. SCIWORA is less common in adults (about 5% of SCIs).

13. **Is magnetic resonance imaging useful in the evaluation of acute spine trauma?**

    Yes. If plain radiographs and CT scans do not explain adequately the extent of injury noted on the neurologic examinations, MRI should be used to evaluate the spine for herniated discs, ligamentous injuries, and evidence of SCI. In addition, MRI is used routinely to further clarify injuries identified on CT imaging.

14. **Fractures of C1 and C2 are visualized best with which view?**
   In the plain radiographs, the **odontoid view** is best, otherwise coronal and sagittal reconstructed CT images. Look for overhang of the lateral mass of C1 off the lateral edges of C2. This occurs in **Jefferson's fractures** (burst fractures of the C1 ring, best seen on axial CT images). Sum total overhang of both C1 lateral masses on C2 of >7 mm may be associated with disruption of the transverse ligament and instability. If you see a C1 fracture, look carefully for a C2 fracture. The three types of odontoid fractures are:
   - Type I occurs in the dens.
   - Type II occurs across the base of the dens where it joins the body of C2.
   - Type III extends into the body of C2.

15. **What is hangman's fracture?**
   Bilateral fractures through the pedicles or pars interarticularis (or "isthmus") of C2 that are caused by a severe hyperextension injury, usually secondary to high-speed motor vehicle accidents. In judicial hangings, the fatal injury is the spinal cord stretch caused by the drop in combination with the C2 fracture. Most patients with hangman's fracture present neurologically intact, and most cases of hangman's fracture can be treated with external immobilization.

16. **Define deficits in complete transverse myelopathy, anterior cord syndrome, central cord syndrome, and Brown-Séquard syndrome.**
   Complete transverse myelopathy may result from transection, stretch, or contusion of the cord. All function below the level of the lesion—motor, sensory, and reflexive—is lost. **Anterior cord syndrome** results from injury of the anterior two thirds of the spinal cord (the distribution of the anterior spinal artery), which carries motor, pain, and temperature tracts. Light touch and proprioception are intact because the posterior columns are preserved.
   Central cord syndrome results from injury to the central area of the spinal cord. Often it is found in patients with preexisting cervical stenosis resulting from spondylotic changes. Characteristically, deficits are more severe in the upper extremities than in the lower extremities, and have been thought to be a result of buckling of thickened posterior ligamentum flavum into the spinal cord, with extension. Pathologically, there is hemorrhage in the center of the spinal cord. Motor function usually is affected more than sensory function.
   Brown-Séquard syndrome characteristically is seen in penetrating injuries, but also may be seen in blunt injury, especially with unilateral, traumatically herniated discs. The syndrome results from injury to half of the spinal cord. Clinically, motor, position, and vibration sense are affected on the side ipsilateral to the injury; these tracts cross in the brainstem. Pain and temperature sensation are abolished contralateral to the lesion; these tracts cross in the cord at or near the level of innervation.

17. **What is the role of methylprednisolone in the treatment of acute cord injury?**
   The results of the Second National Acute Spinal Cord Injury Study (NASCIS II) suggest that high-dose methylprednisolone resulted in a statistically significant improvement in outcome. The dose is a 30-mg/kg load, followed by 5.4 milligrams per kilogram per hour for 23 hours. The NASCIS III trial reported that patients dosed 3 to 8 hours after injury had improved outcomes when treated for 48 hours with the methylprednisolone rather than 24 hours. In patients dosed within 3 hours of injury, no further gains were documented by treating beyond 24 hours. Recent reevaluation of available data has put the value of these steroids in doubt, and the risks may outweigh the benefits. Methylprednisolone is not indicated in the management of penetrating SCI.

18. **Do patients with spinal cord injuries ever undergo acute surgery?**

There are currently no standards on the timing of surgery, in particular with the goal in mind of reversing neurologic deficits. Ideally, unstable spinal injuries (in otherwise systemically stable patients) should be surgically stabilized within 72 hours, so as to facilitate their global care and mobilization of the patient. With regard to urgent surgery to treat neurologic deficits, surgery is usually performed in patients with incomplete injuries or in a patient with SCI and neurologic deterioration. Deterioration may be the result of herniated disc material, epidural hemorrhage, or cord swelling in a narrowed canal, causing cord compression and worsening symptoms. Patients who should not undergo emergent surgery are those with complete injuries >24 hours old and medically unstable patients.

19. **How is the bony injury treated?**
    1. Prevention of further injury using spinal precautions.
    2. Obtaining normal alignment using body position, traction, and bracing.
    3. Open reduction, decompression, and fusion as necessary.

20. **What is the outcome in patients with spinal cord injury?**

With complete lesions (no motor or sensory function below the lesion), the chances of recovery are poor; 2% of patients recover ambulation. The prognosis is markedly better for patients with incomplete lesions: 75% experience significant recovery. Appropriate treatment of bony injuries helps to prevent pain and late neurologic deterioration.

21. **Are cervical spine injuries associated with injuries to the carotid or vertebral arteries?**

Yes. The incidence of blunt vertebral artery injury has been shown to be 0.53% to 1.03% of all blunt trauma admissions. An overall stroke rate of 24% has been observed in all patients diagnosed with blunt vertebral artery injury, regardless of injury grade, and the death rate from blunt vertebral injury was 8%. Risk factors correlated with blunt vertebral artery injury were noted to be cervical fractures involving the foramen transversarium, any fracture involving C1 to C3, and any injury involving subluxation. Screening of patients with these types of injuries 16-slice multidetector computed tomographic angiography (CTA) can identify such vascular injuries, enabling preventative measures such as anticoagulation, before as stroke happens.

22. **Should all patients with spinal cord injuries have inferior vena cava filters placed to prevent pulmonary embolus?**

No, but those patients who do not respond to anticoagulation or have contraindications to anticoagulation should have an inferior vena cava (IVC) filter placed.

KEY POINTS

1. SCI should be suspected in all trauma patients who are unconscious, intoxicated, have distracting injuries, or complain of neck pain or tenderness. Strict spinal precautions should be applied until radiographic and clinical spine clearance.

2. In patients with acute SCI, mean arterial pressure (MAP) should be maintained >90 mm Hg to increase spinal cord perfusion.

3. Patients with cervical spine injuries should be evaluated for carotid and vertebral artery injuries.

4. Patients with SCI who present within 8 hours may be treated with high dose IV methylprednisolone protocol.

WEBSITE

www.asia-spinalinjury.org/

BIBLIOGRAPHY

1. Biffl WL, Egglin T, Benedetto B et al.: Sixteen-slice computed tomographic angiography is a reliable noninvasive screening test for clinically significant blunt cerebrovascular injuries. J Trauma 60(4):745-751, 2006.

2. Bracken MB, Shepard MJ, Holford TR et al.: Administration of methylprednisolone for 24 or 48 hours or tirilazad mesylate for 48 hours in the treatment of acute spinal cord injury: results of the Third National Acute Spinal Cord Injury randomized controlled trial. JAMA 277:1597-1604, 1997.

3. Cothren CC, Moore EE, Biffl WL et al.: Cervical spine fracture patterns predictive of blunt vertebral artery injury. J Trauma 55(5):811-813, 2003.

4. Cortez R, Levi AD: Acute spinal cord injury. Curr Treat Options Neurol March 9(2):115-125, 2007.

5. Fehlings MG, Perrin RG: The timing of surgical intervention in the treatment of spinal cord injury: a systematic review of recent clinical evidence. Spine 31(11 Suppl), S28-S35, 2006.

6. Hadley MN, Walters BC, Grabb PA et al.: Radiographic assessment of the cervical spine in symptomatic trauma patients. Neurosurgery 50(3 Suppl):S36-S43, 2002.

7. Harris MB, Sethi RK: The initial assessment and management of the multiple-trauma patient with an associated spine injury. Spine 31(11 Suppl):S9-S15, 2006.

8. Holmes JF, Akkinepalli R: Computed tomography versus plain radiography to screen for cervical spine injury: a meta-analysis. J Trauma 58(5):902-905, 2005.

9. Rabb CH, Johnson JL, VanSickle D et al.: Are upright lateral cervical radiographs in the obtunded trauma patient useful? A retrospective study. World J Emerg Surg 2-4, 2004.

10. Sliker CW, Mirvis SE, Shanmuganathan K: Assessing cervical spine stability in obtunded blunt trauma patients: review of medical literature. Radiology. 234(3):733-739, 2005.

CHAPTER 19

PENETRATING NECK TRAUMA

C. Clay Cothren, MD, and Ernest E. Moore, MD

1. **Why are penetrating neck wounds unique?**
   Although comprising only a small percentage of body surface area, the neck contains a heavy concentration of vital structures.

2. **What constitutes a penetrating neck wound?**
   Violation of the platysma muscle defines a penetrating neck wound. This investing fascial layer of the neck is superficial to vital structures. If the platysma is not penetrated, the wound is managed as a simple laceration and the patient discharged from the emergency department (ED).

3. **Which side of the neck is more likely to be injured?**
   The left side because most assailants are right handed.

4. **Do gunshot wounds and knife wounds cause the same relative injuries?**
   Gunshot wounds generally tend to inflict more tissue damage (see Table 19-1).

TABLE 19-1. GUNSHOT VERSUS STAB WOUNDS		
Structure	Gunshot Wounds (%)	Stab Wounds (%)
Artery	20	5
Vein	15	10
Airway	10	5
Digestive	20	<5

5. **What are the priorities in the management of penetrating neck trauma?**
   The ABCs (airway, breathing, and circulation) are the first priority in every trauma patient. If indicated, patients should be intubated orally, although cricothyrotomy may be necessary with an extensive neck hematoma or ongoing bleeding into the oropharynx. Although the patient may present with a patent airway, early elective airway control should be performed in patients with expanding hematomas. Based on the trajectory of injury, pneumothoraces, hemothoraces, or great vessel injury should be suspected. External bleeding should be controlled with direct digital pressure, and intravenous (IV) access secured using two large-bore peripheral catheters.

6. **How should bleeding be controlled at the accident scene and in the emergency department?**
Direct digital pressure is almost always successful, even for major arterial injuries. Blindly placing clamps inside a wound risks injury to other vital, uninjured structures, particularly nerves.

7. **Should you explore the neck wound in the trauma bay?**
Although careful visual inspection is warranted, probing the wound (digitally, with a Q-tip, or with a surgical instrument) may dislodge a blood clot, causing marked hemorrhage.

8. **What physical examination findings should be elicited?**
Ongoing hemorrhage from the wound, expanding or pulsatile hematomas, hemoptysis, hematemesis, neurologic deficits, dysphagia, dysphonia, hoarseness, and stridor are indicative of significant injury.

9. **How often do patients with cervical crepitus have a significant injury?**
One third of patients with crepitus have an injury of the pharynx, esophagus, larynx, or trachea. In two thirds of these patients, however, the air has been introduced through the wound entrance site, and there is no significant underlying injury.

10. **What are the three zones of the neck?**
Zone I extends from the sternal notch to the cricoid cartilage.
Zone II extends from the cricoid cartilage to the angle of the mandible.
Zone III comprises the area cephalad to the angle of the mandible (see Fig. 19-1).

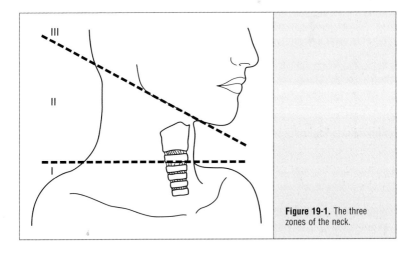

Figure 19-1. The three zones of the neck.

11. **Why are penetrating injuries divided into zones?**
    Each zone has management implications. Because of the technical difficulties of injury exposure and varying operative approaches, a precise preoperative diagnosis is desirable for symptomatic zone I and III injuries. Zone II injuries are more easily evaluated with physical examination (see Fig. 19-2).

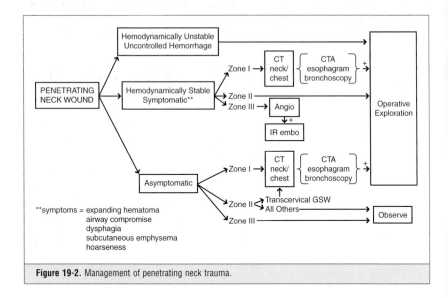

Figure 19-2. Management of penetrating neck trauma.

12. **What are the indications for immediate operative exploration?**
    Hemodynamic instability or external arterial hemorrhage.

13. **What is selective management of penetrating neck trauma?**
    Historically, all zone II injuries violating the platysma were explored operatively. However, as a result of a prohibitive number of negative explorations, this approach lost support. Asymptomatic patients with zone II injuries may be observed for 12 to 24 hours. The exception is patients with transcervial gunshot wounds, who should undergo computed tomographic angiography (CTA) to determine the tract of the missile and need for further diagnostic imaging.

14. **Should arteriography be performed on all patients?**
    Angiography is performed in symptomatic, hemodynamically stable patients with zone I and III injuries. In patients with zone I trauma, angiography identifies great vessel injuries in the thoracic outlet that may require a thoracic operative approach. Angiographic diagnosis of zone III injuries may be followed by angioembolization or endovascular intervention.

15. **What is the value of other diagnostic studies, such as esophagography, esophagoscopy, laryngoscopy, and bronchoscopy?**
    Esophagography, bronchoscopy, and laryngoscopy have been advocated in zone I and selected nonoperatively managed zone II patients, but multislice computed tomography (CT) scanning has limited their role. Esophagoscopy is combined with esophagography if esophageal injury is suspected; if water-soluble contrast material does not show a leak, barium is used.

Missed esophageal injuries can be deadly, with a 20% mortality rate if diagnosis is delayed only 12 hours. Intraoperative endoscopy with insufflation may be used provocatively to show an air leak and associated esophageal injury. Angiography remains the gold standard for diagnosis of arterial injury, and this modality may be therapeutic for zone III injuries; zone III is tough to expose surgically.

16. **Should an asymptomatic patient with a penetrating neck wound be sent home from the emergency department?**
No. Life-threatening penetrating neck wounds initially may be difficult to sort out; the safest policy is to observe all patients in the hospital for at least 24 hours.

KEY POINTS

1. Penetrating injury implies violation of the platysma; management is based on a patient's symptoms and anatomic zones of injury.

2. Immediate operative intervention is indicated in patients with hemodynamic instability or significant ongoing external bleeding.

3. Zone I injuries often have associated great vessel injuries which may necessitate a thoracic approach.

4. Mandatory exploration of all zone II injuries is not necessary; alert and asymptomatic patients can be observed expectantly for 24 hours.

BIBLIOGRAPHY

1. Albuquerque FC, Javedan SP, McDougall CG: Endovascular management of penetrating vertebral artery injuries. J Trauma 53:574-580, 2002.

2. Atteberry LR, Dennis JW, Menawat SS et al.: Physical examination alone is safe and accurate for evaluation of vascular injuries in penetrating zone II neck trauma. J Am Coll Surg 179:657-662, 1994.

3. Biffl WL, Moore EE, Rehse DH et al.: Selective management of penetrating neck trauma based on cervical level of injury. Am J Surg 174:678-682, 1997.

4. Demetriades D, Velmahos G, Asensio JA: Cervical pharygoesophageal and laryngotracheal injuries. World J Surg 25:1044-1048, 2001.

5. Ferguson E, Dennis JW, Vu JH et al.: Redefining the role of arterial imaging in the management of penetrating zone 3 neck injuries. Vascular 13:158-163, 2005.

6. Gracias VH, Reilly PM, Philpott J et al.: Computed tomography in the evaluation of penetrating neck trauma. Arch Surg 136:1231-1235, 2001.

7. Hirshberg A, Wall MJ, Johnston RH et al.: Transcervical gunshot injuries. Am J Surg 167:309, 1993.

8. Inaba K, Munera F, McKenney M et al.: Prospective evaluation of screening multislice helical computed tomographic angiography in the initial evaluation of penetrating neck injuries. J Trauma 61:144-149, 2006.

9. Mazolewski PJ, Curry JD, Browder T et al.: Computed tomographic scan can be used for surgical decision making in zone II penetrating neck injuries. J Trauma 51:315-319, 2001.

10. Woo K, Magner DP, Wilson MT et al.: CT angiography in penetrating neck trauma reduces the need for operative neck exploration. Am Surg 71:754, 2005.

CHAPTER 20

BLUNT THORACIC TRAUMA

Jeffrey L. Johnson, MD, and Ernest E. Moore, MD

1. **How often do patients with isolated blunt chest trauma need an emergent operation?**

   Rarely. In patients who arrive in the hospital alive, operative injuries to pulmonary, vascular, and mediastinal structures are surprisingly rare; only 5% of patients with isolated blunt injury to the chest require thoracotomy.

2. **In a patient with a hemothorax after blunt chest injury, what is the most important guide for the decision to operate?**

   The hemodynamic status of the patient. Hemothorax after blunt injury is most often the result of nonoperative lesions of the lung and chest wall. In a stable patient, therefore, evacuation of the hemothorax, reexpansion of the lung, and correction of coagulopathy, hypothermia and acidosis should be the initial focus. Chest tube output should be noted, but is not the principle consideration.

3. **What is a tension pneumothorax?**

   Air in the pleural space under pressure as a result of a one-way valve mechanism. This is a life-threatening condition because marked elevations in intrapleural pressure produces circulatory collapse from impaired right ventricular filling.

4. **What are the clinical signs of tension pneumothorax?**

   Hypotension, absent breath sounds on the involved side, and distended neck veins. Tension pneumothorax should be treated on clinical suspicion and without delay for radiographic confirmation.

5. **How is tension pneumothorax treated?**

   Make a hole in the chest. For prehospital care, needle decompression via the fifth intercostal space in the midaxillary line or midclavicular line. In the hospital setting, however, an experienced physician can completely decompress the pleural space just as rapidly with a tube thoracostomy.

6. **Does it matter how many ribs are broken?**

   Yes. Six or more fractures indicate a higher risk of pneumonia, adult respiratory distress syndrome (ARDS), and death, particularly in elderly patients.

7. **What is a flail chest?**

   A flail chest occurs when a portion of the thoracic cage loses bony continuity with the rest of the chest. When multiple ribs are fractured in two or more places, the chest wall moves paradoxically ("flails") with respiration.

8. **How does flail chest impact ventilation?**

   In spontaneously breathing patients, the portion of the thoracic cage that has lost bony continuity retracts inward during inspiration. This paradoxical motion can result in impaired ventilation.

9. **Do all patients with a flail segment then need to be put on a ventilator?**
No. The impact of a flail segment on ventilation is not usually profound, and with good analgesia, many patients can maintain their own work of breathing. Standard indications for intubation should be used.

10. **Does flail chest affect oxygenation?**
Flail chest per se has little direct impact on oxygenation. However, virtually all patients with flail chest have an underlying bruise on the lung—pulmonary contusion. The severity of the pulmonary contusion is a more important determinant of outcome and need for intubation than the impaired mechanics of the chest wall. The pathophysiology of blunt injury to the chest with severe bony injury should be thought of as a single process (i.e., flail chest or pulmonary contusion).

11. **What is the natural history of pulmonary contusion?**
It's like a bruise of the lung. Initially, the lung undergoes shearing of parenchyma and rupture of small blood vessels; this tissue injury is followed by edema and inflammation. Thus, like other bruises, patients with pulmonary contusion usually develop clinical deterioration in the first 48 hours. The initial chest radiograph may appear deceptively benign.

12. **What is the most common initial presentation of blunt injury to the thoracic aorta?**
Death. Eighty-five percent of patients with a torn thoracic aorta die of exsanguination before they reach the hospital. Disruption of the heart and great vessels is second only to head injury as a cause of death as a result of blunt trauma.

13. **Of patients surviving to reach the hospital, where is the most common injury to the thoracic aorta?**
A tear across the intima and media just distal to the takeoff of the left subclavian artery. Because the adventitia is intact, the patient does not immediately exsanguinate, and, if the lesion is detected promptly and treated, the survival rate is 85%.

14. **What are the clinical signs of torn thoracic aorta?**
There are no definitive signs. Suspicion must be based on mechanism of injury (rapid deceleration). The physical signs associated with aortic disruption are not commonly observed; they include upper extremity hypertension, unequal upper extremity pressures, loss of lower extremity pulses, and expanding hematoma in the root of the neck.

15. **What findings on chest radiograph are associated with rupture of the descending thoracic aorta?**
Like physical signs, no initial radiographic signs are definitive. The signs that have been associated with torn thoracic aorta include indistinct aortic knob, widened mediastinum (>8 cm at the level of the aortic knob), apical cap, left pleural effusion, depression of the left mainstem bronchus, rightward displacement of the esophagus (look for the nasogastric tube), first rib fractures, displacement of the trachea and loss of the aortopulmonary window. Approximately 15% of patients with torn aorta have a normal mediastinum, and 7% have a completely normal chest radiograph.

16. **In the stable patient with a major mechanism of injury or chest radiographs consistent with aortic injury, how is the diagnosis made?**
Dynamic helical computed tomography (CT) of the chest approaches 100% sensitivity for detecting aortic injury; it is widely available and applicable to all stable patients. Aortography can more precisely identify the site and extent of injury, but has largely been supplanted by CT angiography.

17. **Junior O'Flaherty was hit in the chest with a baseball bat. How can I tell if he has a bruise on his heart (myocardial contusion)?**
You can't unless you are doing his autopsy.

18. **Ok, then, how do I tell if something bad is going to happen to Junior's heart?**
From a practical standpoint, only two things happen to the bruised heart: arrhythmia and pump failure. By far the most common manifestation of blunt cardiac injury is arrhythmia. Patients with an initial electrocardiogram (ECG) that is normal have an exceedingly small chance of developing clinically significant arrhythmias during their hospital course. Any ECG abnormality is an indication for admission and 24 hours of cardiac monitoring. Hemodynamic compromise from blunt cardiac injury is unusual and not subtle; echocardiography should be employed in patients with evidence of impaired contractility. Cardiac enzymes are poor predictors of arrhythmia or pump failure and are not recommended.

19. **Where do blunt injuries to the bronchus usually occur? How do they present?**
Within a few centimeters of the carina. The mainstem bronchi are splayed apart with severe anteroposterior compression of the chest. As the lungs are displaced laterally, the mainstem bronchi may tear near the site where they are fixed at the carina. The typical presentation is subcutaneous air, massive air leak, or failure to reexpand the lung ("dropped lung") after tube thoracostomy.

20. **What are the indications for emergency department thoracotomy after blunt chest injury?**
Cardiovascular collapse after arrival in the emergency department (ED). The outcome, however, is typically dismal; less than 1% of patients survive neurologically intact.

21. **What is traumatic asphyxia?**
Traumatic asphyxia is the result of a protracted crush injury to the upper torso or epigastrium. In such an injury, venous hypertension is transmitted to the valveless veins of the upper body. Patients present with altered sensorium, petechial hemorrhages, cyanosis, and edema of the upper body. Although its initial presentation can be dramatic, with supportive care the outcome is usually good.

KEY POINTS

1. Most blunt chest injuries—even significant ones—can be treated without operation. A chest tube and pain control is usually the most that is needed.

2. Tension pneumothorax is a preterminal event and should be treated immediately with a hole in the chest.

3. Do not bankrupt the hospital searching for a bruise on a patient's heart. Check his ECG and make sure it is pumping.

4. Patients leaking lots of air out of their lungs might have a tear in a major bronchus.

5. Rapid deceleration can result in a tear in the descending thoracic aorta. Despite a normal chest radiograph, patients with this mechanism deserve a CT scan.

BIBLIOGRAPHY

1. Allen GS, Coates NE: Pulmonary contusion: a collective review. Am Surg 62:895, 1996.
2. Branney SW, Moore EE, Feldhaus KM et al.: Critical analysis of two decades of experience with postinjury emergency department thoracotomy in a regional trauma center. J Trauma 45:87, 1998.
3. Bulger EM, Arneson MA, Mock CN et al.: Rib fractures in the Elderly. J Trauma 48:1040, 2000.
4. Demetriades D, Velmahos GC, Scalea TM et al.: Operative repair or endovascular stent graft in blunt traumatic thoracic aortic injuries: the AAST multicenter study. J Trauma 64:561, 2008.

5. Dyer DS, Moore EE, Ilke DN et al.: Thoracic aortic injury: how predictive is mechanism and is chest CT a reliable screening tool? A prospective study of 1500 patients. J Trauma 48:673, 2000.

6. Flagel BT, Luchette FA, Reed L et al.: Half-a-dozen ribs: the breakpoint for mortality. Surgery 138:717, 2005.

7. Gomez-Caro A, Ausin P, Moradiliellos FJ et al.: Role of conservative management of tracheobronchial injuries. J Trauma 61:1426, 2006.

8. Karmy-Jones R, Jrukovich GJ, Nathens AB et al.: Timing of urgent thoracotomy for hemorrhage after trauma: a multicenter study. Arch Surg 136:513, 2001.

9. Kiser AC, O'Brien SM, Detterbeck FC: Blunt tracheobronchial injuries: treatment and outcome. Ann Thorac Surg 71:2059, 2001.

10. Yeong EK, Chen MT, Chu SH: Traumatic asphyxia. Plast Reconstr Surg 93:739, 1994.

CHAPTER 21

PENETRATING THORACIC TRAUMA

Jeffrey L. Johnson, MD, and Ernest E. Moore, MD

1. **How often do patients with penetrating chest wounds need an operation?**
   Most penetrating injuries seen in civilian practice are from knives and low-energy handguns. Consequently, although injuries to the chest wall and lung are common, the vast majority can be treated with tube thoracostomy alone. Formal thoracotomy or median sternotomy is required in less than 15% of isolated penetrating chest injuries.

2. **What are the indications for emergency department thoracotomy after penetrating chest wounds?**
   Patients who arrive within 15 minutes of circulatory collapse (or arrest after arrival) can benefit from an emergency department thoracotomy (EDT). Unlike blunt injury, a treatable cause is more commonly found after penetrating injury (e.g., pericardial tamponade). EDT results in a survival of about 20% in this setting.

3. **What is the "6-hour rule" for chest injuries?**
   An upright chest radiograph with no evidence of pneumothorax after 6 hours makes a delayed pneumothorax or occult injury to an intrathoracic organ unlikely. The 6-hour rule identifies patients who can be safely discharged.

4. **How much blood in the pleural space can be reliably detected by chest radiograph?**
   250 ml or more.

5. **If a stable patient with a penetrating chest wound has a lot of blood coming out of a chest tube, when should I operate?**
   A good rule of thumb is that immediate return of over 1500 ml of blood or ongoing bleeding in excess of 250 ml/hr for 3 consecutive hours should prompt operation. All unstable patients deserve an operation.

6. **What is a "clam shell" thoracotomy?**
   Bilateral anterolateral thoracotomies with extension across the sternum. This procedure allows rapid access to pleural spaces, pulmonary hilae, and the mediastinum.

7. **What is an open pneumothorax?**
   A defect in the chest wall that is open to the pleural space. In penetrating chest injuries, it most often is the result of a close-range shotgun blast.

8. **How is an open pneumothorax treated?**
   The defect in the chest wall should be covered with a dressing that is fixed on only three sides. This temporary fix prevents entry of more air into the pleural space while allowing egress of air under pressure. A chest tube is then inserted. Formal repair of the chest wall can wait until other significant injuries are excluded.

9. **Where is "the box," and why is it important?**

The box describes an area on the anterior chest where a wound should prompt concern about an underlying cardiac injury. Its borders are the midclavicular lines from clavicle to costal margin. Although the typical patient with a penetrating cardiac injury has a wound in the box, the heart also can be reached from the root of the neck, axilla, and epigastrium.

10. **What is Beck's triad? Is it useful in penetrating chest injuries?**

Beck's triad consists of hypotension, distended neck veins, and muffled heart tones. These signs are difficult to appreciate in the trauma patient (particularly muffled heart sounds in a busy resuscitation room) and present in a minority of patients with tamponade from penetrating injuries (less than 40%). The absence of distended neck veins might be expected because most patients have concomitant hypovolemia.

11. **In a stable patient with suspected penetrating cardiac injury, what is the most important initial study?**

After completion of the primary survey (airways, breathing, circulation), bedside ultrasonography should be performed. This rapid, sensitive method for detecting pericardial fluid will identify the results of cardiac injury. Although the initial study may be negative with a small effusion, serial examinations detect virtually all cases.

12. **Junior O'Flaherty just got stabbed in the heart. What is he likely to die of?**

Cardiac tamponade. Knife wounds usually make a slit-like opening in the pericardium, which seals off with clot after the heart bleeds into the pericardial sac. Exsanguination is uncommon; tamponade is the most common threat to life.

13. **What is the initial therapeutic maneuver in the patient with a penetrating cardiac wound who is not yet hypotensive?**

Percutaneous pericardial drainage. One of the early effects of tamponade is subendocardial ischemia, which puts the patient at risk for refractory arrhythmias. Immediate decompression of the pericardium ensures safer transport to the operating room (OR) for definitive repair. Suxiphoid pericardial window is also an option (and popular on television), but ultrasound-guided decompression is the best choice.

14. **In a penetrating chest wound, how do I tell if the diaphragm is also injured?**

At end expiration, the dome of the diaphragm reaches the level of the nipples. In principle, then, any patient with penetrating injury below the level of the nipples may have an injury to the diaphragm. Computed tomography (CT) scanning is not reliable unless it shows obvious herniation of abdominal viscera into the chest. Diagnostic peritoneal lavage (DPL) is the preferred initial procedure. If the DPL fluid comes out a chest tube, there is a hole in the diaphragm. Absent this finding, the red blood cell count can also be used as a guide. Red blood cell counts less than $1000/mm^3$ are negative. Counts >10,000 are positive; for counts of 1000 to 10,000, thoracoscopy or laparoscopy is often used to visualize the hemidiaphragm at risk.

15. **Why is it important to detect a small diaphragmatic laceration?**

Abdominal viscera herniate from the positive-pressure abdominal cavity into the negative-pressure pleural space. The morbidity of a strangulated diaphragmatic hernia is not trivial, often because of delay in diagnosis. It is best to identify the hole at the time of the initial injury!

16. **Junior O'Flaherty was shot all the way through his mediastinum. He seems stable: does he need an operation?**

Probably not. Surprisingly, most wounds that appear to pass completely across the chest do not injure a critical structure. In fact, only about 35% of stable patients require exploration. Junior should be evaluated with history (odynophagia? hoarseness?), physical examination (deep cervical emphysema? expanding hematoma? pulseless extremity?), and CT scan to assess trajectory and evaluate for injury. If the bullet tract indicates critical structures are at risk, follow-up angiography, bronchoscopy, and esophagoscopy may be necessary.

17. Are prophylactic antibiotics warranted to prevent empyema after tube thoracostomy?

Meta-analysis of currently published randomized studies on prophylactic antibiotics for tube thoracostomy suggests a benefit. The number of doses required is unclear; further, the use in patients with blunt multisystem injuries may be questioned because of the risk of emergence of resistance.

18. What is the most important risk factor for posttraumatic empyema?

Persistent hemothorax. Blood is an excellent incubation medium for bacteria; therefore, expedient evacuation of blood from the pleural space via tube thoracostomy or video-assisted thoracoscopic surgery is central in the management of traumatic hemothorax (starve the bugs!).

19. What is a bronchovenous air embolism?

An air embolism occurs when gas under pressure leaks from a lacerated bronchus into an adjacent lacerated pulmonary vein. Air then travels to the left side of the heart and into the coronary arteries. The classic presentation is a patient with a penetrating chest injury who arrests after intubation and application of positive-pressure ventilation.

20. How is bronchovenous air embolism diagnosed and treated?

Diagnosis is based only on the typical history (see question 18). Therapy is directed toward removal of air from the left ventricle and coronary arteries: Trendelenberg (head down) position with right side down, immediate thoracotomy and aspiration of the apex of the left ventricle, the aortic root, and occasionally the coronary arteries.

21. In a penetrating esophageal injury, where may air be evident on physical examination?

The deep subcutaneous tissues of the neck. In the upright position, air in the mediastinum dissects into a plane continuous with the deep cervical fascia.

22. How do penetrating tracheobronchial injuries present?

Laceration of the trachea and major bronchi presents with subcutaneous emphysema, hemoptysis, and dyspnea. Chest radiographs reveal a pneumothorax or pneumomediastinum. After tube thoracostomy, continuous air leak and failure of the lung to reexpand ("dropped lung") should prompt suspicion of a major bronchial injury.

23. What does a blurry bullet on a chest radiograph indicate?

A bullet lodged in the myocardium. Movement of the heart causes the image to be blurry on the radiograph. Beware the blurry bullet.

KEY POINTS

1. Most patients with a hole in their chest do not need an operation. A chest tube is usually the only definitive treatment necessary.

2. If there is not a pneumothorax after 6 hours, the patient is unlikely to have a significant chest injury.

3. If a weapon penetrates the anterior chest in the box, use an ultrasound to look for pericardial blood.

4. Cardiac tamponade is what is likely to kill you after a stab wound to the heart.

5. Diaphragm injuries are important to find, but hard to detect accurately.

6. If a patient with a stab wound to the chest arrests after intubation, a bronchovenous air embolism should be suspected.

BIBLIOGRAPHY

1. Branney SW, Moore EE, Feldhaus KM et al.: Critical analysis of two decades of experience with postinjury emergency department thoracotomy in a regional trauma center. J Trauma 45:87-95, 1998.

2. Cothren CC, Moore EE, Biffl WL et al.: Lung-sparing techniques are associated with improved outcome compared with anatomic resection for severe lung injuries. J Trauma 53:483, 2002.

3. Ibirogba S, Nicol AN, Navsaria PH: Screening helical computed tomography scanning in hemodynamically stable patients with transmediastinal gunshot wounds. Injury 38:48, 2007.

4. Karmy-Jones R, Nathens A, Jurkovich GJ et al.: Urgent and emergent thoracotomy for penetrating chest trauma. J Trauma 56:664, 2004.

5. Mandal AK, Sanusi M: Penetrating chest wounds: 24 years experience. World J Surg 25:1145-1149, 2001.

6. Nagy KK, Lohmann C, Kim DO et al.: Role of echocardiography in the diagnosis of occult penetrating cardiac injury. J Trauma 38:859-862, 1995.

7. Rhee PM, Foy H, Kaufmann C et al.: Penetrating cardiac injuries: a population-based study. J Trauma 45: 366-370, 1998.

8. Stassen AA, Lukan JK, Spain DA et al.: Reevaluation of diagnostic procedures for transmediastinal gunshot wounds. J Trauma 53:635-638, 2002.

CHAPTER 22

BLUNT ABDOMINAL TRAUMA

David J. Ciesla, MD, MS, and Ernest E. Moore, MD

1. **What elements of the history are important in evaluating a patient with suspected blunt abdominal trauma (BAT)?**

   First, the mechanism of injury (e.g., motor vehicle collision, automobile-pedestrian accident, fall) is important. In motor vehicle accidents, note the position of the victim in the car, velocity of impact (high, moderate, or low), type of accident (front, lateral, or rear impact; side swipe; or rollover), and type of restraint used (shoulder restraint, air bag, or lap belt). Information about damage to the vehicle, such as a broken windshield or bent steering wheel, may raise suspicion of cervical and chest injuries. In a fall, it is important to note the distance fallen and the site of anatomic impact. Vertical landing on the feet or in a sitting position causes a different pattern of injury than lateral landing on the side. Serial vital signs and mental status are always important.

2. **Is physical examination accurate in the diagnosis of intraabdominal injury?**

   No. The examination results may be normal in up to 50% of patients with acute intraabdominal bleeding. Signs of intraabdominal injury include abrasions and contusions over the lower chest and abdomen; subcutaneous emphysema or palpable rib fracture; clinically evident pelvic fracture; abdominal pain, tenderness, guarding, or rigidity; blood in the urine or urethral meatus; high-riding prostate or blood on rectal examination; and microscopic hematuria.

3. **Which organs are most frequently injured in BAT?**

Liver, 50%	Colon, 5%
Spleen, 40%	Duodenum, 5%
Mesentery, 10%	Vascular, 4%
Urologic, 10%	Stomach, 2%
Pancreas, 10%	Gallbladder, 2%
Small bowel, 10%	

4. **What diagnostic studies are helpful in BAT?**
   1. **Ultrasound:** reliably identifies peritoneal fluid (blood) and pericardial fluid but may miss up to 25% of isolated solid organ injuries.
   2. **Computed tomography (CT) scan:** identifies the presence and severity of solid organ injury (liver and spleen), detects intraabdominal air and fluid (blood, mucus, urine), and aids in evaluation of pelvic fractures. CT scanning can also identify bowel, pancreatic, renal, and bladder injuries. The sensitivity and specificity of CT scans for diagnosing injury in BAT continues to improve with newer generation scanners.

3. **Diagnostic peritoneal lavage (DPL):** grossly positive DPL (>10 ml blood returned by aspiration of the catheter) indicates significant hemoperitoneum. Positive by cell count after infusion of 1 L of crystalloid fluid (>100, red blood cells/mm^3, presence of bile or fibers) indicates intraabdominal bleeding, injury to hollow viscus, or hepatobiliary system injury. Lavage fluid exiting through a chest tube or urinary catheter indicates diaphragmatic or bladder injury.

5. **How has the availability of ultrasound changed the initial evaluation of BAT?**
The focused abdominal sonography in trauma (FAST) examination has largely supplanted the DPL. The FAST examination can be performed in a hemodynamically unstable patient during the early secondary survey with immediate transfer to the operating room (OR) when hemoperitoneum is identified. CT scan is safe in the hemodynamically stable patient. DPL is still useful when ultrasound (US) is equivocal or not available. DPL is also useful to evaluate for the presence of hollow viscus injury in cases in which free fluid is present on CT scan in the absence of solid organ injury.

6. **How is hollow organ injury diagnosed?**
Hollow organ injury is usually detected by physical examination (peritonitis in the awake patients) or at the time of laparotomy for hemorrhage control. CT findings include peritoneal fluid without solid organ injury, extravasation of oral contrast into the peritoneal cavity, and free intraabdominal air. Suggestive signs include mesenteric stranding and hematoma. Peritoneal lavage results suggestive of hollow organ injury include elevated amylase, alkaline phosphatase, or biliribun levels and the presence of particulate matter.

7. **What are the indications for urgent operation in a patient with BAT?**
Any hemodynamically unstable patient who exhibits significant hemoperitoneum (by US or DPL) requires emergency laparotomy. Other indications for urgent laparotomy include free intraabdominal air and evidence of hollow viscus injury.

8. **How does time in the emergency department (ED) impact the mortality of patients requiring emergent operation for BAT?**
The probability of death from trauma is related to both the extent of hypotension and the interval from the time of injury to definitive surgery. An estimated increase in mortality of 1% is incurred for every 3 minutes spent in the emergency department (ED) up to 90 minutes.

9. **What is the role of angiographic embolization?**
Angiographic embolization may be effective for hemorrhage control in hemodynamically stable patients. Favorable embolization sites include liver, spleen, and kidney injuries; lumbar arteries with retroperitoneal hemorrhage; and pelvic blood vessels associated with pelvic fracture.

10. **What is the "bloody viscus cycle"?**
The bloody viscus cycle is a syndrome of hypothermia, acidosis, and coagulopathy that occurs with profound hemorrhagic shock and massive transfusion. It represents a circular cascade of events in which severe hemorrhagic shock accompanied by metabolic failure provokes a coagulopathy that exacerbates further bleeding.

11. **What is a staged or abbreviated laparotomy (damage control surgery)?**
Staged laparotomy is terminated before all definitive procedures are completed with the intent to return to the OR to complete the operation at a later (and safer) time. The purpose of this approach is to delay additional surgical stress until the patient is in a more favorable physiologic state. The objectives of the initial operation become to (1) arrest bleeding and correct coagulopathy; (2) limit peritoneal contamination and the secondary inflammatory response (to control gastrointestinal [GI] spillage); and (3) enclose the abdominal contents to protect viscera and limit heat, fluid, and protein loss from an open abdomen.

12. **When is staged laparotomy used in trauma patients?**
    - Inability to achieve hemostasis because of recalcitrant coagulopathy (pack the bleeding).
    - Inaccessible major venous injury (retrohepatic caval injury).
    - Demand for control of a life-threatening extraabdominal (e.g., head or thoracic) injury.
    - Inability to close the abdominal incision because of extensive visceral edema.
    - Need to reassess the abdominal contents because of questionable viability at the time of the initial operation.

KEY POINTS: USEFUL DIAGNOSTIC MODALITIES

1. Primary and secondary surveys are crucial, but further diagnostic testing is required in most patients.
2. FAST: reliably identifies intraabdominal and intrapericardial fluid but is poor at hollow viscus evaluation.
3. DPL: effective for evaluation of hemoperitoneum and a useful adjunct along with FAST examination.
4. CT: excellent modality with 99.97% negative predictive value for BAT.

WEBSITE

www.east.org/tpg/bluntabd.pdf

BIBLIOGRAPHY

1. Clarke JR, Trooskin SZ, Doshi PJ et al.: Time to laparotomy for intra-abdominal bleeding from trauma does affect survival for delays up to 90 minutes. J Trauma 52:420, 2002.
2. Davis KA, Fabian TC, Croce MA et al.: Improved success in management of blunt splenic injuries: embolization of splenic artery pseudoaneurysms. J Trauma 44:1008, 1998.
3. Peitzman AB, Harbrecht BG, Rivera L et al.: Failure of observation of blunt splenic injury in adults: variability in practice and adverse consequences. J Am Coll Surg 201:179, 2005.
4. Rodriguez C, Barone JE, Willbanks TO et al.: Isolated free fluid on computed tomographic scan in blunt abdominal trauma: a systematic review of incidence and management. J Trauma 53:79, 2002.
5. Stengal D, Bauwens K, Sehouli J et al.: Emergency ultrasound based algorithms for diagnosing blunt abdominal trauma. Cochrane Database Syst Rev 18:CD004446, 2005.
6. Tien H, Spencer F, Tremblay L et al.: Preventable deaths from hemorrhage at a level 1 Canadian trauma center. J Trauma 62:142, 2007.

CHAPTER 23

PENETRATING ABDOMINAL TRAUMA

C. Clay Cothren, MD, and Ernest E. Moore, MD

1. **Why is the evaluation different for patients with stab wounds versus gunshot wounds?**

   Although one third of stab wounds (SWs) to the anterior abdomen do not penetrate the peritoneum, 80% of gunshot wounds (GSWs) violate the peritoneum. Additionally, of those wounds that penetrate the peritoneum, 95% of GSWs have associated visceral or vascular injuries while only one third of SWs do (see Fig. 23-1).

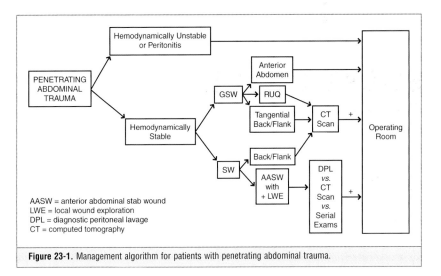

Figure 23-1. Management algorithm for patients with penetrating abdominal trauma.

2. **What are the indications for emergent laparotomy in patients with stab wounds?**

   Hypotension, peritonitis, and obvious signs of abdominal visceral injury (hematemesis; proctorrhagia; palpation of diaphragmatic defect on chest tube insertion; radiologic evidence of injury to the gastrointestinal [GI] tract) mandate immediate exploration. Most authorities also advocated prompt exploration for omental or intestinal evisceration.

3. **What are the indications for immediate laparotomy in patients with gunshot wounds?**

   Because of the high incidence of visceral injury, early exploration is indicated for all GSWs that violate the peritoneum. The exception is penetrating trauma isolated to the right upper quadrant; in hemodynamically stable patients with bullet trajectory confined to the liver by computed tomography (CT) scan, nonoperative observation may be considered. Similarly, in obese patients if the GSW is thought to be tangential through the subcutaneous tissues, CT scan can delineate the tract and exclude peritoneal violation. Laparoscopy is another option to assess peritoneal penetration, and may be followed by laparotomy to repair injuries. If in doubt, it is always safer to explore the abdomen than to equivocate.

4. **When is emergency department thoracotomy indicated for a penetrating abdominal wound?**
   Resuscitative thoracotomy should be considered when a patient presents in cardiac arrest (cardiopulmonary resuscitation [CPR] <15 minutes) or with profound hypotension (systolic blood pressure [SBP] <70 mm Hg) that is refractory to initial resuscitation. Following anterolateral thoracotomy, the descending aorta is cross-clamped to decrease subdiaphragmatic hemorrhage and improve coronary and cerebral perfusion. Open cardiac massage is performed if necessary.

5. **What are the key elements of the secondary survey?**
   Examine the patient systematically; it is easy to overlook synchronous injuries. The examination includes looking for additional entry or exit sites; be sure to look thoroughly in the axilla and perineum as wounds can be hidden in folds of skin. Evaluation for blood in the GI, genitourinary (GU), and gynecologic systems should be done, and associated blunt mechanisms of injury should be considered; some unfortunate patients are assaulted with both knives and fists (see Fig. 23-2).

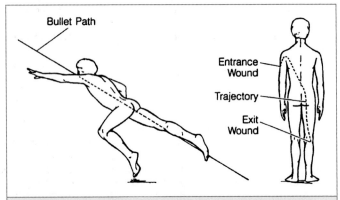

Figure 23-2. An example of how the path of a bullet through a contorted body can produce confusion when the patient is examined in the ED. An entrance wound will be found at the left upper arm and an exit wound at the medial aspect of the right knee. The bullet could have damaged any structure between these two wounds when the patient's body was contorted.

6. **What are the appropriate initial studies?**
   In stable patients, a chest radiograph excludes hemothorax or pneumothorax and determines the position of intravenous (IV) catheters (e.g., endotracheal, nasogastric [NG], and pleural tubes). Biplanar abdominal radiographs are helpful in locating retained foreign bodies (i.e., bullets) and may reveal pneumoperitoneum. The location of entrance and exit wounds, identified with a radiopaque marker applied to the skin, may be helpful in determining the trajectory of missiles. Injuries in proximity to the rectum obligate sigmoidoscopy

(see Chapter 27), and those with proximity to the urinary tract should be evaluated with CT scanning (see Chapter 30).

7. **What is the difference between a penetrating wound to the anterior abdomen versus the flank or back?**
Because the incidence of injury is higher for anterior wounds, and injuries are within the peritoneal cavity, diagnostic evaluation differs.

8. **How is an anterior abdominal stab wound evaluated in asymptomatic patients?**
The first step is local exploration of the wound to determine peritoneal penetration. If the tract clearly terminates superficially, above the fascia, no further evaluation is required and the patient is discharged from the emergency department (ED). If the fascia is penetrated or the peritoneum violated, further evaluation is warranted. The optimal diagnostic approach remains debated between serial examination, diagnostic peritoneal lavage (DPL), and CT scanning.

9. **What constitutes a positive diagnostic peritoneal lavage result after penetrating trauma?**
A grossly positive tap (aspiration of >10 mL; of blood or aspiration of GI or biliary contents) mandates immediate exploration. A negative initial aspirate result is followed by the instillation of 1000 ml of saline (15 ml/kg in children) into the abdomen through a dialysis catheter, followed by gravity drainage of the fluid back into the saline bag. The finding of >100,000/μL red blood cells (RBCs), >500 μL white blood cells (WBCs), amylase >20 IU/L, alkaline phosphatase >3 IU/L, or elevated bilirubin level are also indications for exploration.

10. **How are stab wounds to the flank and back evaluated in asymptomatic patients?**
The incidence of significant injuries is 10% for SWs to the back and 25% for SWs to the flank. SWs to the flank and back should undergo triple-contrast CT to detect occult retroperitoneal injuries of the colon, duodenum, and urinary tract. The most valuable aspect of CT scanning is determining the wound trajectory.

11. **How is a lower chest stab wound evaluated?**
Stab wounds to the lower chest are associated with abdominal visceral injury in 15% of cases, whereas gunshot wounds to the lower chest are associated with abdominal visceral injury in nearly 50% of cases. The lower chest is defined as the area between the nipple line (fourth intercostal space) anteriorly, the tip of the scapula (seventh intercostal space) posteriorly, and the costal margins inferiorly. Because the diaphragm reaches the fourth intercostal space during expiration, the abdominal organs are at risk of injury even after what appears to be an "isolated chest" wound. Thus, wounds to the lower chest should also be managed as abdominal wounds to rule out intraabdominal injury. Occult injury to the diaphragm must be ruled out in patients with SWs to the lower chest. Patients undergoing DPL evaluation have different laboratory value cut-offs than standard anterior abdominal stab wounds. A red blood cell count of more than 10,000/μL is considered positive, and an indication for laparotomy whereas patients with a DPL red blood cell count between 1,000/μL and 10,000/μL should undergo laparoscopy or thoracoscopy.

12. **Which patients with abdominal gunshot wounds are candidates for nonoperative management?**
Hemodynamically stable patients with tangential, subcutaneous missile tracts or those with isolated hepatic trauma. Selective management of GSWs to the back and flank are based on triple-contrast CT scan results.

13. **If abdominal operative exploration is indicated, what is the general approach?**
A midline abdominal incision provides rapid entry and wide exposure; it may be extended as a median sternotomy to access the chest. The aorta should be palpated just below the diaphragm to assess the patient's blood pressure (BP). Liquid and clotted blood is evacuated with multiple laparotomy pads and suction to identify the major source(s) of active bleeding. After localizing the source of hemorrhage, direct digital occlusion (vascular injury) or laparotomy pad packing (solid organ injury) are used to control bleeding. Hollow visceral injuries are temporarily isolated with noncrushing clamps or are rapidly oversewn. The entire abdomen is systematically explored before undertaking extensive repairs so that injuries can be prioritized for definitive treatment.

KEY POINTS

1. GSWs to the abdomen generally require operative exploration; an exception could be right upper quadrant wounds with isolated hepatic injury.

2. Following an SW, patients with hypotension, peritonitis, or evisceration should undergo operative exploration.

3. Anterior abdominal SWs in stable patients are initially evaluated with local wound exploration; penetration of the peritoneum requires further evaluation (serial examination, DPL, or CT scan).

4. Flank and back SWs in stable patients are evaluated with triple-contrast CT scan.

CONTROVERSY

14. **What is the role of laparoscopy and thoracoscopy after penetrating abdominal trauma?**
Although an intriguing diagnostic modality with additional therapeutic capabilities, laparoscopy thus far appears to have limited application after trauma. With the exception of suspected diaphragmatic injury, an isolated solid organ injury, or evaluation for peritoneal penetration, laparoscopy has yet to demonstrate advantages over the algorithm delineated previously. The potential for missed injuries, poor evaluation of the retroperitoneum, and expense are major drawbacks.

BIBLIOGRAPHY

1. Biffl WL, Cothren CC, Brasel KJ et al.: A prospective observational multicenter study of the optimal management of patients with anterior abdominal stab wounds. J Trauma 64:250, 2008.

2. Boyle EM Jr, Maier RV, Salazar JD et al.: Diagnosis of injuries after stab wounds to the back and flank. J Trauma 42:260, 1997.

3. Chiu WC, Shanmuganathan K, Mirvis SE et al.: Determining the need for laparotomy in penetrating torso trauma: a prospective study using triple-contrast enhanced abdominopelvic computed tomography. J Trauma 51:860-868, 2001.

4. Demetriades D, Hadjizacharia P, Constantinou C et al.: Selective nonoperative management of penetrating abdominal solid organ injuries. Ann Surg 244:620, 2006.

5. Freeman RK, Al-Dossari G, Hutcheson KA et al.: Indications for using video-assisted thoracoscopic surgery to diagnose diaphragmatic injuries after penetrating chest trauma. Ann Thorac Surg 72:342-347, 2001.

6. Henneman PL, Marx JA, Moore EE et al.: Diagnostic peritoneal lavage: accuracy in predicting necessary laparotomy following blunt and penetrating trauma. J Trauma 30:1345-1355, 1990.

7. McAnena OJ, Marx JA, Moore EE: Peritoneal lavage enzyme determinations following blunt and penetrating abdominal trauma. J Trauma 31:1161-1164, 1991.

8. Moore EE, Marx JA: Penetrating abdominal wounds: a rationale for exploratory laparotomy. JAMA 253:2705-2708, 1985.

9. Reber PU, Schmied B, Seiler CA et al.: Missed diaphragmatic injuries and their long-term sequelae. J Trauma 44:183-188, 1998.

10. Simon RJ, Rabin J, Kuhls D: Impact of increased use of laparoscopy on negative laparotomy rates after penetrating trauma. J Trauma 53:297-302, 2002.

CHAPTER 24

HEPATIC AND BILIARY TRAUMA

Jarrod N. Keith, MD, and Ernest E. Moore, MD

1. **How often is the liver injured in trauma?**
   The liver is both big and central, so it is vulnerable to blunt trauma and an easy target for penetrating wounds.

2. **Do the liver and spleen respond similarly to injury?**
   No. The liver has a unique ability to establish spontaneous hemostasis even with extensive injuries. For this reason, the majority of liver injuries in hemodynamically stable patients can be managed nonoperatively. In contrast, many splenic fractures continue to bleed; therefore, a greater percentage of patients with splenic injuries require operative intervention.

3. **What are the determinants of mortality after acute liver injury?**
   The mechanism of injury, grade of injury, and the associated abdominal organs injured determine mortality. The mortality for stab wounds (SWs) to the liver is 2%; for gunshot wounds (GSWs), 8%; and for blunt injuries, 15%. The mortality rate for isolated grade III hepatic injuries is 2%; for grade IV, 20%; and for grade V, 65%. Retrohepatic vena cava injuries carry mortality rates of 80% for penetrating trauma and 95% for blunt trauma.

4. **What history and physical signs suggest acute liver injury?**
   Any patient sustaining blunt abdominal trauma (BAT) with hypotension must be assumed to have a liver injury until proven otherwise. Specific signs that increase the likelihood of hepatic injury are contusion over the right lower chest, fracture of the right lower ribs (especially posterior fractures of ribs 9 to 12), and penetrating injuries to the right lower chest (below the fourth intercostal space, flank, and upper abdomen). Physical signs of hemoperitoneum may be absent in as many as one third of patients with significant hepatic injury.

5. **What diagnostic tests are helpful in confirming acute liver injury?**
   Diagnostic peritoneal lavage (DPL) is sensitive for hemoperitoneum (99%), but not specific for liver injury. Ultrasound (US) is highly sensitive in identifying >200 ml of intraperitoneal fluid. It is noninvasive and may be repeated at frequent intervals, but it is relatively poor for staging liver injuries. Abdominal computed tomography (CT) scan currently is used in patients who are hemodynamically stable that are candidates for nonoperative management. Grading of liver injuries by CT scan is useful in determining the success rate of nonoperative management because higher grade injuries are more likely to require intervention.

6. **What is the role of hepatic angiography?**
   Selective hepatic artery embolization is effective therapy for hepatic arterial bleeding, both for avoidance of surgery and for recurrent postoperative bleeding. Embolization should be considered for patients with active contrast extravasation into the peritoneum seen on CT scan because they are less likely to tamponade.

SURGICAL ANATOMY OF THE LIVER

7. **How many anatomic lobes are present in the liver? What is their topographic boundary?**

The liver is divided into two anatomic lobes, the right and the left. Their boundary lies in an oblique plane extending from the gallbladder fossa anteriorly to the inferior vena cava (IVC) posteriorly. The three hepatic veins define the division between the lobar segments and the planes of surgical resection. Lobar segments are numbered I to VIII, according to Couinaud's nomenclature (see Fig. 24-1).

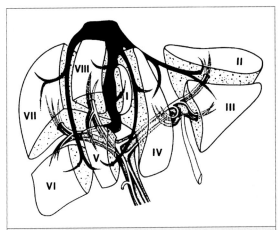

Figure 24-1. The functional division of the liver and the segments according to Couinaud's nomenclature. (From Bismuth H: Surgical anatomy and anatomical surgery of the liver, World J Surg 6:6, 1982, with permission.)

8. **What is the blood supply to the liver and the relative contribution of each structure to hepatic oxygenation?**

The hepatic artery supplies approximately 30% of the blood flow to the liver and 50% of its oxygen supply. The portal vein provides 70% of the liver's blood flow and 50% of its oxygen. The relative significance of arterial flow in cirrhotic patients is greater; therefore, hepatic artery ligation is not recommended in patients with cirrhosis.

9. **What are the most common variations in hepatic arterial supply to the right and left lobes of the liver?**

In most people, the common hepatic artery originates from the celiac axis and divides into right and left hepatic arterial branches within the porta hepatis. Approximately 15% of people have a replaced right hepatic artery (sole arterial supply to the right lobe) that originates from the superior mesenteric artery (SMA). A replaced right hepatic artery always supplies a cystic artery; thus, ligation should be followed by cholecystectomy. A replaced left hepatic artery (approximately 15% of people) arises from the left gastric artery; it may be the sole blood supply to the left lobe or may contribute to blood supply in conjunction with a normal left hepatic artery. In 5% of people, the hepatic arterial supply does not arise from the celiac axis.

In these people, either the right and left hepatic arteries are replaced or a single main hepatic trunk derives from the SMA.

10. **What is the venous drainage of the liver?**
The right, middle, and left hepatic veins are the major venous tributaries and enter the IVC below the right hemidiaphragm.

OPERATIVE MANAGEMENT OF LIVER INJURY

11. **How are acute liver injuries classified?**
Liver wounds are generally graded on a scale of I to VI according the depth of parenchymal laceration and involvement of the hepatic veins or retrohepatic portion of the IVC. Optimal methods of obtaining hemostasis vary with the severity of the injury (see Table 24-1).

TABLE 24-1. LIVER INJURY SCALE

Injury Grade	Subcapsular Hematoma	Lacertion	Parenchymal Hematoma	Vascular
		Description of Injury		
I	<10% surface area	1 cm in depth	—	—
II	10%–50% surface area	1–3 cm in depth	≦10 cm in length	—
III	>50% surface area	>3 cm in depth	>10 cm in length	—
IV	—	25%–75% of the lobe or 1–3 Couinaud segments	—	—
V	—	>75% of the lobe or >3 Couinaud segments	—	Retrohepatic inferior vena cava or major hepatic veins

Data from Moore EE, Cogbill TH, Jurkovich GJ et al.: Organ injury scaling: spleen and liver (1994 revision), J Trauma 38:323-324, 1995.

12. **Do all patients with a traumatic liver injury require surgery?**
No. Nonoperative treatment is the standard for victims of blunt trauma who remain hemodynamically stable (approximately 85% of patients). One third of such patients require blood transfusions, but if the volume exceeds 6 units in the first 24 hours, angiography should be done. CT scan should be repeated in 5 to 7 days for grade IV and V injuries. Complications, including perihepatic infection, biloma, bilhemia, and hemobilia, have been reported in 10% of nonoperative patients.

13. **Which patients are more likely to fail nonoperative management?**
Those patients requiring ongoing fluid resuscitation to maintain hemodynamic stability, pooling or blush of contrast seen on CT scan, and those with injuries to multiple solid organs.

14. **What are the options for temporary control of significant hemorrhage in victims of hepatic trauma?**

Ongoing hemorrhage leads to the vicious cycle of acidosis, hypothermia, and coagulopathy. Manual compression, perihepatic packing, angioembolization, and the Pringle maneuver are the most effective temporary strategies.

15. **What is the Pringle maneuver?**

The Pringle maneuver is a manual or vascular clamp occlusion of the hepatoduodenal ligament to interrupt blood flow into the liver. Included in the hepatoduodenal ligament are the hepatic artery, portal vein, and common bile duct. Failure of the Pringle maneuver to control liver hemorrhage suggests either (1) injury to the retrohepatic vena cava or hepatic vein or (2) arterial supply from an aberrant right or left hepatic artery (see question 9).

16. **What is the finger fracture technique?**

Finger fracture hepatotomy or tractotomy is the method of exposing bleeding points deep within liver lacerations by blunt dissection. Pushing apart the liver parenchyma enables points to be identified and ligated. This method is most commonly required for penetrating injuries.

17. **What is the role of selective hepatic artery ligation in securing hemostasis in patients with a major liver injury?**

Deep lacerations of the right or left hepatic lobe may result in bleeding that cannot be completely controlled by suture ligation of specific bleeding points within the liver parenchyma. In this situation, either the right or left artery can be ligated for control of the bleeding with little risk of ischemic liver necrosis.

18. **Why is retrohepatic vena caval laceration lethal?**

Exposure requires either extensive hepatotomy, extensive mobilization of the right lobe, or right lobectomy, or transection of the vena cava. The large caliber and high flow of the IVC results in massive hemorrhage during surgical exposure, whereas clamping of the IVC often results in hypotension attributable to an abrupt decrease in venous return to the heart.

19. **What is the physiologic rationale for use of a shunt in attempted repair of retrohepatic vena caval injuries?**

Hemorrhage control requires maintenance of venous return to the heart while both antegrade and retrograde bleeding through the laceration is stopped. These requirements are met by shunting blood through a tube spanning the laceration between the right atrium and lower IVC.

20. **What is the intrahepatic balloon tamponading device?**

For transhepatic penetrating injuries, a 1-inch Penrose drain is sutured around a red rubber catheter. This forms a long balloon that is threaded through the bleeding liver injury and inflated with contrast media through a stopcock in the red rubber catheter. The balloon tamponades liver hemorrhage. The catheter is brought out through the abdominal wall, deflated, and removed 24 to 48 hours later.

21. **What are the indications for perihepatic packing?**

Liver packing with planned reoperation for definitive treatment of injuries in patients who have hypothermia, acidosis, and coagulopathies is a life-saving maneuver (damage control laparotomy). Laparotomy pads (>20) are packed around the liver to compress and control hemorrhage. A temporary dressing is then placed over the open abdomen (damage control laparotomy), and the patient's metabolic abnormalities and coagulopathy are corrected with planned reoperation within 24 hours.

22. What is the abdominal compartment syndrome?

The abdominal compartment syndrome is a potentially lethal complication of perihepatic packing or large volume resuscitation. It may occur when intraabdominal pressure exceeds 20 cm H_2O. Intraabdominal pressure increases because of bowel and liver edema secondary to ischemia and reperfusion injury or continued hemorrhage into the abdominal cavity. As pressure increases beyond 20 cm H_2O, venous return, cardiac output (CO), and urine output decrease, but ventilatory pressures increase. Patients must return promptly to the operating room (OR) for decompression of the abdomen. A manometer attached to the Foley catheter is useful in following intraabdominal pressure.

23. What are the common complications related to liver injury?

After blunt injury to the liver, overall, 13% develop hepatic complications. Complications include bleeding, biliary leaks or fistulae, abdominal compartment syndrome, and infection. Complications occur more frequently in higher grades of injury: 5% in grade III, 22% in grade IV, and 52% in grade V.

BILIARY TRACT INJURY

24. Why are complications associated with bile duct leaks?

Bilomas (i.e., collections of bile) frequently become infected and may result in lethal peritonitis. Biliopleural fistula, a communication between the biliary system and pleural cavity, persists because of the relative negative pressure in the thorax and may result in a bile empyema. Bilhemia results from an intrahepatic fistula between the bile ducts and hepatic veins, resulting in severely elevated bilirubinemia. Hemobilia occurs from the rupture of an arterial pseudoaneurysm into the biliary system, resulting in upper gastrointestinal hemorrhage.

25. What is the incidence of bile duct leak?

For patients managed nonoperatively, the leak rate is 3%, and they are rarely seen for grade I, II, or III injuries. Leak rates are higher for those who undergo operations or angioembolization. Perihepatic fluid collections identified by US suggest a leak, however, they are more accurately identified by hepatobiliary iminodiacetic acid (HIDA) scan or endoscopic retrograde cholangiopancreatography (ERCP).

26. What is the initial management of a bile leak?

ERCP is usually quite useful in diagnosing and treating leaks. Biliary stenting with or without sphincterotomy and percutaneous drainage of bilomas frequently allows spontaneous resolution of bile duct injuries. Extensive injuries require hepaticojejunostomy for reconstruction.

KEY POINTS

1. Liver injuries are common following BAT and should be considered in all patients who are hypotensive.

2. Eighty-five percent of patients with liver injuries can be treated nonoperatively. Angioembolization is an important adjunct.

3. Higher grade injuries are more likely to fail nonoperative management and have an increased complication rate.

4. Damage control laparotomy should be considered for severe hepatic injuries.

5. The hepatic artery delivers 30% of blood flow, and the portal vein delivers 70% of blood flow.

6. Biliary injuries can occur with severe hepatic injury, but most are treated by minimally invasive techniques.

WEBSITE

www.acssurgery.com

BIBLIOGRAPHY

1. Croce MA, Fabian TC, Menke PG et al.: Nonoperative management of blunt hepatic trauma is the treatment of choice for hemodynamically stable patients. Ann Surg 221:744-753, 1995.

2. Franklin GA, Casos SR: Current advances in the surgical approach to abdominal trauma. Injury 37:1143-1156, 2006.

3. Hiatt JR, Gabbay J, Busutill RW: Surgical anatomy of the hepatic arteries in 1000: cases. Ann Surg 220:50-52, 1994.

4. Hurtuk M, Reed RL, Esposito TJ et al.: Trauma surgeons practice what they preach: the NTDB story on solid organ injury management. J Trauma 61:243-255, 2006.

5. Kozar RA, Moore FA, Cothren CC et al.: Risk factors for hepatic morbidity following nonoperative management. Arch Surg 141:451-459, 2006.

6. Lui F, Sangosanya A, Kaplan LJ: Abdominal compartment syndrome: clinical aspects and monitoring. Crit Care Clin 23:415-433, 2007.

7. Meredith JW, Young JR, Bowling J et al.: Nonoperative management of adult blunt hepatic trauma: the exception or the rule? J Trauma 36:529-534, 1994.

8. Moore EE: Staged laparotomy for the hypothermia, acidosis, and coagulopathy syndrome. Am J Surg 172:405-410, 1996.

9. Moore EE, Cogbill TH, Malangoni MA et al.: Organ injury scaling. Surg Clin North Am 75:293-303, 1995.

10. Poggetti RS, Moore EE, Moore FA et al.: Balloon tamponade for bilobar transfixing hepatic gunshot wounds. J Trauma 33:694-697, 1992.

11. Tai NR, Boffard KD, Goosen J et al.: A 10-year experience of complex liver trauma. Br J Surg 89:1532-1537, 2002.

12. Velmahos GC, Toutouzas K, Radin F et al.: High success with nonoperative management of blunt hepatic trauma. The liver is a sturdy organ. Arch Surg 138:475-481, 2003.

13. Verous M, Cillo U, Brolese A et al.: Blunt liver injury: From non-operative management to liver transplantation. Injury 34:181-186, 2003.

14. Wahl WL, Brandt MM, Hemmila MR et al.: Diagnosis and management of bile leaks after blunt liver injury. Surgery 138:742-748, 2005.

CHAPTER 25

SPLENIC TRAUMA

Sarah Judkins, MD, and Ernest E. Moore, MD

1. **What is the physiologic role of the spleen?**
   In fetal development, the spleen serves as a major site for hematopoiesis. In early childhood the spleen produces immunoglobulin M (IgM) and tuftsin. The spleen also functions as a filter, allowing resident macrophages to remove abnormal red blood cells (RBCs), cellular debris, and encapsulated and poorly opsonized bacteria.

2. **What injury patterns are associated with splenic trauma?**
   Direct blunt force, deceleration, and compression to the left torso. Think **spleen** after a motor vehicle accident or fall: lower rib fractures, left side-only rib fractures, and high-energy transfer (big hits) increase the probability of splenic injury.

3. **What are the signs and symptoms of splenic injury?**
   The main sign is pain in the left upper quadrant. This is produced by stretching the splenic capsule. Peritoneal irritation (rebound tenderness) is caused by extravasated blood. Vital signs vary depending on associated blood loss and are not specific for injuries to the spleen. Unfortunately, a large number of patients with a significant splenic injury exhibit no signs or symptoms at all.

4. **What studies can help in diagnosing splenic trauma?**
   Ultrasound (US) is routinely performed in the emergency department (ED) and can rapidly identify as little as 200 ml fluid or blood. When US is equivocal, diagnostic peritoneal lavage (DPL) is an accurate and sensitive measure of intraabdominal bleeding. Computed tomography (CT) scanning is the gold standard diagnostic test because it is nearly 100% accurate for identifying splenic injuries but also defines the magnitude of injury and quantifies the amount of intraperitoneal blood.

5. **How are splenic injuries classified, and why is that important?**
   Management is governed by the hemodynamic status of the patient, but therapy is also influenced by the CT grade of splenic injury. Nonoperative management is most successful in grades I to III, whereas operative intervention is often required for grade IV injuries. Grade V injuries demand prompt operative intervention (see Table 25-1).

TABLE 25-1.	GRADES OF SPLENIC INJURY
Grade	**Description**
I	Hematoma: nonexpanding subcapsular <10% surface area Laceration: nonbleeding capsular <1 cm parenchymal depth
II	Hematoma: nonexpanding, subcapsular <50% surface area Nonexpanding intraparenchymal <5 cm diameter Laceration: bleeding, capsular <3 cm parenchymal depth

TABLE 25-1.	GRADES OF SPLENIC INJURY—CONT'D
Grade	Description
III	Hematoma: subcapsular >50% surface area, expanding, ruptured with active bleeding Intraparenchymal >5 cm diameter or expanding Laceration: capsular >3 cm parenchymal depth, involving trabecular vessel
IV	Hematoma: ruptured, intraparenchymal, with active bleeding Laceration: involves segmental or hilar vessels with >25% splenic devascularization
V	Laceration: shattered spleen Vascular: hilar avulsion or complete splenic devascularization

6. **Do splenic injuries require laparotomy?**
   No. Nonoperative management is successful in approximately 95% of patients with grades I to III. Patients who are hemodynamically stable with evidence of ongoing bleeding (requiring transfusion) may be treated by selective arterial embolization if a bleeding site is identified on angiography.

7. **What are contraindications to nonoperative management of splenic injuries?**
   - Hemodynamic instability.
   - Persistent coagulopathy.
   - Additional intraabdominal injury requiring operative intervention.

8. **What is the failure rate of nonoperative management of splenic injury?**
   Any patient with signs of hemodynamic instability, persistent bleeding, worsening pain or tenderness, or progressive injury by CT scanning has failed nonoperative management. Approximately 60% of all splenic injuries can be managed nonoperatively with a failure rate of 12%. Factors that predict nonoperative failure include multiple injuries, grade >III spleen injuries, and need for blood transfusion.

9. **What is delayed rupture of the spleen?**
   This is a rare complication that occurs in <1% of patients with a splenic injury. Delayed splenic rupture should be distinguished from a delay in diagnosis of splenic injury and rupture of a known splenic injury. True delayed splenic rupture occurs >48 hours in a patient with a history of abdominal trauma and no overt clinical evidence of intraabdominal injury on initial presentation.

10. **What are the general principles of operative management of the injured spleen?**
    The first priority is to control bleeding. This can usually be accomplished by packing and manual compression of the spleen. If successful, the abdomen is then thoroughly explored for other injuries. Complete mobilization of the spleen by division of the splenocolic, splenorenal, phrenosplenic, and gastrosplenic ligaments is required for complete assessment of the spleen. The short gastric vessels can be ligated with division of the gastrosplenic ligament. Repair of the spleen can be accomplished by application of hemostatic agents, direct pledgeted suture repair of the splenic parenchyma, partial splenectomy, and construction of a "splenic wrap" using absorbable mesh. If splenectomy is required, the splenic artery and vein should be ligated individually before removing the spleen.

11. **What early complications arise after splenectomy?**
    Recurrent bleeding, acute gastric dilatation, gastric perforation, pancreatitis (the splenic artery courses along the top of the pancreas), and subphrenic abscess.

12. **What is splenic autotransplantation?**
    Autotransplantation is accomplished by implanting splenic tissue parenchymal slices into pouches created in the gastrocolic omentum.

13. **Does splenic autotransplantation preserve splenic function?**
    Autotransplantation after splenectomy is controversial. At least 30% of the original splenic mass is needed to provide normal function. After autotransplantation, immunoglobulin G (IgG) and IgM levels are increased in response to pneumococcal vaccine compared with patients after splenectomy alone.

14. **Does postsplenectomy leukocytosis predict infection?**
    Elevations in white blood cell (WBC) count and platelet count (PC) after splenectomy are a common physiologic event. After the fourth postoperative day, however, a WBC $>15 \times 103$ and a PC/WBC <20 are highly associated with sepsis and should not be confused with the physiologic response to splenectomy.

15. **Should a follow-up computed tomography scan be performed after nonoperative management of splenic injuries before patient discharge?**
    No. Most patients who fail nonoperative management do so within 5 days and will exhibit hemodynamic evidence of ongoing hemorrhage. However, follow-up CT should be performed for grade III and IV injuries at 4 to 6 weeks before getting back to vigorous physical activity.

16. **What is overwhelming postsplenectomy sepsis, and how is it prevented?**
    Overwhelming postsplenectomy sepsis (OPSS) is a devastating bacteremia (typically encapsulated bacteria) that occurs in 2% of patients after splenectomy. The risk of OPSS is greatest when splenectomy is performed during infancy. The most common organisms are pneumococcus (50%), meningococcus, *Escherichia coli, Haemophilus influenzae,* staphylococcus, and streptococcus. Although rare, OPSS carries a mortality rate of 75% and has spurred interest in splenic preservation. OPSS is primarily prevented by postoperative vaccination. Pneumococcal, meningococcal, and *Haemophilus* flu vaccines should be given 2 weeks after splenectomy and are recommended every 5 years. Sepsis can occur despite vaccination; consequently, long-term prophylaxis with oral penicillin is recommended for children.

KEY POINTS: EXPECTANT MANAGEMENT OF SPLENIC INJURIES

1. Nonoperative management is successful in 95% of grades I to III injuries.

2. Eighty percent of all splenic injuries are managed nonoperatively, with a 12% failure or conversion rate.

3. Factors that predict failure or conversion to operative treatment include injury >grade III, and need for blood transfusion.

4. Patients with evidence of ongoing bleeding (e.g., contrast "blush" on CT or ongoing transfusion requirements) may be managed with selective arterial embolization.

WEBSITES

www.east.org/tpg/bluntabd.pdf

www.acssurgery.com/abstracts/acs/acs0506.htm

BIBLIOGRAPHY

1. Bala M, Edden Y, Mintz Y et al.: Blunt splenic trauma: predictors for successful non-operative management. Isr Med Assoc J 9:857-861, 2007.
2. Cadeddu M, Garnett A, Al-Anezi K et al.: Management of spleen injuries in the adult trauma population: a ten year experience. Can J Surg 49:386-390, 2006.
3. Leemans R, Harms G, Rijkers GT et al.: Spleen autotransplantation provides restoration of functional splenic lymphoid compartments and improves the humoral immune response to pneumococcal polysaccharide vaccine. Clin Exp Immunol 17:596-604, 1999.
4. Moore EE, Cogbill TH, Jurkovich GJ et al.: Organ injury scaling: Spleen and liver (1994 revision). J Trauma 38:323-324, 1995.
5. Shatz DV: Vaccination practices among North American trauma surgeons in splenectomy for trauma. J Trauma 53:950-956, 2002.
6. Taylor M, Genuit T, Napolitano L: Overwhelming postsplenectomy sepsis and trauma: time to consider revaccination? J Trauma 59:1482-1485, 2005.
7. Uecker J, Pickett C, Dunn E: The role of follow-up radiographic studies in nonoperative management of spleen trauma. Am Surg 67:22-25, 2001.

CHAPTER 26

PANCREATIC AND DUODENAL INJURY

Jeffry L. Kashuk, MD, FACS

1. **How common are pancreatic and duodenal injuries?**

   Because the duodenum and pancreas are intimately associated with vital structures in a deep and narrow area of the retroperitoneum, affording a significant degree of protection, reported injury frequency is between 7% and 10% for all trauma celiotomies. Blunt duodenal injury occurs in less than 1% of blunt trauma.

2. **What other injuries are typically associated with penetrating pancreatic trauma?**

   Liver injury is the most frequent concomitant injury, with a reported incidence of 50%. Other commonly associated injuries include the stomach (40%), large abdominal vessels such as the aorta and vena cava (40%), spleen (25%), kidney (2%), and duodenum (20%).

3. **How are pancreatic injuries diagnosed preoperatively?**

   Penetrating trauma to the pancreas is usually discovered during exploration for associated injuries. Such patients may present with hemodynamic instability from bleeding, positive focused abdominal sonography in trauma (FAST) examination, or peritonitis. Patients with blunt injury who are hemodynamically stable should undergo abdominal computed tomography (CT) scan, and possible endoscopic retrograde cholangiopancreatography (ERCP). Elevated serum amylase concentrations are nonspecific for pancreatic injury and can be normal in a high proportion of patients.

4. **What are some of the commonly used surgical options for the treatment of pancreatic injuries?**

   Most low-grade penetrating and blunt injuries are adequately treated by closed suction drains placed at surgery. In more severe injuries, the integrity of the main pancreatic duct should be evaluated, either by direct inspection or by intraoperative pancreatography. Distal duct injuries are treated with distal pancreatectomy, with or without splenectomy, and closed drainage of the pancreatic stump. Preservation of the spleen is preferable. Injury to the pancreatic duct in the head or neck may require resection of significant portions of distal pancreas and are usually performed in a delayed manner following damage control procedures.

5. **Describe the common complications of pancreatic injuries.**

   Exsanguination is the most common cause of early death, prompting the use of damage control. For patients who survive their initial operation, the two most common complications are pancreatic fistulas and intraabdominal abscesses. Other late problems are pancreatitis, pancreatic pseudocyst, and pancreatic hemorrhage. Most patients who die after sustaining injuries to the pancreas do so as a result of late complications and not from the pancreatic injury itself.

KEY POINTS: SURGICAL OPTIONS FOR PANCREATIC INJURIES

1. Low-grade injuries are treated with simple closed suction drainage at the time of celiotomy.

2. Associated injuries are common and should be searched for and addressed.

3. Patients who are unstable should undergo debridement of devascularized tissue, hemostatis, and drainage with delayed reconstruction until the patient is stable.

4. If ductal injury is suspected in a stable patient, visualize with ERCP or cholangiogram.

5. If ductal injury is present in the head or neck of the pancreas, ligate proximally and attempt to preserve pancreatic tissue with Roux-en-Y pancreaticojejunostomy.

6. Consider establishing enteral nutritional access by placing a jejunal feeding tube in patients with more than minor injuries.

DUODENUM

6. What is the role of computed tomography scanning in diagnosing blunt duodenal injuries?

Although CT is an excellent tool for visualizing solid injuries, CT is less useful with injuries to hollow organs such as the duodenum. Even the addition of an oral contrast agent to the study has a high specificity but poor sensitivity. Subtle signs of duodenal injury on CT scans include paraduodenal edema, fluid, retroduodenal air, and fat standing with loss of sharp tissue planes, which may usually indicate a duodenal rupture and spillage of small amounts of intralumenal contents into the retroperitoneum. Such subtle findings in a patient with a high-risk mechanism of injury may warrant operative exploration.

7. What is the importance of the Kocher maneuver?

In 1903, Kocher described what has now become a routine maneuver during the exploratory celiotomy to visualize and repair injuries to the duodenum, distal common bile duct, and pancreatic head. The avascular lateral peritoneal attachments to the duodenum are incised sharply; then the duodenal sweep is elevated and reflected medially, allowing for inspection and palpation of its posterior surface as well as of the head of the pancreas.

8. What are the four portions of the duodenum and their surgical relationships?

The **first portion** of the duodenum starts at the pylorus (intraperitoneally) and passes backward (retroperitoneally) toward the gallbladder (the remainder of the duodenum is retroperitoneal). The **second portion** descends 7 to 8 cm and is anterior to the vena cava. The left border of the duodenum is attached to the head of the pancreas, at the site where the common bile and pancreatic ducts enter; it shares a common blood supply with the head of the pancreas through the pancreaticoduodenal arcades. The **third portion** of the duodenum turns horizontally to the left, with its cranial surface in contact with the uncinate process of the pancreas, and passes posterior to the superior mesenteric artery and vein. The **fourth portion** continues to the left, ascending slightly and crossing the spine anterior to the aorta, where it is fixed to the suspensory ligament of Treitz at the duodenojejunal flexure.

9. How are duodenal injuries classified?

An organ injury scale has been adopted that allows for standardized descriptions of duodenal injuries, which extend from grade 1 (less severe) to grade V (most severe). The grading of duodenal injuries assists surgeons in selecting the appropriate surgical procedure for the repair or reconstruction of these frequently complex injuries (see Table 26-1).

TABLE 26-1. GRADES OF PANCREATIC INJURY

Grade	Injury	Description
I	Hematoma	Involving single portion of duodenum
	Laceration	Partial thickness; no perforation
II	Hematoma	Involving more than one portion
	Laceration	Disruption <50% of circumference
III	Laceration	Disruption 50%–75% circumference of D2 or disruption of 50%–100% of D1, D3, or D4*
IV	Laceration	Disruption >75% of D2 or involving ampulla or distal common bile duct
V	Laceration	Massive disruption of duodenopancreatic complex
	Vascular	Devascularization of duodenum

*D1, D2, D3, and D4 refer to the portions of the duodenum (i.e., first through fourth).

10. **What are the main surgical options for penetrating duodenal injuries?**
Most simple lacerations (grade 1 to 2) can be repaired primarily. Complex lacerations (grade 3) with devitalized margins or lacerations that involve >50% of the duodenal circumference require debridement of margins and reanastomosis of the divided ends. If tension on the suture line is anticipated because of extensive tissue loss (grade 3 to 4) adjunctive techniques such as Roux-en-Y duodenojejunostomy or pyloric exclusion are more appropriate. Severe duodenal injuries involving the distal bile duct and pancreatic head (grade 5) may warrant pancreaticoduodenectomy (i.e., Whipple procedure) after damage control procedures. In patients with all but simple repairs, consideration should be given to establishment of enteral access via jejunostomy.

KEY POINTS: SURGICAL OPTIONS FOR DUODENAL INJURIES

1. Associated injuries are common, particularly to the pancreas, and they should be searched for and addressed.

2. Although penetrating injuries are usually discovered at laparotomy for bleeding or peritonitis, blunt injuries are difficult to diagnose even with CT scan, and the decision to operate must include consideration of subtle clinical signs.

3. Thorough exploration requires a Kocher maneuver and full evaluation of all anatomic regions of the duodenum.

4. Operative repair is determined by injury severity classification. Most injuries are managed with simple primary repair, and extensive resections should be delayed in most patients via damage control procedures.

5. Enteral access should be considered in all but the simplest injuries.

BIBLIOGRAPHY

1. Huerta S, Bui T, Porral D et al.: Predictors of morbidity and mortality in patients with traumatic duodenal injuries. Am Surg 71:763, 2005.

2. Kap LS, Bulger EM, Parks DL et al.: Predictors of morbidity after traumatic pancreatic injury. J Trauma 55:898, 2003.

3. Lopez PP, Benjamin R, Cockbum M et al.: Recent trends in the management of combined pancreatoduodenal injuries. Am Surg 71:847, 2005.

4. Moore EE, Cogbill T, Malangoni M et al.: Organ injury scaling II: pancreas, duodenum, small bowel, colon, and rectum. J Trauma 30:1427, 1990.

5. Patel SV, Spencer JA, el-Hansani S et al.: Imaging of pancreatic trauma. Br J Radiol 71:985, 1998.

6. Supramann A, Dente CJ, Feliciano DY: The managing of pancreatic trauma in the modem era. Surg Clin North Am 87:1515, 2007.

7. Takishima T, Sugimoto K, Hirata M et al.: Serum amylase level on admission in the diagnosis of blunt injury to the pancreas: its significance and limitations. Ann Surg 226:70, 1997.

8. Timaran CH, Daley BJ, Enderson BL: Role of duodenography in the diagnosis of blunt duodenal injuries. J Trauma 51:648, 2001.

9. Vassiliu P, Toutouzas KG, Velahos GC: Prospective study of post-traumatic biliary and pancreatic fistuli. The role of expectant management. Injury 35:223, 2004.

10. Velmahos GC, Constantimon C, Kassotakis G: Safety of repair for severe duodenal injury. World J Surg 32:7, 2008.

11. Wales PW, Shuckett B, Kim PC: Long-term outcome after non-operative management of complete traumatic pancreatic transaction in children. J Pediatr Surg 36:823, 2001.

CHAPTER 27

TRAUMA TO THE COLON AND RECTUM

Walter L. Biffl, MD, FACS

COLON TRAUMA

1. **How do most colon injuries occur?**
   Nearly all (>95%) colon injuries are caused by penetrating trauma from gunshot, stab, iatrogenic, or sexual injury. Blunt colonic trauma is rare and usually results from seat belts during motor vehicle crashes.

2. **How are colon injuries diagnosed?**
   They are usually diagnosed during laparotomy for penetrating trauma. For patients in whom the need for laparotomy has not been established, chest and upright abdominal radiographs may reveal free air and detect the location of penetrating objects. Triple-contrast (i.e., oral, intravenous [IV], and rectal) computed tomography (CT) or soluble-contrast radiographs can diagnose retroperitoneal colon injuries. Elevated white blood cell counts or enzyme (amylase, alkaline phosphatase) levels or fecal material in diagnostic peritoneal lavage (DPL) is highly suggestive of a bowel injury.

3. **How are colon injuries graded?**
   Grade I: contusion hematoma without devascularization or partial-thickness laceration.
   Grade II: laceration <50% circumference.
   Grade III: laceration >50% circumference.
   Grade IV: transection of the colon.
   Grade V: transection with segmental tissue loss.

4. **What are three primary surgical options for managing a colon injury?**
   1. **Primary repair:** suturing of simple perforations or resection and primary anastomosis for more complex injuries.
   2. **Colostomy:** injured colon is resected and the proximal colon is brought out as a colostomy or the injury is repaired but a more proximal ileostomy or colostomy is brought out to divert the fecal stream.

5. **What are the advantages and disadvantages of each of these options?**
   1. **Primary repair** is desirable because definitive treatment is carried out at the initial operation, and the patient is spared the morbidity of a colostomy and its reversal. The disadvantage is that suture lines are created in suboptimal conditions, so leakage may occur.
   2. **Proximal colostomy** avoids an unprotected suture line in the abdomen but requires a second operation to close the colostomy. Stomal complications, including necrosis, stenosis, obstruction, and prolapse, may occur.

6. **How are most patients with colon injuries surgically managed?**
   Primary repair is safe and effective in essentially all patients with colon trauma. Handsewn and stapled anastomoses have equal complication rates. Prophylactic antibiotics are administered for no longer than 24 hours postoperatively.

7. **How should the surgical incision and penetrating wound be managed?**
Wounds should be left open (for delayed primary closure) to decrease the incidence of wound infection and fascial dehiscence.

8. **What complications are associated with colonic injury and its treatment?**
   - Wound infection (= 65% if the skin incision is closed primarily; do not be tempted to close a dirty incision).
   - Intraabdominal abscess (20%).
   - Fascial dehiscence (10%).
   - Stomal complications (5%).
   - Anastomotic leak (5%).
   - Mortality (<1%).

RECTAL TRAUMA

9. **How do rectal injuries occur?**
Similar to colon injuries, most rectal injuries result from penetrating trauma as a result of gunshot, stab, iatrogenic, or sexual injury. Blunt pelvic fractures should be assessed with a strong suspicion for rectal (and urethral) injury.

10. **How are rectal injuries diagnosed?**
A thorough examination is crucial, and the diagnosis is suggested by the course of the projectiles and the presence of blood on digital rectal examination. If rectal trauma is suspected, the patient should undergo proctoscopy to look for hematoma, contusion, laceration, or gross blood. If the diagnosis is in question, radiographs with soluble-contrast enemas should be performed.

11. **How are patients with intraperitoneal rectal injuries treated differently from those with extraperitoneal injuries?**
The portion of the rectum proximal to the peritoneal reflection is called the intraperitoneal segment. Injuries of this portion are treated similar to colonic injuries.

12. **What are the four basic principles for managing simple extraperitoneal rectal injuries?**
    1. **Diversion:** either a loop or an end sigmoid colostomy or ileostomy is appropriate.
    2. **Drainage:** a retroanal incision should be used to place Penrose or closed-suction drains near the perforation site.
    3. **Repair:** appropriate when possible, but not mandatory
    4. **Washout:** irrigation of the distal rectum with isotonic solution until the effluent is clear. The role of washout remains controversial, but it may benefit patients whose rectum is full of feces.

    These principles have recently been questioned, but they are still supported by the literature and most expert recommendations.

13. **How are complex extraperitoneal rectal injuries managed?**
In patients with massive pelvic trauma and an associated rectal injury, an abdominoperineal resection may be required for adequate debridement and hemostasis. An abdominoperineal resection is also required in rare instances in which anal sphincters have been destroyed.

14. **What complications are associated with rectal trauma and its treatment?**
They are similar to those in colonic injuries. In addition, pelvic osteomyelitis may occur. In this case, debridement may be necessary, and culture-specific IV antibiotics should be administered for 2 to 3 months.

15. **What is the role of antibiotics in colorectal trauma?**
Antibiotics are important. They should be initiated preoperatively (you need a good blood level at the time you make your incision) and ended quickly (12 to 24 hours postoperatively). Broad-spectrum, combination therapy is superior to single-agent therapy.

KEY POINTS: COLORECTAL TRAUMA

1. Primary repair of colon injuries is safe.

2. Handsewn and stapled anastomoses have equal complication rates.

3. A preoperative dose of antibiotic therapy, to be continued for 24 hours or less, is advantageous.

4. The management of extraperitoneal rectal injuries is evolving. Diversion and drainage is the most conservative strategy.

BIBLIOGRAPHY

1. Curran TJ, Borzotta AP: Complications of primary repair of colon injury—Literature review of 2964 Cases. Am J Surg 177:42-47, 1999.

2. Demetriades D, Murray J, Chan LS et al.: Handsewn versus stapled anastomosis in penetrating colon injuries requiring resection: a multicenter study. J Trauma 52:117-121, 2002.

3. Demetriades D, Murray J, Chan L et al.: Penetrating colon injuries requiring resection: diversion or primary anastomosis? An AAST prospective multicenter study. J Trauma 50:765-775, 2001.

4. Gonzalez RP, Phelan H 3rd, Hassan M et al.: Is fecal diversion necessary for nondestructive penetrating extraperitoneal rectal injuries? J Trauma 61:815-819, 2006.

5. Miller PR, Fabian TC, Croce MA et al.: Improving outcomes following penetrating colon wounds. Ann Surg 235:775-781, 2002.

CHAPTER 28

PELVIC FRACTURES

Steven J. Morgan, MD, FACS, and Wade R. Smith, MD

1. **What are the first steps in the evaluation and treatment of a patient with pelvic trauma?**
   The ABCs (airway, breathing, and circulatory assessment). The answer to this first trauma question is always the same. Trauma patients with displaced pelvic fractures have a high incidence of associated injuries to the head, chest, and abdomen.

2. **What are the sources and potential volume of bleeding in the displaced pelvic fracture?**
   Pelvic fractures bleed from exposed cancellous bone surfaces, pelvic veins, and pelvic arteries. Cadaveric injection studies have demonstrated that 90% of patients with trauma fatalities with pelvic fractures bleed to death from exposed bone and injured veins. Only 10% bleed from arteries. The total volume the pelvis can hold is 4 to 6 L before a tamponade effect slows venous and bone bleeding.

3. **Should a Foley catheter be placed in trauma patients with displaced pelvic fractures?**
   Yes. Contraindications include urethral injuries, which should be suspected when blood is observed at the penile meatus or vaginal introitus. A manual rectal examination in men and a bimanual examination in women are mandatory to exclude an open fracture into the vagina or rectum or a high-riding prostate. If a urethral injury is present, a suprapubic catheter can be easily inserted percutaneously, and both a urethrogram and cystogram are performed.

4. **What is the incidence of urologic injury associated with pelvic fractures?**
   The overall incidence is 16%.

5. **What are the commonly used radiographic classification schemes for pelvic fractures?**
   The mechanistic classification describes pelvic fractures as anteroposterior compression (APC), lateral compression (LC), vertical shear (VS), or combined mechanism (CM). The Tile classification categorizes fractures into three groups, A, B, or C, with numbered subgroups based on increasing severity of ligamentous and bony disruption.

6. **What is an open pelvic fracture?**
   An open fracture has been contaminated via a laceration in the skin, vagina, or rectum. When an open pelvic fracture is suspected, patients should receive a rectal examination with an ano-scope, and a vaginal examination performed bimanually and with a speculum.
   With open fractures, the morbidity and mortality rates are increased both in the acute period (because of hemorrhage) and in the delayed period (because of infection). Open injuries in the rectal or perirectal region often require a diverting colostomy to prevent deep pelvic infection.

7. When is acute mechanical stabilization of a pelvic fracture indicated?

Open-book and vertical shear fractures with displacement may benefit from acute mechanical stabilization. When hemodynamic instability persists in the face of ongoing aggressive resuscitation, pelvic stabilization with a beanbag, external wrap, or external fixation device may help to decrease pelvic bleeding by decreasing pelvic volume (tamponade effect), stabilizing fracture surfaces, and promoting clot formation.

8. What is pelvic packing, and when is it used?

Pelvic packing is the technique of opening the retroperitoneum, either directly through a Pfannenstiel type approach or indirectly through the peritoneal reflection, during emergent laparotomy and placing sponges to absorb and tamponade bleeding. Historically packing was used as a last ditch effort late in the course of failed resuscitations. Recent reports have shown packing to be safe and potentially beneficial in reducing mortality in unstable pelvic trauma patients as long as the procedure is done early in the resuscitation and as part of a multidisciplinary protocol with specific indications and access to emergent angiography.

9. What is the role of angiography in an acute pelvic fracture?

Angiography can identify and embolize arterial bleeding caused by pelvic fractures. But only a low percentage of pelvic bleeding is from arterial injury. Suspicion should be increased when patients with hypotension fail to respond to pelvic ring stabilization and aggressive fluid resuscitation. If retroperitoneal pelvic packing is employed during resuscitation, continued transfusion requirement signals a high likelihood of arterial bleeding and subsequent need for angiography.

10. Why do patients die from pelvic fractures?

Mortality is usually caused by associated injuries rather than the pelvic fracture. Only 2% of patients with a pelvic fracture experience isolated trauma to the pelvis. For example, patients with LC pelvic fractures are more likely to die secondary to associated head injuries rather than from pelvic hemorrhage. However, in pelvic fractures with major bleeding, death is most often as a result of shock and multisystem organ failure (MOF). Limiting blood loss through aggressive resuscitation with 1:1 blood/fresh frozen plasma transfusion, mechanical stabilization, operative treatment of associated injuries, pelvic packing, and angiography for refractory shock are the keys to reducing pelvic fracture mortality.

Mortality overall is high for patients with shock but can be reduced by a multidisciplinary protocol.

11. What is external fixation?

External fixation by the use of pins placed into the iliac wings and connected to a frame or by pins placed into the bone just superior to the acetabulum and connected to a C clamp can be used as a temporary method of fracture reduction and stabilization. External fixation does not prevent vertical and posterior displacement of the pelvis in the case of complete posterior disruption. The fixation device must be placed in a manner that permits abdominal access for laparotomy, diagnostic imaging, and the definitive operative approach for open reduction and internal fixation.

12. Is there a role for pneumatic antishock garments in the treatment of pelvic fractures?

Pneumatic antishock garments (PASGs) are falling out of favor in the treatment of pelvic fractures. Their potential role is limited to emergency transportation and initial stabilization of patients with a complex pelvic fracture. PASGs can reduce displacement of APC fractures but may increase the displacement of a LC fracture. The garment also restricts access to the patient, compromises pulmonary reserve, and is associated with increased risk of compartment syndrome.

13. **When can patients with a pelvic fracture ambulate?**
Patients with fractures involving only the anterior pelvic ring, such as unilateral or bilateral pubic rami fractures, may bear weight immediately. If the fracture pattern involves the posterior structures, such as the sacroiliac joint or iliac wing, patients must not bear weight for 10 weeks.

14. **What is the most common source of arterial bleeding associated with a pelvic fracture?**
The superior gluteal artery.

15. **Which gender and what portion of the urethra is most commonly injured in patients with a displaced pelvic fracture?**
The male urethra is more commonly injured. The urethra passes through the urogenital diaphragm or pelvic floor, transitioning in an abrupt fashion from the membranous to the bulbous urethra. The urethra at this point is attenuated and relatively fixed above, accounting for the large number of injuries at the membranous bulbous junction. The female urethra is much shorter, and the pelvic floor is less well developed, allowing for greater mobility of the female urethra (or perhaps it is because girls are smarter, more cautious, and do not get injured as often). The most common site of urethral injury in girls and women is at the bladder neck.

16. **Describe the mechanism that results in a bladder rupture.**
The bladder is both an intraperitoneal and extraperitoneal structure. Compression of a distended bladder results in an intraperitoneal rupture along the bladder dome. Extraperitoneal rupture, a more common injury, results from the laceration of the bladder by displaced pubic rami fracture fragments.

17. **What are the three radiographic views required to evaluate patients with pelvic fractures?**
    1. Anteroposterior (AP) pelvis view
    2. Inlet view
    3. Outlet view

18. **What is the appropriate insertion location for a diagnostic peritoneal lavage catheter in the presence of a pelvic fracture?**
A supraumbilical location avoids inadvertent decompression of the pelvic hematoma and a false-positive result.

19. **What percent of patients with an unstable pelvic fracture will suffer an associated neurologic injury?**
Associated injuries of the lumbosacral plexus, sacral foramina, and sacral canal are reportedly as high as 50%.

20. **What is a potential pitfall of aggressive blood transfusion of patients with hemodynamically unstable pelvic fracture?**
Coagulopathy. Forty percent of patients with unstable pelvic fractures may require 10 units of blood. Fresh frozen plasma and platelets should be transfused early in the resuscitation.

21. **What is the significance of an L5 transverse process fracture in a patient with a pelvis fracture?**
A transverse process (TP) fracture at the level of L5 may indicate vertical instability of the pelvic fracture. The iliolumbar ligaments attach to.

KEY POINTS: BLOOD LOSS FROM PELVIC FRACTURES

1. Ninety percent of deaths related to pelvic bleeding result from venous and bony bleeding.

2. The remaining 10% are a result of arterial bleeding, most commonly from the superior gluteal artery.

3. Normally the pelvis can hold 4 to 6 L of blood before a tamponade effect occurs.

4. Pelvic wraps or fixation can limit bleeding, reduce bony shear, and promote clot formation.

5. Angiography is therapeutic and diagnostic, but only 10% of injuries are predominantly arterial.

6. Mortality overall is high for patients with shock, but can be reduced by a multidisciplinary protocol.

WEBSITES

www.east.org/tpg/pelvis.pdf

BIBLIOGRAPHY

1. Biffl WL, Smith WR, Moore EE et al.: Evolution of a multidisciplinary key clinical pathway for the management of unstable pelvis fractures. Ann Surg 233:843-850, 2001.

2. Burgess AR, Eastridge BJ, Young JW et al.: Pelvic ring disruptions: effective classification system and treatment protocols. J Trauma 30:848-856, 1990.

3. Cook RE, Keating JF, Gillespie I: The role of angiography in the management of hemorrhage from major fractures of the pelvis. J Bone Joint Surg 84B:178-182, 2002.

4. Ghaemmaghami V, Sperry J, Gunst M et al.: Effects of early use of external pelvic compression on transfusion requirements and mortality in pelvic fractures. Am J Surg 194(6):720-723; discussion 723, 2007.

5. Hauschild O, Strohm PC, Culemann U et al.: Mortality in patients with pelvic fractures: results from the German pelvic injury register. J Trauma 64(2):449-455, 2008.

6. Perez JV, Hughes TM, Bowers K: Angiographic embolization in pelvic fracture. Injury 29:187-191, 1998.

7. Smith W, Williams A, Agudelo J et al.: Early predictors of mortality in hemodynamically unstable pelvis fractures. J Orthop Trauma 21(1):31-37, 2007.

8. Smith WR, Moore EE, Osborn P et al.: Retroperitoneal packing as a resuscitation technique for hemodynamically unstable patients with pelvic fractures: report of two representative cases and a description of technique. J Trauma 59(6):1510-1514, 2005.

9. Starr AJ, Griffin DR, Reinert CM et al.: Pelvic ring disruptions: prediction of associated injuries, transfusion requirement, pelvic arteriography, complications, and mortality. J Orthop Trauma 16:553-561, 2002.

10. Stover MD, Summers HD, Ghanayem AJ et al.: Three-dimensional analysis of pelvic volume in an unstable pelvic fracture. J Trauma 61(4):905-908, 2006.

11. Tötterman A, Madsen JE, Skaga NO et al.: Extraperitoneal pelvic packing: a salvage procedure to control massive traumatic pelvic hemorrhage. J Trauma 62(4):843-852, 2007.

12. Velmahos GC, Toutouzas KG, Vassiliu P et al.: A prospective study on the safety and efficacy of angiographic embolization for pelvic and visceral injuries. J Trauma 53:303-308, 2002.

UPPER URINARY TRACT INJURIES

Fernando J. Kim, MD, FACS, and Mario F. Chammas, Jr., MD

1. **What is the most common type of renal trauma in the United States, blunt or penetrating?**
   Blunt, by far.

2. **Do most renal injuries require surgery?**
   No. Fewer than 2% of blunt injuries require surgery, and many penetrating injuries can also be treated nonoperatively.

3. **Are pediatric kidneys more susceptible to major injury?**
   Yes. Because of children's weaker abdominal muscles, less-ossified thoracic cage, decreased perirenal fat, and increased renal size in relation to the rest of the body, the risk for renal injury is greater in the pediatric population.

4. **When should potential renal trauma be investigated?**
   All blunt trauma patients with gross hematuria or with microscopic hematuria and shock (systolic blood pressure <90 mm Hg) should be closely examined. Penetrating injurious with any degree of hematuria should be imaged. For pediatric patients, liberal use of studies is advisable. When children spill <50 red blood cells per high-powered field (hpf) on microscopic analysis, significant renal injury is rare.

5. **When does one suspect renal trauma?**
   The mechanism of injury, physical examination (i.e., flank ecchymosis, location of penetrating wounds) and associated injuries (e.g., rib fractures) should raise the suspicion of renal trauma. Although the degree of hematuria does not correlate with the degree of renal injury, when hematuria is out of proportion to the history of trauma, it suggests preexisting renal abnormality (e.g., hydronephrosis, ectopic kidney, tumor, cystic disease, vascular malformation). Conversely, renal pedicle injuries (grade 4) may cause little or no hematuria because of arterial interruption.

6. **What imaging study is the best to evaluate renal trauma?**
   Computed tomography (CT) scan of the abdomen and pelvis with and without intravenous (IV) contrast should be performed, but it is pivotal that the perfusion and excretion phases (10 minutes after IV contrast is administered) are obtained during the study.

7. **What is a "single-shot IVP" and when do you perform it?**
   Single-shot IVP is an imaging study were only a single film is taken 10 minutes after intravenous push (IVP) of 2 ml/kg of contrast material. It is performed in situations in which preoperative renal CT staging cannot be performed (i.e., the patient is undergoing immediate exploration and is hemodynamically unstable).

8. **How is renal trauma classified?**
   Grade 1: Contusion. There is subcapsular hematoma, nonexpanding without parenchymal laceration
   Grade 2: Superficial laceration (<1 cm parenchymal depth of renal cortex without urinary extravasation)
   Grade 3: Deep laceration (>1 cm parenchymal depth of renal cortex without collecting system rupture or urinary extravasation)
   Grade 4: Parenchymal laceration extending through renal cortex, medulla, and collecting system or renal artery or vein injury with contained hemorrhage
   Grade 5: Shattered kidney or avulsion of renal hilum

9. **How is the management according to the degree of trauma?**
   A patient who is hemodynamically stable with an injury well staged by CT can usually be managed without renal exploration; indeed, 98% of blunt renal injuries can be managed nonoperatively. Grade IV and V injuries more often require surgical exploration, but even these high-grade injuries can be managed without renal operation if carefully staged and selected.

10. **What are the different types of renal pedicle trauma?**
    The renal pedicle may be interrupted by thrombosis or complete avulsion; both events are characterized by urographic nonvisualization and minimal hematuria. The most common site of arterial interruption is the junction of the proximal and middle thirds of the main renal artery. Although hematuria is often absent, one may see transitory gross hematuria or microhematuria, emphasizing the requirement for urinalysis in all circumstances.

11. **How long can a nonperfused kidney tolerate warm ischemia?**
    Irreversible renal damage may be seen in kidneys after 30 minutes of warm ischemia, and after 8 hours of ischemia, renal salvage is minimal. Recently, single reports of renovascular trauma with intimal tear treated with endovascular stents have been encouraging.

12. **What is the significance of delayed gross hematuria?**
    This occurs 3 to 4 weeks after trauma and may indicate an arteriovenous fistula. Selective embolization is the next step if conservative therapy (bed rest) fails. Rarely, operative intervention, usually for partial nephrectomy, is necessary.

13. **How do you manage an unexpected retroperitoneal bleeding during surgical exploration?**
    A pulsatile hematoma suggests a major vascular injury, and exploration should be preceded by vascular control (both proximal and distal) and preparation for rapid blood replacement. Stable hematomas (above the pelvic brim) may be left undisturbed unless studies (preoperative or intraoperative) disclose severe renal damage. When doubt exists, exploration is justified, with the likelihood of losing a kidney.

14. **How are patients with posttraumatic urine extravasation managed?**
    When urine extravasation is caused by a major laceration into the collecting system and coexists with significant persistent bleeding, surgical correction is advised. Otherwise urine extravasation commonly resolves promptly. Reimaging at 48 to 72 hours defines cases requiring drainage, stenting, or operative repair.

15. **What is included in conservative management of renal trauma?**
    Conservative management includes bed rest until gross hematuria has subsided. Strenuous activities are avoided until microhematuria has subsided (usually within 3 weeks). Patient followed for grade 5 renal trauma should undergo ultrasonography, CT scan of the abdomen and pelvis, or urography at 6 weeks. Hospitalization is not required during these periods.

16. **What is the likelihood of subsequent hypertension?**
Documented posttraumatic hypertension occurs in <2% of patients and is rennin mediated. Onset generally occurs within the first several months of injury. The mechanisms of posttraumatic hypertension may be the result of renal artery stenosis or occlusion, renal parenchymal compression (extravasation of blood or urine), and posttrauma arteriovenous fistula.

KEY POINTS: PRINCIPLES OF URETERAL REPAIR

1. Any level of primary ureteral anastomosis should be performed maintaining adequate ureteral vascular supply during dissection of ureteral ends, tension-free ureteral anastomotic site, over stent with absorbable suture.

2. For a distal injury in the lower third ureter below the iliac vessels, ureteroneocystostomy is recommended. If more ureteral length is needed to keep the anastomosis tension free, a Bohari Flap (bladder flap) and Psoas Hitch may be performed.

3. For middle and proximal third injuries, end-to-end anastomosis is recommended, but anastomosis stricture rate is higher than the proximal or distal ureteral repair.

4. For a proximal injury (uretero-pelvic junction injury), more common in children, immediate laparotomy and surgical repair is needed.

17. **How are most ureters damaged?**
The ureter is the least-often injured genitourinary organ, accounting for less than 1% of all urologic traumas secondary to external violence. Ureteral injury occurs more commonly intraoperatively (80%) than from external violent trauma (20%). Blunt trauma and stab wounds (SWs) rarely result in injury to the ureter. Blunt trauma represents 4.1% and SWs 5.2% of all ureteral traumas. The most common ureteral injuries from external violence are from gunshot wounds (GSWs; 90.7%).

18. **How do you evaluate and identify an ureteral injury?**
The site and mechanism of trauma should prompt the surgeon to suspect ureteral injury. The clinical manifestations are characteristically subtle and often obscured by coexisting injury and complaints. The majority of SWs and GSWs would also injure bowel, colon, liver, spleen, blood vessels, or pancreas. Hematuria is often microscopic, but it may be absent. Extravasation of contrast may be detected with noninvasive (IVP and CT scan) and invasive (anterograde and retrograde ureteropyelogram) imaging studies. If ureteral injury is suspected during laparotomy, indigo carmine (1 vial IV bolus) should be given to identify the site of leakage (blue coloration).

19. **What are the potential consequences of missed ureteral injury?**
Fever, leukocytosis, azotemia, flank pain, ileus, urinoma, or urinary fistula. Presentation is often delayed by several weeks after injury.

20. **Distal ureter is injured and ureteral reimplantation with psoas hitch (tack up the bladder to the psoas muscle) is performed. Postoperatively the patient complains of anterior thigh numbness. What did you do wrong?**
The genitofemoral nerve lies on the anterior aspect of the ileopsoas muscle. You caught this nerve when you synched this to the tendon of the psoas muscle.

WEBSITES

www.east.org/tpg/GUmgmt.pdf

BIBLIOGRAPHY

1. Alsikafi NF, McAninch JW, Elliott SP et al.: Nonoperative management outcomes of isolated urinary extravasation following renal lacerations due to external trauma. J Urol 176(6 Pt 1):2494, 2006.

2. Alsikafi NF, Rosenstein DI: Staging, evaluation, and nonoperative management of renal injuries. Urol Clin North Am 33:13, 2006.

3. Broghammer JA, Fisher MB, Santucci RA: Conservative management of renal trauma: a review. Urology 70:623, 2007.

4. Elliott SP, McAninch JW: Ureteral injuries: external and iatrogenic. Urol Clin N Am 33:55, 2006.

5. Elliott SP, McAninch JW: Ureteral injuries from external violence: the 25-year experience at San Francisco General Hospital. J Urol 170:1213, 2003.

6. Santucci RA, Fisher MB: The literature increasingly supports expectant (conservative) management of renal trauma—a systematic review. J Trauma 59(2):493, 2005.

CHAPTER 30

LOWER URINARY TRACT INJURY AND PELVIC TRAUMA

Mario F. Chammas, Jr., MD, and Fernando J. Kim, MD, FACS

1. **What are the causes of bladder injury?**

   Iatrogenic manipulation and penetrating or blunt trauma. Because of the rich detrussor blood supply, bladder injury is usually accompanied by hematuria. Other signs may include suprapubic pain, inability to void, or incomplete recovery of catheter irrigation.

2. **What types of bladder injury may occur with blunt trauma?**

   Laceration or perforation may be either intraperitoneal or extraperitoneal. Hematuria with a normal cystogram defines bladder contusion in the absence of upper tract injury. Extraperitoneal injuries constitute the majority of bladder trauma and tend to concentrate at the bladder base or parasymphyseal area. These can usually be managed conservatively with urinary catheter for 10 days. Intraperitoneal ruptures typically occur when the bladder is distended at the time of trauma, causing a blowout of the dome of the bladder. Intraperitoneal vesical rupture should be surgically repaired using a two-layer closure with absorbable sutures and placement of suprapubic and urethral catheters.

3. **What is the likelihood of a bladder injury in patients with a fracture pelvis?**

   Extraperitoneal bladder injury occurs in 10% of all pelvic fractures. Conversely, approximately 85% of blunt bladder injury is associated with pelvic fracture. Bladder injuries occur more often with parasymphyseal pubic arch fractures and more often with bilateral than unilateral fractures. Isolated ramus fractures produce bladder laceration in 10% of cases.

4. **How is bladder injury evaluated?**

   Both computed tomography (CT) cystography and retrograde cystourethrography provide great diagnostic accuracy for bladder rupture. The bladder should be filled under gravity with a total of 300 to 400 mL of a 50% dilution of standard radio contrast agent using the Foley catheter. Films should include anteroposterior (AP), lateral, and oblique views. Finally, a postvoid film should be obtained. When renal or distal ureteral injury is suspected, upper tract imaging (intravenous pyelogram [IVP] or CT scan) should precede the cystogram.

5. **What are the retrograde cystourethrographic patterns of bladder injury?**

   Extraperitoneal injury allows contrast agent to scape adjacent to the symphysis, but it is confined to the bladder base by the intact peritoneum. Intraperitoneal extravasation produces a "sunburst" appearance from the bladder dome, which may collect in the paracolic gutters, outline loops of bowel, or pool under the liver or spleen. It is pivotal to obtain postvoid films.

6. **How is bladder rupture managed?**

   Extraperitoneal lacerations can be managed with an indwelling catheter for 7 to 10 days, at which time cystogram usually confirms resolution of extravasation. Intraperitoneal lacerations require operative repair. In selected patients a laparoscopic approach could be an option for these patients. Bladder contusion requires catheter drainage until gross hematuria has subsided.

7. **When should urethral injury be investigated?**
   The mechanism of injury (e.g., crushing or deceleration/impact, straddle injuries) and associated trauma (e.g., pelvic fracture), blood at the meatus, penile or scrotal swelling and ecchymosis, upward prostatic displacement on digital rectal examination, and inability to void or to pass a urethral catheter should be investigated.

8. **When a patient presents with a pelvic fracture, is concomitant urethral injury a major concern?**
   Yes. Urethral trauma occurs in 10% of pelvic fractures; it is more common with anterior disruption of the pelvic ring, including 20% of unilateral and 50% of bilateral parasymphyseal fractures. Posterior (prostatomembranous) avulsion is associated with potential disabling sequelae and requirements for complex and challenging operative corrections. In contrast, more distal urethral injures avoid impotence and incontinence issues and are more surgically accessible.

9. **How is urethral injury best assessed?**
   Retrograde urethrography must always be performed before inserting a Foley catheter. Incomplete urethral transaction produces local contrast dye extravasation and bladder opacification. Total avulsion produces extensive local extravasation, and no contrast dye gets into the bladder. Incomplete transection is more common with anterior (50%) than posterior (10%) urethral injuries.

10. **How is urethral injury managed?**
    For incomplete transection regardless the site, either catheter stenting across the defect (performed by the urologist) or diversion by suprapubic cystostomy permits resolution. With complete urethral transection, the bladder should be decompressed initially via suprapubic cystostomy. Early restoration of continuity by placement of a bridging urethral catheter should be performed endoscopically if possible.

11. **What are the complications of urethral injury?**
    Strictures, incontinence, and impotence (associated with traumatic prostatic displacement). Iatrogenic complications are associated with retropubic dissection during the surgical management of the injury.

12. **What is the differential diagnosis in blunt scrotal trauma?**
    Testicular rupture, hematocele, scrotal hematoma, intratesticular hematoma, and testicular torsion. Ultrasonography helps sort this out.

13. **What is the sonographic sign of testicular rupture?**
    The sign loss of the normal homogenous echo texture of the testicle, with areas of irregular hyperechogenicity or hypoechogenicity.

14. **How are patients with acute testicular rupture managed?**
    Management includes surgical exploration and debridement of extruded, nonviable tubules and evacuation of the hematoma. After proper hemostasis is achieved, the tunica albuginea should be closed with running absorbable sutures.

15. **What is the most common cause of penile fractures?**
    Penile fracture is a rupture of the corpus cavernosum, most commonly associated with sexual intercourse, aggressive masturbation, or an abnormally forced bending of the erect penis. Characteristically the patient hears a popping sound, followed by pain and detumescence.

16. **What are the physical examination findings with a penile fracture?**
    Injury to the tunica albuginea causes formation of hematoma and deviation of the shaft to the opposite side of the injury. If Buck's fascia is intact, the hematoma will be confined to the penis ('eggplant deformity'); disruption of Bucks fascia allows spread of the hematoma under Colle's and Scarpa's fascia onto the perineum and abdominal wall.

17. **How are penile fractures managed?**
    Surgically. Closure of the defect (or defects) along the tunica albuginea and evacuation of hematoma are performed after degloving the penis. A retrograde urethrogram should be performed when urethral injury is suspected because it may occur in approximately 20% of cases.

18. **In penile amputation injuries, how should the amputated portion of the penis be preserved for transport?**
    The amputated portion of the penis should be wrapped in a saline-soaked gauze and placed in a sealed sterile bag, then the bag containing the protected penis is placed in an ice-slush bath (double-bag procedure), the ice should not be in direct contact with the penile skin. The penis should be reimplanted within the first 24 hours after injury.

19. **How is major scrotal skin loss managed?**
    If primary repair is not possible, meshed split-thickness skin grafts may be used to cover the testis. When delayed repair is necessary, thigh pouches should be created until permanent reconstruction is feasible.

20. **A 50-year-old woman complains of urine leakage from her vagina after a hysterectomy. What is the most likely diagnosis?**
    Unrecognized bladder injury during hysterectomy with subsequent urine extravasation into the surgical field and drainage via the vaginal suture line leads to formation of vesicovaginal fistula.

21. **What is the best time to repair a vesicovaginal fistula secondary to an uncomplicated hysterectomy?**
    Although 3 to 6 months after injury has been recommended in the past, early repair can be successful if there is minimal inflammation and there are no complicating factors.

WEBSITE

www.east.org/tpg/GUmgmt.pdf

BIBLIOGRAPHY

1. Chapple C, Turner-Warwick R: Vesico-vaginal fistula. BJU Int 95:193, 2005.
2. Corriere JN Jr, Sandler CM: Diagnosis and management of bladder injuries. Urol Clin North Am 33:67, 2006.
3. Kim FJ, Chammas MF Jr, Gewehr EV et al.: Laparoscopic management of intraperitoneal bladder rupture secondary to blunt abdominal trauma using intracorporeal single layer suturing technique. J Trauma 65(1):234-236, 2008.
4. Kommu SS, Illahi I, Mumtaz F: Patterns of urethral injury and immediate management. Curr Opin Urol 17:383, 2007.
5. Morey AF, Metro MJ, Carney KJ et al.: Consensus on genitourinary trauma: external genitalia. BJU Int 94:507, 2004.
6. Wessells H, Long L: Penile and genital injuries. Urol Clin North Am 33:117, 2006.

CHAPTER 31

EXTREMITY VASCULAR INJURIES

Ashok N. Babu, MD, and Ernest E. Moore, MD

1. **What are the "hard signs" of arterial injury?**
   - Distal circulatory deficit: ischemia or diminished or absent pulses.
   - Bruit.
   - Expanding or pulsatile hematoma.
   - Arterial (pulsatile) bleeding.

2. **What are the four ways in which an arterial injury may present?**
   1. Hemorrhage.
   2. Thrombosis.
   3. Arteriovenous fistula.
   4. Pseudoaneurysm.

3. **What are the "soft" signs of arterial injury?**
   Small- to moderate-sized stable hematoma.
   Adjacent nerve injury.
   Shock not explained by other injuries.
   Proximity of penetrating wound to a major vascular structure.

4. **What are the symptoms of acute arterial occlusion?**
   The six *P*'s: pain, pallor, pulse deficit, paresthesia, paralysis, and poikilothermia (cold).

5. **What initial screening test is used to evaluate an extremity for occult vascular injury?**
   Calculation of arterial pressure indices (APIs).

6. **What are the APIs for the upper extremity and lower extremity called?**
   An API for the upper extremity is the wrist brachial index (WBI).
   An API for the lower extremity is the ankle brachial index (ABI).

7. **How are WBI and ABI measured, and what is considered a normal value?**
   A handheld Doppler and blood pressure cuff are used to measure systolic blood pressure (SBP) in the brachial, radial, ulnar, dorsalis pedis (DP), and posterior tibial (PT) arteries bilaterally. The ABI for each leg is the highest DP or PT divided by the highest brachial pressure. The WBI for each arm is the highest radial or ulnar artery pressure divided by the highest brachial pressure. A value of 1.0 is normal.

8. **What API value raises concern for arterial injury, and what is the sensitivity and specificity?**
   - An API value <0.9 has a sensitivity of 95% and specificity of 97% for major arterial injury.
   - An API >0.9 has a negative predictive value of 99%.

9. **When the API value is <0.9 in an injured extremity, what should be the next diagnostic test?**
CT angiography with follow-up arteriography to establish the diagnosis and plan for operative intervention.

10. **What abnormalities on arteriography determine a positive test result?**
- Obstruction of flow
- Extravasation of contrast
- Early venous filling or arteriovenous fistula
- Wall irregularity or filling defect
- False aneurysm (pseudoaneurysm)

11. **What study should be performed for patients with proximity injury or soft signs (API >0.9)?**
Duplex ultrasonography to rule out occult vascular injury.

12. **What occult vascular injuries can be detected by duplex ultrasonography?**
- Intimal flap.
- Pseudoaneurysm.
- Arteriovenous fistula.
- Focal vessel narrowing.
- Nonoperative observation of these injuries is safe and effective: 89% of them do not require surgery.

13. **What is a pseudoaneurysm?**
It is a disruption of the arterial wall leading to a pulsatile hematoma contained by fibrous connective tissue (but not all three arterial wall layers). (See Figs. 31-1 and 31-2.)

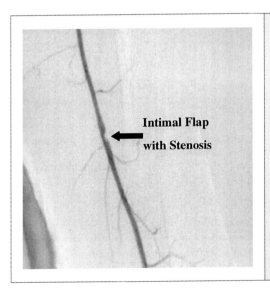

Intimal Flap
with Stenosis

Figure 31-1. Subtraction angiography demonstrating intimal flap with stenosis of superficial femoral artery.

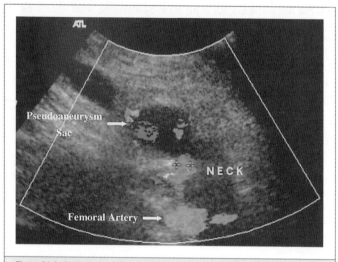

Figure 31-2. Duplex ultrasound of common femoral artery demonstrating pseudoaneurysm sac and associated neck between pseudoaneurysm sac and femoral artery after percutaneous access for angiography.

14. **What is a true aneurysm?**
Dilatation of all three layers of the vessel wall (i.e., intima, media, and adventitia).

15. **What is the most effective way to control arterial bleeding in an injured extremity?**
Direct digital pressure.

16. **What means of controlling vascular injury should be avoided? Why?**
A tourniquet should be avoided because collateral circulation is occluded and leads to increased tissue ischemia.
     Blind clamping should also be avoided because it may cause further vessel damage, making reconstruction more difficult and may injure adjacent nerves.

17. **How should a patient with an extremity vascular injury be prepared and draped in the operating room?**
The entire involved extremity should be in the sterile field. The major arterial trunk proximal to the site of injury (for proximal control) and a portion of lower extremity permitting access to saphenous vein should be included in the sterile field.

18. **What else should be prepared and draped for proximal extremity injuries?**
The chest should be prepped for proximal injuries of the upper extremity. The abdomen should be prepped for proximal injuries of the lower extremity. (Access to the chest or abdomen may be necessary to obtain safe proximal vascular control.)

19. **What are the operative principles relative to repair of vascular injuries?**
   - Perform longitudinal incisions over vessels to be explored.
   - Initial dissection should be away from the site of suspected injury and adjacent hematoma.

- Obtain proximal and distal control of the injured vessel.
- Debride the injured vessel.
- Perform primary repair if tension free (fully extend extremity to ensure tension-free repair).
- Repair with autogenous interposition vein graft if there is inadequate length (tension).

20. **What is the best conduit to use for extremity vascular injuries if primary repair is not possible? Why?**
   Saphenous or cephalic vein from the uninjured extremity because long-term patency rates are better and there is less risk of infection.

21. **Should injuries to major veins of the extremities be repaired?**
   Yes. Repair of a major vein enhances the success of a concomitant arterial repair by improving outflow. This is most applicable to popliteal venous injuries. Late thrombosis often occurs after venous repair, but initial patency helps by allowing collateral circulation to develop. This may also reduce the incidence of postoperative venous insufficiency.

22. **When should injured major veins be ligated?**
   Major veins should be ligated rather than repaired when the patient is hemodynamically unstable or the repair is too complex.

23. **What complications can develop after ligation of major extremity veins?**
   Possible complications include rapid increase in muscle compartment pressure, leading to compromised venous or arterial flow and compartment syndrome. Postoperative venous stasis may also occur, which can be attenuated with intermittent pneumatic calf compression and leg elevation.

24. **What is a compartment syndrome?**
   Development of pathologically elevated tissue pressures (preventing perfusion) within nonexpansile envelopes (inside fascial compartments) of the arm or leg.

25. **What is the most common cause of a compartment syndrome?**
   Ischemia-reperfusion injury when ischemia depletes intracellular energy stores and then reperfusion leads to toxic oxygen radicals, causing cellular swelling and interstitial fluid accumulation.

26. **What is the earliest sign of compartment syndrome after vascular repair of an extremity?**
   Neurologic deficit in the distribution of the peroneal nerve with weak dorsiflexion and numbness in the first dorsal webspace.

27. **Are there any other signs of a developing compartment syndrome of an extremity?**
   - Increased pain with passive motion of the ankle.
   - Pain out of proportion to clinical findings (ischemia hurts).
   - Tense muscle compartments that are tender to palpation.
   - Distal pulses can remain intact.

28. **How is the objective diagnosis of a compartment syndrome made?**
By measuring compartment pressures with a percutaneous needle and pressure transducer. Criteria for compartment syndrome are as follows:
- When diastolic pressure-compartment pressure is $= 20$ mm Hg or
- When mean arterial pressure-compartment pressure is $= 30$ mm Hg.

29. **What is the treatment for compartment syndrome of an extremity?**
Emergent fasciotomy with decompression of the four compartments of the lower leg (anterior, lateral, superficial posterior, and deep posterior) or decompression of the forearm compartments.

30. **What is the result of untreated compartment syndrome?**
Loss of perfusion promotes eventual myoneuronecrosis.

31. **Which are the most commonly injured arteries in the upper extremity?**

Brachial artery	30% (most frequently caused by catheterization for arteriography)
Radial or ulnar artery	20%
Axillary artery	10%
Subclavian artery	5%

32. **Which are the most commonly injured arteries in the lower extremity?**

Superficial femoral artery	20%
Popliteal artery	10%
Common femoral artery	<5%
Anterior, posterior tibial, and peroneal arteries	<5%
Deep femoral artery	2%

33. **Can a patient with an extremity arterial injury have palpable distal pulses?**
Yes. In 20% of proven arterial injuries, a distal pulse is palpable (often because of collateral circulation).

34. **What orthopedic injuries commonly have associated vascular injuries?**
- Supracondylar humerus fractures are associated with brachial artery injuries.
- Knee dislocations are associated with popliteal artery injuries.
- Femur fractures can be associated with injury to the superficial femoral artery.

35. **For an injured extremity with concomitant fracture and vascular injury, which repair should be performed first?**
The vascular repair should be performed first to restore flow and reverse tissue ischemia.

36. **After reducing or fixing an extremity fracture, what must you always do?**
Evaluate the distal pulses to ensure adequate vascular inflow (especially if fixation or any manipulation follows a vascular repair).

37. **What is the likely diagnosis in a patient with repetitive palmar trauma and finger ischemia or necrosis?**
Hypothenar hammer syndrome (HHS). The mechanism is thought to be repetitive palmar trauma in patients with preexisting palmar artery fibrodysplasia. (The arteriogram shows digital artery occlusions with segmental ulnar artery occlusion or "corkscrew" elongation.) (See Fig. 31-3.)

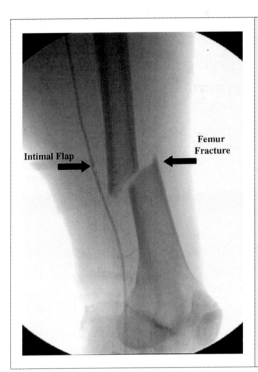

Figure 31-3. Angiography demonstrating intimal flap in superficial femoral artery associated with femur fracture.

38. **What complications can occur after angiography when a percutaneous closure device is used on the femoral artery?**
   - Thrombosis, ischemia, or both when the closure suture involves the posterior wall (back wall) of the artery.
   - Infected pseudoaneurysm.
   - Distal embolization when a hemostatic plug closure device is used.

39. **What are some of the characteristics that make computed tomography angiography an effective alternative to conventional angiography in the evaluation of extremity vascular injury?**
A higher sensitivity (95% to 100%), lower cost, decreased time to diagnosis as compared to angiography, effective even in distal arm and leg vessels, purely diagnostic (no possibility for intervention as with conventional angiography).

KEY POINTS: COMPARTMENT SYNDROME

1. Pathologically elevated tissue pressures in nonexpansile fascial compartments prevent tissue perfusion.

2. The most common cause is ischemia-reperfusion injury following traumatic extremity injuries.

3. The earliest clinical sign is numbness in the first dorsal webspace associated with compromise of the deep peroneal nerve. Other signs: pain with passive joint motion, pain out of proportion to injury, and tense and tender muscle compartments.

4. Distal pulses are evident until late in the diagnosis and should not be used to rule out compartment syndrome.

5. Handheld manometer is used to measure muscular compartments.
   Normal pressure ≤ 10 mm Hg; pathologic pressure ≥ 35 mm Hg.

6. Treatment is emergent fasciotomy.

WEBSITES

www.east.org/tpg/lepene.pdf

www.surgery.ucsf.edu/eastbaytrauma/Protocols/ER%20protocol%20pages/extremity.htm

BIBLIOGRAPHY

1. Ferris BL, Taylor LM Jr, Oyama K et al.: Hypothenar hammer syndrome: proposed etiology. J Vasc Surg 31:104-113, 2000.

2. LeBus GF, Collinge C: Vascular abnormalities as assessed with CT angiography in high-energy tibial plafond fractures. J Orthop Trauma 22(1):16-22, 2008.

3. McCroskey BL, Moore EE, Pearce WH et al.: Traumatic injuries of the brachial artery. Am J Surg 156(6):553-555, 1988.

4. Peng PD, Spain DA, Tataria M et al.: CT angiography effectively evaluates extremity vascular trauma. Am Surg 74(2):103-107, 2008.

5. Rutherford RB, editor: *Vascular surgery*, 5th ed., Philadelphia, 2000, W.B. Saunders.

6. Schwartz SI, editor: *Principles of surgery*, 7th ed., New York, 1999, McGraw-Hill.

CHAPTER 32

FACIAL LACERATIONS

Raffi Gurunluoglu, MD, PhD

1. What distinguishes facial lacerations from other lacerations?

Appearance is clearly of primary importance. Quality of the final result depends on strict adherence to basic principles of wound management and painstaking technique. Copious irrigation, judicious debridement, gentle tissue handling, meticulous hemostasis, and minimization of sutures combined with early stitch removal are critical to an optimal result. Fine suture and sharp instruments should be used; eversion of the wound margin with layered closure, obliteration of dead space, and lack of tension are mandatory.

2. What factors influence treatment for the wound?

The mechanism, location and depth of injury, the clinical assessment of contamination, and the time elapsed since wounding dictate treatment. Soft tissue injuries are of greatest concern when located in the posterior and inferior aspect of the cheek. Within this vital area lies the branches of the facial nerve, the parotid gland and duct, and the masseter muscle. Clean lacerations, heavily contaminated wounds, crush injuries, and bites are treated quite differently.

3. How are clean lacerations repaired?

Clean lacerations are treated with minimal, tension-free, fine monofilament suture placement and early suture removal (3 to 5 days). The use of plain catgut absorbable sutures in children appears to be an acceptable alternative to nonabsorbable suture because the long-term cosmetic outcome seems to be at least as good.

4. How are dirty lacerations repaired?

Heavily contaminated wounds should remain open after irrigation and debridement to undergo delayed closure. Because of cosmetic considerations, however, this approach is unacceptable in the face. For this reason, meticulous debridement of devitalized tissue and removal of all foreign material is essential. The wound should be cultured before copious irrigation, and a broad-spectrum antibiotic should be instituted prophylactically. The patient must be informed of the potential of a postrepair infection.

5. What factors influence suture selection?

Any method of suturing provokes tissue damage, impairs host defense, increases scar proliferation, and invites infection. Presence of a single silk suture in a wound lowers the infective threshold by a factor of 10,000. Therefore, fine, monofilament suture, just strong enough to overcome the resting wound tension, should be used. Use as few sutures as possible. Wounds with little or no retraction may be closed with tape alone.

6. Which wounds are suitable for closure with tissue adhesives and steri strips?

N-butyl-2-cyanoacrylate may suffice for cutaneous closure of low-tension lacerations in children (preferred method) and adults. This adhesive effectively closes low-tension lacerations. This method is fast and relatively painless. It has a low complication rate and produces excellent cosmetic outcomes. In many instances, if initial wound orientation is against Langer's lines, it may, in fact, offer an advantage over conventional manual suturing. Steri strips may also suffice for closure of low-tension simple lacerations both in adults and children and provide similar cosmetic outcomes.

7. **Should eyebrows be shaved when facial lacerations are repaired?**
No. They provide a landmark for realignment of disrupted tissue edges and do not always grow back.

8. **How should crush avulsion injuries with associated skin loss be repaired?**
Nonviable elements must be surgically excised because they predispose to infection and lead to excessive scarring. If viability is in doubt, the wound should be irrigated thoroughly and left open with moist dressings. A delayed closure can be accomplished when the questionable areas have declared themselves. It is often prudent to close facial tissue as it lies; this technique often produces a less obtrusive scar than straight-line debridement and closure.

9. **How should bites be treated?**
Both animal and human bite wounds are heavily contaminated and prone to infection. The wound should be left open and closed in a delayed fashion. However, despite the risk of infection, the wound can be irrigated and primary repair can be undertaken in an attempt to achieve the best cosmetic outcome. Antibiotic prophylaxis is indicated. If the wound becomes infected, the sutures must be removed and the wound allowed to drain and heal. The patient should be informed that a scar revision may be necessary.

10. **Should skin grafts or flaps be used for primary closure of a wound?**
Complicated tissue transfer techniques have no place in the acute treatment of facial wounds. Closure should be achieved in the simplest way possible and complex reconstructive efforts should be deferred until the scar has matured (months). When tissue loss prevents closure, it may be necessary to use a full-thickness skin graft (preferably as a sheet graft) or a skin flap for coverage. Reconstructive options should be considered early in wounds with substance loss (i.e., through and through defects of lip, nose, or ear).

11. **When are antibiotics indicated in the treatment of facial lacerations?**
Copious irrigation, debridement, and gentle tissue handling are more pertinent to the prevention of infection than the use of antibiotics in clean and clean-contaminated wounds. Antibiotic coverage is indicated, however, in crush avulsion injuries, bites, and heavily contaminated injuries.

12. **What determines the quality of the scar?**
Location of the wound, age of the patient, and type and quality of skin determine it. Lesser determinants are the type and quantity of suture material and wound care. Final appearance depends little on the method of suture. Contusion, infection, retained foreign body, improper orientation of laceration, pattern of laceration (e.g., "U" shaped), tension, and beveling of edges predict a poor outcome. Differences among suture materials are negligible; however, the technical factors of suture placement to produce wound eversion and time to removal affect the final result.

13. **When should scars be revised?**
A scar usually has its worst appearance at 2 weeks to 2 months after suturing. Scar revision should await complete maturation, which may take 4 to 24 months. A good rule of thumb is to undertake no revisions for at least 6 to 12 months after initial repair. The maturation of the wound may be assessed by its degree of discomfort, erythema, and induration.

14. **What techniques are available for scar revision?**

Circular or U-shaped scars or those crossing natural skin folds usually benefit from some form of revision involving change in direction, lengthening, or staggering. Surgical techniques include Z-plasty and W-plasty.

CONTROVERSIES

15. **What controversies exist regarding the care and repair of facial lacerations?**

There is little controversy about the care and repair of facial lacerations. Attention to basic principles of wound care usually produces a satisfactory scar. Because of the cosmetic considerations in facial trauma, primary repair in some instances is undertaken for the sake of appearance despite the risk of infection that would be deemed unacceptable in other areas of the body. A good example would be an animal or human bite wound that may be repaired primarily following copious irrigation and debridement of nonviable tissues.

KEY POINTS: FACIAL LACERATIONS

1. Appearance and function are of paramount importance.

2. Clean lacerations are treated with minimal, tension-free, fine monofilament suture placement and early suture removal (3 to 5 days).

3. N-butyl-2-cyanoacrylate (Dermabond) or steri strips are preferably used to repair pediatric facial lacerations, particularly with low tension.

4. Heavily contaminated wounds are irrigated, debrided, and repaired with administration of antibiotics.

BIBLIOGRAPHY

1. Hochberg J, Ardenghy M, Toledo S et al.: Soft tissue injuries to face and neck: early assessment and repair. World J Surg 25:1023-1027, 2001.

2. Holger JS, Wandersee SC, Hale DB: Cosmetic outcomes of facial lacerations repaired with tissue-adhesive, absorbable, and non-absorbable sutures. Am J Emerg Med 22:254-257, 2004.

3. Karounis H, Gouin S, Eisman H et al.: A randomized, controlled trial comparing long-term cosmetic outcomes of traumatic pediatric lacerations repaired with absorbable plain gut versus nonabsorbable nylon sutures. Acad Emerg Med 11:730-735, 2004.

4. Leach J: Proper handling of soft tissue in the acute phase. Facial Plast Surg 17:227-238, 2001.

5. Mattick A, Clegg G, Beattie T et al.: A randomized, controlled trial comparing a tissue adhesive (2-octylcyanoacrylate) with adhesive strips (steristrips) for pediatric repair. Emerg Med J 19:405-407, 2002.

6. Mcheik JN, Vergnes P, Bondonny JM: Treatment of facial dog bite injuries in children: a retrospective study. J Pediatr Surg 35:580-583, 2000.

7. Mitchell RB, Nanez G, Wagner JD et al.: Dog bites of the scalp, face, and neck in children. Laryngoscope 113:492-495, 2003.

8. Moscati RM, Mayrose J, Reardon RF et al.: A multicenter comparison of tap water versus sterile saline for wound irrigation. Acad Emerg Med 14:404-409, 2007.

9. Schalamon J, Ainoedhofer H, Singer G et al.: Analysis of dog bites in children who are younger than 17 years. Pediatrics 117:374-379, 2006.

10. Singer AJ, Quinn JV, Clark RE et al.: Closure of lacerations and incisions with octylcyanoacrylate: a multicenter randomized controlled trial. Surgery 131:270-276, 2002.

11. Singer AJ, Quinn JV, Thode HC et al.: Determinants of poor outcome after laceration and surgical incision repair. Plast Reconstr Surg 110:429-435, 2002.

12. Stefanopoulos PF, Tarantzopoulou AD: Facial bite wounds: management update. Int J Oral Maxillofac Surg 34:464-472, 2005.

13. Valente JH, Forti RJ, Freundlich LF et al.: Wound irrigation in children: saline or tap water? Ann Emerg Med 41:609-616, 2003.

14. Zempsky WT, Parrotti D, Grem C et al.: Randomized controlled comparison of cosmetic outcomes of simple facial lacerations closed with steri strip skin closures or dermabond tissue adhesive. Pediatr Emerg Care 20:519-524, 2004.

CHAPTER 33

BASIC CARE OF HAND INJURIES

Kagan Ozer, MD, and Laura DiMatteo, MD

1. **How are hand fractures and hand injuries splinted?**
   Injury specific immobilization should include splinting the joint above and below the injury. For example, a fracture of the metacarpal bone should be immobilized at the wrist and metacarpal phalangeal joint.
   Volar wrist splint: Ideal resting splint for the hand after burn and soft tissue injuries.
   Thumb spica splint: Ideal for injuries located on the radial side of the hand including tendinitis of the first dorsal compartment (de Quervain's).
   Ulnar gutter splint: Commonly used for the fractures of the fourth and fifth metacarpals (boxer's fracture).
   Stack splint: Used for mallet finger injuries and nail bed trauma. It allows proximal interphalangeal joint (PIP) flexion preventing the development of any contracture.

2. **What are the signs of flexor tenosynovitis?**
   Kanaval signs: flexed posture of the digit, circumferential swelling, tenderness along the flexor tendon sheath, and pain with passive extension of the digit.

3. **How is flexor tenosynotivitis treated?**
   Urgent decompression of the tendon sheath in the operating room (OR), culture specific antibiotics, and wound care.

4. **How and where should hand injuries be explored?**
   Hand wounds should be explored under tourniquet control with adequate analgesia using delicate instruments in a well-lighted surgery suite. Visual magnification is usually mandatory.

5. **How is emergency hemostasis of injured hands achieved?**
   In the acute setting (outside the operating suite), no tourniquet should be applied; and there should be no blind clamping or suture tying of any structures. Hemostasis may be achieved by elevation of the extremity and with direct compression of the wound for 10 minutes. This approach prevents injury to delicate underlying structures that are tough to see.

6. **How are fingertip injuries treated?**
   If <1 cm of pulp is disrupted, the wound will heal spontaneously with daily cleansing and dressing with nonadherent, moist gauze. Larger defects may require a skin graft, which can often be provided by defatting the amputated piece. Bone exposure necessitates flap coverage if digital length is to be maintained. Digital nerves cannot be repaired distal to the distal interphalangeal (DIP) joint.

7. **What is the classification system for fingertip amputations?**
   Classification for fingertip amputations is based on the amount of remaining sensate volar skin. Although the favorably angulated amputation commonly removes some nail and bone, the volar skin is available for easy coverage. This amputation type is "favorable" for treatment by

dressings only, allowing wound repair by contraction and epithelialization. The volarly angulated amputation angle is "unfavorable" for conservative management and usually requires a reconstructive procedure (see Fig. 33-1).

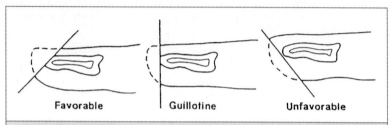

Figure 33-1. Fingertip amputations. Image from Ditmars DM Jr: Fingertip and nail bed injuries. In Kasdan ML, editor: *Occupational hand and upper extremity injuries and disease*. Philadelphia, 1991, Hanley & Belfus, 1991, with permission.)

8. **How are nail bed injuries repaired?**
Repair of the disruption of the germinal matrix must be meticulously approximated under magnification; and the nail bed splinted, preferably with the avulsed part. Subungual hematomas should be evacuated by a hot-tipped paperclip or battery-powered electric cautery. Repair of the disruption of the sterile eponychial fold must be maintained for 3 weeks with Xeroform gauze or with the original nail. Often, nail bed disruption cannot be diagnosed without removal of the nail.

9. **What is the initial management of flexor tendon laceration?**
Flexor tendon laceration is not an emergency, and repair should not be undertaken in the emergency department (ED). If a hand surgeon is unavailable, the wound should be copiously irrigated and sutured and prophylactic antibiotics instituted. This injury can be repaired primarily in 3 weeks.

10. **What is the proper management of an open fracture?**
Open fractures should be cleaned and dressed in the ED, but not probed or cultured. A first-generation cephalosporin, such as Ancef, should be administered; tetanus immunization should be updated; a saline-soaked dressing applied over the wound; and the hand should be splinted in the position of function with a bulky dressing. The wound and fracture should be urgently taken to the operating room (OR) for formal irrigation, debridement, and wound closure if possible. Wounds meeting the criteria of a Gustilo and Anderson open fracture should also receive Penicillin and an aminoglycoside, such as Gentamicin.

11. **What is the proper treatment for hand infection?**
The extremity should be immobilized and elevated, and parenteral antibiotics should be given. The patient should be immediately referred for possible surgical drainage.

12. **What is the proper management of human and animal bites?**
After cleansing of the wound, a radiograph should be taken. The wound should be left open; never closed. Antibiotics should be started, and the wound should be rechecked at 24 and 48 hours. If evidence of infection is present, parenteral antibiotics should be instituted

and referred for possible surgical drainage. In human bites, the most common microorganism is *Eikenella Corrodens* and is best treated with penicillinase resistant penicillin, such as amoxicillin/clavulanate. In animal bites, *Pasteurella Multocida* is the most common organism and should be treated with amoxicillin/clavulanate. The so-called fight bite occurs over the metacarpophalangeal (MCP) joint or proximal interphalangeal joint when a clenched fist is impaled on the front teeth of an adversary. This often inoculates the MCP joint with anaerobic streptococci. When infection is diagnosed, immediate arthrotomy and lavage should be performed.

13. **How are injection injuries treated?**
   Despite their innocuous appearance, injection injuries may cause profound destruction of hand structures. Any such injury requires immediate hospitalization with prompt and extensive decompression, drainage, and debridement.

14. **What are the most preventable causes of deformity in hand injuries?**
   Edema and infection lead to increased scarring and restricted function. Prolonged immobilization in a poor position also impairs function, as does delayed skin closure. Failure to obtain a radiograph leads to a missed diagnosis with delay in recognition of an injury.

15. **What is the proper emergency department treatment of the patient with an amputated part?**
   First the patient should be treated in accordance with the advanced trauma life support (ATLS) protocol. Once the patient condition is stabilized, tetanus immunization and prophylactic antibiotics should be administered. Broad-spectrum antibiotics should be given if the wound is heavily contaminated or if the patient is diabetic or immunocompromised. For further evaluation of the patient with a potentially replantable part, the following tests should be ordered: radiographs of the injured extremity and the amputated part, hemoglobin/hematocrit content, blood type and screening, and other tests as indicated (blood glucose for diabetics, etc.). While these tests are pending, a replantation center should be contacted for transfer. Because prolonged ischemia of the amputated part results in complete loss of the part and the function, once agreed, the transfer should be instituted as soon as possible. For a digit, replantation is usually possible up to 12 hours. However, parts containing muscle (forearm, arm) may not be replanted after 6 hours.

16. **How should the amputated part be transported to the replantation center?**
   First, the part should be placed on a wet gauze with normal saline. Then it should be placed in a sealed plastic bag which should then be placed in a container with ice saline maintaining the temperature of 4° C. Direct contact to ice should be avoided to prevent freezing. Hypotonic and hypertonic solution should not be used to prevent osmotic damage to the part.

17. **What is acute carpal tunnel syndrome?**
   Acute compression of the median nerve in the carpal tunnel. Associated with trauma to the hand, wrist, or forearm; for example, a distal radius fracture. Diagnosed clinically and presents with worsening wrist pain and sensory changes in the median nerve distribution. Sensory changes typically include parasthesias in the volar thumb, index, middle, and half of the ring finger. The best test is 2-point discrimination with less than 5 mm at the finger tips in normal hands.

18. **How is acute carpal tunnel treated?**
   Emergent operative decompression of median nerve by incising the transverse carpal ligament which is the fascial roof of the carpal tunnel.

KEY POINTS: ACUTE VERSUS CHRONIC CARPAL TUNNEL SYNDROME

1. Both are compression neuropathies.

2. Chronic form has predilection to women after 40, acute carpal tunnel syndrome can be seen at any age.

3. Acute form is related to a trauma whereas chronic form is seen more commonly in repetitive manual workers.

4. Pain is the predominant symptom in acute carpal tunnel syndrome followed by numbness and tingling. In chronic form, numbness, tingling and night awakenings are the dominant symptoms.

WEBSITE

www.ninds.nih.gov

Search: carpal tunnel

BIBLIOGRAPHY

1. Dunn R, Watson S: Suturing versus conservative management of hand lacerations. Hand lacerations should be explored before conservative treatment. Br Med J 325:299, 2002.

2. Goldner RD, Urbaniak JR: Replantation. In Green DP, editor: *Green's operative hand surgery*, 5th ed., Philadelphia, 2005, Elsevier.

3. Gustilo RB, Anderson JT: Prevention of infection in the treatment of one thousand and twenty-five open fractures of long bones: retrospective and prospective analyses. J Bone Joint Surg Am 58(4):453-458, 1976.

4. Hansen TB, Carstensen O: Hand injuries in agricultural accidents. J Hand Surg [Br] 24B:190-192, 1999.

5. Irvine AJ: Suturing versus conservative management of hand lacerations. Incisions are not lacerations. Br Med J 325(7359):299, 2002.

6. Jebson PJL, Louis DS, editors: Hand infections. Hand Clin 14(4):511-711, 1998.

7. Lee SJ, Montgomery K: Athletic hand injuries. Orthop Clin North Am 33:547-554, 2002.

8. Mack GR, McPherson SA, Lutz RB: Acute median neuropathy after wrist trauma. The role of emergent carpal tunnel release. Clin Orthop Relat Res 300:141-146, 1994.

9. Martin C, Gonzalez Del Pino J: Controversies in the treatment of fingertip amputations: conservative versus surgical reconstruction. Clin Orthop Relat Res 353, 63-73, 1998.

10. Riaz M, Hill C, Khan K et al.: Long-term outcome of early active mobilization following flexor tendon repair in zone 2. J Hand Surg 24B:157-160, 1999.

11. Taras JS, Lamb MJ: Treatment of flexor tendon injuries: surgeons' perspective. J Hand Ther 12:141-148, 1999.

12. VanderMolen AB, Matloub HS, Dzwierzynski W et al.: The hand injury severity scoring system and Workers' Compensation cases in Wisconsin, USA. J Hand Surg 24B:184-186, 1999.

CHAPTER 34

BURNS

Janeen R. Jordan, MD, and Walter L. Biffl, MD, FACS

1. **Where do burn injuries occur?**
   Eighty percent of burn-related injuries occur in the home, mostly in low-income, multifamily dwellings.

2. **Who is at risk of suffering burns?**
   The incidence of burn injuries and deaths in the United States is substantially higher than that of the rest of the industrialized world. The male-to-female ratio for burn injuries is roughly 2:1. Work-related burn injuries account for most of the disparity between males and females, with accidents in the petrochemical and transportation industries responsible for a significant proportion. Alcohol abuse and illicit drug activity also increase the risk of burn injury and death. The death rate for children younger than 5 years and adults age 65 or older is 5 to 6 times higher than for the rest of the population.

3. **What factors influence burn outcomes most profoundly?**
   The overall mortality risk of burns is 7.6%. Pediatric burn centers record mortalities between 2% and 3%, whereas mortality for those older than 50 years is more than 3 times higher than the national mean, and above 70 years of age, mortality exceeds 33%. Three major risk factors have been identified, with essentially equal weight in predicting mortality: burn size of >40% total body surface area (TBSA), patient age >60 years, and the presence of inhalation injury to the lungs. The cumulative probability of death when one or more of these factors is presented in Table 34-1.

TABLE 34-1. MORTALITY RATES ASSOCIATED WITH BURN INJURY	
Number of Risk Factors Present	Mortality
0	0.3%
1	3%
2	33%
3	90%

4. **Do any other variables influence survival?**
   Ethanol abuse and illicit drug abuse can be added to the three factors listed previously, increasing the risk of death by a factor of 2 to 4 times.

5. **As a single mode of injury, why do burns pose such a devastating challenge and threat to victims?**
   - Extensive damage to the skin (considered the largest single organ in the body and consuming almost 20% of the cardiac output [CO]) sets the stage for bacterial invasion.

- Because humans are almost 70% water, enclosed by a complex integumentary system, serious derangements in fluid homeostasis occur when the skin envelope is destroyed.
- Heat-induced denaturation of integumentary proteins enter the circulation. Systemic infection or sepsis remains the dominant precipitant of organ failure and death; this points to a burn injury-related immune dysfunction or failure.

6. What happens locally in burn injury?

The injury site may be divided into three zones by standard light microscopy: an inner zone of necrosis, a middle zone of stasis, and an outer zone of hyperemia. In the **zone of necrosis,** all proteins are denatured; all microvascular and macrovascular structure and function are destroyed. Surrounding this central zone is a **zone of stasis.** Here, cellular morphology is intact but cells are swollen with microstructural changes with extravasation of leukocytes and red blood cells into the interstitial space, increased interstitial fluid, and capillary stasis. A third **zone of hyperemia** then gently transitions into the adjacent normal tissues where no abnormalities are seen.

7. What changes occur systemically?

Systemic events become clinically significant beyond an injury size of 10% TBSA. Two important abnormalities occur: (1) a trend to fluid retention with generalized edema, caused by an increased systemic microvascular permeability of rapid onset (minutes to hours) and (2) a definite and reproducible decrease in CO that gradually resolves over 12 to 36 hours to evolve into an ensuing cardiovascular hyperdynamism at 36 hours postinjury. To summarize, the pump is failing, and the microvasculature is leaking.

8. How can burn victims be managed in a rational way from the time of injury?

Five phases of care can be identified:
1. Burn first aid.
2. Prehospital care.
3. Emergency department (ED).
4. Transport to burn unit.
5. Stabilization in burn unit or patient room.

9. What can first responders do when witnessing a burn injury?

First, do no harm. No ice, butter, dry ice, or any other substance should be applied to the wound after extinguishing the fire. If the burn is minor (<10% TBSA), running tepid tap water over the burn with a handheld shower for 20 minutes is beneficial. Applying wet towels appears to provide no benefit and may provoke hypothermia. If stranded in a remote area, encourage oral fluid intake and cover the wound with clean towels. Aspirin or ibuprofen may benefit the patient and the wound. Elevate any burned extremities and encourage full range of motion of all joints.

10. What actions are needed from prehospital providers (i.e., after the prehospital crew arrives, what are their priorities)?

The American College of Surgeons' Committee on Trauma (ACS-COT) advises that all ambulance crews follow "scoop and run" procedure guidelines for all burn victims within 60 minutes of an appropriate hospital (level I or II trauma center or burn facility). Attempt to place an intravenous (IV) line en route, but this is not essential if the travel time is <60 minutes. Lines may be placed through burned skin, preferably in antecubital veins.

11. How does the hospital-based emergency department contribute to the care of the patients with major burns?

Urgency in caring for the victim, not the wound, is pivotal for the ultimate survival of the victim:
- A. Airway. Look for soot in the pharynx and for extensive facial burns.
- B. Breathing. Identify hoarseness or stridor. Listen for breath sounds on both sides.

C. Circulation. Place two peripheral IV lines, start fluids as lactated Ringer's solution; calculate the Parkland formula = 4 ml × kg body weight × % body burn [half of volume in first 8 hours; other half over 16 hours].

D. Neurologic deficit. Examine central nervous system (CNS) and cranial nerves; assess the neurologic status of burned extremities.

E. Expose and examine the skin, log roll and meticulously determine burn size on the posterior body, and then cover and preserve body heat. The patient's environment should be heated to 90° F.

F. Fluid therapy should be assessed for effect as demonstrated by 1 ml of urine output per kilogram of body weight every hour.

Pain management and psychoemotional support are also vitally important. Avoid overdosing with narcotics.

12. How are burns sized?

This determination is done clinically, with the aid of three important clinical tools:

1. The **volar surface of the victim's opened hand** (including fingers) = 0.8% to 1.0% of TBSA; most useful for the sizing of small, scattered wound areas

2. **Rule of nines:** most commonly used; easy to memorize; not accurate; usually overestimates

   Adult head = 9%

   Total upper extremity = 2 × 9%

   Total anterior lower extremity = 2 × 9%

   Total posterior lower extremity = 2 × 9%

   Anterior torso = 2 × 9%

   Posterior torso including buttocks = 2 × 9%

   Genitals = 1%

   Note that adults and children differ significantly by the difference in the relative size of the head (9% in adults, 15% in infants). By contrast, a thigh in an infant is much smaller than in adults (6% versus 10%).

3. **Lund and Browder chart:** more accurate; time consuming; requires practice; not easy to memorize

13. Besides the actual skin injury, what other associated injuries may occur?

Inhalation injury is diagnosed in 10% of all hospitalized burn victims. Other physical trauma is frequently associated with explosions or merely the attempts to escape the fire. Awareness of associated trauma justifies the importance of a careful Advanced Trauma Life Support (ATLS) trauma evaluation.

14. How is inhalation injury defined?

In contrast to the visible and somewhat quantifiable external burn injury to the skin, the inhalation of heat, carbon monoxide, cyanide, and other toxic or noxious vapors is less visible and less quantifiable, yet quite dangerous. Four separate mechanisms of injury to the airways are sometimes incorrectly grouped as inhalation injury:

1. Carbon monoxide intoxication.

2. Heat damage to upper airways.

3. Inhalation of toxic smoke components that are produced by the combustion of modern synthetic materials used in the interior decoration of houses, buildings, and cars.

4. **Cyanide poisoning:** The combustion of many synthetic materials also produces cyanide gas, which binds to the cytochrome enzyme system and inhibits mitochondrial function and cellular respiration. Blood cyanide levels should be assessed in all patients with carbon monoxide levels >10%.

15. **How is inhalation injury diagnosed?**
    1. Obvious hoarseness or stridor.
    2. Substantial head and neck or facial burns.
    3. Entrapment in enclosed space or direct proximity to an explosion.
    4. Extensive total body burns (>50% in young adults; less in elderly individuals).
    5. Event history of superheated steam.

16. **What treatment has most influenced the outcome of burn victims over the past 100 years?**
    Adequate and timely fluid resuscitation.

17. **Why should fluid be resuscitated, and by what route?**
    All patients with burns >10% TBSA should receive fluid. Fluid resuscitation through the gastrointestinal (GI) tract with an orogastric tube is used quite often in pediatric burn centers. In adults, the IV route is mandatory.

18. **How is fluid therapy managed?**
    The fluid management plan has two components. First, determine the burn wound size and the patient's weight in kilograms, calculate the hourly fluid rate by the Parkland formula, and administer lactated Ringer's solution at the hourly rate calculated.

    The second component of the plan is just as important. Monitor the effectiveness of your fluid therapy plan and adjust it promptly when indicated. Our goals is a patient who is hemodynamically normalized, with a urine output of 0.5 to 1.0 ml of urine per kilogram body weight per hour.

19. **What should be done if this treatment algorithm fails to achieve clinical improvement and patient stabilization?**
    Failure to respond to the Parkland formula is indicative of a poor prognosis. However, some additional measures may be beneficial but are not currently considered as part of the standard of care. These include the use of hypertonic saline solutions in massive burns, early use of colloids in massive burns, and the early use of inotropes (dopamine is preferred in most burn texts).

20. **How are fluid requirements calculated when there has been a delay in the initiation of therapy?**
    Sometimes delay is unavoidable. In an attempt to address a perceived backlog of fluid resuscitation, current teaching is to proportionally increase the fluid volume in an attempt to get the desired total volume for 8 hours into the patient before the 8-hour period elapses. This remedy does require some common sense; one should not apply this guideline if the patient arrives at the resuscitation site later than 3 hours after the injury. Instead, administer fluids based on blood pressure (BP), pulse, and urine output.

21. **What is the best way to care for burn wounds initially?**
    Early on, these wounds need simple coverage with a surgically clean or, if available, sterile sheet or surgical drape. The ACS-COT burn and trauma guidelines state that definitive wound care need not occur up to 24 hours postinjury. No ointment or specific antibacterial treatment is initially required. The patient should be kept warm because exposure precipitates systemic hypothermia.

    For definitive wound care, the entire patient is washed or showered, and residual debris and damaged epidermis are removed. Then the extent of the injury is mapped, usually on a

Lund and Browder chart, along with preliminary attempts to determine the depth of the injury. A burn wound is usually a mosaic of different areas injured to varying degrees (depths). All burn wounds deepen to some extent over the first 48 to 96 hours, so a better prediction of which areas require grafting will come with time.

22. **Why and how is the depth of a burn injury graded?**
    This depends on the presence of skin appendages (hair follicle and sweat gland) that carry the germinal layer deep into the dermis, from which reepithelialization can occur. On the day of injury, the visual ability to differentiate burn wound that will heal from that which will not is poor (50% accurate). Over time (next 3 to 7 days), the accuracy of clinical prediction will improve somewhat ($\approx$90%). Table 34-2 helps to elucidate these aspects.

    Fourth-degree burns involve damage to structures deeper than the dermis (e.g., fat, muscle, bone, tendon, nerve, joint capsule). Burns are designated as fifth degree when tissue is lost, blown off, or vaporized by the burn or blast.

TABLE 34-2. DEPTH OF INJURY WITH CLINICAL SIGNS AND PROBABLE OUTCOME

Depth of Injury	Clinical Signs and Symptoms	Outcome
First degree (superficial injury limited to epidermis)	Erythema of the skin with mild to moderate discomfort.	Wounds heal spontaneously in 5–10 days; damaged epithelium peels off, leaving no residual effects.
Second degree Superficial (involves entirety of epidermis and superficial portion of dermis) Deep (involves deeper dermis, but viable portions of epidermal appendages remain)	Wounds are blistered or weeping, erythematous, and painful. Skin is desiccated, blistered, white eschar often seen. Wounds are occasionally moist and difficult to distinguish from third-degree burn.	Wounds heal spontaneously within 2–3 weeks without residual scarring and with good-quality skin; pigmentation may be altered. Wounds heal spontaneously beyond 3–4 weeks; hypotrophic scarring often occurs and, occasionally, unstable epithelium. For best results, remove eschar by tangential excision and cover with split-thickness skin graft.
Third degree (all epidermal appendages destroyed)	Avascular, waxy, white, leathery brown or black, insensate eschar.	Unless small in size (<2 cm in diameter), wounds require removal of eschar and coverage with skin graft for healing.

23. **When should surgical excision of the burn wound begin?**
    It should start as soon as possible, but it should be blended with common sense and pragmatism, which implies a patient who is hemodynamically "normalized" with no signs of sepsis or other contraindication to major surgery. This can be as soon as 24 hours after injury in small to moderate size burns ($\approx$30% depending on age) but may take up to 4 to 10 days in unstable, septic, or frail patients.

24. **How is the excised area managed?**

    A significant advance in burn management occurred in the early 1970s when Janzekovic demonstrated that excised wounds should be immediately grafted with skin. This remains the goal. If donor sites are insufficient, cadaver skin, pigskin, or biosynthetic products (e.g., Integra, Biobrane, or Transcyte) can be used for wound coverage. These areas require autografting subsequently. Cultured autologous keratinocytes are an attractive theoretical alternative, but they still lack consistent high-percentage engraftment when used on large areas.

25. **What is the impact of a severe burn injury on the body?**

    A big burn is on the top of the list of diseases or injuries that are best avoided. The metabolic response peaks at 2.5 times the basal metabolic rate (BMR) in all burns >50% TBSA. This maximal acceleration of the body's metabolism by burn injury leads to rapid and severe catabolism, further aggravated by periods of septicemia and heat loss through increased evaporation.

26. **How can we best supply fuel to the metabolic furnace of the body?**

    Nutritional support of the burn victim is paramount. Total enteral nutrition may have the added benefit of maintaining the intestinal barrier function, which is purported to reduce septic events by preventing bacterial translocation.

27. **What is the role of antibiotics in burn care?**

    Antibiotics are never administered prophylactically for burn injuries. However, early and appropriate antibiotic therapy is a critically important and life-saving tool in the management of established infections in burn patients.

28. **How are chemical burn injuries approached?**

    Brush off all chemicals that remain in powdered form on the victim. Thereafter, immediate and prolonged irrigation (30 minutes) of the contaminated skin should be done with running tap water; in the case of alkali burns, irrigate for 60 minutes. Some chemicals may be absorbed; therefore, immediate contact with a toxicology center is indicated.

29. **How are patients with electrical burns managed?**

    An injury caused by electricity may either be an electrical **flash** burn or **contact or conduction** injury. In electrical flash injury, the air or atmosphere is ionized by the electrical discharge, without conduction of current through the body. Thus, the injury is only cutaneous. A true electrical flash burn most frequently heals without much grafting. Airway compromise is rare. In electrical conduction injury, however, tissue is damaged through the actual transfer of electrical energy through the patient from entry point to exit. Thermal energy is generated within the tissues because of the relative resistance to the conduction of current, with resultant protein denaturation and cell death. Different structures (e.g., bone, skin, muscle, nerve, tendon, and lung) exhibit different electrical conductivity, resulting in unpredictable conduction pathways. Thus, the skin is often only minimally involved at the entry and exit sites, with extensive muscle, nerve, tendon, and even bone necrosis in erratic patterns. Neurologic injury, compartment syndrome, and myoglobinuria are frequent complications. Rapid tissue decompression (i.e., fasciotomy) is essential with early and repeated reexploration to remove necrotic tissue. The goal of fluid therapy should be to achieve high urine volumes (>1.0 to 1.5 milliliters per kilogram per hour). Alkalinization of the urine is also beneficial.

30. **After burn injuries have healed, what important issues remain to be addressed in the rehabilitation period?**

    The rehabilitation of a burn victim must begin on the day of admission and is a total team effort that involves physiatrists, plastic surgeons, occupational therapists, physical therapists, nutritionists, psychologists, social workers, pulmonologists, microbiologists, pharmacists, speech therapists, and nurses. Rehabilitation of the mind and body must occur in concert.

KEY POINTS: FACTORS STRONGLY ASSOCIATED WITH MORTALITY AFTER BURN INJURY

1. Burn size >40% TBSA.

2. Patient age >60 years.

3. Presence of inhalation injury.

4. One risk factor: 3% mortality rate; all three risk factors: 90% mortality rate.

WEBSITE

www.ameriburn.org/

BIBLIOGRAPHY

1. Blumetti J, Hunt JL, Arnoldo BD et al.: The Parkland formula under fire: is the criticism justified? J Burn Care Res 29:180, 2008.

2. Demling RL: Burn care in the immediate resuscitation period. In *American College of Surgeons: Surgery: Principles and Practice*, Chicago, 2002, American College of Surgeons.

3. Gibbons J: Prevention. In Gibbons J, editor: *Fire! 38 Lifesaving tips for you and your family*, Seattle, 1995, Ballard Publishing.

4. Heyland DK, Novak F, Drover JW et al.: Should immuno nutrition become routine in critically ill patients? *JAMA* 29:944, 2001.

5. Krzywiecki A, Ziora D, Niepsuj G et al.: Late consequences of respiratory system burns. J Physiol Pharmacol 58 (Supp 5):319, 2007.

6. McDonald-Smith GP, Saffle JR, Edelman L et al.: *National Burn Repository 2002 Report*, Chicago, 2002, American Burn Association.

7. McGill V, Kahn S, Gamelli RL et al.: The impact of substance use on mortality and morbidity from thermal injury. J Trauma 38:931, 1995.

8. Mustonen KM, Vuola J: Acute renal failure in intensive care burn patients. J Burn Care Res 29(1):227-237, 2008.

9. Pruitt BA, Goodwin CW, Mason AD Jr: Epidemiological, demographic and outcome characteristics of burn injury. In Herndon DN, editor: *Total burn care*, 2nd ed., Philadelphia, 2002, W.B. Saunders.

10. Ryan CM, Sheridan RL, Tompkins RG et al.: Objective estimates of the probability of death from burn injuries. N Engl J Med 338:362-368, 1998.

CHAPTER 35

PEDIATRIC TRAUMA

Jonathan P. Roach, MD, and David A. Partrick, MD

1. **What is the leading cause of death in children in the United States?**
   Injuries cause more death and disability in children from ages 1 to 18 years than all other causes combined. Unintentional injury deaths account for 65% of all injury deaths in children under 19 years of age. Each year, approximately 20,000 children and teenagers die as a result of injury and 50,000 children suffer permanent disabilities. Each year, nearly 1 in 4 children receives medical treatment for an injury. The estimated annual cost is $15 billion.

2. **What age groups are at particular risk for traumatic death?**
   Infants younger than age 2 years have a consistently higher mortality rate for the same level of injury. During adolescence, however, injury takes the greatest toll, accounting for nearly 80% of deaths.

3. **What primary mechanisms account for pediatric traumatic injuries?**
   Blunt (90%), penetrating (9%), and crush injuries (<1%). Motor vehicle accidents are the most common cause of injury (50%) and death in childhood.

4. **What is the incidence of injuries by body region?**
   Multiple (50%), extremities (20%), head and neck (15%), abdomen (3%), face (2%), and thorax (1%).

5. **What is the overall mortality from injury in children?**
   Two percent of all injured children, and 3% of hospitalized injured children.

6. **What is the mortality rate of injuries by mechanism?**

Mechanism	Mortality (%)
Beating	13
Gunshot wound (GSW)	8
Motor vehicle accident	5
Pedestrian	5
Motorcycle	3
Bicycle	2
Sport	1
Fall	1
Other	3

7. **Are boys and girls equally susceptible to injury?**
   No. Boys are injured twice as often as girls. Boys and men are at a 4 times greater risk for "successful" suicide (although boys try it less often), 3 times greater risk for drowning, 2.5 times greater risk for homicide, and 2 times greater risk for motor vehicle-related trauma. The second X chromosome is clearly protective.

8. **How is a child's airway different from an adult's?**
   Children are at increased risk of airway obstruction because of their large tongue; floppy epiglottis; increased lymphoid tissue; and short, small-diameter trachea. Uncuffed endotracheal tubes are appropriate in children younger than age 8 years to minimize vocal cord trauma, subglottic edema, and ulceration. The narrowest part of a child's airway is the cricoid ring, which functions as a seal for the uncuffed endotracheal tube.

9. **What is the appropriate size of endotracheal tube to place in a child?**
   The endotracheal tube should be the same size as the child's small finger. For newborns, use a 3-mm tube; children in first year of life, 4-mm tube; children older than 1 year, internal diameter of the endotracheal tube = 18 + patient's age in years ÷ 4 (but, in an urgent situation do not resort to extensive calculations; simply look at the child's pinky).

10. **What if oral endotracheal intubation cannot be accomplished?**
    A needle cricothyrotomy is preferable to surgical cricothyrotomy and can be performed with a 14-gauge catheter. Conceptually, this is the same as jet insufflation in adults. Surgical cricothyrotomy is much more difficult in small children and has a high association with secondary subglottic stenosis.

11. **What is a child's total blood volume?**
    It is 80 ml/kg (8% of body weight).

12. **What is the first sign of significant blood loss in children?**
    Tachycardia. Young children are incredibly tough and have a remarkable tolerance to blood loss. Hemorrhage of 30% of blood volume may result in no blood pressure (BP) change, but such blood loss does cause a rapid increase in heart rate. A child's cardiac output (CO) depends largely on heart rate (HR); unlike adults, children have a limited capacity to increase stroke volume.

13. **What are signs of hypovolemic shock in children?**
    Tachycardia (progressing to bradycardia), altered mental status, respiratory compromise, delayed capillary refill (>2 sec), and decreased or absent peripheral pulses.

14. **Is hypotension a reliable indicator of blood loss in children?**
    No. Fewer than half of injured children with documented hypotension have an identifiable insult resulting in significant volume loss. Hypotension is often associated with an isolated closed head injury, especially in children younger than age 6 years.

15. **Why are children at increased risk for hypothermia during resuscitation?**
    The child's surface area is large relative to internal body mass; an unclothed child can lose heat fast. Cold intravenous (IV) fluids and inhaled gases can exacerbate hypothermia, leading to hypoxemia, which causes pulmonary hypertension and progressive metabolic acidosis. Particularly vulnerable are infants <6 months of age, who lack significant subcutaneous fat and an effective shivering mechanism.

16. **What sites are preferred for venous access in children?**
    Two large-bore IV catheters should be inserted percutaneously in the upper extremities. The second choice is percutaneous access to the distal saphenous vein (or a cutdown).

17. **What if you cannot establish an intravenous line?**
    The intraosseous route is safe and actually requires less time than a venous cutdown. The anteromedial surface of the proximal tibia is used most commonly, with the needle placed 3 cm distal to the tibial tuberosity. The proximal femur, distal femur, and distal tibia are other

potential sites. Saline, glucose, blood, bicarbonate, atropine, dopamine, epinephrine, diazepam, antibiotics, phenytoin, and succinylcholine have been administered successfully via the intraosseous route. Complications are rare and result primarily from infection or extravasation. Intraosseous volume resuscitation facilitates subsequent cannulation of the venous circulation.

18. **What are the appropriate crystalloid and blood resuscitation volumes in children?**

Administer 20 ml/kg of Ringer's lactate solution or normal saline by bolus. A response is a decrease in HR and an increase in urinary output. The 20-ml/kg bolus should be repeated if assessment reveals inadequate tissue perfusion. If evidence of shock persists after two bolus infusions of crystalloid solution, 10 ml/kg of packed red blood cells (type specific if available or O-negative) should be administered. Unfortunately, a favorable response to resuscitation does not exclude a big abdominal or thoracic injury.

19. **Why are head injuries more common in children than adults?**

Until age 10 years, children's heads are larger in relation to the body than heads of adults. Central nervous system (CNS) injury is the leading cause of death among injured children and, thus, is the principal determinant of outcome.

20. **What types of head injuries are more common in children?**

Epidural hemorrhage is the most common; subdural hemorrhage is relatively rare. However, mortality from subdural hemorrhage is 40% versus 4% for an epidural bleed. Pediatric patients also tend to sustain injuries that produce diffuse edema rather than focal, space-occupying lesions.

21. **Can children have significant chest trauma without rib fractures?**

Absolutely. The chest wall is much more compliant in children than in adults; thus, kinetic energy is transmitted more readily to structures within the thorax. A child with significant blunt chest trauma is at increased risk of life-threatening contusion to the lungs or heart even with no or relatively few rib fractures. Furthermore, pneumothorax may prove rapidly fatal in children because of a more mobile mediastinum. When present, rib fractures in children reflect nonaccidental trauma. Thoracic injury is the second leading cause of death (after head trauma) in children.

22. **What types of thoracic injuries are common or uncommon in children?**

Pulmonary contusion, traumatic asphyxia, and tracheobronchial injuries are common. Traumatic aortic rupture, flail chest, diaphragmatic rupture, and open pneumothorax are unusual.

23. **What is the frequency of abdominal organ injury in blunt trauma?**

In decreasing order of frequency, they are spleen, liver, kidneys, intestine, pancreas, urinary bladder, and major blood vessels. Approximately one third of children with major trauma have significant intraperitoneal injuries that must be recognized and treated expeditiously.

24. **How accurate is physical examination in the evaluation of pediatric blunt abdominal trauma?**

Poor. Physical examination is misleading in ≈50% of injured children.

25. **What are the advantages and disadvantages of diagnostic peritoneal lavage in children?**

Diagnostic peritoneal lavage (DPL) is 96% accurate in detecting intraabdominal injury. However, it may lead to nontherapeutic laparotomy rates of 15%.

26. **What are the advantages and disadvantages of computed tomography in children?**
Abdominal computed tomography (CT) scan is safe, noninvasive, and can assess retroperitoneal structures and identify specific organ injuries. CT is critical in the decision to manage children nonoperatively. Disadvantages include insensitivity for hollow visceral injury and the need for IV and enteral contrast agents. In addition, CT is time consuming (spiral CT may prove better) and requires patient transport and sedation. A trip to the scanner leaves patients vulnerable and unmonitored. Thus, CT is risky in unstable patients.

27. **Is ultrasonography effective in the evaluation of children with abdominal trauma?**
Yes. It is simple, fast, readily available, and can be performed at the bedside. In addition, it is noninvasive and easily repeatable. The sensitivity and specificity of a focused abdominal sonography in trauma (FAST) examination exceeds 95%. Abdominal ultrasound is best used as a triage tool to detect significant intraperitoneal fluid, thus identifying hemodynamically unstable patients who might benefit from a laparotomy.

28. **Is there a reliable method to diagnose hollow visceral injury in children?**
No. Serial physical examinations remain the gold standard. Repeat physical examination by the trauma surgical team is mandatory.

29. **What are the "soft signs" of pediatric intraabdominal injury?**
   - Lap-belt ecchymosis corresponds to a high incidence of solid organ injury, hollow viscus injury, and lumbar spine injury.
   - Gross hematuria has a 30% risk for significant intraabdominal injury not even involving the genitourinary system.
   - Elevation of the liver enzymes aspartate aminotransferase (>250 U/L) or alanine aminotransferase (>450 U/L) corresponds to a 50% risk for liver injury.
   - Children with documented pelvic fracture have at least a 20% risk for associated intraabdominal injury.
   - Children with severe neurologic impairment (Glasgow Coma Scale score <8) frequently suffer concurrent intraabdominal injury.

30. **What should be suspected in children with seat belt or handlebar injuries?**
The **seat-belt complex** consists of ecchymosis of the abdominal wall, a flexion-distraction injury to the lumbar spine (Chance fracture), and intestinal injury. Approximately 30% of children with the seat-belt sign have an associated intestinal injury. A **handlebar injury** classically causes disruption of the pancreas at the junction of the body and tail, where the pancreas crosses the vertebral column and is vulnerable to anterior blunt compression.

31. **Does the presence of hemoperitoneum in children require laparotomy?**
No. Unlike in adults, <15% of children with hemoperitoneum require laparotomy for control of bleeding or repair of an injury.

32. **Do all children with solid organ injuries require operative repair?**
No. As with adult patients, selective nonoperative management of solid organ injuries has revolutionized the management of pediatric trauma. In fact, most patients sustaining a Grade I to IV liver or spleen injury will not require an operation.

33. **When is nonoperative management of solid organ injury in children appropriate?**
When the vital signs remain stable, 50% or less of the blood volume is replaced, and no other significant intraabdominal injuries are present. The decision for nonoperative management versus laparotomy should be based on the child's physiologic condition and not on the extent of injury as documented radiographically.

34. **What are the long-term consequences of nonoperative management of a splenic injury in children?**

   Vascular pseudoaneurysm and splenic cyst are known sequelae of splenic trauma. However, in pediatric patients these complications are exceedingly rare (<1%). Up to 15% of children (depending on grade of injury) may experience prolonged pain >4 weeks after injury. In almost all cases, though, this pain is related to the healing process or is entirely unrelated to the spleen.

35. **What are the indications for operative intervention for solid organ injuries?**

   Massive bleeding on presentation and transfusion of >50% of blood volume (40 ml/kg) within 24 hours of injury.

36. **What is SCIWORA?**

   SCIWORA stands for spinal cord injury without radiologic abnormalities. It is a problem unique to children. A child's spine has increased elasticity, shallow and horizontally oriented facet joints, anterior wedging of the vertebral bodies, and poorly developed uncinate processes. The spinal cord can be completely disrupted in young children without apparent disruption of the vertebral elements. However, most patients have evidence of spinal cord injury (SCI) on magnetic resonance imaging (MRI). Two thirds of SCIWORA cases are seen in children ≈8 years of age.

37. **What is the hallmark of SCIWORA?**

   A documented neurologic deficit that may have changed or resolved by the time the child arrives in the emergency department (ED). The danger is that immediate reinjury of the same area may produce permanent disability. Many children with SCIWORA tend to develop neurologic deficits hours to days after the reported injury. Therefore, spinal immobilization should continue, and thorough neurosurgical evaluation is essential in any child with reliable evidence of even a transient neurologic deficit.

38. **What percentage of pediatric deaths attributed to injury are caused intentionally?**

   Twenty-five percent. More than 80% of deaths from head trauma in children younger than 2 years are caused by intentional abuse.

39. **What signs are suspicious for nonaccidental trauma (NAT)?**
   - History of failure to thrive.
   - Delay in obtaining medical care.
   - Multiple previous injuries.
   - Absent or uninterested caregiver.
   - Fluctuating or conflicting histories.
   - History inconsistent with the injury or developmental level of the victim.

   Suspicious physical findings include bite, pinch, slap, or cord marks or bruises in various stages of healing; multiple or bilateral skull fractures; a skull fracture in a fall <4 feet; retinal hemorrhages (from shaking), rib fractures, and perineal burns or linear burn borders (from "dipping" the child into scalding liquid).

40. **List the characteristics of shaken baby syndrome.**
   - Retinal hemorrhage.
   - Subdural or subarachnoid hemorrhage.
   - Little evidence of external trauma.
   - Age <2 years.

41. **What fracture patterns are suspicious for NAT?**
    - Multiple rib fractures of different ages.
    - Extremity fractures such as metaphyseal "chip" or "bucket-handle" fractures.
    - Diaphyseal spiral fracture in children <9 months of age.
    - Transverse midshaft long-bone fracture.
    - Femur fracture in infants <2 years of age.
    - Fracture of the acromion process of the scapula.
    - Proximal humerus fracture.

42. **What percentage of NAT cases involves burn injuries? What are their characteristics?**
    Twenty percent of abuse cases involve burns. Scalding by hot water is the most common. Specific patterns of injury may raise suspicion of abuse, including burns involving the buttocks and perineum (bathing trunk distribution), back, dorsum of the hand, and stocking-glove distribution. Cigarette burns look like circular punched-out ulcers of similar size.

43. **What are the necessary steps in evaluation of children with suspected NAT?**
    Any child with suspected NAT should have a detailed physical examination with thorough documentation (drawings and photographs can be quite helpful) of all injuries, head CT scan, skeletal survey (babygram), and retinal fundoscopic examination. The appropriate child protective services should be contacted immediately.

44. **How common is postinjury multiple organ failure in children?**
    It is rare. With equivalent injury severity, multiple organ failure (MOF) in children is much lower than in adults and carries a much lower mortality.

45. **Does the blood glucose level in pediatric trauma patients matter?**
    Yes. While this intensive care unit (ICU) issue has been given great attention in the adult trauma population, only recently have the beneficial effects of tight glycemic control been examined in the pediatric trauma population. Euglycemia (glucose 90 to 130 mg/dl) is associated with decreased rate of infection, decreased hospital length of stay, and increased survival.

KEY POINTS: PEDIATRIC HEMODYNAMICS

1. Blood volume: 80 ml/kg.
2. The first sign of hypovolemia is tachycardia, which progresses to bradycardia.
3. Hypotension is *not* a reliable indicator of blood loss; children can lose 30% of blood volume without detectable change in BP.
4. Preferred IV access routes in order: (1) two large-bore upper extremity IVs; (2) distal saphenous vein or cutdown; (3) intraosseous access.
5. Resuscitation fluid is lactate Ringer's, 20 ml/kg × 2; then packed red blood cells (10 ml/kg) if instability continues.

BIBLIOGRAPHY

1. Calkins CM, Bensard DD, Moore EE et al.: The injured child is resistant to multiple organ failure: a different inflammatory response? J Trauma 53:1058, 2002.
2. Dare AO, Dias MS, Li V: Magnetic resonance imaging correlation in pediatric spinal cord injury without radiographic abnormality. J Neurosurg 97(1 suppl):33, 2002.

3. Kristoffersen KW, Mooney DP: Long-term outcome of nonoperative pediatric splenic injury management. J Pediatr Surg 42:1038, 2007.

4. Holmes JF, Gladman A, Chang CH: Performance of abdominal ultrasonography in pediatric blunt trauma patients: a meta-analysis. J Pediatr Surg 42:1588, 2007.

5. Mazzola CA, Adelson PD: Critical care management of head trauma in children. Crit Care Med 30(11 suppl): S393, 2002.

6. Mehall JR, Ennis JS, Saltzman DA et al.: Prospective results of a standardized algorithm based on hemodynamic status for managing pediatric solid organ injury. J Am Coll Surg 193:347, 2001.

7. Partrick DA, Bensard, DD, Janik JS et al.: Is hypotension a reliable indicator of blood loss from traumatic injury in children? Am J Surg 184:555, 2002.

8. Roaten JB, Partrick DA, Nydam TL et al.: Nonaccidental trauma is a major cause of morbidity and mortality among patients at a regional level I pediatric trauma center. J Pediatr Surg 41:2013, 2006.

9. St. Peter SD, Keckler SJ, Spilde TL et al.: Justification for an abbreviated protocol in the management of blunt spleen and liver injury in children. J Pediatr Surg 43:191, 2008.

10. Stafford PW, Blinman TA, Nance ML: Practical points in evaluation and resuscitation of the injured child. Surg Clin North Am 82:273, 2002.

11. Tuggle DW, Kuhn MA, Jones SK et al.: Hyperglycemia and infections in pediatric trauma patients. Am Surg 74:195, 2008.

APPENDICITIS

CHAPTER 36

Laurel R. Imhoff, MD, MPH, and Alden H. Harken, MD

1. **What is the classic presentation of acute appendicitis?**
   Periumbilical pain that migrates to the right lower quadrant (RLQ) in a patient who is anorexic. Associated symptoms include: nausea, vomiting, and bowel changes.

2. **What is the pathophysiology of appendicitis?**
   The appendix is susceptible to luminal obstruction, via lymphoid hyperplasia, a retained fecalith, tumor, foreign body, or kink. Any of these processes may result in lymphatic and venous obstruction that increases intraluminal pressure and causes distention of the appendiceal lumen. Consequently, an acute inflammatory response develops that leads to ischemia, bacterial overgrowth and eventually necrosis. Unless surgically removed, the gangrenous appendix will perforate, releasing the appendiceal contents into the peritoneal cavity. Subsequently a phlegmon, intraperitoneal abscess, or local peritonitis develops.

3. **What is the mechanism of the periumbical pain?**
   The intestines are insensitive to touch or inflammation unless the enclosing peritoneum is involved. Epigastric pain results from a distended section of intestine. This pain is referred along midline.

4. **Where is McBurney's point?**
   One third the distance between the anterosuperior iliac spine and the umbilicus.

5. **What is McBurney's point?**
   The point of maximal tenderness in acute appendicitis. It results from local inflammation of the parietal peritoneum.

6. **Was McBurney a cop from Boston?**
   Probably. Another McBurney was a surgeon from New York who, in collaboration with a surgeon named Fitz, coined the term *appendicitis* in classic papers published in 1886 and 1889.

7. **What are the typical laboratory findings of a patient with appendicitis?**
   - White blood cell (WBC) count: 12,000 to 14,000
   - Negative urinalysis results (no WBCs)
   - Negative pregnancy test result

8. **What layers does the surgeon encounter on exposing the appendix through a Rockey-Davis incision?**
   Skin, subcutaneous fat, aponeurosis of the external oblique muscle, internal oblique muscle, transversalis abdominus muscle, tranvsersalis fascia, and peritoneum.

9. **Other possible signs in appendicitis include:**
   Rovsings sign: pain in the RLQ with palpation of the left lower quadrant (LLQ).
   Dunphy's sign: increased pain with coughing (a cough jostles the inflamed peritoneum).

Psoas sign: pain on passive extension of the right thigh. It is present when the inflamed appendix is retrocecal and overlying the right psoas muscle.

Obturator sign: pain on passive internal rotation of the hip when the right knee is flexed. It is present when the inflamed appendix is in contact with the obturator internus muscle.

10. Who was Rockey-Davis?

Rockey-Davis was a pair of surgeons—A.E. Rockey and G.G. Davis—who developed RLQ transverse, muscle-splitting incisions that extend into the rectus sheath.

11. What is the blood supply to the appendix and right colon?

The ileocolic and right colic arteries, which come off the superior mesenteric artery.

12. Does surgery for appendicitis involve a risk of mortality?

No surgical procedure is devoid of risk.

Mortality rate	
Nonperforated appendix	$<0.1\%$
Perforated appendix	$\approx5.0\%$

13. What patient groups are at higher risk of death from perforated appendicitis?

1. Very young patients (younger than 2 years).
2. Elderly patients (older than 70 years) who exhibit diminished abdominal innervation and present late.
3. Diabetic patients, who present late because of diabetic visceral neuropathy.
4. Patients taking steroids; steroids mask everything.

14. What is a "white worm"?

A normal appendix.

15. What is the differential diagnosis of right lower quadrant pain?

Meckel's diverticulum	Tubo-ovarian abscess (TOA)
Diverticulitis	Pelvic inflammatory disease (PID)
Ectopic pregnancy	Carcinoid tumor
Crohn's disease	Cholecystitis
Ovarian torsion	Ruptured ovarian cyst

16. What is an acceptable negative appendectomy rate?

This is a controversial topic currently being debated in surgical literature. Traditionally up to a 20% negative appendectomy rate was considered acceptable. Now with the adjunct of imaging (ultrasound [US] and computed tomography [CT]) lower negative rates are expected.

17. What is the role of imaging in the diagnosis of acute appendicitis?

US and CT can be both negatively and positively helpful. They may eliminate alternative diagnoses such as ectopic pregnancy or TOA when a perfectly normal right fallopian tube and ovary is seen. They may establish the diagnosis when an inflamed, edematous appendix is visualized. CT is particularly useful in visualizing periappendiceal tissue and may reveal that the appendix has already perforated by showing a phlegmon or abscess.

18. What are sonographic and CT findings suggestive of appendicitis?

1. An appendix of 7 mm or greater in anteroposterior diameter.
2. The presence of an appendicolith.
3. Periappendiceal fluid or mass.

19. **Is laparoscopic appendectomy replacing the traditional approach?**
In the hands of a skilled laparoscopic surgeon both the normal appendix and the inflamed, perforated appendix can be removed safely with the laparoscope. Also when the diagnosis is in question, the laparoscope can be used to help identify the correct pathology. Occasionally conversion from laparoscopic to open appendectomy is indicated.

KEY POINTS: APPENDICEAL CARCINOID

1. Sixty percent of carcinoid tumors occur in the appendix; 0.03% of appendectomies reveal incidental carcinoid.

2. This malignant but slow tumor spreads to lymph nodes, liver, and right heart.

3. If tumor size is <2 cm and does not involve the base of the appendix, appendectomy alone may suffice; however, bowel should be assessed because of 30% chance of synchronous lesion.

4. If tumor size is >2 cm or involves the base of the appendix, right hemicolectomy is necessary.

---

20. **What is a Meckel's diverticulum?**
Meckel's diverticulum is a congenital omphalomesenteric mucosa remnant that may contain ectopic gastric mucosa. It is found in 2% of the population, 2 feet upward from the ileocecal valve. It becomes inflamed in 2% of patients (i.e., the rule of 2's).

21. **Can chronic diverticulitis masquerade as appendicitis?**
Yes. Fifty percent of patients aged 50 years and older have colonic diverticula. The appendix is just a big cecal diverticulum. Thus, it makes sense that appendicitis and diverticulitis should look, act, and smell alike.

22. **Can a woman with a negative pregnancy test present with an ectopic pregnancy?**
Yes. The fallopian tube must be inspected for a walnut-sized lump. Appropriate surgical therapy is a longitudinal incision to "shell out" the fetus with subsequent repair of the tube. This approach (as opposed to salpingectomy) is designed to preserve fertility. Methotrexate also may precipitate spontaneous evacuation.

23. **Can Crohn's disease initially present as appendicitis?**
Yes; this presentation is typical. Crohn's disease is boggy, edematous, granulomatous inflammation of the distal ileum. Traditional surgical dictum suggests that it is appropriate to remove the appendix in patients with Crohn's disease unless the cecum at the appendiceal base is involved.

24. **Is it possible to confuse appendicitis with a TOA?**
Of course. An ovarian abscess buried deep in an inflamed, edematous, matted right adnexa can be treated successfully with intravenous (IV) antibiotics alone. Do not drain pus into the free peritoneal cavity; this will only make the patient sicker.

25. **Can pelvic inflammatory disease resemble appendicitis?**
PID can look exactly like appendicitis except for a positive "chandelier sign." On pelvic examination, manual tug on the cervix moves the inflamed, painful adnexae, and the patient hits the chandelier. Patients with PID should be treated with antibiotics (either orally or intravenously, depending on how sick the patient is).

26. **How does one deal with an appendiceal carcinoid tumor?**

    Carcinoid tumors may present anywhere along the gastrointestinal (GI) tract; 60%, however, are in the appendix. An obstructing carcinoid tumor, much like a fecalith, can lead to appendicitis; and in 0.3% of appendectomies, carcinoid tumors are the culprit. Most carcinoid tumors are small (<1.5 cm) and benign; 70% are located in the distal appendix. They are effectively treated with appendectomy alone. A large carcinoid tumor (>2.0 cm) at the appendiceal base, especially with invasion into the mesoappendix, must be considered malignant and mandates a right hemicolectomy.

27. **Can appendicitis be mistaken for acute cholecystitis?**

    Occasionally, yes. Both entities reflect acute, localized, intraperitoneal inflammation. Laboratory studies may be identical: WBC count of 12,000 to 14,000, negative urinalysis result, and negative pregnancy test result. Thus, if one is thinking "appendicitis," the major difference may be only right upper quadrant pain versus RLQ pain. Laparoscopic cholecystectomy is possible for acute cholecystitis, but conversion to an open procedure should be more frequent.

WEBSITES

www.websurg.com (lectures, videos, excellent photos of laparoscopic surgery)

www.pmppals.org/appendiceal_carcinoid.htm

BIBLIOGRAPHY

1. Cope Z, Rev. by Silen W: *Cope's early diagnosis of the acute abdomen*, 19th ed., New York, 1996, Oxford University Press.
2. Fitz RH: Perforating inflammation of the vermiform appendix with special reference to its early diagnosis and treatment. Trans Assoc Am Physicians 1:107, 1886.
3. Flum DR, McClure TD, Morris A et al.: Misdiagnosis of appendicitis and the use of diagnostic imaging. J Am Coll Surg 201(6):933-939, 2005. Epub Oct 13, 2005.
4. Guss DA, Behling CA, Munassi D: Impact of abdominal helical computed tomography on the rate of negative Appendicitis. J Emerg Med 34:7-11, 2008. Epub Dec 26, 2007.
5. Huynh V, Lalezarzadeh F, Lawandy S et al.: Abdominal computed tomography in the evaluation of acute and perforated appendicitis in the community setting. Am Surg 73(10):1002-1005, 2007.
6. Meakins JL: Appendectomy and appendicitis. Can J Surg 42:90, 1999.
7. Pokala N, Sadhasivam S, Kiran RP et al.: Complicated appendicitis—is the laparoscopic approach appropriate? A comparative study with the open approach: outcome in a community hospital setting. Am Surg 73(8): 737-741; discussion 741-742, 2007.
8. Rockey AE: Transverse incisions in abdominal operations. Med Rec 68:779, 1905.
9. Samuel M: Pediatric appendicitis score. J Pediatric Surg 37:877-881, 2002.
10. Urbach DR, Cohen MM: Is perforation of the appendix a risk factor for tubal infertility and ectopic pregnancy? An appraisal of the evidence. Can J Surg 42:101-108, 1999.

CHAPTER 37

GALLBLADDER DISEASE

Walter L. Biffl, MD, FACS

1. **What is the prevalence of gallstones in western society for women and men 60 years of age?**
   Women, 50%; men, 15%, although there is formidable ethnic predilection with gallstones endemic in American Indians.

2. **What is the difference between cholelithiasis, cholecystitis, choledocholithiasis, and cholangitis?**
   Cholelithiasis refers to the presence of gallbladder stones. Symptomatic cholelithiasis is the most common indication for cholecystectomy. Cholecystitis is an inflammatory condition of the gallbladder, usually initiated by gallstone impaction in the gallbladder neck with obstruction of the cystic duct. Choledocholithiasis is the presence of stones in the common bile duct (CBD). Cholangitis is an infection of the biliary tree, generally as a result of obstruction, usually secondary to choledocholithiasis.

3. **What percentage of asymptomatic gallstones becomes symptomatic?**
   Ten percent at 5 years, 15% at 10 years, and 18% by 15 years.

4. **Should patients with asymptomatic gallstones undergo cholecystectomy?**
   No. The risk of observation of patients with asymptomatic gallstones is less than or equal to the risk of operation.

5. **In what groups of patients with asymptomatic gallstones is prophylactic cholecystectomy beneficial?**
   - Patients with congenital hemolytic anemia who have gallstones at the time of splenectomy.
   - Obese patients undergoing bariatric surgery who have already developed gallstones.

6. **What is the optimal timing for laparoscopic cholecystectomy in acute cholecystitis?**
   "Cooling the gallbladder down" and delaying surgery for 6 weeks is associated with recurrent cholecystitis in 20% of patients. Prospective randomized studies have consistently found that early cholecystectomy allows shorter hospital stays, with no difference in morbidity or mortality, compared with delayed cholecystectomy. Procedures performed within the first 24 hours generally are easier because the area of dissection is not yet maximally inflamed, and fibrosis and increased blood vessel proliferation have not yet occurred.

7. **What is the conversion rate from laparoscopy to the open approach in acute cholecystitis and in symptomatic cholelithiasis?**
   Ten percent to 15% for acute cholecystitis and <5% for symptomatic cholelithiasis.

8. **What is the incidence of acalculus cholecystitis?**
   Ten percent of all cases of cholecystitis.

9. **What organisms require antibiotic coverage in biliary infections?**
   Escherichia coli, Klebsiella species, *Streptococcus faecalis, Clostridium welchii, Proteus* species, *Enterobacter* species, and anaerobic *Streptococcus* species.

10. **What is the incidence of CBD injury in open and laparoscopic cholecystectomy?**
    It is 0.2% to 0.3% for open and 0.4% to 0.6% for laparoscopic cholecystectomy.

11. **How does laparoscopic intraoperative ultrasound compare with laparoscopic intraoperative cholangiography?**
    The sensitivity of laparoscopic intraoperative ultrasound (LUS) is high (90%) and comparable to that of laparoscopic intraoperative cholangiography (LIOC). Potential advantages of LUS include less time and less dissection than LIOC.

12. **Does LUS or LIOC prevent CBD injuries during cholecystectomy?**
    In population-based studies, there are fewer CBD injuries among patients undergoing LIOC; however, there is no level I evidence that the LIOC was preventive. LIOC does, however, identify injuries at the time they occur. Advocates of LUS argue that identifying the anatomy before a duct is transected (and LIOC catheter inserted) *may* prevent CBD injuries.

13. **What percentage of patients undergoing cholecystectomy have unsuspected choledocholithiasis?**
    About 2%. However, if the patient has no history of jaundice and a CBD <6 mm in diameter, there is no role for routine laboratory screening. The vast majority of these stones will pass spontaneously.

14. **When, if ever, should laparoscopic cholecystectomy be performed during pregnancy?**
    Most attacks of acute biliary colic during pregnancy resolve spontaneously. To avoid a surgically induced abortion, cholecystectomy should be performed after delivery. If surgery is necessary, however, the second trimester is preferred for any surgical intervention.

15. **What is the prevalence of gallbladder carcinoma found incidentally during cholecystectomy?**
    Open, 1%; laparoscopic, 0.1%.

16. **Why is cholecystectomy increasing in the pediatric population?**
    Gallstone identification has increased because of the more liberal use of ultrasonography in patients with abdominal pain.

KEY POINTS: GALLBLADDER DISEASE

1. Overall incidence in United States: women >60 years old, 50%; men >60 years old, 15%.
2. Fifteen percent to 20% of patients with gallstones become symptomatic.
3. Patients with acute cholecystitis should have surgery as soon as possible after the onset of symptoms.
4. Routine LUS may identify CBD stones and may help avoid CBD injuries.

BIBLIOGRAPHY

1. Adamsen S, Hansen OH, Funch-Jensen P et al.: Bile duct injury during laparoscopic cholecystectomy: A prospective nationwide series. J Am Coll Surg 184:571-578, 1997.

2. Biffl WL, Moore EE, Offner PJ et al.: Routine intraoperative laparoscopic ultrasonography with selective cholangiography reduces bile duct complications during laparoscopic cholecystectomy. J Am Coll Surg 193:272-280, 2001.

3. Fletcher DR, Hobbs MST, Tan P et al.: Complications of cholecystectomy: Risks of the laparoscopic approach and protective effects of operative cholangiography. A population-based study. Ann Surg 229:449-457, 1999.

4. Ghumman E, Barry M, Grace PA et al.: Management of gallstones in pregnancy. Br J Surg 84:1646-1650, 1997.

5. Machi J, Tateishi T, Oishi A et al.: Laparoscopic ultrasonography versus operative cholangiography during laparoscopic cholecystectomy: review of the literature and a comparison with open intraoperative ultrasonography. J Am Coll Surg 188:361-367, 1999.

6. Robinson TN, Biffl WL, Moore EE et al.: Routine preoperative laboratory analyses are unnecessary before elective laparoscopic cholecystectomy. Surg Endosc 17:438-441, 2003.

7. Siddiqui T, MacDonald A, Chong PS et al.: Early versus delayed laparoscopic cholecystectomy for acute cholecystitis: a meta-analysis of randomized clinical trials. Am J Surg 195:40-47, 2008.

CHAPTER 38

PANCREATIC CANCER

Martin D. McCarter, MD

1. What is the magnitude of the problem?

For the most recent year in which statistics are available, there were approximately 37,000 new cases of pancreatic cancer in the United States, and more than 33,000 deaths, making this arguably one of the most lethal tumors. It is the fourth most common cause of cancer death in the United States for both men and women.

2. What are the histologic types of pancreatic cancer?

Adenocarcinoma is far and away the most common (and lethal) type. Neuroendocrine tumors make up approximately 1% of cases generally have a more indolent course. Other rare tumor types such as sarcoma, lymphoma, peusdopapillary and intraductal papillary mucinous (IPMN) tumor can occur as well.

3. What are the presenting signs of pancreatic cancer?

- Painless jaundice: 40% of patients.
- Pain (epigastric, right upper quadrant, back) with jaundice: 40%.
- Metastatic disease (e.g., hepatomegaly, ascites, lung nodules) with or without jaundice: 20%.

Most patients also have other nonspecific gastrointestinal (GI) symptoms such as bloating, food intolerance or pancreatic insufficiency, and weight loss.

4. What is the estimated survival for pancreatic cancer patients?

Overall 5-year survival for those undergoing a complete resection ranges from 5% to 20%.

Stage	At Diagnosis	Estimated Median Survival
Resectable	10%–20%	18 months
Locally Advanced	40%–45%	9–12 months
Metastatic	40%–45%	6–9 months

5. Why is there such a high rate of advanced disease at diagnosis?

The pancreas is retroperitoneal, relatively insensate, and symptoms of disease do not manifest themselves until local obstruction of duodenum, pancreatic or biliary duct forms. About 80% arise in the head of the gland, 10% arise in the body, and 10% in the tail.

6. A previously healthy 73-year-old patient presents with pruritus, dark urine, and icteric sclerae after recent overseas travel. What is a reasonable differential diagnosis?

1. Gallstones.
2. Cancer of the extrahepatic bile ducts.
3. Cancer of the pancreas.
4. Hepatitis.

7. **What is the first step in evaluating the patient?**
The first step is liver function tests (LFTs) to determine the degree of jaundice and hepatic dysfunction. Then ultrasound (US) is done to determine whether the cause is intrahepatic (normal bile ducts) or extrahepatic (dilated bile ducts). US can detect stones in the gallbladder or common duct with about 95% accuracy. Thus, if a jaundiced patient has normal bile ducts on US, the problem is intrahepatic cholestasis, probably from hepatitis.

8. **What if an ultrasound shows dilated extrahepatic bile ducts?**
Proceed to endoscopic retrograde cholangiopancreatography (ERCP) or transhepatic cholangiogram to determine whether the obstruction is high or low in the common bile duct (CBD) and to determine its likely cause (stricture, stone, tumor). The biliary tract can be decompressed with an internal stent at this time, allowing liver function to improve before major surgery. If stones are present, endoscopic sphincterotomy should be performed, allowing the stones to pass and simplifying future surgery.

9. **What, if any, other imaging is indicated?**
Generally the most useful study is a fine cut, multiple phase computed tomography (CT) scan of the abdomen. This provides information about possible metastatic disease and helps assess local vascular involvement (portal vein, superior mesenteric vein, celiac axis, hepatic artery, superior mesenteric artery). Endoscopic ultrasound (EUS) can be helpful if the mass is not clear and a tissue diagnosis is needed. Positron emission tomography (PET) or CT scans are often obtained to help rule out metastatic disease but its additional benefit (some studies suggest new findings in 20% of patients) is still being debated. Likewise, as imaging has improved, the role of routine laparoscopy to assess resectability has diminished.

10. **What is the significance of a "double-duct" sign?**
This refers to the presence of a dilated pancreatic and biliary ductal system identified on CT scan or ERCP. In the absence of a biliary stone, this nearly always implies the presence of an underlying cancer as the etiology.

11. **What in the world is CA19-9?**
CA 19-9 stands for carbohydrate antigen 19-9. It is a tumor marker associated with pancreatic and biliary tumors, which is measured in the patient's serum. It is non-specific (may be elevated in inflammation and other benign conditions) but may be helpful in monitoring a patient's progress/response to therapy.

12. **In this case, ultrasound, ERCP, and CT scan show dilated extrahepatic bile ducts, a mass in the head of the pancreas, and no obvious cause other than cancer. The tumor seems separate from the portal vein, and there are no liver metastases. What should be done next?**
Make an assessment of operative risk. If the patient is a poor operative risk, one should consider percutaneous or endoscopic US-guided fine-needle aspiration (FNA) to document cancer, if possible, and endoscopic stenting of the bile duct; surgery probably is not a good option. If the patient is a good operative risk, the next step is surgery. The clinical picture is accurate in at least 90% of cases, and FNA adds no useful information at this time. If no malignant tissue is obtained, surgery is still indicated because the needle may have missed the lesion, sampling only the pancreatitis that surrounds all such tumors.

13. **We are in the operating room, the abdomen is open, and the discussion revolves around taking out the tumor. What is a Whipple procedure?**
Pancreaticoduodenectomy involves the removal of the gallbladder, distal common duct, duodenum, gastric antrum, and the portion of pancreas to the right of the portal vein; in essence, a proximal pancreatectomy.

14. **What is distal pancreatectomy? A total pancreatectomy?**

    Distal pancreatectomy removes the portion of gland to the left of the portal vein, along with the spleen. Total pancreatectomy combines both procedures, again, with antrectomy in some centers.

15. **Why remove gallbladder, duodenum, and stomach if the problem is in the pancreas?**

    After the ampulla of Vater is removed, the gallbladder does not function well and forms gallstones. The second and third portions of the duodenum share a blood supply with the head of the pancreas and are usually devascularized when the head is removed. Historically, the gastric antrum was removed to improve resection margins. Vagotomy was added to reduce the incidence of marginal ulceration at the anastomosis between the gastric remnant and jejunum.

    Removing the antrum adds little to the scope of the operation, however, and marginal ulceration can be prevented by placing the gastrojejunostomy downstream from where bile and pancreatic secretions enter the gut. Thus, many surgeons now perform a pylorus-preserving Whipple procedure whenever possible, preserving the vagus nerve as well. A pylorus preserving "Whipple" has the same overall survival, is associated with decreased operative time and blood loss but it has been difficult to prove any physiologic benefit.

16. **How does one determine whether to perform a Whipple procedure, distal pancreatectomy, or total pancreatectomy? What is the cure rate?**

    Whipple procedures are used for mobile tumors in the head without signs of lymph node metastases at the celiac axis or root of mesentery. Distal pancreatectomy is used for lesions of the body and tail unaccompanied by signs of spread. Total pancreatectomy is generally reserved for a few rare situations in which a diffuse cancer involves most of the gland but nowhere else; this is a rare event. Median survival with each procedure is about 20 months, and 5-year survival is about 15%. This procedure has about 1% to 3% operative mortality and 25% to 40% morbidity in centers with extensive experience; in other settings, the operative risk and complication rate can be much higher.

17. **What should be done if there are nodal metastases at the celiac axis or root of mesentery?**

    The patient cannot be cured with surgery, so the goal is palliation. If obstructive jaundice is present, a biliary-enteric bypass should be performed. If a tumor obstructs the duodenum, a gastroenterostomy should also be carried out. Some surgeons believe gastroenterostomy should be done routinely for cancers of the pancreatic head, regardless of whether duodenal compromise is present, because up to 20% of patients without this problem at the time of surgery may require intervention for poor gastric emptying in the future.

18. **Do any other signs of inoperability exist?**

    General contraindications to resection include metastatic disease, invasion of the inferior vena cava (IVC), or major local arteries (celiac axis, hepatic artery, superior mesenteric artery). Relative contraindications to resection include invasion of the portal or superior mesenteric vein. Resection of the portal vein and reconstruction can be done with less morbidity than in the past but this technical exercise has not led to improved survival.

19. **A patient is found to have unsuspected spread to the celiac axis. You carry out a biliary and gastric bypass. Is there anything else you can offer the patient, either surgically or nonsurgically?**

    Some of these patients, if suffering from preoperative back pain, can be relieved of this by intraoperative alcohol celiac ganglion block. Alternatively, such treatment can be carried out postoperatively by an interventional radiologist. Palliative chemotherapy and radiation therapy can also provide pain relief but generally do not improve survival.

20. **Are there any other treatments (chemotherapy, radiation therapy, pet therapy) that improve outcomes in pancreatic cancer?**

Not yet. This is not as a result of a lack of interest or effort. There is some evidence that chemotherapy (gemcitabine) or a combination of chemotherapy, radiation therapy, and immunotherapy may add a few months to overall survival following resection (at some cost to quality of life) however, the vast majority of trials have failed to make a significant difference in overall survival. Here is a genuine opportunity for bright students such as the present reader to make a difference!

21. **With high morbidity and low cure rates, why are surgeons so eager to do Whipple procedures?**

Unfortunately, this represents the only chance for cure. In addition, pancreatic resection—when carried out safely—probably offers the best long-term palliation in those destined to die of their disease. Finally, future advances in adjuvant therapy may provide hope for improvement in overall survival.

KEY POINTS: DIAGNOSTIC WORK-UP OF A PATIENT WITH JAUNDICE

1. LFTs: determine degree of jaundice (obstructive versus nonobstructive) and hepatic dysfunction.

2. US of right upper quadrant: rules out gallstones, evaluates intrahepatic versus extrahepatic ductal dilatation.

3. If hepatic ducts are dilated: ERCP or percutaneous transhepatic cholangiography to delineate site of mechanical obstruction.

4. CT: evaluates size of tumor if present, degree of regional spread, or liver metastases.

WEBSITES

www.nccn.org/

www.cancer.org

BIBLIOGRAPHY

1. Diener MK, Knaebel HP, Heukaufer C et al.: A systematic review and meta-analysis of pylorus-preserving versus classical pancreaticoduodenectomy for surgical treatment of periampullary and pancreatic carcinoma. Ann Surg 245:187-200, 2007.

2. Garofalo M, Flannery T, Regine W: The case for adjuvant chemoradiation for pancreatic cancer. Best Pract Res Clin Gastroenterol 20:403-416, 2006.

3. Goldin SB, Bradner MW, Zervos EE et al.: Assessment of pancreatic neoplasms: review of biopsy techniques. J Gastrointest Surg 11:783-790, 2007.

4. Jemal A, Siegel R, Ward E et al.: Cancer statistics, 2007. CA Cancer J Clin 57(1):43-66, 2007.

5. Kalra MK, Maher MM, Mueller PR et al.: State-of-the-art imaging of pancreatic neoplasms. Br J Radiol 76 (912):857-865, 2003.

6. Ryan DP, Willett CG: Management of locally advanced adenocarcinoma of the pancreas. Hematol Oncol Clin North Am 16:95-103, 2002.

7. Siriwardana HP, Siriwardena AK: Systematic review of outcome of synchronous portal-superior mesenteric vein resection during pancreatectomy for cancer. Br J Surg 93:662-673, 2006.

8. Sohn TA, Lillemoe KD: Surgical palliation of pancreatic cancer. Adv Surg 34:249-271, 2000.

9. Stojadinovic A, Hoos A, Brennan MF et al.: Randomized clinical trials in pancreatic cancer. Surg Oncol Clin N Am 11:207-229, 2002.

10. Ujiki MB, Talamonti MS.: Guidelines for the surgical management of pancreatic adenocarcinoma. Semin Oncol, 34:311-320, 2007.

11. Varadhachary GR, Tamm EP, Abbruzzese JL et al.: Borderline resectable pancreatic cancer: definitions, management, and role of preoperative therapy. Ann Surg Oncol 13:1035-1046, 2006.

CHAPTER 39

ACUTE PANCREATITIS

Adam H. Lackey, MD, and C. Clay Cothren, MD

1. **What are the common causes and incidence of acute pancreatitis?**
   Gallstones (45%), alcohol (35%), and other (20%). Acute pancreatitis is estimated to be responsible for 210,000 hospital admissions in the United States per year.

2. **What are the uncommon causes?**
   Hyperlipidemia, hypercalcemia (hyperparathyroidism, multiple myeloma), iatrogenic factors (up to 15% of patients undergoing endoscopic retrograde cholangiopancreatography [ERCP] may experience pancreatitis), drugs (didanosine, thiazide diuretics, H2 blockers, tetracycline, azathioprine, salicylates, valproic acid), infections (mumps, coxsackievirus), pancreas divisum, and scorpion bites, and autoimmune pancreatitis. Approximately 10% of cases are considered truly idiopathic.

3. **What are the characteristic symptoms?**
   Acute onset of severe epigastric pain that is boring in nature and often radiates to the back. Pain is frequently accompanied by nausea and vomiting.

4. **What may be found on physical examination?**
   Diffuse abdominal tenderness, abdominal distention, "board-like" abdominal guarding, and hypoactive bowel sounds. Patients may be febrile, tachycardic, and dehydrated. Evidence of jaundice or identification of gallstones on right upper quadrant ultrasound (US) indicates a biliary cause of pancreatitis. Severe pancreatitis may result in retroperitoneal bleeding, leading to periumbilical or flank discoloration (called Cullen's sign and Grey Turner sign, respectively).

5. **What is the appropriate therapy for mild to moderate pancreatitis?**
   The critical component of supportive therapy is adequate fluid resuscitation to maintain urine output (place a Foley catheter); patients may require up to 10 L of crystalloid as a result of the extensive amount of third spacing in the abdomen. Appropriate treatment also includes pain medications, alcohol withdrawal prophylaxis, nasogastric (NG) decompression for persistent emesis, and avoidance of oral intake. Patients are started on a regular diet once their laboratory markers are decreasing or normal, their abdominal pain is resolving, and they have bowel sounds.

6. **Which is the better laboratory test, amylase or lipase?**
   Serum amylase levels tend to peak sooner than lipase levels, which may remain elevated for 4 to 5 days. Up to 30% of patients have normal amylase levels, most notably alcoholics with chronic "burned-out" pancreatitis. Serum lipase has a greater sensitivity and specificity than amylase levels, with 3 times the normal limit being diagnostic of pancreatitis.

7. **What other disease states cause hyperamylasemia?**
   Perforated peptic ulcers, small bowel obstruction, parotid gland inflammation or tumor, renal failure, and ovarian tumors are associated with elevated amylase levels.

8. **What is the significance of hypoxemia early in the course of pancreatitis?**
   Patients with necrotizing pancreatitis may develop respiratory failure requiring mechanical ventilation, which may progress to multiple organ failure (MOF). Hypoxemia is an ominous sign, as are infiltrates on admission chest radiograph.

9. **What is the Ranson score?**

Ranson indices are 11 measurements that are useful in indicating the severity and predicting the outcome of pancreatitis. A score of 3 or higher is considered severe disease.

On admission	After the initial 48 hours
Age >55 years	Rise in blood urea nitrogen (BUN) >5 mg/dl
White blood cell count >16,000 μl	Decrease in hematocrit level >10%
Glucose >350 mg/dl	Calcium <8 mg/dl
Lactate dehydrogenase >350 U/L	Partial pressure of oxygen (PaO$_2$) <60 mm Hg
Aspartate aminotransferase (AST) > 250 μ/L	Base deficit >4 mmol/L
Fluid sequestration >6 L	

10. **How do Ranson's indices relate to mortality?**

Number of criteria	Mortality rate (%)
0–2	5
3–4	15
5–6	50
7–8	100

11. **What is the limitation of using the Ranson score for predicting severity of pancreatitis?**

A true Ranson score cannot be calculated until after 48 hours of inpatient treatment. Other predictive indices include the acute physiology and chronic health evaluation II (APACHE II) scoring system and the Balthazar scoring system. The APACHE II scoring system achieves positive and negative predictive values that are comparable to the Ranson's criteria for predicting the severity and expected mortality of acute pancreatitis. The Balthazar score, based on findings from computed tomography (CT) scanning (amount of inflammation, presence and extent of necrosis, and presence of fluid collections), is also acceptable for evaluation of expected morbidity and mortality.

12. **What is necrotizing pancreatitis?**

The inflammation and edema of acute pancreatitis may progress with subsequent devitalization of pancreatic and peripancreatic tissue. Pancreatic necrosis occurs in approximately 20% of acute episodes.

13. **Why is it important to differentiate acute pancreatitis from necrotizing pancreatitis?**

The presence and extent of necrosis are key determinants of the clinical course. Approximately 10% to 20% of patients with pancreatic necrosis develop infected pancreatic necrosis. Infection accounts for 80% of all deaths from pancreatitis, and surgical debridement is the current standard of care. Although there is interest in conservative treatment of biopsy-proven, infected pancreatic necrosis, no studies have shown this to be a safe clinical strategy.

14. **What is the optimal method for diagnosing pancreatic necrosis with or without associated infection?**

Dynamic CT scans with intravenous contrast allow visualization and differentiation of healthy, perfused parenchyma from patchy, poorly perfused necrotic tissue. Sensitivity of CT imaging increases in the days following presentation, with optimal identification of necrosis occurring >4 days. Therefore, a CT scan should be obtained in patients that do not clinically improve in response to fluid resuscitation and supportive treatment. CT-guided aspiration of the necrotic tissue may be performed to determine the presence of infection.

15. **When is surgery indicated in patients with acute pancreatitis?**

Infected pancreatic necrosis is the only absolute indication for surgery. Open drainage is best accomplished via a bilateral subcostal incision, placement of the greater omentum over the transverse colon to prevent enteric fistulas, and removal of necrotic material from the lesser sac. The patient may require multiple trips to the operating room (OR) for repeated debridement; typically, the abdomen is not formally closed until only viable tissue remains. Operative intervention for sterile pancreatic necrosis is controversial. The only absolute indications for surgery in sterile pancreatic necrosis are 1) abdominal compartment syndrome, 2) suspected enteric perforation, or 3) bleeding (splenic artery pseudoaneurysms can complicate the disease). Although there is a high incidence of infection in patients with >50% necrosis, "preemptive" debridement is associated with a high morbidity and mortality.

16. **When should antibiotic therapy be added?**
Antibiotics do not alter the course of pancreatitis or decrease septic complications of the disease; therefore, patients with mild cases of pancreatitis should be treated with supportive measures. The literature is confusing regarding antibiotic use in patients with necrotizing pancreatitis. Despite a paucity of class I evidence supporting the use of prophylactic antibiotics, many institutions continue to administer them. In patients with signs of sepsis, treatment with empiric antibiotics is reasonable while a source of infection is sought (i.e., CT-guided aspiration of pancreatic necrosis).

17. **What is the most common complication of acute pancreatitis?**
Pancreatic pseudocysts. Patients with pseudocysts typically present with persistent abdominal pain, nausea and vomiting, or an abdominal mass. CT scan imaging is diagnostic. Intervention is indicated in symptomatic patients or those asymptomatic patients with documented increase in pseudocyst size by serial CT scans. Operative (cyst-gastrostomy or cyst-jejunostomy) or endoscopic transmural drainage can be performed 6 to 12 weeks after the acute presentation, once the pseudocyst is "mature."

18. **What is the natural history of cholelithiasis following gallstone pancreatitis?**
Cholecystectomy is curative and should be performed before patient discharge in the 80% of patients with uncomplicated, acute edematous pancreatitis. Cholecystectomy is performed when the patient's pain is resolved, vital signs have normalized, and laboratory markers are decreasing. Cholecystectomy should be accompanied by an intraoperative cholangiogram or laparoscopic ultrasonography; if a retained stone is seen in the common bile duct (CBD), laparoscopic common duct exploration or ERCP should be performed before discharge.

19. **What is the natural history of alcoholic pancreatitis?**
Attacks recur. Abstinence from alcohol should be encouraged because many patients develop chronic pancreatitis.

KEY POINTS

1. Causes: gallstones (45%), alcohol (35%), other (10%), idiopathic (10%).

2. Symptoms: acute onset of epigastric pain that radiates to back with associated nausea or emesis.

3. Lab tests: elevated amylase and/or lipase (more sensitive).

4. Imaging: CT scan diagnoses pancreatic necrosis, peripancreatic fluid collections, and pseudocysts.

5. Treatment: crystalloid resuscitation, bowel rest, and NG decompression (if persistent emesis); 10% of cases progress to necrotizing pancreatitis, which requires operative debridement if infected.

BIBLIOGRAPHY

1. Banks PA, Freeman ML: Practice guidelines in acute pancreatitis. Am J Gastroenterology 101:2379-2400, 2006.
2. Dellinger EP, Tellado JM, Soto NE et al.: Early antibiotic treatment for severe acute necrotizing pancreatitis. A randomized, double-blind, placebo-controlled study. Ann Surg 245:674-683, 2007.
3. Gotzinger P, Sautner T, Kriwanek S et al.: Surgical treatment for severe acute pancreatitis: extent and surgical control of necrosis determine outcome. World J Surg 26:474-478, 2002.
4. LeMee J, Paye F, Sauvanet A et al.: Incidence and reversibility of organ failure in the course of sterile or infected necrotizing pancreatitis. Arch Surg 136:1386-1390, 2001.
5. Morton JM, Brown A, Galanko JA et al.: A national comparison of surgical versus percutaneous drainage of pancreatic pseudocysts: 1997–2001. J Gastrointest Surg 9:15, 2005.
6. Nealon WH, Bawduniak J, Walser EM: Appropriate timing of cholecystectomy in patients who present with moderate to severe gallstone-associated acute pancreatitis with peripancreatic fluid collections. Ann Surg 239:741, 2004.
7. Rosing DK, de Virgilio C, Yaghoubian A et al.: Early cholecystectomy for mild to moderate gallstone pancreatitis shortens hospital stay. J Am Coll Surg 205:762-766, 2007.
8. Uhl W, Warshaw A, Imrie C et al.: IAP guidelines for the surgical management of acute pancreatitis. Pancreatology 2:565, 2002.
9. Vriens PW, van de Linde P, Slotema E et al.: Computed tomography severity index is an early prognostic tool for acute pancreatitis. J Am Coll Surg 201:497-502, 2005.
10. Whitcomb DC: Clinical practice. Acute pancreatitis. N Engl J Med 354(20):2142-2150, 2006.

CHAPTER 40

DIAGNOSIS AND THERAPY OF CHRONIC PANCREATITIS

Adam H. Lackey, MD, and C. Clay Cothren, MD

1. What is chronic pancreatitis?
The classic syndrome consists of smoldering abdominal pain and evidence of pancreatic insufficiency. Histologically, chronic inflammation results in destruction of the functioning endocrine and exocrine pancreatic cells.

2. What is the most common cause?
Alcohol abuse accounts for over 70% of cases. Other known causes include posttraumatic strictures, pancreas divisum, genetic mutations, autoimmune disorders, and metabolic disorders (hypertriglyceridemia and hypercalcemia). The overall incidence is estimated to be 3 to 10 per 100,000 people.

3. Is chronic pancreatitis the result of acute pancreatitis?
Patients may not have had acute pancreatitis, although alcoholism is common to both. One hypothesis is the inflammation from recurrent bouts of acute pancreatitis causes interstitial acinar fibrosis with secondary dilatation of the main pancreatic duct. Paradoxically, the average age for chronic pancreatitis is 13 years less than for acute disease.

4. What are the signs of pancreatic insufficiency?
Insulin-dependent diabetes mellitus (found in up to 30% of patients) and steatorrhea (in 25%). The form of diabetes associated with chronic pancreatitis is termed IIIc; it can be particularly difficult to manage because of the destruction of both the insulin and glucagon producing cells.

5. How much of the pancreas must be destroyed before diabetes develops?
Approximately 90%.

6. What is steatorrhea? How does one confirm the diagnosis?
Steatorrhea is soft, greasy, foul-smelling stools. A 72-hour fecal fat analysis may be done to confirm the diagnosis. The D-xylose test shows normal results, and the Schilling test is not sensitive for pancreatic insufficiency. Patients with steatorrhea are treated with a variable combination of low-fat diets, pancreatic enzymes, antacids, and cimetidine. The presence of steatorrhea indicates that lipase production is >10% below normal levels.

7. Is serum amylase elevated in patients with chronic pancreatitis?
No. The serum amylase level is usually normal in cases of "burned-out" pancreatitis.

8. What are the complications of chronic pancreatitis?
Pancreatic pseudocyst, abscess, or fistula may occur. Obstruction of the biliary tree with resultant jaundice may be caused by areas of fibrosis. Malnutrition and narcotic addiction are more likely to coexist than actual complications of pancreatic insufficiency.

9. **What is a possible source of upper gastrointestinal bleeding in a patient with chronic pancreatitis?**
Although gastritis and peptic ulcer disease are more common causes of upper gastrointestinal bleeding (UGIB), splenic vein thrombosis with associated gastric varices and hypersplenism should also be considered. (Your attending will love this answer!)

10. **What is the "chain of lakes"?**
During endoscopic retrograde cholangiopancreatography (ERCP), contrast dye is injected into the pancreatic duct; sequential areas of narrowing followed by dilatation of the duct cause the appearance of a "string of beads" or "chain of lakes."

11. **What are the treatment options for chronic pancreatitis?**
Initially, medical therapy includes pain medications, a low-fat diet, abstinence from alcohol, and pancreatic enzyme replacement or insulin therapy as indicated. Patients with evidence of pancreatic insufficiency and persistent abdominal pain requiring repeated hospitalizations should consider more invasive therapeutic options. For patients with a proximal pancreatic duct stricture and upstream ductal dilation, endoscopic treatment (sphincterotomy, stricture dilation, stone extraction, stent placement) may be successful. The remainder of patients with refractory symptoms may undergo surgical intervention.

12. **What are the indications for surgery?**
There are no steadfast rules. Relative indications include unabating pain refractory to medical management, a dilated main pancreatic duct, biliary or gastric outlet obstruction, pancreas divisum, symptomatic or enlarging pseudocyst, and suspicion of malignancy.

13. **Which operative procedures are commonly performed?**
A Roux-en-Y lateral pancreaticojejunostomy (i.e., a Peustow procedure) provides pain relief through ductal drainage while preserving pancreatic parenchyma. The entire "chain of lakes" pancreatic duct is opened from head-to-tail, and the Roux jejunal limb is sutured to the pancreatic capsule around the "filleted" duct to provide a drainage route. Pancreaticoduodenectomy (i.e., a Whipple procedure) may be performed for patients with an inflammatory mass in the head of the pancreas. The Frey procedure entails "coring out" the pancreatic head combined with draining both the pancreatic head ducts and the length of the pancreatic duct. Distal pancreatectomy may be used for isolated distal disease or retrograde drainage into a pancreaticojejunostomy.

14. **What is the result of operative intervention?**
Pain relief occurs in approximately 70% of patients at the end of 1 year and in 50% of patients at the end of 5 years. Although associated morbidity ranges from 6% to 50% based on the type of operation, overall mortality from these procedures is 1% to 3%.

KEY POINTS

1. Causes: alcohol (70%), other/idiopathic (30%).

2. Symptoms: smoldering abdominal pain and pancreatic insufficiency (diabetes, steatorrhea).

3. Lab tests: none.

4. Imaging: computed tomography (CT) scan diagnoses pancreatic masses, ductal dilation, calcifications, and pseudocysts; ERCP evaluates the pancreatic duct including strictures.

5. Treatment: pain medications, a low-fat diet, abstinence from alcohol, pancreatic enzyme replacement and insulin therapy; unabating pain, refractory to medical management, may be treated with endoscopic or surgical intervention.

BIBLIOGRAPHY

1. American Gastroenterological Association: AGA technical review: treatment of pain in chronic pancreatitis. Gastroenterology 115:765-776, 1998.

2. Cahen DL, Gouma DJ, Nio Y et al.: Endoscopic versus surgical drainage of the pancreatic duct in chronic pancreatitis. N Engl J Med 356(7):676-684, 2007.

3. Fernandez-del Castillo C, Rattner DW, Warshaw AL: Standards for pancreatic resection in the 1990s. Arch Surg 130:295-300, 1995.

4. Heiko W, Apte MV, Volker K et al: Reviews in basic and clinical gastroenterology, chronic pancreatitis: challenges and advances in pathogenesis, genetics, diagnosis, and therapy. Gastroenterology 132:1557-1573, 2007.

5. Jordan Jr PH, Pikoulis M: Operative treatment for chronic pancreatitis pain. J Am Coll Surg 192:498-509, 2001.

6. Schnelldorfer T, Lewin DN, Adams DB: Operative management of chronic pancreatitis: long term results in 372 patients, J Am Coll Surg 204:1039-1047, 2007.

7. Steer ML, Waxman I, Freedman S: Chronic pancreatitis, N Engl J Med 332:1482-1490, 1995.

CHAPTER 41

PORTAL HYPERTENSION AND ESOPHAGEAL VARICES

Ramin Jamshidi, MD, and Gregory V. Stiegmann, MD

1. **Describe the blood supply to the liver.**

   Total hepatic blood flow is roughly 1500 ml/min or 25% of cardiac output (CO). The hepatic artery normally supplies about 30% of blood flow, and the portal vein contributes 70%. However, the hepatic artery and portal vein each supply 50% of the liver's oxygen. With portal hypertension, portal flow decreases and the relative contribution of the hepatic artery necessarily increases.

2. **How is portal hypertension defined?**

   The portal venous pressure is normally 5 to 10 mm Hg; >20 mm Hg is defined as portal hypertension. Direct measurement is risky, so the hepatic venous pressure gradient (HVPG) is used instead. This is the change in hepatic vein pressure when flow is occluded by wedging a balloon catheter into it (analogous to the estimation of left atrial pressure by wedging a pulmonary artery). A normal HVPG is 2 to 6 mm Hg; >12 mm Hg is considered portal hypertension.

3. **What is hepatopetal flow?**

   Physiologic portal blood flow into the liver is termed *hepatopetal flow*. Reversal of flow in the portal vein can occur with greatly increased hepatic vascular resistance and is called *hepatofugal flow*. In this case, the hepatic artery must provide the dominant perfusion of the liver.

4. **What are the most common causes of portal hypertension?**
   - In the world: schistosomiasis.
   - In the United States: chronic hepatitis C virus (HCV) infection or alcoholic cirrhosis (Laennec's disease).
   - In children: extrahepatic portal venous occlusion (as in portal vein thrombosis) or biliary atresia.

5. **What are schistosomiasis and Katayama fever?**

   Infection by a freshwater blood fluke that causes an initial dermatitis ("swimmer's itch") and rash followed after 1 to 2 months by fever, myalgias, abdominal pain, and bloody diarrhea (Katayama fever). As these parasites mate and lay eggs in the venous system, the resulting inflammation causes chronic obstructing fibrosis of organs and vessels, which is manifested by portal hypertension. Katayama fever lasts a few weeks and is second only to malaria as a cause of chronic tropical illness. Treat with praziquantel.

6. **How can the causes of portal hypertension be classified anatomically?**

   Presinusoidal:
   - Extrahepatic: portal or splenic vein thrombosis, congenital biliary atresia, extrinsic compression (e.g., tumor).
   - Intrahepatic: primary biliary cirrhosis, schistosomiasis, hepatic metastases, polycystic disease, sarcoidosis.

   Sinusoidal: hepatic cirrhosis (e.g., viral infection, alcohol, hemochromatosis).

   Postsinusoidal: Budd-Chiari syndrome, inferior vena cava (IVC) obstruction, right-sided heart failure.

7. **List the four major anatomic connections between the portal and systemic venous systems.**
   1. Left gastric (coronary) vein to the esophageal vein (potential esophageal varices).
   2. Inferior mesenteric vein through the superior hemorrhoidal veins to the hypogastric vein (potential rectal varices).
   3. Portal vein to umbilical vein to superficial veins of the abdominal wall (potential caput medusae).
   4. Mesenteric veins to perilumbar veins of Retzius into the IVC (potential retroperitoneal hemorrhage).

   Note that the reason these anastomoses can shunt blood (around the liver) is that splanchnic veins lack one-way valves.

8. **Define sinistral portal hypertension.**
   Derived from *sinister* (Latin for "left") this is "left-sided" portal hypertension specifically caused by splenic vein thrombosis or obstruction. This causes shunting from the short gastric branches of the splenic vein to the left gastric vein, resulting in gastric varices. Splenectomy is the definitive treatment.

9. **What are the common complications of portal venous hypertension?**
   - Ascites and spontaneous bacterial peritonitis.
   - Hemorrhage from esophageal varices (the major cause of mortality).
   - Hypersplenism.
   - Rectal varices (hemorrhoids).
   - Portosystemic encephalopathy.
   - Portal hypertensive gastropathy and colopathy.

10. **What impact can portal hypertension have on other organ systems?**
    - Hyperdynamic circulation (decreased systemic vascular resistance with increased CO and low blood pressure).
    - Hepatorenal syndrome.
    - Hepatopulmonary syndrome or portopulmonary hypertension.

11. **Liver function is classified according to what system?**
    The modified Child-Turcott-Pugh system defines three classes of liver disease based on mortality; the points should be totaled from Table 41-1.
    Class A (5 to 6 points): 100% 1-year survival
    Class B (7 to 9 points): 80% 1-year survival
    Class C ($\geq$ 10 points): 45% 1-year survival

TABLE 41-1. CHILD-TURCOTT-PUGH SYSTEM OF SCORING LIVER DISEASE

Parameter	1 Point	2 Points	3 Points
Albumin (g/dl)	>3.5	2.8–3.5	<2.8
Bilirubin (mg/dl)	<2	2–3	>3
International normalized ratio (INR)	<1.7	1.7–2.2	>2.2
Ascites	None	Moderate	Severe
Encephalopathy	None	Moderate	Severe

12. **What is MELD?**

    The **M**ayo **e**nd-stage **l**iver **d**isease score is a completely objective measure of disease calculated with international normalized ratio (INR), bilirubin, and creatinine. In 2002, MELD was adopted by the United Network for Organ Sharing (UNOS) for determining liver transplantation priority.

13. **How is MELD calculated?**

    $$\text{MELD} = 10 \times [0.957 \times \ln(\text{creatinine mg/dl}) + 0.378$$
    $$\times \ln(\text{bilirubin mg/dl}) + 1.120 \times \ln(\text{INR})]$$

    Maximum creatinine entered is 4.0. Result is rounded to the nearest integer.

14. **How common are esophageal varices?**

    At time of diagnosis of cirrhosis, approximately 30% of patients have esophageal varices, and the incidence of new varix formation in patients with known cirrhosis is roughly 6% per year. There is a 50% point prevalence of varices in cirrhotic patients. However, bleeding occurs in only about one third of patients with varices.

15. **Is upper gastrointestinal bleeding in cirrhotic patients with documented varices always variceal?**

    Honed test-taking skills tell you the answer must be no. Twenty percent of these patients bleed from another source (e.g., alcoholic gastric ulcerations, peptic ulcer disease). This includes patients with ascites, spider angiomata, and asterixis.

16. **Are gastric varices a common bleeding source in patients with portal hypertension?**

    No. Only about 5% of variceal bleeds in cirrhotic patients are caused by gastric varices. Portal hypertension with gastric varices and no esophageal varices is usually associated with splenic vein thrombosis. Gastric varices bleed much less frequently—but more severely—than their esophageal counterparts.

17. **What factors are predictive of variceal bleeding?**

    - Size of varices (the most important factor), which increases vessel wall tension.
    - Red wale markings on the varices (longitudinal "whip marks") from decreased wall thickness.
    - Severity of liver disease.
    - Active alcohol abuse.

    All told, variceal hemorrhage occurs in 30% of patients within 2 years of varix documentation.

18. **Does the degree of portal hypertension predict bleeding?**

    Surprisingly, no. Bleeding risk correlates poorly with the magnitude of portal pressure. However, bleeding rarely occurs with HVPG <12 mm Hg; this threshold pressure is considered necessary but not sufficient for hemorrhage.

19. **An initial variceal bleed is associated with what mortality and rebleeding risk?**

    Forty percent of these patients rebled within 6 weeks, with 40% occurring in the first 5 days. If untreated, up to 75% of patients rebleed within the first year and roughly 50% die.

20. **Should selective or nonselective β-blockers be used in the treatment of esophageal varices?**

    Nonselective β-blockade best minimizes bleeding by lowering blood pressure and reducing splanchnic flow. β_1-adrenergic antagonism causes splanchnic vasoconstriction by reflex activation of α-receptors and decreases myocardial contractility. β_2-blockade prevents splanchnic and peripheral vasodilation. Nadolol is the drug of choice.

21. **What are the major components of acute variceal bleed management?**
    - Fluid or blood product resuscitation (be careful not to worsen ascites).
    - Pharmacologic agents to lower portal pressure and flow.
    - Endoscopy to confirm diagnosis and treat by banding or sclerotherapy.
    - Antibiotic prophylaxis.
    - Lactulose catharsis (gastrointestinal [GI] bleeding increases protein load—blood is protein-rich—and may worsen encephalopathy).
    - Tamponade, surgery, or transjugular intrahepatic portosystemic shunting (TIPS) if refractory or an early recurrent bleed.

22. **What pharmacologic treatments are used in acute variceal bleeding?**
    Vasopressin (start at 0.2 U/min intravenously [IV] and increase the level while watching the electrocardiogram [ECG]) decreases splanchnic perfusion and thus portal pressure. Be careful; systemic vasoconstriction can cause myocardial or mesenteric ischemia and infarction.
    Terlipressin (2 mg IV every 4 hours) is a synthetic vasopressin analog with fewer side effects and simpler dosing. It has shown clear promise in randomized controlled trials but is not yet available in the United States outside of clinical trials.
    Octreotide (50 μg IV bolus, then 25 μg/h IV) is a synthetic somatostatin analog that decreases portal blood flow by selective splanchnic vasoconstriction, so side effects are limited. Octreotide acts through vasoactive peptides substance P and glucagon.

23. **What endoscopic treatments are used in acute variceal bleeding?**
    - Endoscopic band ligation (EBL): direct strangulation of varices with rubber bands, similar to hemorrhoid banding.
    - Sclerotherapy: intravariceal injection of a sclerosing chemical.
    Either technique typically controls acute bleeding in ≈90% of variceal bleeding, but although sclerotherapy can be easier in the face of a large bleed, EBL is safer (less chance of perforation) and tends to require fewer retreatments (see Fig. 41-1).

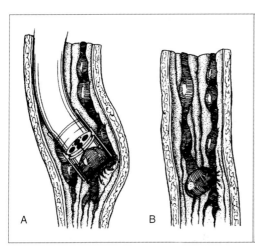

Figure 41-1. Endoscopic band ligation. **A,** The endoscope is positioned over a varix and suction is applied to draw it into the ligator. A rubber band is then ejected over the base of the lesion. **B,** The band strangulates the varix, which sloughs off and passes through the body in about 5 to 7 days.

24. **Why should antibiotics be given to cirrhotic patients admitted for GI bleeding?**
    These patients have almost twice the risk of developing bacterial infections while hospitalized than do cirrhotic patients admitted for other reasons (nosocomial infection rates approach 50%). Spontaneous bacterial peritonitis, bacteremia, and pneumonia are the most common

infections. Short-term antibiotic prophylaxis decreases infection incidence and early rehemorrhage with a resultant increase in survival. Oral norfloxacin (400 mg twice daily for 7 days), is a proven regimen; intravenous ceftriaxone (1 g once daily for 7 days) is superior for patients with hypovolemic shock.

25. **What is a Sengstaken-Blakemore tube?**
   A large nasogastric (NG) tube with two inflatable balloons that can be used to tamponade both the esophagus and the gastric cardia. The gastric balloon is inflated in the stomach (insert 150 ml of saline plus 25 ml of Gastrografin so that you can confirm appropriate positioning by radiograph) and pull this inflated balloon gently up against the gastroesophageal junction. Most bleeds occur in the distal 5 cm of esophagus, so if bleeding continues, the esophageal balloon should be inflated as well. To prevent balloon-induced esophageal ischemia or rupture, do not inflate this balloon to >30 mm Hg (exceeds portal venous pressure) and limit use to 24 hours. Half of patients rebleed after balloon deflation, and 10% to 25% suffer aspiration pneumonia (see Fig. 41-2).

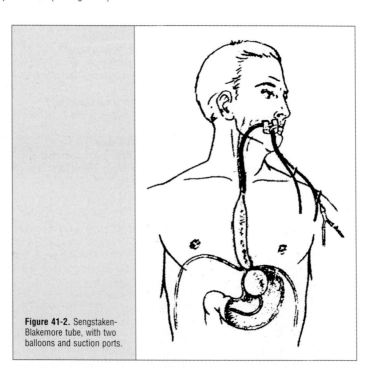

Figure 41-2. Sengstaken-Blakemore tube, with two balloons and suction ports.

26. **What are the options for preventing recurrent variceal bleeds?**
   Without treatment, 75% of patients rebleed within 1 year. β-blockers reduce this to 40%; when combined with sclerotherapy, the rate is 35%, and when combined with EBL, the rate is reduced to 25%. The lowest rebleeding rates are thus accomplished with EBL and chronic nadolol. Interestingly, EBL with β-blockade has demonstrated no difference in 2-year survival when compared with β-blocker and nitrate treatment alone. Shunt surgery and TIPS are slightly better than all these options at 15% rebleeding per year, but these invasive interventions are also more morbid.

27. **How should a patient with recurrent variceal bleeds be treated?**
Primary treatment should be EBL combined with β-blockade. Failing this treatment, the second-line option is to decompress the portal venous system by shunting blood away with a portosystemic anastomosis. The decision of open versus radiologic shunting is based on the urgency and the patient's fitness for surgery.

28. **What is transjugular intrahepatic portosystemic shunting?**
TIPS is a percutaneous radiologic technique for diverting portal venous blood directly into the IVC. Under fluoroscopy, a stent is placed through the hepatic parenchyma to link the hepatic and portal veins. Although TIPS relieves ascites and is superior to EBL in lowering variceal bleed risk, it also exacerbates encephalopathy without any decrease in mortality. New or worsened encephalopathy occurs in at least 25% of patients after TIPS. Stent stenosis and dysfunction occurs in 30% by 1 year and 50% by 2 years (Fig. 41-3).

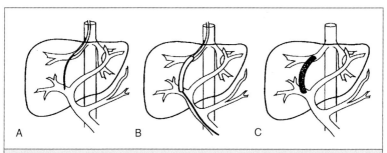

Figure 41-3. TIPS placement. **A,** From a hepatic vein, a needle punctures through the liver to reach a portal vein. **B,** The tunnel is widened with a balloon catheter. **C,** A permanent stent is placed. (From McNally PR, editor: *GI/Liver Secrets*, 2nd ed., Philadelphia, 2001, Hanley & Belfus.)

29. **Describe the basic options for surgical shunting.**
Nonselective (central) shunt: portovacal and mesocaval shunts nonselectively decompress the portal venous system, thus risking hepatofugal flow and worsening hepatic failure. Large amounts of portal blood (not detoxified in the liver) in the systemic circulation worsen encephalopathy. Creating a smaller diameter conduit (partial shunt) helps preserve some anterograde portal flow and limits this effect.
Selective splenorenal (Warren) shunt: anastomosis of the distal splenic vein to the left renal vein with ligation of the left gastric. This does not decompress as thoroughly, and therefore, this technique enjoys a lower risk of encephalopathy.
As a rule, the more central the shunt site, the more extensive the portal decompression, but the tradeoff is the increased risk of encephalopathy (as demonstrated by TIPS).

30. **How can you estimate operative mortality for elective portosystemic shunting?**
Perioperative mortality correlates well with Child-Pugh class (this was the original purpose of the classification). Classes A, B, and C demonstrate up to 5%, 10%, and 40% mortality, respectively, at 30 days.

31. **Is there a definitive treatment for recurrent variceal bleeding?**
Liver transplantation provides portal decompression and restores hepatic function. Listing criteria are strict, and the psychological assessment of the "reformed alcoholic" is particularly arduous. Prior TIPS or shunting operations are not contraindications to transplant.

CONTROVERSY

32. How should a patient with known esophageal varices be treated to prevent an initial variceal bleed?

The combination of β-blocker and nitrate is used for primary prophylaxis, but EBL is at least equivalent to pharmacotherapy without the side effects (one third of patients cannot tolerate β-blockers because of fatigue or bronchospasm, and 20% cannot tolerate nitrates secondary to pounding headaches). These treatments reduce the incidence of an initial bleed from 30% to <10% and the mortality of a bleed from 30% to 20%. EBL was previously suggested for prophylaxis only in class C disease, but mounting evidence suggests that EBL is at least as effective as pharmacotherapy in all patients.

KEY POINTS: PORTAL HYPERTENSION

1. Portal venous pressure >20 mm Hg (normal = 5 to 10 mm Hg).

2. Most common causes in the United States are hepatitis C and alcoholism.

3. Anatomic causes characterized as presinusoidal, sinusoidal, or postsinusoidal.

4. Complications include ascites, esophageal varices, encephalopathy, hypersplenism, and hemorrhoids.

5. Initial management is medical and endoscopic; surgery is reserved for refractory cases.

BIBLIOGRAPHY

1. Abraldes JG, Bosch J: The treatment of acute variceal bleeding. J Clin Gastroenterol 41:S312-S317, 2007.

2. Albillos A: Preventing first variceal hemorrhage in cirrhosis. J Clin Gastroenterol 41:S305-S311, 2007.

3. deFranchis R, Dell'Era A, Iannuzzi F: Diagnosis and treatment of portal hypertension. Dig Liver Dis 36:787-798, 2004.

4. Hayes PC: Primary prophylaxis of variceal hemorrhage: a randomized controlled trial comparing band ligation, propranolol, and isosorbide mononitrate. Gastroenterology 123:735-744, 2002.

5. Jensen DM: Endoscopic screening for varices in cirrhosis: findings, implications, and outcomes. Gastroenterology 122:1620-1630, 2002.

6. Lo GH, Chen WC, Chen MH et al.: Banding ligation versus nadolol and isosorbide mononitrate for the prevention of esophageal variceal rebleeding. Gastroenterology 123:728-734, 2002.

7. Lui HF, Stanley AJ, Forrest EH et al.: Gastroesophageal variceal hemorrhage. N Engl J Med 345:669-681, 2001.

CHAPTER 42

GASTROESOPHAGEAL REFLUX DISEASE

Michael E. Fenoglio, MD, and Lawrence W. Norton, MD

1. What symptoms suggest gastroesophageal reflux disease (GERD)?

Substernal burning after meals or at night, associated occasionally with regurgitation of gastric juices, is one symptom. Discomfort is relieved by standing or sitting. Dysphagia, a late complication of GERD, is caused by mucosal edema or stricture of the distal esophagus. However, no symptom is specific for GERD, and therapeutic decisions should not be made on symptoms alone.

2. What is the difference between heartburn and GERD?

Heartburn is a lay term for mild, intermittent reflux of gastric content into the esophagus without tissue injury. It is relatively common among adults. GERD implies esophagitis with varying degrees of erythema, edema, and friability of the distal esophageal mucosa. It occurs in 10% of the population.

3. What causes GERD?

The underlying abnormality of GERD is functional incompetence of the lower esophageal sphincter (LES), which allows gastric acid, bile, and digestive enzymes to damage the unprotected esophageal mucosa. Achalasia, scleroderma, and other esophageal motility disorders are sometimes associated with GERD.

4. Is hiatal hernia an essential defect in patients with GERD?

No. Not all patients with GERD have a hiatal hernia, and not all patients with a hiatal hernia have GERD. A total of 50% of patients with GERD have an associated hiatal hernia.

5. What studies are useful to diagnose GERD?

Endoscopy with biopsy is essential in diagnosing GERD. Barium swallow with or without fluoroscopy can diagnose reflux but cannot identify esophagitis. Twenty-four-hour esophageal acid-base balance (pH) testing associates reflux with symptoms and is useful in some patients. Gastric secretory or gastric emptying tests are occasionally helpful. Manometry of the esophagus and LES is required whenever an esophageal motility disorder is suspected and before any surgical intervention.

6. What is the initial management of a patient suspected of having GERD?

- Change diet to avoid foods known to induce reflux (e.g., chocolate, alcohol, and coffee).
- Avoid large meals before bedtime.
- Stop smoking.
- Do not wear tight, binding clothes.
- Elevate the head of the bed 4 to 5 inches.
- Take antacids when symptomatic.
- Weight loss can be quite effective in reducing GERD symptoms.

7. If initial treatment fails, what should be recommended?

About 50% of patients show significant healing with H2 blockers, but only 10% of these patients remain healed 1 year later. Metoclopramide promotes gastric emptying but rarely relieves symptoms consistently in the absence of acid reduction.

KEY POINTS: DIAGNOSTIC WORK-UP OF GASTROESOPHAGEAL REFLUX DISEASE

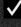

1. Underlying anatomic abnormality may cause functional incompetence of the LES.

2. Endoscopy and biopsy are paramount in diagnosis.

3. Swallow studies delineate possible anatomic causes.

4. Twenty-four-hour pH monitoring can link reflux to patient's symptoms.

5. Manometry of the LES is required if esophageal motility disorder is suspected.

8. What is the role of proton pump inhibitor (PPI) in GERD?

PPIs (omeprazole and others) irreversibly inhibit the parietal cell hydrogen ion pump and are >80% successful in healing severe erosive esophagitis. Two thirds of patients who continue the medication remain healed. A concern in prolonged PPI therapy is hypergastrinemia secondary to alkalinization of the antrum. Gastrin is trophic to gastrointestinal (GI) mucosa, but the initial fear of induced neoplasia has not been borne out by follow-up studies.

9. When should operation for GERD be recommended?

Failure of nonoperative (medical) therapy is the primary indication for surgery. Noncompliance with prescribed treatment is a frequent cause of failure and even stricture unresponsive to dilation. With PPIs, most patients' symptoms can be controlled for long periods of time. Current recommendations for surgical intervention include: (1) failed medical therapy (e.g., intractable disease, intolerance or allergy to medications, noncompliance, and recurrence of symptoms while on medical therapy), (2) complications (e.g., stricture, respiratory symptoms, medicosocial changes, and premalignant mucosal changes), (3) patient preference (e.g., cost—long-term medical prescriptions can be expensive—or lifestyle issues).

10. What is the goal of surgical treatment?

Operations for GERD attempt to prevent reflux by mechanically increasing LES pressure and, in most procedures, to restore a sufficient length of distal esophagus to the high-pressure zone of the abdomen. Hiatal hernia, when present, is reduced simultaneously.

11. What procedures can accomplish this goal and how do they do it?

- In the **Nissen fundoplication,** which is used in >95% of patients, the fundus of the stomach is mobilized, wrapped around the distal esophagus posteriorly, and secured to itself anteriorly (i.e., 360-degree wrap). The procedure alters the angle of the gastroesophageal junction and maintains the distal esophagus within the abdomen to prevent reflux. The operation is performed transabdominally by either laparotomy or laparoscopy (see Fig. 42-1).

- The **Belsey Mark IV operation** accomplishes the same anatomic changes but is done via a thoracotomy (see Fig. 42-2).

- The **Hill gastropexy** restores the esophagus to the abdominal cavity by securing the gastric cardia to the preaortic fascia (see Fig. 42-3).

- The **Toupet (partial) fundoplication** is used in patients who have associated motility disorders. Because the wrap is not circumferential, the incidence of postoperative dysphagia is significantly reduced with this partial wrap compared with a full 360-degree wrap (Nissen fundoplication). However, long-term durability may not be as good as with a Nissen fundoplication. This operation can be done transabdominally by either laparotomy or laparoscopy (see Fig. 42-4).

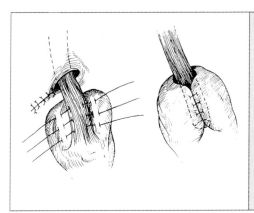

Figure 42-1. In the Nissen fundoplication, which is used in >95% of patients, the fundus of the stomach is mobilized, wrapped around the distal esophagus posteriorly, and secured to itself anteriorly (i.e., 360-degree wrap). The procedure alters the angle of the gastroesophageal junction and maintains the distal esophagus within the abdomen to prevent reflux. The operation is performed transabdominally by either laparotomy or laparoscopy.

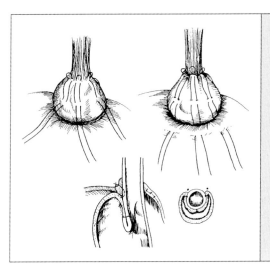

Figure 42-2. The Belsey Mark IV operation accomplishes the same anatomic changes as the Nissen fundoplication but is done via a thoracotomy.

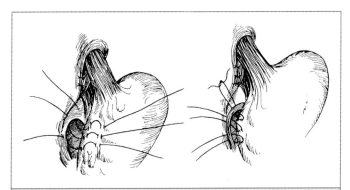

Figure 42-3. The Hill gastropexy restores the esophagus to the abdominal cavity by securing the gastric cardia to the preaortic fascia.

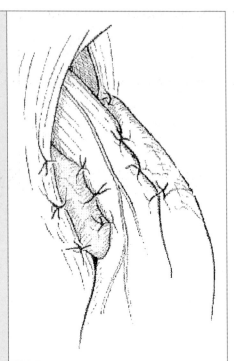

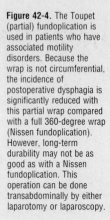

Figure 42-4. The Toupet (partial) fundoplication is used in patients who have associated motility disorders. Because the wrap is not circumferential, the incidence of postoperative dysphagia is significantly reduced with this partial wrap compared with a full 360-degree wrap (Nissen fundoplication). However, long-term durability may not be as good as with a Nissen fundoplication. This operation can be done transabdominally by either laparotomy or laparoscopy.

12. **What are the success rates for such procedures?**
    All of the procedures described in question 11 eliminate GERD in almost 90% of patients who are followed for 10 years. But the Nissen fundoplication wins in comparison studies. Recurrent symptoms should be thoroughly worked up because they are frequently associated with other disorders and not recurrent GERD.

13. **What are the long-term complications of such procedures?**
    The repair may fail, with recurrence of reflux, after any of these operations. Incorrect placement or slippage of the stomach wrap can complicate Nissen fundoplication and the Belsey Mark IV procedure. Dysphagia and the inability to belch (i.e., gas-bloat syndrome) result from too tight a wrap.

14. **How can stricture from GERD be managed?**
    Pliable (unfixed) strictures can be dilated. Fixed strictures require surgical repair. A Thal patch expands the stricture by interposing a piece of stomach.

CONTROVERSIES

15. **Is GERD better treated in the long term by PPI therapy or Nissen fundoplication?**
    PPIs really work in resolving esophagitis and eliminating symptoms of GERD, but the long-term side effects are not fully known. Fundoplication potentially frees the patient from daily medicine (this has been challenged recently) and may cause morbidity in ≈10% of patients.

16. Should a Nissen fundoplication be performed by laparoscopy or laparotomy?

The same procedure can be accomplished by either approach. Postoperative morbidity and mortality is comparable. The distinct advantages of laparoscopy are less postoperative pain, shorter hospitalization, and earlier return to work.

17. Can this disease be treated by other minimally invasive means?

Yes. Other endoscopic methods include:

- Endoluminal suturing.
- Radiofrequency treatment of the LES.
- Injection of bulk-forming agents around the LES.

WEBSITE

www.emedicine.com/med/topic857.htm

BIBLIOGRAPHY

1. Anand O, Wani S, Sharma P: Gastroesophageal reflux disease and Barrett's esophagus. Endoscopy 40:126-130, 2008. Epub Dec 4, 2007.
2. Bremner RM, DeMeester TR, Crookes F et al.: The effect of symptoms and nonspecific motility abnormalities on outcomes of surgical therapy for gastroesophageal reflux. J Thorac Cardiovasc Surg 107:1244-1250, 1994.
3. DeMeester TR, Peters JH, Bremner CG et al.: Biology of gastroesophageal reflux disease: pathophysiology relating to medical and surgical treatment. Annu Rev Med 50:469-506, 1999.
4. Hinder RA, Filipi CJ, Wetscher G et al.: Laparoscopic Nissen fundoplication is an effective treatment for gastroesophageal reflux disease. Ann Surg 220:472-481, 1994.
5. Lagergren J, Bergstrom R, Lindgren A et al.: Symptomatic gastroesophageal reflux as a risk factor for esophageal adenocarcinoma. N Engl J Med 340:825-831, 1999.
6. Lord RV, Kaminski A, Oberg S et al.: Absence of gastroesophageal reflux disease in a majority of patients taking acid suppression medications after Nissen fundoplication. J Gastrointest Surg 6:3-9, 2002.
7. Peters JH, DeMeester TR, editors: *Minimally invasive surgery of the foregut.* St. Louis, 1994, Quality Medical Publishing.
8. Roy-Shapira A, Stein HJ, Scwartz D et al.: Endoluminal methods of treating gastroesophageal reflux disease. Dis Esophagus 15:132-136, 2002.
9. Spechler SJ: Comparison of medical and surgical therapy for complicated gastroesophageal reflux disease in veterans. N Engl J Med 326:786-792, 1992.
10. Spechler SJ, Lee E, Ahnen D et al.: Long-term outcome of medical and surgical therapies for gastro-esophageal reflux disease: follow-up of a randomized controlled trial. JAMA 285:2331-2338, 2001.
11. Spivak H, Lulcuk S, Hunter JG: Laparoscopic surgery of the gastroesophageal junction. World J Surg 23:356-367, 1999.
12. Strate U, Emmermann A, Fibbe C et al.: Laparoscopic fundoplication: Nissen versus Toupet two-year outcome of a prospective randomized study of 200 patients regarding preoperative esophageal motility. Surg Endosc 22:21-30, 2008. Epub Nov 20, 2007.
13. Triadafilopoulos G, DiBaise JK, Nostrant TT et al.: The Stretta procedure for the treatment of GERD: 6 and 12 month follow-up of the U.S. open label trial. Gastrointest Endosc 55:149-156, 2002.
14. Trus TL, Laycock WS, Waring JP et al.: Improvement in quality of life measures after laparoscopic antireflux surgery. Ann Surg 229:331-336, 1999.
15. Watson DI, Jamieson JG, Pike GK et al.: Prospective randomized double-blind trial between laparoscopic Nissen fundoplication and anterior partial fundoplication. Br J Surg 86:120-130, 1999.

CHAPTER 43

ESOPHAGEAL CANCER

Ricardo J. Gonzalez, MD

1. What are the risk factors for developing esophageal cancer?

Both alcohol and tobacco increase the risk of carcinoma of the esophagus by a factor of 10. Additional risk factors include Barrett's esophagus with dysplasia, carcinogen exposures (e.g., nitrosamines in the Eastern world), vitamin and trace element deficiencies, and Plummer-Vinson syndrome.

2. What is the epidemiology of carcinoma of the esophagus?

Esophageal cancer accounts for 1% of all cancers and 2% of cancer-related deaths. Generally, it is 3 times more common in men and occurs most commonly in the seventh decade of life. Worldwide, 95% of all esophageal cancers are of squamous cell origin; however, in the Western world, the relative incidence of adenocarcinoma has increased dramatically over the past 20 years because of the comparable increase in the incidence of Barrett's esophagus.

3. What is Barrett's esophagus, and how does it relate to esophageal cancer?

Chronic reflux of gastric contents into the esophagus may lead to Barrett's esophagus, which is characterized by replacement of the normal squamous esophageal mucosa with a glandular columnar mucosa resembling the stomach. This is also called intestinal metaplasia. If Barrett's esophagus progresses to high-grade dysplasia, patients have a fortyfold increased risk of esophageal adenocarcinoma. Patients with high-grade dysplasia are traditionally treated by esophagectomy; however, photodynamic therapy (PDT) may eliminate dysplastic Barrett's mucosa, obviating surgical resection. PDT remains unapproved and experimental.

4. What are the most common presenting symptoms of esophageal cancer?

Dysphagia occurs in 85% of patients. Others symptoms include weight loss (60%), chest or epigastric pain (25%), regurgitation of undigested food (25%), hoarseness caused by recurrent laryngeal nerve involvement (5%), cough or dyspnea (3%), and hematemesis (2%).

5. What is the diagnostic work-up for patients presenting with these symptoms?

1. History and physical examination.
2. Upper gastrointestinal (GI) series (contrast study of the upper GI tract).
3. Upper endoscopy with biopsies of all concerning luminal structures.
4. Computed tomography (CT) scan of chest and abdomen to define nodal and potential metastatic disease.
5. Endoscopic ultrasound (EUS) to define the T stage (i.e., size) of the primary mass and regional lymph node involvement with possible fine-needle aspiration (FNA) biopsy.
6. Positron emission tomography (PET) scan to define distant metastatic spread.

6. What is the anatomic distribution of esophageal cancer?

The esophagus is divided into three anatomic segments: upper, middle, and lower thirds. Fifteen percent of esophageal cancers arise in the upper third, 50% in the middle third, and 35% in the lower third.

7. **What is neoadjuvant chemotherapy? What are its advantages and disadvantages?**

   This is chemotherapy, radiation therapy, or both to the primary lesion before surgical resection. The advantages include:
   - Potential downstaging (to shrink the tumor or treat locoregional lymph node involvement).
   - Early treatment of micrometastatic disease.
   - Treatment is better tolerated before surgical stress.
   - Calibrates the patient's ability to tolerate major surgery.
   - Verification of primary tumor's sensitivity to the chemotherapy or radiation therapy so as to plan for effective adjuvant therapy.

   The disadvantages include:
   - Delay in treatment of the primary lesion, particularly when the primary tumor progresses despite neoadjuvant therapy.
   - Selection for chemoresistant cell lines.

8. **What are the surgical options for treatment of carcinoma of the esophagus?**

   Surgery alone or combined with chemoradiotherapy offers the only hope for cure. The surgical approaches include: (1) transabdominal resection of lesions located at the gastroesophageal junction; (2) resection with intrathoracic anastomosis by left thoracoabdominal (Sweet procedure) or combined midline laparotomy and right thoracotomy (Ivor-Lewis procedure); and (3) transhiatal esophagectomy with cervical anastomosis. Laser therapy, esophageal stenting procedures, and dilatation are reserved for palliation.

9. **What are the risks of surgery?**

   Anastomotic leak.
   Anastomotic stricture.
   Death.
   Dysphagia.
   Hemorrhage.
   Empyema and sepsis.
   Local recurrence of cancer.

10. **What is the natural history of esophageal cancer?**

    In a collected series of almost 1000 untreated patients, the 1- and 2-year survival rates were 6.0% and 0.3%, respectively. Untreated patients typically succumb to progressive malnutrition complicated by aspiration pneumonia, sepsis, and death. Formation of a fistula between the aorta or pulmonary artery and the esophagus or pulmonary tree is a somewhat more dramatic (or perhaps merciful) mode of exit. Treated or untreated, esophageal cancer is a bad disease.

11. **Describe the stages of esophageal cancer and the respective 5-year survival rate after esophagectomy.**

    Stage I is cancer confined to the inner layer (muscularis mucosae or submucosa), and 5-year survival is as high as 80%. **Stage II** describes tumors that are confined to the layers outside the submucosa with local lymph node involvement, and 5-year survival can be as high as 35%. **Stage III** tumors have either invaded surrounding structures (lung, aorta, or trachea) irrespective of regional lymph node involvement or go through the wall of the esophagus with nodal involvement. The 5-year survival is typically <10%. **Stage IV** esophageal cancer has spread to nonregional lymph nodes (supraclavicular or celiac nodes) or distant organs (lung, liver, or bone). Essentially, all patients with stage IV disease die within 2 years of diagnosis.

12. **What is an "R0" (or "R zero") resection, and how does it impact survival?**

    All gross disease is removed, and microscopically, the margins of resection are negative for tumor. Achieving an R0 resection is the surgeon's goal and is the most robust predictor of a favorable outcome after surgery for esophageal cancer. An R1 resection represents removal of all gross disease, yet resection margins are microscopically positive for tumor. The overall 5-year survival (any stage) for patients with microscopically positive margins decreases by an order of magnitude (e.g., 30% down to 3%).

KEY POINTS: ESOPHAGEAL CARCINOMA

1. Most common in older patients with dysphagia (85% of cases) and weight loss (60% of cases).

2. Major causative factors are alcohol and tobacco (tenfold increase in risk).

3. Diagnosis is made by upper GI endoscopy and biopsy.

4. Most common variant is adenocarcinoma; second most common is squamous cell cancer.

5. Radiographic work-up is necessary to stage disease.

WEBSITES

www.emedicine.com/med/topic741.htm

www.acssurgery.com/abstracts/acs/acs0309.htm

BIBLIOGRAPHY

1. Alexiou C: Survival after esophageal resection for carcinoma: the importance of histologic cell type. Ann Thorac Surg 82:1073-1077, 2006.
2. Cordero JA: Self-expanding esophageal metallic stents in the treatment of esophageal obstruction. Am Surg: 66:958-959, 2000.
3. Hofstetter W: Treatment outcomes of resected esophageal cancer. Ann Surg 236:376-384, 2002.
4. Kato H: Comparison of PET and computerized tomography in the use of the assessment of esophageal carcinoma. Cancer 15:921-928, 2002.
5. Kelsen DP: Long-term results of RTOG trial 8911 (USA Intergroup 113): a random assignment trial comparison of chemotherapy followed by surgery compared with surgery alone for esophageal cancer. J Clin Oncol 25: 3719-3725, 2007.
6. Malaisrie SC: The addition of induction chemotherapy to preoperative, concurrent chemoradiotherapy improves tumor response in patients with esophageal adenocarcinoma. Cancer 107:967-974, 2006.
7. Oesophageal Cancer Group: Surgical resection with or without preoperative chemotheraphy in oesophageal cancer. Lancet 359:1727-1733, 2002.
8. Overholt BF: Photodynamic therapy in the management of Barrett's esophagus with dysplasia. J Gastrointest Surg 4:129-130, 2002.
9. Reed C: Techniques of esophageal surgery. Chest Surg Clin North Am 5:379-574, 1995.
10. Shumaker DA: Potential impact of preoperative EUS on esophageal cancer management and cost. Gastrointest Endosc 56:391-396, 2002.
11. Swaroop VS: Re: Practice guidelines for esophageal cancer. Am J Gastroenterol 94:2319-2320, 1999.
12. Urba S: Combined modality therapy for esophageal cancer-standard of care? Surg Oncol Clin North Am 11:377-386, 2002.
13. Walsh T: A comparison of multimodal therapy and surgery for esophageal adenocarcinoma. N Engl J Med 335:462-467, 1996.

CHAPTER 44

ACID-PEPTIC ULCER DISEASE

Erik D. Peltz, DO, and Thomas N. Robinson, MD

DUODENAL ULCER DISEASE

1. What is the risk of duodenal ulcer disease?

The lifetime risk for duodenal ulcer is about 1 in 14. It usually occurs between ages 20 and 60 years, with peak incidence in the fourth decade of life. It is more common in males. Hemorrhage is the most common cause of hospital admission. The annual number of deaths in the United States is about 10,000 deaths caused by duodenal ulcers.

2. What is the role of *Helicobacter pylori* in duodenal ulcer?

H. pylori, a gram-negative bacillus, is strongly associated with peptic ulcer disease. It is isolated from antral mucosa in 80% of patients with peptic ulcer disease. Ulcers may occur in the absence of *H. pylori.* These ulcers occur in the setting of hyperacid secretion, normal acid secretion, or after acid reduction operations such as vagotomy. Recurrent or multiple ulcerations may indicate an underlying endocrine disease. The breakdown of the duodenal mucosal barrier probably also contributes to ulcerogenesis.

3. Is acid hypersecretion necessary for peptic ulcer disease?

No. Gastric hypersecretion of acid and pepsin plays an important role in ulcer formation; however, only 40% of ulcer sufferers manifest acid hypersecretion.

4. What are the clinically important complications of *H. pylori* infection?

Peptic ulcer disease: As noted, *H. pylori* is present in 80% of peptic ulcers. Conversely, 50% of the general population harbors this organism. In individuals infected with *H. pylori,* the lifetime risk of developing a peptic ulcer is 10% to 20%. *H. pylori* may be part of the indigenous human gastric flora; antigens were detected in pre-Columbian Central American mummies whose last meal was 1700 years ago.

Gastric carcinoma: *H. pylori* is strongly linked to gastric cancer and is now classified as a group I carcinogen. It may also cause mucosa-associated lymphoid tissue (MALT) lymphoma.

Barrett's esophagus is a possible *H. pylori*-associated disease, although it is more commonly associated with chronic gastroesophageal reflux.

H. pylori probably synergizes with nonsteroidal anti-inflammatory drug (NSAID) use.

5. What is the most commonly used test for *H. pylori*?

The **CLO test** detects the presence of *H. pylori*. *H. pylori* releases urease, which breaks down urea to ammonia and bicarbonate, thus increasing the acid-base balance (pH). The CLO test can be performed at the time of endoscopy by obtaining scrapings from the antral mucosa.

If endoscopy is not available, the **enzyme-linked immunosorbent assay** (ELISA) may be used to detect anti-*H. pylori* immunoglobulin A (IgA) and immunoglobulin G (IgG) antibody titers.

Direct culture of the organism should be reserved for cases in which antibiotic resistance becomes the issue.

6. **What other risk factors are associated with duodenal ulcer disease?**
   - Cigarette smoking is a major risk factor; its cessation is a key component of ulcer therapy.
   - Blood group O is associated with higher incidence of duodenal ulcer, as are leukocyte antigens HLA-B5, B12, and BW35.
   - NSAIDs promote ulcer formation by suppressing systemic prostaglandin production.
   - Chronic pancreatitis, cirrhosis, emphysema, and α_1 antitrypsin deficiency are also associated with the condition.

7. **Which endocrine disorder is associated with severe ulcer disease?**
   Patients with multiple endocrine neoplasia (MEN) type I have a 75% incidence of gastrinoma with severe ulcer diathesis.

8. **What other endocrine disorders should be screened?**
   Pituitary tumor and hyperparathyroidism should be suspected when MEN type I is considered.

9. **What are the clinical presentations of peptic ulcer disease?**
   - Pain is usually epigastric in origin, although radiation to the back may indicate pancreatic involvement. It is often relieved by food or antacid ingestion. Nausea and vomiting may occur.
   - Upper gastrointestinal (GI) bleeding. (Peptic ulcers are responsible for 28% to 59% of all upper GI bleeding)
   - Gastric outlet obstruction (GOO) may result from pyloric spasm, inflammatory mass constriction, duodenal scarring, or fibrosis.
   - Perforation is a surgical emergency with a mortality rate as high as 10%. Perforation may occur without a history of peptic ulcer disease, especially if the ulcer is situated on the anterior surface of the duodenum.

10. **How does the location of the ulcer affect its clinical presentation?**
    Anterior wall ulcers (usually first portion of duodenum) may perforate and cause peritonitis with free air in the abdomen. Posterior ulcers may erode into the gastroduodenal artery or pancreas.

11. **What are the differential diagnoses of epigastric pain?**
    In addition to peptic ulcer disease, gastroesophageal reflux disease (GERD), gastritis, gastric carcinoma, biliary tract disease, pancreatitis or pancreatic carcinoma, aortic aneurysm, intestinal angina (ischemia), and myocardial ischemia should be considered.

12. **What initial test should be performed when evaluating epigastric pain of presumed gastrointestinal origin?**
    Flexible esophagogastroduodenoscopy (EGD) is preferred, although the upper GI contrast study with barium may be acceptable. The CLO test can be performed at the time of the EGD if indicated. Ultrasound (US) should be performed if gallbladder or vascular diseases are suspected. A lateral-view angiogram for intestinal angina, computed tomography (CT) scan for aneurysm, and a baseline electrocardiogram (ECG) should be obtained because ischemic heart disease is always possible.

13. **How are patients with duodenal ulcer treated?**
    - **Diet:** Aspirin and NSAIDs must be discontinued. Alcohol and nicotine should be avoided.
    - **Antacids:** Neutralizing gastric pH may alleviate symptoms, but its impact on ulcer healing is not well defined.
    - **H2 receptor antagonists:** The use of cimetidine or ranitidine prevents gastric acid secretions by blocking the H2 histamine receptor.

- **Sucralfate:** A protective-barrier medicine adheres to the ulcer base, providing a protective coating. Medications that decrease acid secretion should not be used at the same time because sucralfate requires an acidic environment to be activated.
- Proton pump inhibitors (PPIs): Omeprazole blocks the hydrogen-potassium adenosine triphosphatase pump in the gastric parietal cells and inhibits hydrogen ion release. It usually is reserved for failures of first-line therapy (i.e., H2 receptor antagonists).
- ***H. pylori* eradication:** If *H. pylori* infection is diagnosed, the combination of triple therapy (bismuth, tetracycline, and metronidazole) with an H2 receptor antagonist regimen appears to provide a 90% cure rate. Erythromycin, amoxicillin-omeprazole, or erythromycin-omeprazole may be added for initial failures.

14. **What are the recurrence rates after medical therapy?**
    Approximately 80% of duodenal ulcers heal in 6 weeks. The recurrence rate within 1 year of treatment is 70%; thus, repeated treatment may be necessary.

15. **What complications are associated with medical therapy?**
    H2 receptor antagonists may induce mental status changes and gynecomastia. Cimetidine, in particular, may affect hepatic metabolism of warfarin, phenytoin, theophylline, propranolol, and digoxin, leading to abnormal serum levels. Omeprazole may cause hypergastrinemia by blocking gastric acid secretion. *H. pylori* resistance to antibiotics may develop, especially to metronidazole; therefore, a triple combination of at least two antimicrobials with an acid inhibitory drug is recommended as initial therapy.

16. **How should recurrent or multiple ulcers be evaluated?**
    In addition to the previously mentioned work-up, serum gastrin levels should be obtained to evaluate for possible endocrine disorder. Patients should not be taking omeprazole when gastrin levels are measured. In Zollinger-Ellison syndrome, gastrin hypersecretion from the pancreatic islet tumor results in multiple or intractable ulcers (normal serum gastrin, <200 pg/ml; Zollinger-Ellison syndrome, usually >500 pg/ml).

17. **How do you evaluate a borderline serum gastrin value (200 to 500 pg/ml)?**
    The secretin stimulation test may be used to diagnose Zollinger-Ellison syndrome. An intravenous (IV) bolus of secretin (2 U/kg) should result in an increase of gastrin of 150 pg/ml within 15 minutes if the patient has this syndrome.

18. **What are the indications for operative treatment of duodenal ulcers?**
    Failure of medical management to control pain, bleeding (<6 units of packed red blood cell transfusions in 24 hours or, better yet, two thirds of the patient's calculated blood volume loss in 24 hours), and obstruction are the usual indications. Perforation of the ulcer is usually treated surgically unless the patient presents 24 hours after the event without peritonitis and the Gastrografin upper GI series confirms that the perforation has been well sealed (usually with omentum).

19. **What operations are used to treat duodenal ulcers?**
    - Truncal vagotomy and pyloroplasty (V and P) or gastrojejunostomy.
    - Truncal vagotomy and antrectomy with Billroth I or II anastomosis.
    - Subtotal gastrectomy with Billroth I or II anastomosis.
    - Selective vagotomy (just the vagal branches to the parietal cells in the stomach).
    - Total gastrectomy.

20. **What are Billroth I and Billroth II anastomoses?**
    The **Billroth I** operation is an anastomosis between the duodenum and the gastric remnant (gastroduodenostomy). The **Billroth II** operation is constructed by sewing a loop of jejunum to the gastric remnant (gastrojejunostomy). Either method is acceptable.

21. **Which procedure is preferred, Billroth I or Billroth II?**

Billroth I has the advantages of eliminating the duodenal stump and requiring only one suture line instead of two (as in Billroth II). Duodenal stump blowout is a critical surgical emergency that requires immediate laparotomy. Afferent loop syndrome (i.e., sludging of stuff in the loop that is not in the enteric stream) is also a complication of Billroth II. Bile reflux gastritis may occur in both procedures. Billroth I is more physiologic; thus, it results in better protein and fat digestion. Billroth I is more susceptible to gastric outlet obstruction with ulcer or tumor recurrence; therefore, a Billroth I hook-up is not recommended for patients with gastric carcinoma.

22. **What is afferent loop syndrome?**

Postprandial abdominal pain often is relieved by bilious vomiting. A narrowing at the junction of the stomach and duodenal side of a Billroth II anastomosis leads to biliary and pancreatic fluid buildup within the afferent limb of the intestine. Pain is relieved when the fluid content is emptied into the stomach, which may result in bilious vomiting and severe reflux gastritis.

23. **How is afferent loop syndrome prevented?**

Prevention requires avoidance of a long or twisted afferent limb with too narrow an anastomosis during Billroth II construction. A Billroth I procedure eliminates this possible problem.

24. **Who was Billroth?**

Christian Albert Theodor Billroth (1829–1894) was an Austrian surgeon credited with performing the first successful gastric resection in 1881 and introducing innovations to intestinal bypass surgery. The father of modern U.S. surgery, William Halsted, was once an apprentice to Billroth in Vienna.

25. **How does alkaline or bile reflux gastritis occur?**

Reflux of bile and pancreatic secretions into the stomach after a Billroth II (sometimes Billroth I) anastomosis may cause marked gastric irritation, leading to chronic postprandial pain. Persistent pain should be evaluated with endoscopy, and surgical reconstruction should be considered, usually with a Roux-en-Y gastrojejunostomy from a 40-cm efferent jejunal limb.

26. **What is selective vagotomy?**

In this limited proximal vagotomy, the gastric parietal cells are selectively denervated. Fibers to antrum, pylorus, liver, biliary tract, and the rest of the intestinal tract are left **intact,** thereby precluding the need for a gastric emptying procedure. Recurrence of ulcer disease may be 10% or greater, but its side effects, namely dumping (caused by resection of the pylorus) or diarrhea (caused by the vagotomy), are minimized to 2%.

27. **What is dumping syndrome?**

Resection of the pylorus can lead to uncontrolled, rapid emptying of hyperosmolar gastric contents into the proximal small bowel. The osmotic and glucose load in the intestine sucks intravascular volume into the gut, making the patient transiently hypovolemic. The physiologically appropriate adrenergic response to this volume shift produces tachycardia, sweating, flushing, weakness, nausea, abdominal cramps, and even syncope. Ingesting a small, dry, low-carbohydrate meal (to limit the available osmols) may prevent this syndrome. Anticholinergic drugs also may help. As many as 20% of patients experience the dumping syndrome in the early postoperative period, but only 2% develop chronic problems.

28. **What must accompany truncal vagotomy?**

Truncal vagotomy denervates the stomach, resulting in gastric hypomotility. Some gastric emptying procedure such as a pyloroplasty or a side-to-side gastroduodenostomy should be performed.

29. **What is a Heinecke-Mikulicz pyloroplasty?**
A pyloduodenal incision along the longitudinal axis followed by a transverse closure flops the pylorus open and promotes gastric emptying.

30. **What is a Finney pyloroplasty?**
A side-to-side gastroduodenal anastomosis that transects and defunctionalizes the pylorus and promotes gastric emptying.

31. **What is a Jaboulay pyloroplasty?**
This gastric emptying procedure comprises a side-to-side gastroduodenal anastomosis that does not transect the pylorus. It is ideal if severe pyloric scarring is present.

32. **What are the rates of ulcer recurrence after surgical treatment?**
Vagotomy and pyloroplasty: 10%.
Vagotomy and antrectomy: 2%.
Highly selective vagotomy: 10%.
Subtotal gastrectomy: 1%.
Total gastrectomy: <1%.

33. **What is the mortality rate of these operations?**
Vagotomy and pyloroplasty: 1%.
Vagotomy and antrectomy: 2%.
Highly selective vagotomy: 0.1%.
Subtotal gastrectomy: 2%.
Total gastrectomy: 5%.

34. **How are patients with perforated duodenal ulcers treated?**
The patient must be resuscitated first, following the ABCs of airway, breathing, and circulation. The stomach contents are emptied via nasogastric (NG) tube. Surgical closure by omental patch (Graham closure) is widely practiced. For hemodynamically stable patients, oversewing of the ulcer followed by a selective vagotomy is appropriate. Antrectomy with vagotomy to remove the ulcer is appropriate if the patient has an intractable peptic ulcer.

35. **What (ulcer-specific question) should you always ask before you proceed to the operating room?**
Past history of ulcer disease. Choice of operation will depend on acute versus chronic ulcer disease.

36. **What is the long-term result after Graham closure of a perforated ulcer?**
One third of patients remain asymptomatic, one third have symptoms controlled by medical treatment, and one third require an additional ulcer operation.

37. **What are the complications of surgery for duodenal ulcers?**
Duodenal stump leakage may occur within the first week after antral resection and Billroth anastomosis. Treatment consists of prompt reoperation to drain and control the leak. Total parenteral nutrition may be required as a "bowel rest" adjunct.
Gastric retention may occur because of edema at the anastomosis or atony of the stomach after vagotomy. It usually resolves spontaneously in 3 to 4 weeks.
Bleeding may occur from a suture line, a missed ulcer, or other gastric mucosal lesions. Most postgastrectomy bleeding ceases spontaneously, but endoscopy may be necessary in some cases.

38. **Where do ulcers recur after operation?**
Ulcers usually recur adjacent to the gastric anastomosis on the intestinal side (i.e., jejunum, duodenum).

39. **Why do they recur?**
   The responsible factors are inadequate gastric resection, incomplete vagotomy, inadequate drainage of the gastric remnant (stasis of gastric contents proximal to the anastomosis), or retained gastric antrum (gastrin-producing cells) after a Billroth II procedure.

40. **How do you treat pyloric stenosis?**
   Fluid resuscitation and NG tube decompression should be initiated. Metabolic alkalosis may result from prolonged vomiting (loss of hydrogen ions) and should be corrected with normal saline infusion. Either vagotomy with gastrojejunostomy or resection of the stenosis with a Billroth II bypass is acceptable. Partial gastrectomy is required less often.

GASTRIC ULCER DISEASE

41. **What is the most important factor in managing gastric ulcers?**
   All gastric ulcers must be evaluated for malignancy. The incidence of malignancy is about 10%.

42. **How is gastric ulcer evaluated?**
   Biopsy is mandatory. EGD with multiple biopsies (typically, six) of the ulcer crater is the best method. Upper GI series may be helpful, but biopsy is not possible. The CLO test can be performed at the time of the EGD to detect *H. pylori*. Benign ulcers usually heal by 12 weeks. Intractability should arouse suspicion for malignancy.

43. **In patients with bleeding peptic ulcers what are the endoscopic findings suggestive of rebleeding?**

Endoscopic Finding	Risk of Rebleeding (%)	Forrest Classification
Active bleeding	90%	IA
Active oozing	55%	IB
Nonbleeding visible vessel	50%	IIA
Adherent clot	33%	IIB
Red or blue spot on surface	7%	IIC
Clean base	3%	III

44. **How are gastric ulcers classified?**

Type I	At the incisura or most inferior portion of the lesser curvature
Type II	Gastric ulcer + duodenal ulcer
Type III	Prepylorus
Type IV	Gastroesophageal junction or proximal cardia
Type V	Any ulcer from NSAID or aspirin use.

45. **Which is the most common type of gastric ulcer?**
   Type I.

46. **How do benign gastric ulcers differ from duodenal ulcers?**
   Benign gastric ulcers are difficult to treat and have a higher rate of recurrence and complications. Gastric ulcer disease and gastric carcinoma have a probable common etiologic factor, which is atrophic gastritis induced by *H. pylori*. By contrast, factors associated with duodenal ulcer may protect against gastric cancer.

47. **How is *H. pylori* related to gastric ulcer disease?**
   H. pylori colonization induces chronic active gastritis, which is associated with ulcer formation, although a direct cause-and-effect link has not been clearly established. Other

factors such as focal defect in acid neutralization that allows acid diffusion into the stomach mucosa or hypersecretion of acid (in cases of type II and III ulcers) may play important roles.

48. What is a "trial of healing"?

A combination of H2 receptor antagonists or hydrogen pump inhibitors with anti-*H. pylori* medications, if indicated, may be tried for 6 to 12 weeks. A second EGD should be performed to evaluate the ulcer. An additional trial of 12 weeks is acceptable provided that the biopsy results for malignancy are negative.

49. What is the aim of *H. pylori* eradication in the setting of gastric ulcer?

Therapy aimed at *H. pylori* eradication is associated with increased ulcer healing and decreased ulcer relapse. Several series have shown decreases in recurrences from 50% to <10% with *H. pylori* eradication. *H. pylori* is strongly linked to gastric cancer and is now classified as a group I carcinogen. It also may cause MALT lymphoma.

50. How are patients with *H. pylori* infection treated?

They should be given a triple therapy of bismuth, metronidazole, and tetracycline, usually supplemented with acid-reducing medications.

51. Does gastric ulcer healing guarantee a benign ulcer?

No. Gastric ulcers with foci of malignancy may heal completely on medical therapy.

52. What are the indications for operative therapy of benign gastric ulcers?

Hemorrhage, perforation, obstruction, and intractability (the same as duodenal ulcers).

53. What is the definitive procedure used for benign gastric ulcers?

Hemigastrectomy or antrectomy (including the ulcer) without vagotomy for types I and IV ulcers is the standard procedure. Type I and IV ulcers have low or normal acid levels. For types II and III, vagotomy should be added.

54. What are the options under emergent (i.e., hemorrhage or perforation) conditions?

Hemodynamically stable: truncal vagotomy and distal gastrectomy. Hemodynamically stable patients with upper GI bleed from peptic ulcers may also be treated with endoscopic management. EGD with use of cautery, endoclips, or injection with vasoconstrictors or sclerosing agents is effective in up to 90% of bleeding peptic ulcers. The risk of rebleeding after endoscopic therapy is 15% to 20% and management decision making requires surgical evaluation. Rebleeding after a second endoscopic attempt at hemostasis is an absolute indication for surgical intervention.

Unstable: truncal vagotomy and drainage procedure with biopsy followed by excision and oversewing of ulcer.

55. What is the rebleeding rate if the ulcer is left in situ?

It is 33%.

56. What is giant gastric ulcer?

An ulcer >3 cm in diameter, usually located along the lesser curvature. The malignancy risk is about 30% and increases with the diameter. Early surgical resection is indicated because of the risk of malignancy. Vagotomy may be added.

57. What is Cushing's ulcer?

A stress ulcer found in patients who are critically ill with central nervous system (CNS) injury. Typically, single, deep, and with tendency to perforate.

58. What is Curling's ulcer?

A stress ulcer found in patients who are critically ill with burn injuries.

59. What is Dieulafoy's ulcer?

Erosion of the gastric mucosa overlying a vascular malformation, which often leads to hemorrhage. Chronic inflammation is not associated with this lesion.

60. What is a marginal ulcer?

An ulcer found near the margin of the gastroenteric anastomosis, usually on the small bowel side.

61. When does stress gastritis occur? Why?

Sixty percent of them occur within 24 to 48 hours after trauma, shock, or sepsis. Usually, mucosal erosions begin proximally in the stomach and travel distally. These are eventually seen in nearly all patients who are critically ill. The integrity of cellular barrier in the lamina propria is compromised, probably from decreased blood supply, leading to back diffusion of acid; erosion of submucosa; and, finally, bleeding.

62. How are patients with bleeding stress gastritis treated?

Blood clots should be removed from the stomach lumen by NG tube suction and lavage. Fibrinolysins from clots increase bleeding. Stomach pH should be kept above 4.0 with acid-reducing medications.

KEY POINTS: *HELICOBACTER PYLORI*

1. *H. pylori* is a gram-negative urease-producing bacillus.

2. It has a strong association with peptic ulcer disease (80% of ulcer patients).

3. It is linked to development of MALT lymphoma.

4. It is associated with development of gastric carcinoma.

5. *H. pylori* infection is diagnosed by EGD biopsy and CLO test.

6. Treatment includes triple antibiotic therapy supplemented with acid-reduction medication (90% cure rate).

WEBSITE

www.emedicine.com/med/topic1776.htm

BIBLIOGRAPHY

1. Aabakken L: Current endoscopic and pharmacological therapy of peptic ulcer bleeding. Best Pract Res Clin Gastroenterol 22(2):243-259, 2008.

2. Calam J, Baron JH: ABC of the upper gastrointestinal tract: pathophysiology of duodenal and gastric ulcer and gastric cancer. Br Med J 323:980, 2001.

3. Correa P, Willis D, Allison MJ et al.: *Helicobacter pylori* in pre-Columbian mummies. Gastroenterology 114(suppl 4): A956, 1998.

4. Hansson LE, Nyren O, Hsing AW et al.: The risk of stomach cancer in patients with gastric or duodenal ulcer disease. N Engl J Med 335:242, 1996.

5. Kokoska ER, Kauffman GL: *Helicobacter pylori* and the gastroduodenal mucosa. Surgery 130:13, 2001.

6. Leung WK, Graham DY: Ulcer and gastritis. Endoscopy 33:8, 2001.

7. Palmer K: Acute upper gastrointestinal haemorrhage. British Med Bull 83:307, 2007.

8. Rollhauser C, Fleischer DE: Nonvariceal upper gastrointestinal bleeding. Endoscopy 34:111, 2002.

9. Rosin D, Rosenthal RJ, Bonner G et al.: Gastric MALT lymphoma in a *Helicobacter pylori*-negative patient: a case report and review of literature. J Am Coll Surg 192:652, 2001.

10. Schwesinger WH, Page CP, Sirinek KR et al.: Operations for peptic ulcer disease: paradigm lost. J Gastrointest Surg 5:438, 2001.

11. Talamini G, Tommasi M, Vantini I et al.: Risk factors of peptic ulcer in 4943 inpatients. J Clin Gastroenterol 42(4):373-380, 2008.

12. van Lanschot JJ, van Leerdam M, van Delden OM et al.: Management of bleeding gastroduodenal ulcers. Dig Surg 19:99, 2002.

13. van Leerdam M: Epidemiology of acute upper gastrointestinal bleeding. Best Pract Res Clin Gastroenterol 22(2):209-224, 2008.

CHAPTER 45

SMALL BOWEL OBSTRUCTION

Elizabeth L. Cureton, MD, and Joyce A. Majure, MD

1. **Name three mechanisms of bowel obstruction, and give examples and incidence of each type.**
   1. **Extrinsic compression:** adhesions (60%), malignancy (20%), hernias (10%), volvulus and others (5%).
   2. **Internal blockage** of the lumen by abnormal materials (obturation): bezoars, gallstone, worms, or foreign body (usually obstructs at the ileocecal valve).
   3. **Mural disease** encroaching on the lumen (inflammatory bowel disease [5%]), fibrous stricture secondary to trauma, ischemia, or radiation, intussusception).

2. **What are the most common symptoms of small bowel obstruction (SBO)?**
   1. **Abdominal pain:** initially nonspecific, often colicky, coinciding with waves of peristalsis trying to pass the point of obstruction.
   2. **Bloating:** the more distal the obstruction, the more severe the abdominal distention caused by proximal bowel dilatation.
   3. **Vomiting:** bilious, frequent, and profuse with proximal obstruction, less frequent but larger volume and often feculent with distal obstruction.
   4. **Obstipation:** failure to pass gas or stool; occasionally, the patient has a few loose stools early on, as the bowel distal to the obstruction empties.

3. **What are the pertinent questions in the patient's history?**
   - Any previous abdominal or pelvic surgery?
   - Any previous SBO?
   - Any history of cancer? What type, and how treated? Any radiation?
   - Any previous abdominal infections or inflammation (include pelvic inflammatory disease [PID], appendicitis, diverticulitis, inflammatory bowel disease, perforation, and trauma)?
   - Any history of gallstones?
   - Current medications, particularly anticoagulants, anticholinergics, chemotherapy, or diuretics?

4. **What are the findings on physical examination?**
   The patient is often dehydrated and may have a low-grade fever, postural hypotension, and abdominal distention. Bowel sounds may be hyperactive with "tinkles and rushes" or may be totally silent if the patient has delayed seeking treatment. Percussion usually reveals diffuse tympani, and thin, elderly patients may even have visible loops of distended small bowel. Palpation may increase the abdominal pain, but localized tenderness or peritoneal signs indicate likely strangulation or another diagnosis.

5. **Is a rectal examination necessary?**
   Absolutely. The rectal examination may reveal signs of cancer, such as a rigid rectal shelf from carcinomatosis, and blood on hemoccult examination may herald ischemia or strangulation or may indicate inflammatory bowel disease. An obturator hernia can best be palpated transrectally or transvaginally.

6. **Where should the examiner look for obstructing hernias?**

   Examine the groins near the pubic tubercle and along the inguinal floor, check the femoral triangles for bulging or tenderness, do a rectal examination to look for obturator hernia (see question 5), and palpate all existing incisions. Check all trocar sites from previous laparoscopic surgeries.

7. **What is the most inexpensive way to confirm the diagnosis?**

   The "four-way abdominal series" (flat and upright abdominal films, plus posterolateral [PA] and lateral chest radiographs) is diagnostic about 75% of the time. Look for:
   - Air-fluid levels in dilated small intestine (also known as "stair steps" or "string of pearls" sign).
   - Absent or minimal air in the distal colon and rectum.
   - "Ground glass" appearance and obscuring of the psoas shadows by extraperitoneal fluid.
   - Sometimes a single distended loop of small bowel with a "beak" at each end, indicating a closed loop obstruction in an otherwise gasless abdomen or a single fixed loop that remains in the same location on both supine and upright films.
   - Chest radiographs may demonstrate an infiltrate, with accompanying ileus, rather than SBO. The lateral chest radiograph is the most sensitive for identifying free air in the abdomen; this necessitates an urgent laparotomy for perforated viscus.

8. **What other imaging studies can be used?**

   Oral contrast studies with water-soluble contrast (Gastrografin) help to distinguish partial from complete obstruction, intraluminal tumor or foreign body, and inflammatory bowel disease; they may also define the point of obstruction. Gastrografin may actually help resolve partial obstructions by its osmotic effect.

   Computed tomography (CT) and **magnetic resonance imaging (MRI)** can both help delineate bowel obstructions. MRI has the advantage of speed (6 to 10 minutes using the HASTE [half Fourier single shot turbo spin echo] technique), no need for contrast agent, and a higher accuracy rate. A recent Mayo Clinic series also claims superior accuracy (95% versus 71%). Ultrasound (US) has not proven useful.

9. **Which laboratory studies are indicated?**

   1. **Complete blood cell count (CBC)** to check for leukocytosis or unexpected anemia
   2. **Urinalysis** to look for urinary tract infection (which may also cause an ileus and present with a similar picture to SBO) and to assess hydration (urine-specific gravity)
   3. **Chemistry panel** to check for electrolyte abnormalities such as hypokalemic or hypochloremic metabolic alkalosis (associated with vomiting of acid gastric contents), hyponatremia, and prerenal azotemia (elevated blood urea nitrogen [BUN] and creatinine levels).
   4. **Amylase** and **lipase** to rule out pancreatitis; amylase can also be elevated, although not as high, with SBO or ischemic bowel.

10. **What are the initial steps in treatment?**

    Nasogastric (NG) suction and intravenous (IV) fluids should be instituted to restore electrolyte and fluid balance, and a Foley catheter should be placed to monitor urine output. As soon as resuscitation is complete, prompt surgical intervention is mandatory for complete obstructions and for anyone with signs and symptoms of strangulation.

11. **How can I distinguish between a complete and partial obstruction?**

    - **Clinically:** If partial, the patient may continue to pass small amounts of gas or stool. Pain and distention decreases rapidly with nasogastric suction.
    - **Radiographically:** Radiographs show gas moving into the colon (partial obstruction).
    - **With oral contrast studies:** Barium or water-soluble contrast agent given via the NG tube passes into the colon in partial obstructions.

12. **What conditions should be included in the differential diagnosis?**
Ileus from other causes (e.g., as urinary tract infection [UTI], pneumonia, hypokalemia), viral gastroenteritis, appendicitis (usually with perforation), ureteral stone, diverticulitis, mesenteric thrombosis, and obstructing colon cancer should be included.

KEY POINTS: SMALL BOWEL OBSTRUCTION

1. Most common cause is adhesive disease, followed by hernias.
2. Malignancy must be considered as a possible cause.
3. Treatment involves NG decompression, fluid and electrolyte repletion, and expectant management.
4. Surgical intervention is required if strangulation or closed loop obstruction is suspected.

13. **What are the three types of SBO, based on bowel viability?**
    1. **Simple obstruction:** Nothing passes the point of obstruction, but the vascular supply is not compromised. It may be partial and resolve with nonoperative management.
    2. **Strangulated obstruction:** The mesentery is twisted or there is so much dilation of the bowel that arterial or venous flow is cut off and the bowel becomes ischemic. Urgent surgery is mandatory.
    3. **Closed loop obstruction:** The bowel is obstructed proximally and distally, usually for a short segment, and that segment becomes massively dilated and susceptible to strangulation and perforation. Urgent surgery is mandatory.

14. **What are the "five classic signs" of strangulation? How accurate are they?**
    1. Continuous pain (not colicky).
    2. Fever.
    3. Tachycardia.
    4. Peritoneal signs (localized guarding or tenderness, rebound tenderness).
    5. Leukocytosis.
These signs usually indicate irreversible ischemia. Persistent pain, progressive fever, and leukocytosis are indications for surgery.

15. **What is the mortality rate of SBO?**
    - **Simple obstruction:** Mortality ≈5% if operated within 24 hours.
    - **Strangulated obstruction:** Mortality rate ≈25%. The mortality depends on the patient's resiliency (comorbid disease); but strangulation escalates the mortality by fivefold.

16. **What operative interventions may be needed for treatment of SBO?**
    - Open or laparoscopic lysis of adhesions at the point of obstruction.
    - Reduction and repair of hernia.
    - Resection of obstructing lesions with primary anastomosis.
    - Resection of strangulated segment with primary anastomosis.
    - Bypass of obstructing lesions (used mostly for carcinomatosis).
    - Placement of long tube down through the duodenum and into the small bowel (a Baker tube is the most commonly used).

17. **Describe criteria for distinguishing viable from dead bowel at the time of operation.**

    Pink color, peristalsis, and arterial pulsations are the most obvious way to identify viable intestine. In questionable cases, Doppler US can detect arterial pulsations, but the most reliable is the IV injection of fluorescein dye with use of a Wood's lamp. Viable bowel fluoresces purple.

18. **What is the risk of development of SBO after initial laparotomy? After previous laparotomy for SBO? Which operations are associated with high rates of SBO?**

    Approximately 15% of all patients undergoing laparotomy eventually develop an SBO. About 12% of patients with a prior SBO develop another. The more recurrences, the higher the recurrence rate. Total or subtotal colectomy has a 1-year rate of 11% and a 30% rate at 10 years. Hysterectomy also carries a high rate of SBO: about 5% for routine procedures and up to 15% after radical hysterectomy.

19. **What can surgeons do to decrease the risk of SBO?**
    - Use powderless gloves or wash off glove powder from gloves.
    - Avoid suturing through the peritoneum at closure.
    - Use barrier film between the incision and small intestine.

20. **What is the role of laparoscopy in SBO?**

    Laparoscopic lysis of adhesions is usually reserved for patients who have not had multiple previous laparotomies. Approximately one third of them can be treated successfully by laparoscopy alone, one third require a minimal laparotomy ("lap-assisted"), and about one third require a full open laparotomy. Recent series claim more than 80% success.

21. **What should I consider if the patient has had Roux-en-Y gastric bypass (RYGB)?**

    The most common causes of SBO after RYGB are internal hernias (42%), adhesive disease (22%), jejunojejunostomy stenosis (15%), and incisional hernia (9%). Internal hernias can occur through the transverse mesocolon, small bowel mesentery at the jejunojejonostomy, and between the jejunal mesentery and the mesocolon (Peterson's hernia). Evaluation for SBO should include upper GI studies or CT scan, keeping a low threshold for operative exploration.

22. **What can be done for patients with multiply recurrent bowel obstructions for adhesions?**

    Long tube placement, either via NG, gastrostomy, or jejunostomy with the tube advanced through to the ileocecal valve, can be done. The long tube is left in position for approximately 7 days and reportedly allows the bowel to reform adhesions in more gentle curves. Many other techniques have been tried and abandoned, including Noble plication (i.e., suturing the bowel in orderly loops) and adding various irrigants (e.g., heparin, Dextran, saline) to the peritoneal cavity before closure.

23. **Name five complications associated with surgery for SBO.**
    1. Enterotomy.
    2. Prolonged ileus.
    3. Wound infection.
    4. Abscess.
    5. Recurrent obstruction.

24. **Name products purported to decrease adhesion formation.**
    - Oxidized cellulose (Interceed).
    - Sodium hyaluronate and carboxymethylcellulose (Seprafilm).
    - Icodextrin (Adept; investigational).
    - 0.5% Ferric hyaluronate gel (Intergel; investigational).

BIBLIOGRAPHY

1. Beall DP, Fortman BJ, Lawler BC et al.: Imaging bowel obstruction: a comparison between fast magnetic resonance imaging and helical computed tomography. Clin Radiol 57:719-724, 2002.

2. Beck DE, Opelka FG, Bailey HR et al.: Incidence of small-bowel obstruction and adhesiolysis after open colorectal and general surgery. Dis Colon Rectum 42:241-248, 1999.

3. Choi HK, Chu KW, Law WL: Therapeutic value of Gastrografin in adhesive small bowel obstruction after unsuccessful conservative treatment: a prospective randomized trial. Ann Surg 236:1-6, 2002.

4. DeCherney AH, diZerega GS: Clinical problem of intraperitoneal postsurgical adhesion formation following general surgery and the use of adhesion prevention barriers. Surg Clin North Am 77:671-688, 1997.

5. Hayanga AJ, Bass-Wilins K, Bulkley GB: Current management of small-bowel obstruction. Adv Surg 29:1-33, 2005.

6. Helton WS, Fisichella PM: Intestinal obstruction. In *ACS Surgery: Principles and Practice*, New York, 2008, WebMD Inc.

7. Koppman JS, Li C, Gandsas A: Small bowel obstruction after laparoscopic Roux-en-Y gastric bypass: a review of 9.527 patients, J Am Coll Surg 206(3):571-584, 2008.

8. Zerey M, Sechrist CW, Kercher KW et al.: The laparoscopic management of small-bowel obstruction. Am J Surgery 194(6):882-888, 2007.

CHAPTER 46

INTESTINAL ISCHEMIA

Thomas F. Rehring, MD, FACS

1. **What is the arterial supply to the gut?**

   The foregut (stomach and duodenum) receives its blood supply from the celiac artery, the midgut (jejunum to the proximal descending colon) from the superior mesenteric artery (SMA), and the hindgut (the remainder of the intraperitoneal gut) from the inferior mesenteric artery (IMA).

2. **Name the potential collateral pathways between the celiac axis and SMA? SMA and IMA? Iliac and IMA?**

   The pancreaticoduodenal arteries form the major collaterals between the celiac artery and the SMA. The gastroduodenal artery gives off the superior pancreaticoduodenal artery that encircles the head of the pancreas and anastomoses with the inferior pancreaticoduodenal artery, the first branch of the SMA.

   The SMA and IMA have two main connections. The marginal artery of Drummond lies within the mesentery of the colon and is made up of branches of the ileocolic, right, middle, and left colic arteries. The arc of Riolan (meandering mesenteric artery) is more central and connects the middle colic branch of the SMA and the left colic branch of the IMA.

   The internal iliac artery gives rise to the middle rectal artery, which can provide flow to the superior rectal and thus the IMA.

3. **For extra credit, for whom is the marginal artery of Drummond named? What about the arc of Riolan?**

   Hamilton **Drummond,** a British surgeon, proved the anastomotic connection that bears his name by ligating the origins of the right, middle, and left colic arteries and demonstrating flow to the sigmoidal arteries in 1913 and 1914.

   Jean **Riolan** (1577–1657) was a well-known French anatomist who (ironically) opposed Harvey's theory of circulation but is acknowledged to be the first person to point out the communication between the SMA and IMA.

4. **Name the common causes of acute intestinal ischemia.**

   Acute SMA embolism (50% of all cases), acute SMA thrombosis, nonocclusive mesenteric ischemia (NOMI), mesenteric venous thrombosis, vasculitis, and iatrogenic causes (e.g., inotropic agents, aortic surgery).

5. **What is the mortality rate of patients with acute mesenteric ischemia?**

   Although the prognosis of embolic occlusion is somewhat better because of the dramatic presentation, the diagnosis of acute mesenteric ischemia is often made after infarction. The result is a high mortality rate (60% to 80%), regardless of cause. Despite advances in diagnosis, intervention and critical care, this figure has gone unchanged for more than 50 years.

6. **What is a "paradoxical embolus"?**

   A paradoxical embolus occurs in the setting of a venous thrombus embolizing to the arterial circulation via a cardiac defect (typically an atrial septal defect allowing right-to-left shunting).

7. **What is the diagnostic triad of acute embolic intestinal ischemia?**
   Sudden onset of (1) severe abdominal pain, (2) bowel evacuation (vomiting or diarrhea), and (3) a history of cardiac disease (arterial emboli). An additional hallmark is pain out of proportion to physical findings.

8. **How does the presentation of patients with acute thrombotic occlusion differ?**
   Thrombotic occlusion typically presents in elderly patients with diffuse atherosclerotic occlusive disease or in patients with a history consistent with chronic mesenteric ischemia (see question 25). Particularly in the former group of patients, acute embolic occlusion may be indistinguishable from thrombotic occlusion.

9. **Which laboratory value is diagnostic of acute intestinal ischemia? Is acidosis?**
   No laboratory values are diagnostic for acute intestinal ischemia. Metabolic acidosis is a late finding and implies advanced ischemia or infarction. Similarly, elevated lactate and elevated phosphate levels are nonspecific and frequently late findings. Although leukocytosis is found in the majority of patients, no laboratory studies are specific. The diagnosis is pursued on clinical suspicion alone.

KEY POINTS: DIAGNOSTIC TRIAD OF ACUTE EMBOLIC INTESTINAL ISCHEMIA

1. Sudden onset of severe abdominal pain out of proportion to physical examination.
2. Sudden bowel evacuation (vomiting or diarrhea).
3. History of cardiac disease (e.g., atrial fibrillation that accounts for embolic source).
4. No laboratory findings (e.g., lactate level) are diagnostic; metabolic acidosis is a late finding.
5. Emergent arteriography is indicated.

10. **When acute intestinal ischemia is suspected, what study is diagnostic?**
    Emergent arteriography is diagnostic. It is important to include lateral views of the aorta to visualize the visceral vessels. In many institutions, multidetector computed tomography angiography (CTA) is rapidly supplanting arteriography. For this indication, it has the distinct advantages of speed, accessibility, and evaluation for other sources in the differential diagnosis of acute abdominal pain.

11. **How do the operative findings differ in patients with atherosclerotic occlusion and patients with SMA embolism?**
    An SMA embolus usually lodges 3 to 4 cm distal to its origin, and thus beyond the proximal jejunal and middle colic arteries. Therefore, the proximal 6 to 10 inches of jejunum are usually spared. Thrombotic occlusion occurs directly at the ostia, where the atherosclerotic narrowing is most severe, causing ischemia of the entire midgut.

12. **What is the appropriate management of an SMA embolus? Is there a role for thrombolysis?**
    Immediate heparinization, urgent exploration, embolectomy, assessment of bowel viability, and resection of any infarcted bowel. Postoperative anticoagulation is essential to avoid further embolization.
    Thrombolysis currently has little or no role in the treatment of acute mesenteric ischemia. Revascularization of bowel must be pursued rapidly, and bowel viability must be ascertained directly.

13. **How is visceral ischemia of thrombotic origin managed?**
The general management follows that of an embolism; however, mesenteric ischemia from thrombotic occlusion is the end stage of progressive atherosclerotic occlusion. Therefore, thrombectomy alone is not sufficient; bypass or endarterectomy of the proximal diseased vessel or vessels is necessary. Again, bowel viability is assessed after reperfusion.

14. **Which intraoperative tests help surgeons determine bowel viability?**
Both systemic intravenous (IV) infusion of fluorescein, which is evaluated using a Wood's lamp, and intraoperative Doppler examination of the bowel are helpful, but ultimately the decision is based on clinical judgment.

15. **When the extent of bowel viability is in question, what should be done?**
All nonviable and necrotic bowel should be resected. The surgeon should schedule a second-look operation 12 to 24 hours later to evaluate the bowel of marginal viability. Some segments that were initially questionable may become clearly viable or necrotic during this period.

16. **How much small intestine is required to maintain adequate nutrition?**
About 100 cm of small intestine is required to maintain adequate nutrition. The distal ileum and ileocecal valve are the most important segments to retain for vital bowel absorption and function.

17. **Should a second-look operation be canceled because a patient improves?**
Never. The decision is made in the operating room (OR) based on findings at the time of surgery. No clinical parameters within the ensuing 12 to 24 hours accurately indicate the status of the bowel in question.

18. **What is NOMI?**
Nonocclusive mesenteric ischemia (NOMI) accounts for approximately 20% of acute ischemic cases. This typically occurs in patients who are critically ill with systemic hypoperfusion. In such low-flow states, splanchnic blood flow is reduced in an attempt to preserve perfusion to cardiac and cerebral beds. Pharmacologic agents such as ergot alkaloids, digitalis, cocaine and vasoconstrictors may also predispose to NOMI.

19. **How is NOMI diagnosed and managed?**
Angiography documents vasospasm in the absence of an anatomic occlusion. The right colon is most commonly affected because of its less consistent collateral blood flow. It is associated with (and may be exacerbated by) the concomitant use of digitalis in patients with systemic hypoperfusion. In severe cases associated with multisystem organ failure (MOF), the mortality rate approaches 75%. Treatment consists of hemodynamic optimization, weaning of inotropes, and selective arterial infusion of vasodilators (papaverine) through the angiogram catheter. Surgical intervention is reserved for intestinal infarction or perforation.

20. **If mesenteric vein thrombosis (MVT) is suspected, which test is best?**
The signs and symptoms of MVT are similar to those of acute intestinal ischemia, but they are often subtler. Delay in diagnosis is thought to contribute to the reported high mortality rate of 50%. Contrast-enhanced computed tomography (CT) scan remains the gold standard for diagnosis.

21. **What are the risk factors for MVT? How is it treated?**
Approximately half of patients with MVT have an underlying hypercoagulable state. Other causes include splenectomy, portal hypertension, visceral infections, pancreatitis, malignancy, and blunt abdominal trauma.

Treatment of MVT includes anticoagulation, broad-spectrum antibiotics, treatment of the underlying cause and supportive measures. Surgery is reserved for resection of nonviable bowel. Venous thrombectomy has not proven to be of effective long-term benefit. The use of thrombolytic agents has been explored but only in anecdotal reports. Furthermore, access to the splanchnic venous circulation for directed lysis is difficult.

22. **What is the primary cause of chronic mesenteric ischemia?**
    Atherosclerosis. As the collateral circulation to the gut is robust, symptoms generally do not occur unless two of the three major arteries (celiac, superior mesenteric and inferior mesenteric) are narrowed or occluded.

23. **What is the one unique risk factor for chronic mesenteric ischemia that differs from other atherosclerotic phenomena?**
    It occurs more frequently in women.

24. **What are the clinical features of patients with chronic mesenteric ischemia?**
    Weight loss is the most consistent sign of chronic mesenteric ischemia. Patients gradually and sometimes unknowingly become afraid to eat (food fear) because of postprandial pain (intestinal angina). In the absence of weight loss, the diagnosis of chronic intestinal ischemia is unlikely. Conversely, in patients with severe atherosclerosis and weight loss of unknown cause, mesenteric ischemia should be strongly considered. An epigastric bruit is an important sign suggestive of mesenteric occlusive disease.

25. **How should patients with chronic mesenteric ischemia be evaluated?**
    Noninvasive ultrasound (US) duplex scanning may provide important physiologic information about the celiac axis and SMA. However, this procedure is technician dependent and not widely available. If unavailable or equivocal, mesenteric angiography should be performed. If surgical intervention is considered, arteriography is essential. Although controversial, multidetector CTA is rapidly supplanting traditional angiography as it is fast, noninvasive and widely accessible.

26. **What are the goals of arterial bypass in chronic mesenteric ischemia?**
    Resolution of symptoms, improved nutrition, and prevention of visceral infarction.

27. **If mesenteric revascularization is entertained, what five essential decisions must be considered?**
    - Surgical approach (transabdominal, retroperitoneal, thoracoabdominal).
    - Which and how many vessels to revascularize.
    - Endarterectomy, reimplantation, or bypass.
    - If bypass, antegrade or retrograde.
    - If bypass, what type of conduit (vein versus prosthetic).

    See also questions 31 and 32.

28. **What is ischemic colitis?**
    Ischemic colitis is circulatory insufficiency of the colon that may result from occlusive, nonocclusive, and pharmacologic (e.g., cocaine, nonsteroidal anti-inflammatory drugs [NSAIDs]) causes. Seven percent of all patients having nonemergent abdominal aortic aneurysm surgery and as many as 60% of patients who survive a ruptured abdominal aortic aneurysm suffer from ischemic colitis. Most cases are mild, typically involving only the mucosa and resulting in abdominal pain and bloody diarrhea. Severe disease (15% of cases) is characterized by transmural gangrenous infarction that presents with clear signs of peritonitis and bloody diarrhea.

29. **How is ischemic colitis diagnosed and treated? What are its prognostic implications?**

The diagnosis is made by endoscopy. In idiopathic cases, angiography demonstrates patent large vessels because the responsible emboli or lesions are believed to involve peripheral, end-arterial vessels. Mild disease is typically treated conservatively with bowel rest, vigorous hydration, and broad-spectrum antibiotics. Severe disease requires surgical resection.

Overall mortality rates are about 50%, but in patients requiring colon resection, the mortality rate may exceed 85%. The high mortality in the latter group is attributed to endotoxemic shock and MOF.

CONTROVERSIES

30. **What is celiac compression syndrome (Dunbar's syndrome)?**

Celiac compression is a rare and controversial disorder most commonly described in women (female-to-male ratio is 4:1) between the ages of 20 and 50 years. Also known as median arcuate ligament syndrome, these patients appear to suffer from chronic mesenteric ischemia without angiographic evidence of atherosclerotic disease. The mechanical compression is believed to be caused by the left crus of the diaphragm (i.e., median arcuate ligament), and diagnosis occasionally is confirmed by demonstrating transient celiac compression during expiration. The associated pain is the result of a complicated and still heavily debated redirection of flow (foregut steal) away from the SMA. Effective treatment has required not only release of the compression but also bypass to improve the likelihood of pain resolution.

31. **Which is the preferred treatment for chronic mesenteric ischemia, antegrade or retrograde visceral artery bypass? Is it necessary to reconstruct more than one mesenteric vessel?**

As they apply to intestinal bypass, the terms antegrade and retrograde refer to the origin of the graft from the aorta as either proximal to the celiac axis or distal to the SMA, respectively. The stated advantages of antegrade bypass are less kinking of the graft and possibly better blood flow characteristics. The disadvantages are that supraceliac exposure is technically more difficult and clamping may result in renal or spinal cord ischemia. Retrograde bypass grafts are more difficult to position to avoid kinking.

Recent series suggest that the results for single- or multiple-vessel reconstruction in either antegrade or retrograde fashion are excellent, with symptom-free survival rates >90% at 5 years.

32. **What is the role of percutaneous transluminal angioplasty in chronic mesenteric ischemia?**

The endovascular treatment of chronic mesenteric ischemia is a relatively new technique. The obvious avoidance of surgery is an important advantage, but the rare complications of dissection and embolus can be devastating in arterial beds without adequate collaterals. Success rates approximate 70%; restenosis and recurrent symptoms are reported in 50% of patients. No prospective trials have compared PTA with arterial bypass; however, retrospective reviews suggest that initial results with either technique are similar with regard to morbidity, death, and recurrent stenosis. However, symptom recurrence rates are higher with PTA.

WEBSITE

www.emedicine.com/emerg/topic311.htm

BIBLIOGRAPHY

1. Brown DJ, Schermerhorn ML, Powell RJ et al.: Mesenteric stenting for chronic mesenteric ischemia. J Vasc Surg 2005;42(2):268-274.

2. Fisher DF Jr, Fry WJ: Collateral mesenteric circulation. Surg Gynecol Obstet 164(5):487-492, 1987.

3. Gewertz BL, Schwartz LB: Mesenteric ischemia. Surg Clin North Am 77(2):275-502, 1977.

4. Kasirajan K, O'Hara PJ, Gray BH et al.: Chronic mesenteric ischemia: open surgery versus percutaneous angioplasty and stenting. J Vasc Surg 33(1):63-71, 2001.

5. Kazmers A: Operative management of acute mesenteric ischemia. Part 1, Ann Vasc Surg 12(2):187-197, 1998.

6. Kazmers A: Operative management of chronic mesenteric ischemia. Ann Vasc Surg 12(3):299-308, 1998.

7. Oldenburg WA, Lau LL, Rodenberg TJ et al.: Acute mesenteric ischemia: a clinical review. Arch Intern Med 164 (10):1054-1062, 2004.

8. Seeger JM: The management of splanchnic vascular lesions and disorders. In: Rutherford RB, editor, *Vascular surgery*, 6th ed, Vol. 2, Philadelphia, 2005 Elsevier.

9. Shih MC, Hagspiel KD: CTA and MRA in mesenteric ischemia: part 1, Role in diagnosis and differential diagnosis. AJR 188(2):452-461, 2007.

10. Sivamurthy N, Rhodes JM, Lee D et al.: Endovascular versus open mesenteric revascularization: immediate benefits do not equate with short-term functional outcomes. J Am Coll Surg 202(6):859-867, 2006.

CHAPTER 47

DIVERTICULAR DISEASE OF THE COLON

Alexander Q. Ereso, MD, Elizabeth L. Cureton, MD, and Gregory P. Victorino, MD

1. What is a colonic diverticulum?

A protrusion of mucosa and submucosa through the muscular layers of the bowel wall. It has no muscular covering. Because diverticula do not involve all layers of the bowel wall, they are really "false" diverticula. Diverticulum formation may be related either to weakness of the bowel wall at the sites of vessel perforation or to increased intraluminal pressure caused by low dietary fiber and constipation.

2. What is the difference between diverticulosis and diverticulitis?

Diverticulosis is colonic diverticula without associated inflammation. Diverticulitis is inflammation and infection. Only 15% of patients with diverticulosis develop diverticulitis.

3. How does a diverticulum cause pain?

Pain apparently results from perforation of the diverticulum The resulting leakage may be scant and contained within pericolic fat or extensive, involving the mesentery, other organs, or the peritoneal cavity. Sigmoid diverticulitis typically causes pain in the left lower quadrant.

4. Where in the colon are diverticula usually located?

In the United States, 95% of all diverticula occur in the left colon, primarily in the sigmoid colon. Diverticula, however, may occur anywhere in the colon. In Asia, right colonic diverticula are more common.

5. At what age is diverticulitis most common?

The sixth or seventh decade of life. Patients younger than 50 with diverticulitis tend to have more complications. Younger patients are more likely than older patients to have right colonic diverticulitis.

6. What strategy may decrease diverticulitis in patients with diverticula?

A diet high in fiber. Large bulk in the colon decreases segmentation and intraluminal pressure.

7. What is the best imaging test for diagnosing acute diverticulitis?

Computed tomography (CT) scan, which can also diagnose local complications of diverticulitis.

8. What complications can result from perforation of a colonic diverticulum?

- Inflammatory phlegmon or abscess in the bowel mesentery.
- Peritonitis.
- Intraabdominal abscess.
- Internal fistula.
- Bowel obstruction.

9. **Can diverticular disease cause bleeding?**
   Yes. Diverticulosis (not *-itis*) is a common cause of lower gastrointestinal (GI) bleeding. Bleeding from diverticulitis is uncommon.

10. **How can the site of diverticular bleeding be localized?**
    It is localized with angiography performed via the inferior mesenteric artery (IMA) and, if necessary, the superior mesenteric artery (SMA). Tagged red blood cell studies are less useful. Colonoscopy is rarely helpful.

KEY POINTS: LOCALIZATION OF LOWER GASTROINTESTINAL BLEEDING

1. Common causes: diverticulosis, cancer, angiodysplasia.

2. Proctosigmoidoscopy without prep is helpful in ruling out rectal source of bleeding (more proximal bleeding limits the use of endoscopy).

3. Tagged red blood cell nuclear scans are useful for slower GI bleeding (detects bleeding at 0.2 to 0.5 ml/min).

4. Arteriography is the preferred imaging modality because it can be therapeutic and detects bleeding at 0.5 to 2 ml/min.

5. Start arteriography with the IMA, then the SMA, then the celiac axis if necessary; administer vasopressin or embolize (85% success rate).

11. **When should an operation be performed for a bleeding colonic diverticulum?**
    Replacement of 5 to 6 units of blood (two thirds of a patient's blood volume) within 24 hours and rebleeding during hospitalization are standard indications for resection of the segment of colon containing a bleeding diverticulum.

12. **If bleeding is life threatening but cannot be localized within the colon, what treatment is required?**
    Subtotal colectomy with ileostomy and closure of the distal sigmoid colon at the peritoneal reflection (Hartmann's operation) or total abdominal colectomy with ileorectal anastomosis is required.

13. **Which three procedures may be used when perforation of the diverticulum results in an abscess? Which has the lowest operative mortality rate?**
    1. Diverting colostomy and abscess drainage (first of three stages).
    2. Resection of involved colon with proximal colostomy and distal mucous fistula or closure by Hartmann's operation (first of two stages).
    3. Resection with primary anastomosis (one stage).
    Operative mortality is lowest after resection and proximal colostomy for fecal diversion. Despite reports of success with the one-stage procedure, most surgeons favor a safer two-stage approach for perforated diverticulitis (this strategy requires a second operation after 3 months for colostomy takedown and colonic re-anastomosis).

14. **What is the clinical evidence of a vesicocolic or ureterocolic fistula after diverticular perforation?**
    Pneumaturia, fecaluria, and chronic urinary tract infections (polymicrobial).

15. What procedure is required to repair a vesicocolic fistula?
A staged procedure was the standard until recently. Now most patients can be treated with a single procedure that includes sigmoid resection, colonic anastomosis, and primary repair of bladder defect with absorbable suture. A Foley catheter is usually left in place for 10 days after surgery. Some viable tissue should be placed between the colonic and bladder repairs to prevent a recurrent fistula.

BIBLIOGRAPHY

1. Bouillot JL, Berthou JC, Champault G et al.: Elective laparoscopic colonic resection for diverticular disease: results of a multicenter study in 179 patients. Surg Endosc 16:1320-1323, 2002.

2. Constantinides VA, Heriot A, Remzi F et al.: Operative strategies for diverticular peritonitis: a decision analysis between primary resection and anastomosis versus Hartmann's procedures. Ann Surg 245:94-103, 2007.

3. Frattini J, Longo WE: Diagnosis and treatment of chronic and recurrent diverticulitis. J Clin Gastroenterol 7(Suppl 3):S145-149, 2006.

4. Guller U, Jain N, Hervey S et al.: Laparoscopic vs open colectomy: outcomes comparison based on large nationwide databases. Arch Surg 138:1179-1186, 2003.

5. Richter S, Lindemann W, Kollmar O et al.: One-stage sigmoid colon resection for perforated sigmoid diverticulitis (Hinchey stages III and IV). World J Surg 30:1027-1032, 2006.

6. Salem L, Veenstra DL, Sullivan SF et al.: The timing of elective colectomy in diverticulitis: a decision analysis. J Am Coll Surg 199:904-912, 2004.

7. Simpson J, Scholefield JH, Spiller RC: Pathogenesis of colonic diverticula. Br J Surg 89:546-554, 2002.

8. Wolff BG, Devine RM: Surgical management of diverticulitis. Am Surg 66:153-156, 2000.

CHAPTER 48

ACUTE LARGE BOWEL OBSTRUCTION

Erik D. Peltz, DO, and Elizabeth C. Brew, MD

1. **What are the mechanical causes of large bowel obstruction?**
   The most common mechanical causes are carcinoma (50%), volvulus (15%), adhesions (15%), and diverticular disease (10%). Extrinsic compression from metastatic carcinoma is another cause of obstruction. Less frequent causes include, hernia, intussusception, benign tumor, and fecal impaction.

2. **How is the diagnosis made?**
   1. The patient complains of crampy abdominal pain and bloating. Nausea and vomiting occur later in LBO and may be feculent. An acute onset of symptoms is more consistent with volvulus compared with the gradual development of obstructive complaints from patients with colon carcinoma.
   2. Physical examination reveals abdominal distention and high-pitched bowel sounds. Rectal examination may reveal an obstructing rectal cancer or evidence of fecal impaction. Absence of bowel sounds and localized tenderness may be signs of peritonitis. Progression of symptoms accompanied by a high fever or tachycardia requires immediate operative attention.
   3. Flat and upright abdominal radiographs reveal dilated colon proximal to the obstruction. An upright chest radiograph may show free air under the diaphragm if a perforation has occurred.

3. **How is the diagnosis confirmed?**
   A contrast enema (barium or water-soluble contrast) is necessary to delineate the level and nature of an obstruction. A volvulus can be identified by a "bird's beak" narrowing at the neck of the volvulus. Sigmoidoscopy or colonoscopy is an essential part of the evaluation; it allows visualization of the colon and may be therapeutic in the case of a sigmoid volvulus.

4. **What is the role of computed tomography (CT) scanning in the diagnosis of large bowel obstruction?**
   Modern fast acquisition helical multidetector CT (MDCT) imaging is beginning to replace contrast enema for confirming the diagnosis of LBO in many patients. MDCT has a reported sensitivity and specificity of 96% and 94%, respectively, in the diagnosis of LBO. Computed tomography (CT) scans may distinguish between mechanical obstruction or pseudo-obstruction and can help with the diagnosis of diverticulitis or colon carcinoma. CT avoids the risk of perforation with instrumentation during enema or endoscopy and may be of benefit in elderly or frail patients who cannot cooperate with or tolerate other diagnostic procedures.

5. **Why is tenderness in the right lower quadrant (RLQ) important?**
   The cecum is the area that is most likely to perforate. When the cecum reaches 15 cm at its widest diameter, the tension on the wall is so great that decompression is essential to prevent perforation. The larger diameter of the cecum causes more tension of the cecal wall at the same intraluminal pressure (law of Laplace). The other area at risk for perforation is the site of a primary colon cancer.

6. **Where is the obstructing cancer usually located?**
   Most obstructing colorectal carcinomas occur in the splenic flexure, descending colon, or hepatic flexure. In contrast, lesions of the right colon usually present with occult bleeding. Cecal and rectal cancers are uncommon causes of obstruction.

7. **What is a volvulus? Where is it located?**
   A volvulus is an abnormal rotation of the colon on an axis formed by its mesentery and occurs either in the sigmoid colon (75%) or cecum (25%). **Sigmoid volvulus** occurs in an older population when chronic constipation causes the sigmoid colon to elongate and become redundant. **Cecal volvulus** requires a hypermobile cecum as a result of incomplete embryologic fixation of the ascending colon.

8. **When is surgery indicated?**
   Surgery is performed early in colon obstruction. Urgent laparotomy is necessary in patients with suspected perforation or ischemia. Danger signs are quiet abdomen, RLQ tenderness, and increasing pain. The patient's cardiopulmonary status should be assessed and optimized preoperatively. It is essential to correct dehydration and administer perioperative antibiotics. Marking of possible stoma sites and deep venous thrombosis (DVT) prophylaxis are other important preoperative considerations.

9. **Which operation should be performed for a large bowel obstruction?**
   The traditional procedure for a LBO has been a decompressing colostomy. However, careful assessment of the patient's condition, viability of the bowel, location of the obstruction, and absence of intraabdominal contamination often allow resection with or without a primary anastomosis. In fact, an initial diverting colostomy has not been shown to have any survival advantage and incurs the risk of further surgeries.

   An **obstructing carcinoma** may be resected satisfactorily under emergency conditions in 90% of patients. Carcinomas of the right and transverse colon (proximal to the splenic flexure) are routinely treated with resection and primary anastomosis. Recently, obstructing cancers of the descending colon have been treated either with resection and colostomy or intraoperative lavage followed by resection and primary anastomosis. Techniques for nonoperative decompression of the colon, such as balloon dilation, laser therapy, and stent placement, are under investigation. Theoretically, these techniques will allow palliation, bowel preparation, and elective colon resection.

   A **volvulus** should be reduced and resected. Reduction of a sigmoid volvulus can be achieved nonoperatively by sigmoidoscopy or hydrostatic decompression with a contrast enema. The recurrence rate of volvulus after simple nonoperative reduction is 75%. Surgical therapy includes detorsion with colopexy or sigmoid colectomy. Cecal volvulus can be treated similarly with nonoperative decompression, cecopexy, or surgical resection.

   The optimal treatment of **diverticular disease** is initial bowel rest; intravenous (IV) antibiotics; and percutaneous abscess drainage, if necessary. Colon resection and primary anastomosis can be performed after adequate bowel preparation.

10. **What is the role of endoluminal stenting for acute large bowel obstruction?**
   Colorectal stent placement may be useful for colonic decompression, bowel cleansing, and medical optimization before definitive surgical resection. In this preoperative setting colorectal stenting may allow for a single-stage surgical resection. Endoluminal stents may also be useful as an alternative to colostomy for palliative decompression in patients with unresectable malignant obstruction. Complications of stent placement include stent occlusion and migration, inadequate decompression, and bowel perforation. At this time their limited application to a select group of patients requires careful evaluation.

11. What are the nonmechanical causes of large bowel obstruction?
Paralytic ileus (i.e., colonic pseudo-obstruction) or toxic megacolon.

12. What is Ogilvie's syndrome?
Ogilvie's syndrome is an acute paralytic (adynamic) ileus or pseudo-obstruction (i.e., enormous dilation of the colon without a mechanical distal obstructing lesion). Patients present with a massively dilated abdomen and a small amount of pain. Nonoperative management, including bowel rest, IV fluids, and gentle enemas, is the therapy of choice. Gastrografin enema or colonoscopy is diagnostic and therapeutic. Neostigmine is another treatment modality in patients with colons >10 cm in diameter.

13. What is toxic megacolon?
Toxic megacolon is dilatation of the entire colon secondary to acute inflammatory bowel disease. The disease is manifested by acute onset of abdominal pain, distention, and sepsis. Initial therapy includes IV fluid resuscitation, nasogastric (NG) decompression, and broad-spectrum antibiotics. If symptoms do not resolve within a few hours, the patient requires an operation to avoid perforation. Surgical therapy most often consists of an emergency abdominal colectomy with formation of an ileostomy.

KEY POINTS: CAUSES OF LARGE BOWEL OBSTRUCTION

1. Carcinoma: most common cause: 50%.

2. Volvulus: 15%.

3. Adhesions 15%.

4. Diverticular disease: 10%.

5. Other causes: hernia, intussusception, fecal impaction.

WEBSITE

www.emedicine.com/emerg/topic65.htm

BIBLIOGRAPHY

1. Adler DG, Baron TH: Endoscopic palliation of colorectal cancer. Hematol Oncol Clin North Am 16:1015, 2002.
2. Beattie GC, Peters RT, Guy S et al.: Computed tomography in the assessment of suspected large bowel obstruction. ANZ J Surg 77:160-165, 2007.
3. Dauphine CE, Tan P, Beart RW Jr et al.: Placement of self-expanding metal stents for acute malignant large-bowel obstruction: a collective review. Ann Surg Oncol 9:574, 2002.
4. Frager D: Intestinal obstruction: role of CT. Gastroenterol Clin North Am 31:777-799, 2002.
5. Jost RS et al.: Colorectal stenting: an effective therapy for preoperative and palliative treatment. Cardiovasc Intervent Radiol 30:433-440, 2007.
6. Lopez-Kostner F, Hool GR, Lavery IC: Management and causes of acute large-bowel obstruction. Surg Clin North Am 77:1265-1290, 1997.

7. Markogiannakis H, Messaris E, Dardamanis D et al.: Acute mechanical bowel obstruction: clinical presentation, etiology, management and outcome, World J Gastroenterol 13(3):432-437, 2007.

8. Murray JJ, Schoetz DJ, Coller JA et al.: Intraoperative colonic lavage and primary anastomosis in nonelective colon resection, Dis Colon Rectum 34:527, 1991.

9. Paran H, Silverberg D, Mayo A: Treatment of acute colonic pseudo-obstruction with neostigmine, J Am Coll Surg 190(3):315-318, 2000.

10. Tan SG, Nambiar R, Rauff A et al.: Primary resection and anastomosis in obstructed descending colon due to cancer, Arch Surg 126:748, 1991.

CHAPTER 49

INFLAMMATORY BOWEL DISEASE

David E. Stein, MD, and Jeffry L. Kashuk, MD, FACS

1. **What two clinical entities encompass the diagnosis of inflammatory bowel disease?**

   Crohn's disease and ulcerative colitis.

2. **Although the two diseases often overlap, they usually can be distinguished by clinical criteria. What are the major clinical differences?**

   Rectal bleeding is unusual in Crohn's disease but common in ulcerative colitis (UC). An abdominal mass, a history of anorectal diseases (fissures, fistulas, abscesses) are commonly found in Crohn's disease.

3. **What are the major radiologic differences between the two diseases?**

   Computed tomography (CT) scans may show terminal ileal thickening, skip areas, strictures and internal fistulas with associated phlegmons in Crohn's disease. Colon wall thickening can be seen in UC.

4. **What are the major histological differences?**

   Granulomas in the intestinal wall and adjacent lymph nodes can occur in 60% of patients with Crohn's disease. In UC, the inflammation is limited to the mucosa, whereas in Crohn's disease it can be full thickness inflammation. Crypt distortion and paneth cell metaplasia are common histopathologic findings in UC. Severe UC can have ulcerations and erosions from the mucosa into the submucosa and can be confused with Crohn's disease.

5. **Although Crohn's disease may affect the gastrointestinal (GI) tract from the pharynx to the anus, what are the most common clinical patterns of GI involvement?**

   Small bowel only: 28%; both ileum and colon (ileocolitis): 41%; and colon only: 27%. Crohn's involvement of the colon is also called *Crohn's colitis* or *granulomatous colitis*.

6. **Crohn's colitis and ulcerative colitis are often difficult to distinguish clinically. What are the major differences seen at colonoscopy?**

   Crohn's colitis is focal and predominantly right sided. Apthous ulcerations are the earliest lesions seen in Crohn's disease. As the disease progresses, they may form linear or serpiginous ulcers (bear claw ulcerations) in affected areas. When these large ulcerations migrate transversely, islands of normal mucosa appear, known as cobble stoning. In UC, disease begins in the rectum and progresses proximally. Skip areas are more common in Crohn's disease, but be aware that UC patients treated with rectal suppositories or enemas may have a normal appearing rectum. Endoscopic findings in UC may range from simple edema of the mucosa to indurated, friable tissue that bleeds on contact.

7. **What are the major indications for surgery in Crohn's disease?**

   It depends on the site of involvement and significance of symptoms. The guiding principle is to only operate when the disease is affecting the physiology of the patient. A patient with mild diarrhea and an entero-enteric fistula does not need surgery and should be treated medically. A patient with an entero-rectal fistula with profound diarrhea and weight loss, or a patient with a bowel obstruction as a result of a stricture needs surgical intervention. Perianal disease with abscess needs urgent drainage.

8. **What are the major indications for surgery in ulcerative colitis?**
   Medical intractability (including failure to thrive in children, diarrhea, weight loss, and repeated flares), inability to tolerate medications (steroid psychoses, pancreatitis) acute toxic colitis with or without perforation, dysplasia (premalignant cells on surveillance colonoscopy), or colorectal cancer are the indications for surgery in UC.

9. **What is the surgical treatment of ulcerative colitis?**
   A total procto-colectomy provides a surgical cure for UC. Most patients do not want a permanent ileostomy, so a reconstruction to create a neo-rectum is performed. A pouch made out of the patient's small intestine can be fashioned and anastomosed to the anal sphincters providing fecal continence.

10. **What is the surgical procedure for an ileal stricture? What is the procedure for multiple strictures?**
    Because surgery for Crohn's disease is not curative, bowel preservation is important as repeated procedures can lead to short gut syndrome. For an isolated stricture, resection and anastomosis is the procedure of choice. One should anastomose grossly normal ileum to grossly normal colon. For those patients with multiple strictures, a procedure called a strictureplasty is performed. A longitudinal incision is made along the stricture and extended into normal bowel wall. Then the opening is closed transversely, opening the lumen so enteric contents may pass.

11. **How do you evaluate the placement of a stoma (ostomy)?**
    The location of a stoma is a major factor in patient morbidity and maintaining an acceptable quality of life. Placement is optimal when the bowel is brought through the rectus sheath above the umbilicus. This provides the strongest fascia for anchoring the ostomy. One way to identify this area is draw a line from the anterior superior iliac spine to the umbilicus. It is important for the stoma site to be marked preoperatively with the patient lying down, sitting, and standing. Try to identify where the patient wears belts, and avoid this area, and skin folds and creases.

12. **How does one monitor a patient with UC for dysplasia?**
    After an index colonoscopy when the patient is diagnosed, surveillance colonoscopy should begin after 8 to 10 years of disease. Four quadrant biopsies every 10 cm are standard to achieve at least 35 specimens. This provides adequate sample size to detect dysplasia.

13. **Does IBD have a genetic basis?**
    There are five confirmed genetic linkages (meaning significant linkage found in one study and replication of the linkage with a nominal P value <0.01 in an independent study) for inflammatory bowel disease (IBD) that have been identified: (1) linkage between Crohn's disease and a locus on chromosome 16 (the IBD1 locus); (2) linkage between IBD (especially UC) and a locus on chromosome 12q (the IBD2 locus); (3) linkage between IBD (especially Crohn's disease) and a locus on chromosome 6p (the IBD3 locus); (4) linkage between Crohn's disease and a locus on chromosome 14q (the IBD4 locus); and (5) linkage between IBD (especially Crohn's disease) and a locus on chromosome 3p21. There are four other significant linkages to IBD that have not yet been confirmed in independent study populations.

14. **What are some of the medical therapies for inflammatory bowel disease?**
    Many first-line treatments involve the use of antiinflammatory medications that can be delivered orally or rectally. These 5-ASA compounds have minimal toxicities. Other modalities include

immuno-modulating medications. Steroids are the mainstay of treatment for flares or exacerbation of disease symptoms. Immunosuppressive medications, such as azathioprine, its metabolite 6-mercaptopurine and even cyclosporine have been used in IBD. The newest class of medications used, biologics, are antibodies to specific targets (infliximab and adalimumab) such as tumor necrosis factor-α (TNF-α). Antibiotics may also be used in long-term therapy of Crohn's disease patients with fistulas.

15. **What is a Brooke ileostomy?**
The Brooke ileostomy is the "rosebud" or full-thickness ileostomy folded over on itself for approximately 1 cm above the skin. This allows an adequate seal between the stoma appliance and the opening of the bowel. This prevents spillage of bowel contents onto the skin, which can cause significant skin irritation and inflammation.

16. **What is pouchitis, and which patients are likely to get it?**
Pouchitis is defined as an inflammation of the small intestinal pouch. Of all patients who undergo a total procto-colectomy with an ileal-anal pouch 27% will have at least one episode of pouchitis in their lifetime. Although no cause has been found, research has focused on autoimmune possibilities, bacterial overgrowth of the small bowel and a lack of the appropriate bacteria usually found in the colon. Most episodes are treated with antibiotics such as fluoroquinolones and metronidazole. Refractory cases are rare, and may require antiinflammatory medications or even immunosuppressive medications. Pouchitis rarely requires pouch excision. It is interesting to note that it is not seen in patients who have a pelvic pouch for other diseases, such as familial adenomatous polyposis, lending credence to theory that pouchitis may be the result of the same mechanism as IBD.

CONTROVERSIES

17. **Should all patients with entero-enteral fistulas secondary to Crohn's disease have surgery when the fistula is discovered?**
For: Such patients ultimately do poorly, develop further intraperitoneal septic complications and eventually require surgery.
Against: Many of these patients do well without operative treatment with medical management. Surgery is not a cure, so why subject the patient to unnecessary risk. If symptoms worsen we can offer surgery.

18. **Should all patients with ulcerative colitis that is documented for 10 years, whether the disease is active or not, undergo a procto-colectomy to avoid the risk of carcinoma of the colon and rectum?**
For: The risk of colon cancer in ulcerative colitis increases by approximately 1% per year after 8 to 10 years of disease, so this can eliminate their risk of cancer.
Against: Using surveillance colonoscopy and biopsy, we can determine patients who are at high risk for cancer, so why subject many normal patients to surgery?

19. **Is ileorectal anastomosis an acceptable operation after colectomy for ulcerative colitis?**
For: These patients will have more normal bowel habits and avoid the higher complication rate of pelvic surgery.
Against: At least 50% of patients eventually require reoperation for recurrence of disease symptoms. The remaining rectum also may be a site for the development of cancer.

20. **Should we offer a total procto-colectomy and ileal pouch for patients with Crohn's colitis?**

For: With the use of newer medications, these patients can be stoma free for many years.

Against: The rate of fistula formation and pouch failures make this surgery too risky in Crohn's disease.

BIBLIOGRAPHY

1. Duerr RH: The genetics of inflammatory bowel disease. Gastroenterol Clin North Am 31:63-76, 2002.

2. Farouk R: Functional outcomes after ileal pouch-anal anastomosis for chronic ulcerative colitis. Ann Surg 231:919-926, 2000.

3. Fazio V: Current status of surgery for inflammatory bowel disease. Digestion 59:470-480, 1998.

4. Heuschen UA, Hinz U, Allemeyer EH et al.: One or two stage procedures for restorative proctocolectomy: rationale for a strategy in ulcerative colitis. Ann Surg 234:788-794, 2001.

5. Hurst RD, Michelassi F: Strictureplasty for Crohn's disease: techniques and long term results. World J Surg 22:359-363, 1998.

6. Konda A, Duffy MC: Surveillance of patients at increased risk of colon cancer: inflammatory bowel disease and other conditions. Gastroenterol Clin 37:191-213, 2008.

7. Mathew CG, Lewis CM: Genetics of inflammatory bowel disease: progress and prospects. Hum Mol Genet 13(Review Issue 1):R161-R168, 2004.

8. Present DH, Rutgeerts P, Targan S et al.: Infliximab for the treatment of fistulas in patients with Crohn's disease. New Engl J Med 340:1398-1405, 1999.

9. Solomon MJ, Schmirz M: Cancer and inflammatory bowel disease: bias, epidemiology, surveillance and treatment. World J Surg 22:352-358, 1998.

10. Stocchi L, Pemberton JH: Pouch and pouchitis. Gastroenterol Clin North Am 30:223-241, 2001.

11. Sugarman HJ: Ileal pouch-anal anastomosis without ileal diversion. Ann Surg 232:530-541, 2000.

12. Wolff BG: Factors determining recurrence following surgery for Crohn's disease. World J Surg 22:364-369, 1998.

CHAPTER 50

UPPER GASTROINTESTINAL BLEEDING

G. Edward Kimm, Jr., MD, and Allen T. Belshaw, MD

1. **What is upper gastrointestinal bleeding?**
   Bleeding from proximal to the ligament of Treitz (the transition point between duodenum and jejunum).

2. **What are the most common causes of upper gastrointestinal bleeding?**
   In descending order of frequency, they are peptic ulcer disease, esophagogastric varices, vascular malformations, and Mallory-Weiss tears. All other causes account for <5% of cases.

3. **What is the overall mortality rate of upper gastrointestinal bleeding?**
   Approximately 10% for all patients. Mortality is much higher with comorbid factors such as cardiac, pulmonary, hepatic, and renal disease as well as advanced age (>60 years) and large transfusion requirements (>5 units of blood).

4. **What is the most common presentation of upper gastrointestinal bleeding?**
   Eighty percent of patients present with **melena** (blood is a cathartic, and patients pass black, tarry, or maroon-colored stools) or **hematochezia** (bright red blood in the rectum). **Hematemesis** (bright red or coffee-ground emesis) is diagnostic of an upper source of gastrointestinal (GI) bleeding. **Occult bleeding** may present only with guaiac-positive stool.

5. **How much gastrointestinal blood loss is necessary to cause melena?**
   As little as 50 to 100 ml. Occult bleeding (guaiac- or Hematest-positive) can be detected with as little as 10 ml of blood loss.

6. **A 45-year-old man presents to the emergency department with massive hematemesis, tachycardia, and hypotension. What should the Initial approach be?**
   Acute GI hemorrhage requires a prompt and systematic approach. As in all patients who are critically ill, initially assess the ABCs (airway, breathing, and circulation). Start two large-bore intravenous (IV) lines, and give 1 L of Ringer's lactate while monitoring the patient. Place a nasogastric (NG) tube and Foley catheter and irrigate the NG tube with saline. Send blood for type and cross-match and coagulation and liver function tests (LFTs).

7. **This patient stabilizes after your interventions. Is a medical history of any value in determining a cause of the bleeding?**
   Yes. The following are pertinent:
   - Previous symptoms of peptic ulcer disease or nonsteroidal antiinflammatory drug (NSAID) use: bleeding duodenal or gastric ulcer.
   - History of gastroesophageal reflux disease (GERD): esophagitis.
   - Heavy alcohol use: gastritis or bleeding varices.
   - Recent retching or vomiting: Mallory-Weiss tear.
   - Weight loss: upper GI malignancy.

8. **What physical finding may be helpful in establishing the source of bleeding?**
Physical examination is generally not helpful. The stigmata of liver disease (jaundice, caput medusa, ascites, muscle wasting) raise the suspicion of variceal bleeding or multiple superficial gastric erosions.

9. **What percentage of patients with known esophageal varices are bleeding from the varices on presentation?**
Only 50%.

10. **Does bilious or clear NGT aspirate rule out an upper GI source of hemorrhage?**
No. Although NG tube aspiration can be useful in directing the search for a bleeding site, one should keep in mind that the false-negative rate may be as high as 20%.

11. **What studies can be used to determine the source of bleeding?**
Esophagogastroduodenoscopy (EGD) is the first and best test. Barium studies may miss a significant source of upper GI bleeding, such as erosive gastritis, and interfere with other more definitive tests, especially arteriography. Nuclear scans are of limited value in acute upper GI hemorrhage.

12. **What is the sensitivity of EGD?**
EGD identifies the source of bleeding in up to 95% of cases. EGD has the advantage of directly visualizing the source of blood loss and provides the opportunity to biopsy a lesion and perform therapeutic maneuvers.

13. **How can EGD be used to control nonvariceal bleeding?**
Injection, thermal, and mechanical (e.g., clips) interventions can be used. A recent meta-analysis showed that dual endoscopic therapy was significantly superior to epinephrine injection alone.

14. **What amount of bleeding is required to see a "Blush" on arteriography?**
Less than 5 ml/min. Although angiography is the most invasive of these tests, the catheter can be left in place and used for delivery of therapeutic vasopressin or embolization.

15. **What treatment options are available to control variceal bleeding?**
Upper endoscopy with band ligation is more effective than sclerotherapy. In experienced hands, placement of a Sengstaken-Blakemore tube (a double balloon tube that permits direct tamponade of both gastric and esophageal varices) temporarily controls bleeding in 90% of cases. Intravenous (IV) infusion of vasopressin or octreotide should decrease blood flow to the varices but is less successful in patients with more severe liver disease.

16. **What are the indications for surgery in patients with upper gastrointestinal hemorrhage?**
About 10% of patients eventually require surgery. Indications include:
   - Persistent hypotension or shock (failure of resuscitative therapy).
   - Recurrent bleeding while on maximal medical therapy.
   - High-risk patients with significant comorbid disease.
   - Large transfusion requirements (transfusion of more than two thirds of the patient's blood volume in 24 hours).

17. **What is the surgical approach to an unstable patient with a nonlocalized upper gastrointestinal bleed who does not respond to initial resuscitation?**
At laporotomy start with a generous gastroduodenotomy centered over the pylorus. If this does not reveal a source of bleeding, proceed with a proximal gastrotomy.

18. **A patient presents with hematemesis and has a remote history of an abdominal aortic aneurysm repair. What uncommon cause of upper gastrointestinal bleeding needs to be considered?**

    Aortoduodenal fistula. Any patient with a history of aortic surgery and evidence of GI bleeding should be aggressively worked up for aortoenteric fistula. The study of choice is endoscopy.

19. **What is a Dieulafoy's ulcer?**

    A gastric vascular malformation with an exposed submucosal artery, usually within 2 to 5 cm of the gastroesophageal junction. It presents with painless hematemesis, often massive (fortunately, this is uncommon).

20. **A patient recently admitted with a traumatic liver laceration is treated nonoperatively and later develops painless hematemesis. What do you suspect? How should you treat this patient?**

    Hemobilia, another rare cause of upper GI bleeding, usually occurs after liver trauma or hepatic resection. Treatment consists of angiographic embolization.

21. **What are other rare causes of upper gastrointestinal bleeding?**

    Watermelon stomach, portal hypertensive gastropathy, upper GI neoplasm, duodenal diverticulum, and pancreatitis (resulting in erosion into the splenic artery or splenic vein thrombosis with portal hypertension).

KEY POINTS: UPPER GASTROINTESTINAL BLEEDING

1. Upper GI bleeding is defined as bleeding proximal to the ligament of Treitz.

2. The most common causes are gastritis, duodenal ulcer, esophageal varices, benign gastric ulcer, esophagitis, and Mallory-Weiss tear.

3. Eighty percent of patients present with melena or hematochezia.

4. EGD identifies the source of bleeding in 95% of cases.

BIBLIOGRAPHY

1. Conrad SA: Acute upper gastrointestinal bleeding in critically ill patients: causes and treatment modalities. Crit Care Med 30:365-368, 2002.

2. Fallah MA, Prakash C, Edmundowitz S: Acute gastrointestinal bleeding. Med Clin North Am 84:1183-1208, 2000.

3. Jamieson GG: Current status of indications for surgery in peptic ulcer disease. World J Surg 24:256, 2000.

4. Kwan V, Norton ID: Endoscopic management of non-variceal upper gastrointestinal haemorrhage. ANZ J Surg 77:222-230, 2007.

5. Marmo R, Rotondano G, Piscopo R et al.: Dual therapy versus monotherapy of high-risk bleeding ulcers: a meta-analysis of controlled trials. Am J Gastroenterol 102:279-289, 2007.

6. Savides TJ, Jensen DM: Therapeutic endoscopy for nonvariceal gastrointestinal bleeding. Gastroenterol Clin North Am 29:465-487, 2000.

CHAPTER 51

LOWER GASTROINTESTINAL BLEEDING

Kathleen R. Liscum, MD

1. **Describe the initial treatment of a patient who presents with massive lower gastrointestinal (GI) bleeding.**
   Treatment begins with resuscitation. Place two large-bore intravenous (IV) catheters in the upper extremities. Obtain hemoglobin and hematocrit levels, blood type, and cross-match. A Foley catheter should be placed to help monitor volume status.

2. **What is the next step in evaluating the patient?**
   A nasogastric (NG) tube should be placed to rule out an upper GI source. If the aspirate is bilious, the examiner can be fairly certain that the source is distal to the ligament of Treitz. However, if the aspirate reveals no bile, the patient may still be bleeding in the duodenum with a competent pylorus.

3. **What are the two most common causes of massive lower GI bleeding?**
   Diverticular hemorrhage (diverticulosis) and bleeding vascular ectasias. Diverticular disease was previously thought to be the most common cause of lower GI bleeding, but vascular ectasias are now quite frequent.

4. **What are other potential causes of blood from the rectum?**
   Colon cancer
   Inflammatory bowel disease
   Polyps
   Anorectal disorders (e.g., hemorrhoids, fissure)
   Ischemic colitis
   Meckel's diverticulum
   Infectious colitis

5. **After a thorough history and physical examination, what is the first step toward identifying the specific site of bleeding?**
   Anoscopy and rigid proctosigmoidoscopy to rule out anorectal sources. Before proceeding with extensive work-up of the intraperitoneal colon the clinician should feel certain that the etiolgy is not in the most distal portions of the gastrointestinal tract.

6. **Name four options for localizing lower GI bleeding.**
   1. Tagged red blood cell scan.
   2. Sulfur colloid scan.
   3. Angiography.
   4. Colonoscopy.

7. **Discuss the differences between sulfur colloid scan and tagged red blood cell scan.**
   The *sulfur colloid* scan can be accomplished quickly and detects bleeding as minimal as 0.1 ml/min. The radio-labeled sulfur colloid is cleared quickly by the liver and spleen, which may

obscure the bleeding site if it is located in the hepatic or splenic flexure. The test is complete within 20 minutes of administration of the radionuclide.

The *tagged red blood cell* scan requires a 60-minute delay while the autologous red blood cells are labeled with isotope. The test detects bleeding as slow as 0.5 ml/min. Because the tagged cells stay in the patient's system, it is also helpful in identifying the source when the patient is bleeding intermittently. The study can be repeated with if bleeding recurs within 24 hours. The study takes at least 2 hours to perform.

8. What is the role of angiography?

This study is the optimal next step for patients who have significant persistent bleeding and are hemodynamically stable enough to not require an emergent laparotomy.

Angiography detects bleeding rates of 0.5 to 1.0 ml/min but only if the patient is actively bleeding. When a bleeding site is identified, the angiographic appearance may provide further insight into the cause of the bleeding. Whereas diverticular bleeding is often seen as extravasation of contrast, vascular ectasias may be identified by a vascular tuft or early filling vein.

9. What therapeutic options are available with angiography?

(1) Infusion of vasopressin (Pitressin) into a selected vessel and (2) embolization of the bleeding vessel.

10. What role should colonoscopy play in the evaluation of patient with lower gastrointestinal bleeding?

For patients with fairly minor intermittent bleeding colonoscopy is a good study to localize the source. There is a bit more controversy about the role of colonoscopy for patients with larger volume blood loss who continue to bleed. A few studies show a shorter length of stay associated with early endoscopy in this group of patients, whereas another study showed that colonoscopy was more likely to identify the source of bleeding but this identification did not result in any reduction in mortality or transfusion requirements.

KEY POINTS: LOWER GASTROINTESTINAL BLEEDING

1. The most common causes of massive lower GI bleeding are diverticular hemorrhage and bleeding vascular ectasias.

2. The most common cause of lower GI bleeding in children is Meckel's diverticulum.

3. After a thorough history and physical examination, the first steps in identifying the specific site of bleeding are anoscopy and rigid proctosigmoidoscopy.

4. Tagged red blood cell scan, sulfur colloid scan, colonoscopy, and angiography are four options for localizing lower GI bleeding.

5. Indications for surgery include patients who have received 6 U of blood without resolution of bleeding and patients who continue to bleed after vasopressin or embolization or who are too unstable to undergo any localization procedure.

11. Which patients should have angiographic embolization of the bleeding site?

Most surgeons believe that embolization should be reserved for patients who are poor operative risks in that a 15% complication rate is associated with the procedure. Patients may perforate or develop a stricture as a result of bowel wall ischemia.

12. **What is the role of vasopressin infusion?**

Vasopressin is only a temporizing measure. Control of the bleeding with vasopressin allows time for resuscitation and essentially converts an emergent case into an urgent one. Vasopressin occasionally may be used as the only treatment for diverticular bleeding. If the patient has a repeated episode of bleeding after weaning from vasopressin, the surgeon must decide between embolization and surgery.

13. **Do lower GI hemorrhages ever spontaneously resolve?**

Spontaneous resolution occurs in 75% of patients with vascular ectasias, and 90% of patients with diverticular bleeding.

14. **What are the indications for operative intervention?**

When the patient has received 6 units of blood (two thirds of the patient's blood volume in 24 hours) without resolution of bleeding. Any patient who continues to bleed or has recurrent bleeding after vasopressin or embolization should undergo resection.

15. **What is the role of blind subtotal colectomy in the management of patients with massive lower GI bleeding?**

Blind subtotal colectomy is limited to the small group of patients in whom a specific bleeding source cannot be identified. The procedure is associated with a 16% mortality rate. Younger patients tend to tolerate the procedure better than elderly patients. Older patients often suffer with severe diarrhea, urgency, and incontinence. However, blind segmental colectomy is associated with an even higher mortality rate (40%) and a 50% rebleeding rate.

16. **What is the most common cause of lower GI hemorrhage in the pediatric population?**

Meckel's diverticulum.

BIBLIOGRAPHY

1. Biondo S, Kreisler E, Millan M et al.: Differences in patient postoperative and long-term outcomes between obstructive and perforated colonic cancer. Am J Surg 195:427-432, 2008.

2. Cynamon J, Atar E, Steiner A et al.: Catheter-induced vasospasm in the treatment of acute lower gastrointestinal bleeding. J Vasc Interv Radiol 14:211-216, 2003.

3. Green, BT, Rockey, DC, Portwood G et al.: Urgent colonoscopy for evaluation and management of acute lower gastrointestinal hemorrhage: a randomized controlled trial. Am J Gastroenterol 100:2395, 2005.

4. Lee YS, Lee IK, Kang WK et al.: Surgical and pathological outcomes of laparoscopic surgery for transverse colon cancer, Int J Colorectal Dis 23:669-673, 2008. Epub Apr 1, 2008.

5. Mallant-Hent RC, Van Bodegraven AA, Meuwissen SG et al.: Alternative approach to massive gastrointestinal bleeding in ulcerative colitis: highly selective transcatheter embolization. Eur J Gastroenterol Hepatol 15:189-193, 2003.

6. Schmulewitz N, Fisher DA, Rockey DC: Early colonoscopy for acute lower GI bleeding predicts shorter hospital stay: a retrospective study of experience in a single center. Gastrointest Endosc 58:841, 2003.

7. Setya V, Singer JA, Minken SL: Subtotal colectomy as a last resort for unrelenting, unlocalized, lower gastrointestinal hemorrhage: experience with 12 cases. Am Surg 58:295-299, 1992.

8. Strate LL: Lower GI bleeding: epidemiology and diagnosis. Gastroenterol Clin North Am 34:643-664, 2005.

9. Strate LL, Syngal S: Timing of colonoscopy: impact on length of hospital stay in patients with acute lower intestinal bleeding. Am J Gastroenterol 98:317, 2003.

10. Zuccaro G: Management of the adult patient with acute lower gastrointestinal bleeding. Am J Gastroenterol 93:1202, 1998.

CHAPTER 52

COLORECTAL POLYPS

Christina L. Roland, MD, and Carlton C. Barnett, Jr., MD

1. **What are polyps?**
   A polyp is an elevation of the mucosal surface that can occur anywhere in the gastrointestinal (GI) tract. Two thirds of polyps occur in the rectosigmoid and descending colon.

2. **What are the major types of polyps?**
   Polyps are classified by their morphologic features; either pedunculated or sessile.
   Pedunculated polyps have a head attached by a stalk to the mucosa of the colon or rectum. The stalk is usually covered with normal mucosa and <1.5 cm.
   Sessile polyps rest on a broad base.
   In either type, the muscularis mucosa is an important landmark for differentiating invasive from noninvasive lesions. Lymphatics and veins do not extend across the muscularis mucosa. Submucosal lesions, such as carcinoids and lipomas, may resemble colorectal polyps.

3. **At what age do polyps develop?**
   Adenomatous colorectal polyps occur infrequently under the age of 30 years. The incidence increases with age. However, autopsy series report a microscopic frequency as high as 75% in patients older than age 45 years. The clinical incidence is up to 40% for persons older than age 60 years.

4. **Which polyps have no malignant potential?**
   Hyperplastic (metaplastic) polyps are small (1 to 5 mm) and are 10 times more common than adenomas. Unlike adenomatous polyps, hyperplastic polyps are caused by a failure of mucosal cells to spread over the mucosal lumen. These cells accumulate on the luminal surface, forming a polyp of thickened mucosa.
   Hamartomas are benign tumors in an organ (colon) composed of tissue elements normally found at that site but grow in a disorganized mass.
   Inflammatory polyps are common in diseases such as ulcerative colitis (UC), Crohn's disease, and schistosomiasis. They represent islands of healed or healing mucosal epithelium that are not permanent. The appearance of inflammatory polyps actually reflects the severity of the underlying disease.

5. **Which polyps have malignant potential?**
   Adenomatous polyps may be precursors for cancer. There are three histologic types of adenomatous polyps. Polyps containing >75% glandular elements are called tubular. Those containing >75% villous elements are termed villous, and those containing >25% of both glandular and villous are tubulovillous.
   In general, 65% to 80% of all adenomatous polyps removed are tubular; 10% to 25% are tubulovillous; and only 5% to 10% are pure villous adenomas. Tubular adenomas are usually pedunculated and villous adenomas are usually sessile, but all histologic types can be seen in each type of polyp.

6. **Are some types of polyps more frequently associated with adenocarcinoma?**
   Yes. Villous polyps are "bad actors." Coutsoftide and colleages reported 5.6%, 16%, and 41% incidences of adenocarcinoma in tubular, villotubular and villous adenomas, respectively.

7. **What is the relationship between polyp size and risk of adenocarcinoma?**
   Polyps <2 cm have a 2% risk of containing cancer, 2 cm polyps have a 10% risk, and polyps >2 cm have a cancer risk of 40%. Sixty percent of villous polyps are >2 cm, and 77% of tubular polyps are <1 cm at the time of discovery.

8. **What are juvenile polyps?**
   Juvenile polyps are cystic dilations of glandular structures within the lamina propria and occur in the colon and rectum of infants, children, and adolescents. The cause of these polyps is unclear. They may represent a response to inflammation. Juvenile polyps are the most common cause of GI bleeding in children or may serve as lead points for intussusception. They should be left alone unless they cause trouble, at which point endoscopic polypectomy is usually sufficient treatment.

9. **How are colorectal polyps diagnosed?**
   Fecal occult blood test (FOBT) is the most common test in the United States that leads to the discovery of polyps. Sigmoidoscopy and colonoscopy confirm the diagnosis. Colonoscopy has the advantage of being both diagnostic and potentially therapeutic.

10. **What are the risks of colonoscopy?**
    Bleeding and perforation. For diagnostic colonoscopy, these risks are extremely low, 1.0% and 0.2%, respectively. Both risks are still <1% for therapeutic colonoscopy. Bleeding usually stops on its own and rarely necessitates laparotomy.

11. **How can one determine whether endoscopic polypectomy is adequate treatment?**
    In general, if a margin >1 mm can be obtained, there is no invasion of the muscularis mucosa and the histologic grade of the lesion is I or II (well to moderately well differentiated), the patient should be offered endoscopic polypectomy. Polyps with margins <1 mm, invasion into vessels or lymphatics, and histologic grade III (poorly differentiated) lesions should undergo colon resection, unless comorbid medical conditions contraindicate surgery.

12. **What are the screening recommendations to detect polyps?**
    The American Cancer Society and the American Gastoenterological Association recommend that men and women with average risk of colon cancer follow one of the subsequent schedules: Yearly FOBT with screening sigmoidoscopy every 5 years, double-contrast barium enema every 5 years, or colonoscopy every 10 years. All positive tests should be followed up with colonoscopy. Patients with increased risk (personal history of colon cancer or polyps, strong family history, history of inflammatory bowel disease [IBD] or family history of hereditary colorectal cancer syndromes) should begin screening at age 40 years, or 10 years earlier that the youngest cancer diagnosis in the family, whichever comes first.

    The sensitivity and specificity for FOBT is 40% and 96%, respectively, for colorectal polyps. Sigmoidoscopy and colonoscopy are 90% sensitive and 96% specific for polyps. Sigmoidoscopy, however, does not allow for evaluation of the proximal colon, thus lowering the overall effectiveness of this screening technique. Although colonoscopy is highly effective, it must be performed by trained individuals and carries the risk of anesthesia, thus, compromising its value as a screening tool.

13. **What are the screening recommendations for patients with known polyps?**
    Patients with low risk (1 or 2 tubular adenomas <1 cm with low grade dysplasia) should have repeat colonoscopy at 5 to 10 years. If patients are found to have multiple polyps or high-grade lesions, they should undergo colonoscopy at more frequent intervals (2 to 3 years). If patients are found to have no new lesions after one screening cycle, screening can be extended to every 5 years.

14. **Which clinical syndromes are associated with colorectal polyps?**
    Familial adenomatous polyposis (FAP) or **adenomatous polyposis coli** (APC) is inherited as an autosomal dominant trait characterized by multiple adenomatous polyps throughout the GI tract. Diagnosis is made clinically by observing at least 100 adenomatous polyps in the colon; more than 1000 are found in many cases. FAP is caused by the loss of the APC tumor suppressor gene on the long arm of chromosome 5. Multiple family members are often diagnosed with colorectal cancer, generally at a young age. Bleeding, diarrhea, and abdominal pain are common presenting symptoms. FAP is associated with a nearly 100% risk of cancer. FAP is also associated with small bowel, especially periampullary polyps or cancer and mandibular osteoma.
    Gardner syndrome is also associated with the loss of the APC gene. Patients have polyposis, as do patients with FAP, but they also have osteomas of the skull, epidermoid cysts, retinal pigmentation abnormalities, and multiple soft tissue tumors (desmoids).
    Turcot syndrome is also associated with APC mutations and is characterized clinically with central nervous system (CNS) tumors and multiple adenomatous polyps.
    Peutz-Jeghers syndrome consists of multiple hamartomatous polyps throughout the alimentary tract. These polyps are associated with cutaneous melanotic spots on the lips, within the oropharynx, and the dorsum of the fingers and toes. The malignant potential is quite low.

15. **What is the natural history of *adenomatous polyposis coli*?**
    A review of more than 1000 cases of APC showed that the mean age at diagnosis of polyps was 34 years, and the mean age at diagnosis of colorectal cancers was 40 years. The mean age of death was 43 years. It is now recommended that patients with APC undergo at least near total colectomy at age 25 years. Patients are also at risk for the late development of foregut adenocarcinoma, necessitating the need for upper endoscopy every 3 to 5 years. Despite prophylactic colectomy, this group of patients will not have a normal life expectancy.

16. **What are the surgical treatment options for *adenomatous polyposis coli*?**
    Treatment options include total proctocolectomy with permanent ileostomy, abdominal colectomy with rectal preservation, abdominal colectomy with ileorectal anastomosis and ileal pouch-anal anastomosis. In patients in whom the rectum is preserved, yearly endoscopic surveillance is necessary.

17. **What role do genetic defects play in the progression of colorectal polyps to adenocarcinoma?**
    The progression of adenomatous polyps to colorectal cancer is believed to involve an accumulation of genetic defects via the activation of proto-oncogenes and/or the activation of tumor suppressor genes. Colon polyps have provided the best available model of genetic mutations in the progression of normal tissue to cancer. Vogelstein and others have provided an elegant description of genetic events that polyps accumulate alterations of a tumor suppressor gene on chromosome 18, and carcinomas are associated with inactivation of the tumor suppressor gene TP53 with loss of function of the p53 protein.

18. **What role do oncogenes play in the development of adenocarcinoma from adenomatous polyps?**
    Oncogenes are copies of normal cellular genes that have been activated by mutation. Activating mutations of one allele of an oncogene can disrupt normal cell growth and differentiation and

increase the likelihood of neoplastic transformation. The Ki-ras gene is the most commonly mutated oncogene in sporadic colonic neoplasia. Point mutations in the K-ras gene have been observed in approximately 40% of sporadic colorectal adenomas and carcinomas. Analysis of mutations in DNA from cells shed into the stool has been proposed as a potentially useful way to screen for colorectal cancer. In addition, activation of the tyrosine kinase of the c-src gene product pp60c-src is frequent in polyps of high malignant potential; the activity of tyrosine kinase is significantly elevated above the level of primary tumors in liver metastases.

KEY POINTS: COLORECTAL POLYPS

1. A polyp is an elevation of the mucosal surface that can occur anywhere in the GI tract.

2. Hyperplastic polyps are small and constitute >90% of polyps in the colon and rectum.

3. Polyps containing >75% glandular elements are called *tubular;* those with >75% villous elements are termed *villous;* and those containing >25% of both glandular and villous elements are called *tubulovillous.*

4. FOBT is the most common test in the United States that leads to the discovery of polyps.

BIBLIOGRAPHY

1. Ahnen DJ, Feigl P, Quan G: Ki-ras mutation and overexpression predict the clinical behavior of colorectal cancer: a Southwest Oncology Group study. Cancer Res 58:1149-1158, 1998.

2. Brosens LA, van Hattem WA, Jansen M et al.: Gastrointestinal polyposis syndromes. Curr Mol Med 7:29-46, 2007.

3. Levine JS, Ahnen DJ: Adenomatous polyps of the colon. N Engl J Med 355:2551-2557, 2006.

4. Duffy MJ, van Dalen A, Haglund C et al.: Tumour markers in colorectal cancer: European Group on Tumour Markers (EGTM) guidelines for clinical use. Eur J Cancer 43:1348-1360, 2007.

5. Fukami N, Lee JH: Endoscopic treatment of large sessile and flat colorectal lesions. Curr Opin Gastroenterol 22:54-59, 2006.

6. Gallagher MC, Phillips RK, Bulow S: Surveillance and management of upper gastrointestinal disease in Familial Adenomatous Polyposis. Fam Cancer 5:263-273, 2006.

7. Hahn WC, Weinberg RA: Rules for making human tumor cells. N Engl J Med 347:1593-1602, 2002.

8. Hassan C, Zullo A, Winn S et al.: The colorectal malignant polyp: scoping a dilemma. Dig Liver Dis 39:92-100, 2007.

9. Nivatvongs S, Rojanasakul A, Reimann HM et al.: The risk of lymph node metastasis in colorectal polyps with invasive adenocarcinoma. Dis Colon Rectum 34:323-328, 1991.

10. Ransahoff DF, Sandler RS: Screening for colorectal cancer. N Engl J Med 346:4044, 2002.

11. Shih IM, Wang TL, Traverso G: Top-down morphogenesis of colorectal tumors. Proc Natl Acad Sci USA 27:2640-2645, 2001.

12. Winawer S, Fletcher R, Rex D et al.: Colorectal cancer screening and surveillance: clinical guidelines and rationale—update based on new evidence. Gastroenterology 124:544-560, 2003.

13. Winawer SJ, Zauber AG, Fletcher RH et al.: Guidelines for colonoscopy surveillance after polypectomy: a consensus update by the US Multi-Society Task Force on Colorectal Cancer and the American Cancer Society. CA Cancer J Clin 56:143-159, 2006.

14. Coutsoftides T, Lavery I, Benjamin SP, Sivak MV Jr.: Malignant polyps of the colon and rectum: a clinicopathologic study. Dis Colon Rectum 22(2):82-86, 1979.

CHAPTER 53

COLORECTAL CARCINOMA

Kathleen R. Liscum, MD

1. **What are the top three causes of cancer deaths in the United States?**
   Lung, breast or prostate, and colon cancer.

2. **List a few of the presenting symptoms of patients with colorectal cancer.**
   Intermittent rectal bleeding, vague abdominal pain, fatigue secondary to anemia, change in bowel habits, constipation, tenesmus, and perineal pain.

3. **What options are available to evaluate a patient who has guaiac-positive stools?**
   To evaluate the entire colon and rectum, one may perform a barium enema and proctoscopy or a colonoscopy. Colonoscopy is 10 times more expensive but is more sensitive for lesions <1 cm.

4. **List at least five risk factors for colorectal cancer.**
   Prior adenomatous polyps, family history of colorectal cancer, age older than 40 years, chronic ulcerative colitis (UC), Crohn's colitis, history of colon cancer, exposure to pelvic radiation for prostate or cervical cancer, and familial polyposis. Hamartomatous polyps (Peutz-Jeghers syndrome), inflammatory polyps, and hyperplastic polyps are not considered premalignant.

5. **What are the current screening recommendations of the American Cancer Society for colorectal cancers?**
   A yearly digital rectal examination with testing for occult blood for patients age 40 years and older. Additionally, for patients older than age 50 years, a flexible sigmoidoscopy is recommended every 3 to 5 years.

6. **In what part of the colon or rectum are most cancers found?**
   Historically, there has been a higher incidence of cancers in the rectum and left colon. However, over the past 50 years, there has been a gradual shift toward an increased incidence of right colon cancers. This change in pattern may reflect improvement in early detection.

7. **Surgical options for colorectal cancer are dependent on the tumor location. What operation should be performed for a patient with a lesion at 25 cm from the anal verge?**
   A sigmoid colectomy.

8. **What about a lesion at 9 cm from the anal verge?**
   A low anterior resection (LAR).

9. **What about a lesion at 4 cm from the anal verge?**
   An abdominoperineal resection (APR). This requires a permanent colostomy.

10. **What is the significance of finding adenomatous polyps in a patient's colon?**
This patient is 6 times more likely to develop colorectal cancer than a patient without polyps. Evidence suggests that most colon cancers arise from adenomatous polyps. The "adenoma-carcinoma sequence" describes this transformational process. Patients with familial adenomatous polyposis (FAP) typically harbor more than 100 polyps, which cover the colonic mucosa. If these patients go untreated, they will, without exception, develop adenocarcinoma of the colon by age 40 years.

KEY POINTS: COLORECTAL CARCINOMA

1. Presenting symptoms may include intermittent rectal bleeding, vague abdominal pain, fatigue secondary to anemia, change in bowel habits, constipation, tenesmus, and perineal pain.

2. The current recommendations of the American Cancer Society for screening are a yearly digital rectal examination with testing for occult blood at age 40 years and for patients over 50 a flexible sigmoidoscopy every 3 to 5 years.

3. Patients with lymph node involvement should receive chemotherapy postoperatively to treat micrometastases.

11. **How does the surgeon prepare the patient's colon for an operation?**
Bowel preparation includes both a mechanical cleansing and appropriate antimicrobial prophylaxis. This combination has resulted in significant decrease in morbidity and mortality from colon surgery. Mechanical cleansing can be accomplished by lavage with polyethylene glycol (Go-Lytely) or a combination of cathartics and enemas (Fleet's Prep).
   Antimicrobial prophylaxis should cover the expected aerobic and anaerobic flora of the gut. Significant controversy exists over whether the antibiotics should be given enterally (e.g., neomycin, 1 g, and metronidazole [Flagyl], 1 g, 3 times orally at 4-hour intervals the evening before surgery) or parenterally (e.g., cefotetan, 2 g intravenously [IV] within 1 hour before surgery). Many physicians give both to obtain both intraluminal and systemic protection.

12. **What is Dukes' staging system?**
In 1932, Dr. Cuthbert Dukes described a staging system for rectal cancer. He originally described the following:

Dukes' A	Tumor confined to bowel wall.
Dukes' B	Tumor invading through the bowel wall.
Dukes' C	Tumor cells found in the regional lymph nodes.

   Since his original article was published, this classification has been modified several times. One of the most commonly used modifications is the inclusion of Dukes' D stage, which indicates distant metastases. While this system is often easier for the patients to understand, research and publications rely on the TNM staging system.

13. **Which patients with colorectal cancer require adjuvant (postoperative) therapy?**
Patients with lymph node involvement (Dukes' C) Stage III should receive chemotherapy postoperatively to treat micrometastases. Two large studies have documented a survival advantage for these patients. However, no studies have documented a survival advantage for patients with Dukes' B Stage II disease treated with chemotherapy.

Patients with rectal cancer with a significant chance of local recurrence (Dukes' B and C) should be treated with radiation therapy. This may be given preoperatively, postoperatively, or with a combined "sandwich" technique.

WEBSITE

www.nejm.org

BIBLIOGRAPHY

1. Alvarez JA, Baldonedo RF, Bear IG et al.: Emergency surgery for complicated colorectal carcinoma: a comparison of older and younger patients. Int Surg 92:320-326, 2007.

2. Colorectal Cancer Collaborative Group: Adjuvant radiotherapy for rectal cancer: a systematic overview of 22 randomized trials involving 8507 patients. Lancet 358:1291-1304, 2001.

3. Jass JR: Pathogenesis of colorectal cancer. Surg Clin North Am 82:891-904, 2002.

4. Levin B, Brooks D, Smith RA, Stone A: Emerging technologies in screening for colorectal cancer: CT colonography, immunochemical fecal occult blood tests, and stool screening using molecular markers. CA Cancer J Clin 53:44-55, 2003.

5. Lynch HT, de la Chapelle A: Hereditary colorectal cancer. N Engl J Med 348:919-932, 2003.

6. Nakamura T, Mitomi H, Ihara A et al.: Risk factors for wound infection after surgery for coloretal cancer. World J Surg 32:1138-1141, 2008. Epub Apr 11, 2008.

7. Ransohoff DF: Screening colonoscopy in balance issues of implementation. Gastroenterol Clin North Am 31:1031-1044, 2002.

8. Salz LB, Minsky B: Adjuvant therapy of cancers of the colon and rectum. Surg Clin North Am 82:1035-1058, 2002.

9. Scarpa M, Erroi F, Ruffolo C et al.: Minimally invasive surgery for colorectal cancer: quality of life, body image, cosmesis, and functional results. Surg Endosc [Epub ahead of print] Apr 4, 2008.

10. US Multisociety Task Force on Colorectal Cancer: Colorectal cancer screening and surveillance: Clinical guidelines and rationale-update based on new evidence. Gastroenterology 124:544-560, 2003.

CHAPTER 54

ANORECTAL DISEASE

Jeffry L. Kashuk, MD, FACS

GENERAL QUESTIONS

1. **What aspect of the initial patient encounter is most important in the diagnosis of anorectal disease?**
   Clinical history, including duration of complaints, exacerbating or alleviating issues, precipitating events, dietary and bowel habits, current or previous treatments, and lifestyle choices.

2. **What is the most common cause of painless, bright red blood per rectum?**
   Internal hemorrhoids.

3. **What are the proximal and distal anatomic landmarks of the anal canal? What is its average length?**
   The anal canal starts at the anorectal junction, which is the upper border of the internal sphincter muscle or puborectalis muscle, and ends at the anal verge. The average length is only 3 to 4 cm. The midpoint of the anal canal is called the dentate line.

4. **What is the anatomic and surgical significance of the dentate line?**
   The dentate line is the location of the anal crypts that drain the intramuscular and intersphincteric anal glands, which are the site of anorectal abscesses and fistulas in ano. Above the dentate line, the anal canal receives visceral innervation (involuntary control), is covered by columnar epithelium, and is the origin of internal hemorrhoids. Below the dentate line, the anal canal receives somatic innervation (voluntary control), is lined with squamous epithelium, and is the location of external hemorrhoids.

5. **What is the most common cause of anorectal abscess?**
   Ninety percent result from cryptoglandular infection.

6. **What are the four potential anorectal spaces used to classify anorectal abscesses?**
   1. Perianal (area of the anal verge).
   2. Ischiorectal (area lateral to the external sphincter muscles, extending from the levator ani muscles to the perineum).
   3. Intersphincteric (area between the internal and external sphincter muscles, continuous inferiorly with the perianal space and superiorly with the rectal wall).
   4. Supralevator (area superior to the levator ani muscles, inferior to the peritoneum, and lateral to the rectal wall).

7. **Define fistula in ano.**
   A fistula is an abnormal communication between any two epithelial lined surfaces. The internal opening of the fistula in ano involves the anoderm, most commonly in the region of the dentate line, whereas the external orifice is located most commonly at the anal margin.

8. **What is the incidence of fistula in ano after appropriate surgical incision and drainage of acute anorectal abscesses?**
   It is 50%.

9. **What is the most important factor leading to the successful surgical eradication of anorectal abscesses and fistulae?**
   Knowledge of the anorectal anatomy, including the potential spaces involved (memorize the answers to the preceding questions), and establish adequate drainage, identifying the fistula's complete course.

10. **What is Goodsall's rule?**
    The location of the internal opening of an anorectal fistula is based on the position of the external opening. An opening posterior to a line drawn transversely across the perineum originates from an internal opening in the posterior midline. An external opening, anterior to this line originates from the nearest anal crypt in a radial direction.

11. **What is a seton?**
    A seton is a foreign body (such as a heavy suture) placed through the fistulous tract that is then serially tightened, allowing slow, controlled transaction of the sphincter and extrusion of the foreign body. The associated fibrous reaction maintains sphincter integrity. Although associated pain is a limiting factor in its use, the technique can effectively avoid sphincter injury with minimal risks of associated incontinence.

ANAL FISSURE

12. **What is the most common location for idiopathic anal fissure?**
    Ninety percent are posterior, and 10% are anterior.

13. **What are the most common symptoms of anal fissure?**
    Tearing anal pain and bleeding with bowel movements.

14. **What is the underlying pathophysiology of fissure in ano?**
    Cyclic local trauma to the anal canal, internal anal sphincter dysfunction, and ischemia.

15. **What is the differential diagnosis for anal fissure, especially if atypical in location?**
    Anorectal abscess, thrombosed hemorrhoid, inflammatory bowel disease (IBD), or rarely, malignancy.

16. **How do you best diagnose anal fissure?**
    By clinical history and visual inspection; *not* by digital rectal examination or anoscopy (which serves only to turn a friendly patient into an irate one).

17. **What are the nonoperative treatment options?**
    High fiber diet; stool bulking agents; increased hydration, frequent warm sitz baths, and topical agents containing antiinflammatory agents, local anesthetics, and vasodilators (nitroglycerin). Injection of botox (botulin toxin) has also been reported to be effective by relaxation of the sphincter muscles.

18. **What is the most common operation performed to treat intractable fissure in ano?**
    Lateral internal sphincterotomy with or without fissurotomy.

HEMORRHOIDS

19. **What are hemorrhoidal tissues, and what are their normal functions?**
Hemorrhoids are cushions of vascular tissue that contribute to anal continence and protect the sphincter mechanism during defecation. Hemorrhoids are not veins, but sinusoids. Bleeding originates from presinusoidal arterioles, thus explaining the bright red bleeding.

20. **What is the most common cause of pathological hemorrhoids?**
Constipation, prolonged straining, pregnancy, internal sphincter dysfunction, and variceal disease associated with hepatic portal hypertension.

21. **What is the most important difference between internal and external hemorrhoids?**
Internal hemorrhoids are above the dentate line with visceral innervation, whereas external hemorrhoids are below this region with somatic innervation. Ablation of internal hemorrhoids causes a pressure sensation with an urge to defecate, but a similar approach to external hemorrhoids leads to excruciating pain.

22. **What are the most common complaints associated with pathologic internal hemorrhoids?**
Bleeding, mucus discharge, and prolapse.

23. **What are the most common complaints associated with external hemorrhoids?**
Pain, inflammation, thrombosis, and anal hygiene difficulties.

24. **Are there any treatment options for symptomatic internal hemorrhoids based on identifiable physical characteristics?**
Yes: Treatment is based on the degree of prolapse:
Grade 1: Diet, stool-bulking agents.
Grade 2: Spontaneous reduction; in addition to grade 1 measures, rubber band ligation, injection sclerotherapy, cryotherapy, infrared ablation, anal dilatation, and electrocautery.
Grade 3: Manual reduction, and same as grade 2 measures
Grade 4: Irreducible, same as grade 3 measures or operative hemorrhoidectomy, including stapling procedures for extensive disease.

PILONIDAL DISEASE

25. **What is the most common clinical presentation of a pilonidal sinus?**
Pain and swelling in the sacrococcygeal region, which typically is associated with one or more chronic draining sinus tracts.

26. **How is acute pilonidal abscess treated?**
Incision and drainage of the abscess as an outpatient, with later attention to the fistula tract.

27. **What is definitive therapy for pilonidal disease?**
Excision of the entire pilonidal cavity and associated sinus tracts down to the fascia.

28. **How is the best way to treat the wound?**
Small wounds can be closed primarily, whereas large defects may require broad openings or flap closures.

29. **Why is pilonidal disease rare after age 40?**
Changes in body habitus is one theory.

KEY POINTS: ANO-RECTAL DISEASE

1. Perform a careful history and physical with particular attention to bowel habits before examining a patient with ano-rectal complaints. If a fissure is suspected, perform a limited visual inspection.

2. Be particularly familiar with the anorectal anatomy when dealing with conditions of this region.

3. Always keep in mind the location of the anal sphincter when approaching anorectal disease operatively; use a seton when in doubt.

4. Be conservative when treating hemorrhoidal disease, reserving operative therapy in most cases for the last resort.

5. Pilonidal disease should be aggressively eradicated down to the fascia at the initial operative intervention.

BIBLIOGRAPHY

1. Beck OE, Wexner SC, editors: *Fundamentals of anorectal surgery*, Philadelphia, 1999, W.B. Saunders.

2. Brisinda G, Cadeddu F, Brandara F et al.: Randomized clinical trial comparing botulinum toxin injections with 0.2 % nitroglycerin ointment for chronic anal fissure. Br J Surg 94:162, 2007.

3. Cintron JR, Park JJ, Orsay CP et al.: Repair of fistulas-in-ano using fibrin adhesive: long-term fellowship. Dis Colon Rectum 43:944, 2000.

4. Felt-Bersma RJ: Endoanal ultrasound in perianal fistulas and abscesses. Dig Liver Dis 38:537, 2006.

5. Ky AJ, Sylla P, Steinhagen R et al.: Collagen fistula plug for the treatment of anal fistulas. Dis Colon Rectum 51:838-843, 2008.

6. Mattana C, Coco C, Manno A et al.: Stapled hemorrhoidectomy and Milligan Morgan hemorrhoidectomy in the cure of fourth degree hemorrhoids. Dis Colon Rectum 50:1770, 2007.

7. McCallum I, King PM, Bruce J: Healing by primary versus secondary intention after surgical treatment for pilonidal sinus. Cochrane Database Reviews Issue 4 Art: D006213, 2007.

8. Thornton MJ, Kennedy ML, King DOV: Manometric effect of topical glyeryl trinitrate and its impact on chronic anal fissure healing. Dis Colon Rectum 48:1207, 2005.

CHAPTER 55

INGUINAL HERNIA

Elizabeth L. Cureton, MD, Alexander Q. Ereso, MD, and Gregory P. Victorino, MD

1. **"Groin" hernia refers to which three hernias?**
   Direct and indirect inguinal hernias and femoral hernias.

2. **Francois Poupart, a French surgeon and anatomist (1616–1708), described a ligament that bears his name. What is the anatomic name of the Poupart ligament?**
   Inguinal ligament, which is a key element in most groin hernia repair.

3. **Franz K. Hesselbach, a German surgeon and anatomist (1759–1816), described a triangle that is the common site of direct hernias. What are the anatomic margins of Hesselbach's triangle?**
   The triangle is defined inferiorly by the inguinal ligament, superiorly by the inferior epigastric vessels, and medially by the rectus fascia. The transversalis fascia forms the floor of the triangle. The original description used Cooper's ligament as the inferior limit, but because of the common use of the anterior approach to hernias, the more apparent inguinal ligament was substituted as the inferior limit of the triangle. With the increasing use of preperitoneal approaches to hernia repair, Cooper's ligament is again much more apparent and useful as an anatomic touchstone.

4. **Sir Astley Paston Cooper, an English surgeon and anatomist (1768–1841), described a ligament bearing his name. What is the anatomic name for the ligament and the proper name of Cooper's ligament repair?**
   The anatomic name of Cooper's ligament is iliopectineal ligament. The Cooper's ligament repair or McVay repair was popularized by Chester McVay (1911–1987). With Barry Aston, professor of anatomy at Northwestern University, McVay provided the modern description of the groin anatomy.

5. **Antonio de Gimbernat, a Spanish surgeon and anatomist (1734–1816), had his interesting name attached to the lacunar ligament, which marks the medial margin of a groin area opening. What is the opening? What hernia protrudes into this opening?**
   The opening is the femoral canal, which is defined medially by the lacunar ligament, anteriorly by the inguinal ligament, posteriorly by the pectineal fascia, and laterally by the femoral vein. A femoral hernia protrudes into the femoral canal.

6. **Indirect inguinal hernia (particularly in children) and hydrocele are associated with which congenital abnormality?**
   Persistence of an open processus vaginalis, in the case of a hernia, allows descent of bowel into the inguinal canal. With fluid accumulation, partial obstruction presents as a hydrocele of the spermatic cord.

7. **What are the diagnostic criteria for hernia in an infant or child?**
   - Inguinal, scrotal, or labial lump that may or may not be reducible.
   - History of a lump seen by a healthcare provider.

- History of a lump seen by the mother.
- The "silk sign" (the feeling of rubbing together two surfaces of silk cloth when gently rubbing together the two surfaces of a hernia sac).
- An incarceration sometimes felt on rectal examination.

8. What can be done to reduce an incarcerated hernia in an infant or child?
The four-point program is easier said than done, but it is worth the effort:
1. Sedate the patient.
2. Place the patient in the Trendelenburg position.
3. Apply a cold pack (over petroleum gauze to avoid skin injury) in inguinal area.
4. In the absence of spontaneous reduction—and if the patient is quiet—use gentle manipulation.

9. How often can incarceration be successfully reduced? What should be done next?
About 80% of incarcerated hernias can be reduced in children; in adults, the percentage is lower. Despite the fact that 80% to 90% of inguinal hernias occur in boys, most incarcerations occur in girls. The hernia should be repaired electively within a few days after incarceration. The 20% of hernias that are still incarcerated are operated immediately.

10. What is a Bassini repair?
The Bassini repair sutures together the conjoined tendon and the shelving edge of the inguinal ligament up to the internal ring (Fig. 55-1). This classic procedure, introduced in 1887 at the Italian Society of Surgery in Genoa, revolutionized hernia repair. Until recently, it has been the standard of repair. After graduation from medical school and while fighting for Italian independence, Eduardo Bassini (1844–1924) was bayoneted in the groin and, as a prisoner, was hospitalized for months with a fecal fistula.

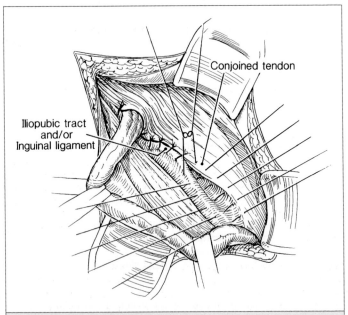

Figure 55-1. The standard right inguinal hernia repair using the conjoined tendon and inguinal ligament.

Conjoined tendon

Iliopubic tract and/or Inguinal ligament

11. **What is the recurrence rate with indirect and direct hernias that have been repaired with classic Bassini repair technique?**
Over a follow-up period of 50 years, the recurrence rate of adult indirect hernias is 5% to 10%; of direct hernias, 15% to 30%.

12. **Describe a McVay hernia repair.**
The line of interrupted sutures starts at the pubic tubercle and joins the tendinous arch of the transversus abdominis muscle to Cooper's ligament up to the femoral canal. At this point, two or three transitional sutures are placed from Cooper's ligament to the anterior femoral fascia, effectively closing the medial extreme of the femoral canal. The final set of sutures joins the transversus abdominis arch and the anterior femoral fascia. The stitches usually incorporate the inguinal ligament at the upper limit of the repair, the site of the new internal inguinal ring and cord structures. About 15 years ago, McVay described lying in a mesh patch and stitching it, at its periphery, to the same anatomic structures. This application of mesh closely resembles the Lichtenstein repair (see question 17), except that it uses Cooper's ligament.

13. **For what type of hernias is the McVay Cooper's ligament repair most useful?**
Femoral and direct hernias.

14. **What is the Shouldice repair?**
The Shouldice repair, popularized at the Shouldice Clinic near Toronto, imbricates or overlays the transversalis fascia and conjoined tendon with four continuous lines, using two fine-wire sutures. The suture tract runs from the pubic tubercle to a new internal ring. Care is taken with the inferior epigastric vessels. The result is layered approximation of the conjoined tendon to the inguinal ligament tract.

15. **What is the reported recurrence rate for the Shouldice repair?**
The recurrence rate is 1%, the lowest reported rate for nonmesh repairs of inguinal hernias in adults.

16. **For what type of groin hernia is the Shouldice repair not appropriate?**
Femoral hernia.

17. **Describe the Lichtenstein repair.**
The Lichtenstein repair consists of a sutured patch of polypropylene mesh (Marlex, C.R. Bard, Inc., Covington, GA) that covers Hesselbach's triangle and the indirect hernia area. It is considered a tension-free repair because the mesh is sutured in place without pulling ligaments or tissues together as in all other repairs. The mesh is divided at its upper end to wrap closely around the spermatic cord and its associated structures in the normal position of the internal inguinal canal. The Lichtenstein procedure is rapidly becoming the most widely used repair of adult inguinal hernia. The reported recurrence rate is <1%.

18. **What are the advantages of using the Marlex mesh?**
Central to acceptance and success of the Lichtenstein hernia repair has been the development of and experience with the Marlex mesh. The monofilament mesh is strong, inert, and resistant to infection. The interstices are rapidly and completely infiltrated with fibroblasts, and the mesh is not subject to deterioration, rejection, or fragmentation (see Fig. 55-2).

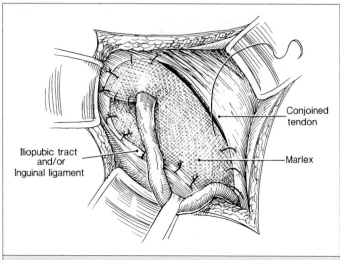

Figure 55-2. The Marlex mesh repair of a right inguinal hernia. Note that the same structures are used but not brought together; thus, the name of the "tension-free" repair.

19. **For what groin area is the Lichtenstein repair not appropriate?**
Femoral hernia.

20. **Which type of repair is acceptable for the femoral hernia?**
Several different repairs can be used. Mesh in the form of a plug can be inserted into the femoral canal and fixed in place. A McVay Cooper's ligament repair can be done. A preperitoneal approach to the hernia can be used to suture or plug the defect. A suture repair or a sartorius facial flap applied from below the inguinal ligament in a femoral approach also may be used. The preperitoneal approach is increasingly used for complicated inguinal and femoral hernias.

21. **What is the preperitoneal or Stoppa procedure?**
The preperitoneal or Stoppa procedure is a groin hernia repair on the internal side of the abdominal wall between the peritoneum and fascial surfaces that do not open into the peritoneal cavity. The anatomic landmarks are quite different and initially quite challenging to surgeons accustomed to the external abdominal wall approach. The technique is suited for recurrent hernias in which scarring and obliterated anatomy increase the risk of cord injury and recurrence. Other problems such as large hernias and femoral hernias are corrected with this approach. Conceptually, the laparoscopic hernia repair uses the same approach (see Fig. 55-3).

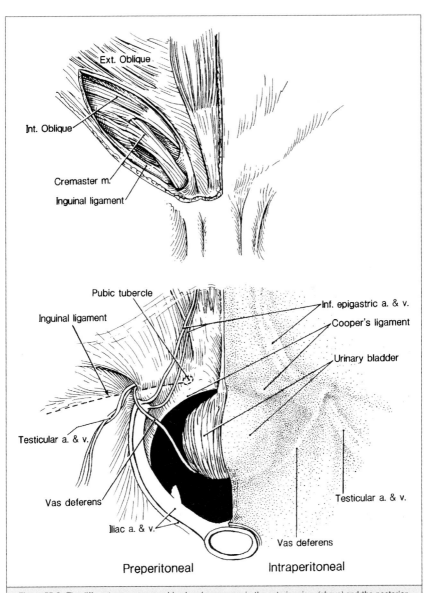

Figure 55-3. The different appearance and landmarks are seen in the anterior view *(above)* and the posterior view *(below)* of the inguinal-femoral area. In the posterior view the importance of the inferior epigastric vessels, bladder, and Cooper's ligament as anatomic landmarks is apparent.

22. **Where are the spaces of Retzius and Bogros? Why are they increasingly important?**
Retzius' space is between the pubis and the urinary bladder. Bogros' space is between the peritoneum and the fascia and muscle planes on the posterior aspect of the abdominal wall below the umbilicus and down to Cooper's ligament. Laterally, the space goes to the iliac spines. In either the open Stoppa procedure or the laparoscopic preperitoneal repair, the spaces of Retzius and Bogros are developed for mesh placement and surgical exposure.

23. **How tight around the spermatic cord should a surgically fashioned, internal inguinal ring be?**
About 5 mm, which is less than a fingertip and more than a forceps tip.

24. **What is the common fascial defect of larger indirect and all direct inguinal hernias?**
Weakness or attenuation of the transversalis fascia.

25. **On examination, the femoral hernia may be confused with what other inguinal hernia?**
The femoral hernia may be confused with a direct inguinal hernia because of the tendency of the femoral hernia to present at the lateral edge of the inguinal ligament.

KEY POINTS: TYPES OF INGUINAL HERNIA REPAIR

1. The Bassini repair sutures together the conjoined tendon and the shelving edge of the inguinal ligament up to the internal ring.

2. The McVay repair is most useful for femoral and direct hernias.

3. The Shouldice repair imbricates the transversalis fascia and conjoined tendon with four continuous lines, using two fine-wire sutures (not appropriate for femoral hernias).

4. The Lichtenstein repair consists of a sutured patch of polyprolene mesh that covers Hesselbach's triangle and the indirect hernia sac.

26. **What is the difference between an incarcerated and a strangulated hernia?**
Incarcerated: structures in the hernia sac still have a good blood supply but are stuck in the sac because of adhesions or a narrow neck of the hernia sac.
Strangulated: herniated structures, such as bowel or omentum, have lost their blood supply because of anatomic constriction at the neck of the hernia. The herniated, ischemic tissue is, therefore, in various stages of gangrenous changes. Strangulated hernias are surgical emergencies.

27. **What operation is done for an uncomplicated indirect infant hernia?**
High ligation of the hernia sac.

28. **What operation is done for an uncomplicated indirect hernia in young adults?**
The appropriate operation consists of high ligation and possibly one or two stitches in the transversalis fascia to tighten the internal ring. This is the basic Marcy technique, developed by Henry Orlando Marcy (1837–1924); it is smaller and more anatomically focused than the Bassini repair.

29. **What operation is done for an uncomplicated but sizable direct hernia in elderly adults?**

Traditionally, the Bassini or McVay repair was chosen. More recently, because of the low recurrence rate, the Shouldice or Lichtenstein repair is favored.

30. **What organ systems should be reviewed with particular care in the work-up of patients with hernia (especially elderly patients with recent onset of hernia)?**

The gastrointestinal (GI), urinary, and pulmonary systems should be reviewed with particular care. One is looking for causes of chronic strain or sudden forces that may have induced the hernia. Straining during defecation or urination, unusual coughing, or difficulty with breathing, if corrected, may be of great value to the patient and reduce the chance of recurrent hernia.

31. **What is a sliding hernia?**

A sliding hernia is formed when a retroperitoneal organ protrudes (herniates) outside the abdominal cavity in such a manner that the organ itself and the overlying peritoneal surface constitute a side of the hernia sac.

32. **What organs can be found in sliding hernias?**

Colon
Bladder
Cecum
Fallopian tubes
Appendix
Uterus (rare)
Ovary

33. **What are common operative and postoperative complications of hernia repairs?**

Intraoperative complications:
- Injury to the spermatic cord, especially in children.
- Injury to the spermatic vessels, resulting in atrophy or acute necrosis of testes.
- Injury to the ilioinguinal nerve, genitofemoral nerve, and lateral femoral cutaneous nerve (the lateral femoral cutaneous nerve is uniquely vulnerable in laparoscopic and properitoneal procedures).
- Injury to the femoral vessels.

Postoperative complications:
- Infection: high risk in children with diaper rash and patients with bowel injury or necrosis.
- Hematoma: should resolve in time.
- Nerve injury: the nerve is not always divided and, with time, may improve. If pain persists, try lidocaine block for both diagnosis and treatment. If a nerve block is not successful, one may consider reexploration to free the nerve from scar or to excise a postsurgical neuroma.

34. **What are the common sites of hernia recurrence?**

Direct hernias often recur at the pubic tubercle. Indirect hernias recur at the internal ring. The cause is usually related to poorly placed or insufficient stitches. Other possible causes include infection, poor tissue, poor collagen formation, or too much tension at the surgical suture line. A single line of repair under moderate tension fails in a significant number of patients, regardless of adequacy of repair or healing process. Tension is almost always bad in surgery.

35. How long should the patient avoid heavy lifting after a hernia repair?

The standard advice for decades has been 6 weeks. The current advice varies from no limitation with the Lichtenstein or preperitoneal repairs to 6 weeks for a Bassini repair. The self-limitation of pain is an excellent guide.

CONTROVERSIES

36. What are some of the anatomic issues related to inguinal hernias?

At issue is the **iliopubic tract,** which is central to the Anson/McVay anatomic description of the inguinal area and featured in the McVay Cooper's ligament repair. Although the McVay repair is used in England, the iliopubic tract is not referred to or described in English anatomic texts.

The term **conjoined tendon,** although commonly used, is considered by many to be anatomically inaccurate and misleading. The internal oblique and transversus abdominis muscles that make up the conjoined tendon are obvious and can be used surgically either alone or together. The tendinous edge of the transversus abdominis muscle and the tendinous edge of the internal oblique muscle start at their insertion on the pubic tubercle and course laterally and superiorly to the medial edge of the internal ring. At this point, the tendinous elements diminish, leaving only muscle tissues, and continue laterally and superiorly to their origins.

Whether the lacunar ligament or the iliopubic tract defines the medial border of the femoral canal is controversial. The compromise position is that the iliopubic tract is the border whereas in the normal unstretched state, the lacunar ligament (Gimbernat's ligament) is the border in the presence of hernia (stretched state). At surgery it is enough to say that a palpable, visible curved ligament is present and used in some femoral repairs.

37. Do all hernias require urgent repair?

Maybe not. Acute incarceration or strangulation of abdominal contents in a hernia is a surgical emergency. Patients with chronic discomfort benefit from elective repair. However, recent data on men with asymptomatic or minimally symptomatic hernias indicates it may be safe to wait to operate until symptoms worsen. As with any surgical procedure, an individual's risk factors and baseline function need to be considered along with the risk of an operative or nonoperative approach. In the case of hernias, a small percentage of asymptomatic patients for whom elective repair is deferred will develop acute hernia incarceration at some time in the future.

38. What are some surgical issues in the repair of inguinal hernias?

Controversy exists over the use of the laparoscope for hernia repair. Data suggests that laparoscopic repair results in less pain and quicker return to normal activities though longer operative times and higher risk of visceral and vascular complications. Laparoscopic repair requires a much longer learning period to achieve recurrence rates comparable to tension-free open repair with mesh.

BIBLIOGRAPHY

1. Avisse C, Delattre JF, Flament JB: The inguinal rings. Surg Clin North Am 80:49-69, 2000.
2. Avisse C, Delattre JF, Flament JB: The inguinofemoral area from a laparoscopic standpoint. History, anatomy, and surgical applications. Surg Clin North Am 80:35-48, 2000.
3. Bendavid R, Howarth D: Transversalis fascia rediscovered. Surg Clin North Am 80:25-33, 2000.
4. EU Hernia Trialists Collaboration: Repair of groin hernia with synthetic mesh: meta analysis of randomized controlled trials. Ann Surg 235:322-332, 2002.
5. Fitzgibbons RJ Jr, Giobbie-Hurder A, Gibbs JO et al.: Watchful waiting vs repair of inguinal hernia in minimally symptomatic men: a randomized clinical trial. JAMA 295:285-292, 2006.
6. Neumayer L, Giobbie-Hurder A, Jonasson O et al.: Open mesh vs laparoscopic mesh repair of inguinal hernia. N Engl J Med 350:1819, 2004.

CHAPTER 56

BARIATRIC SURGERY

Jeffrey L. Johnson, MD

1. **My patient weighs 250 pounds (114 kg). Is he or she morbidly obese?**
   Maybe. The most widely used definition of morbid obesity uses the concept of body mass index (BMI), which is weight (kg) divided by the height squared (m). This is simply a description of how heavy a patient is for his or her height. A BMI of 40 is considered morbidly obese. A patient who weighs 250 pounds and is 5'6" tall is morbidly obese (BMI = 40), but a patient who weighs 250 pounds and is 6'6" tall is simply overweight (BMI = 29).

2. **Is morbid obesity alone really all that morbid?**
   Yes. Even without overt comorbidities (such as diabetes and hypertension), individuals who are morbidly obese are at substantial risk. Many critical organ systems are affected. For example, in the cardiopulmonary system, obstructive sleep apnea, chronic hypoventilation, and pulmonary hypertension are a common finding. This translates into a higher likelihood of poor outcome after medical or surgical treatment of a wide variety of conditions. Patients who are morbidly obese have a measurably shorter life span. In many ways, it is a potentially lethal condition.

3. **What is "metabolic syndrome"?**
   Metabolic syndrome describes a set of changes in physiology that are associated with high cardiovascular risk. Obesity is a central feature, along with insulin resistance, elevated triglycerides, elevated low-density lipoprotein (LDL) cholesterol, and hypertension.

4. **My patient has a BMI of 40. Because he or she appears so well fed, is it safe to assume his or her nutritional status and wound healing are normal?**
   No. Although their *total caloric intake* is high, it is not uncommon for patients who are morbidly obese to have poor protein intake, poor protein stores, and vitamin deficiencies. Furthermore, concomitant diabetes may contribute to impaired wound healing.

5. **So, if patients who are morbidly obese are sick and do not heal well, why would an otherwise rational surgeon choose to do weight loss operations?**
   Because it works so well. There are few behavioral, pharmacologic, or combined approaches to the treatment of morbid obesity that are proven to promote even short-term weight loss. More pills, programs, and press have *not* resulted in a thinner population. Further, these nonsurgical approaches do not even approximate the amount, or durability of weight loss seen in patients who undergo bariatric surgery. The weight loss after bariatric surgery is substantial and appears to be maintained for at least 15 years.

6. **Do patients who undergo bariatric surgery actually get healthier as they get thinner?**
   Yes. The majority of patients with diabetes, hypertension, urinary incontinence, and obstructive sleep apnea are essentially cured of these ills as they lose weight. Ask an internist when they last cured (not palliated. . .) any of these conditions.

7. **If patients who are morbidly obese have decreased life expectancy, do patients who get bariatric surgery actually live longer?**

It appears so. Two large studies have shown improved survival in patients undergoing surgery to promote weight loss.

8. **Some bariatric operations (like jejunoileal bypass) were abandoned because of metabolic complications. Are there some operations that actually work and are considered safe?**

Yes. The Roux-en-Y gastric bypass (RYGB) has the best long-term safety and efficacy data. Other options include the vertical banded gastroplasty, the sleeve gastrectomy, the laparoscopic adjustable gastric band (lap band), and the duodenal switch.

9. **A Roux-en-Y gastric bypass sounds complicated. What does it entail?**

It is not complicated. The proximal stomach is completely divided to produce a proximal pouch about 50 ml in size. The remainder of the stomach is simply left in place. The proximal small intestine (the roux limb, or alimentary limb) is then divided and attached to the pouch. The small bowel is then reconnected downstream.

10. **Why do patients lose weight after gastric bypass?**

There are three basic reasons. First, the patients cannot eat much at one time. Stop. Reflect for a second . . . 50 ml is 10 teaspoons. This is how much the patients can initially eat (or drink) at a time. It actually becomes *work* to get *enough* protein, calories, and fluids in. Second, the patients cannot (at first), tolerate concentrated sweets. The alimentary limb is made of small intestine that will react to high osmolar loads with dumping syndrome. . . an unpleasant combination of abdominal pain, nausea, sweating, and diarrhea. Thus there is a significant disincentive to "cheating" after gastric bypass. Third, because food in the alimentary limb does not get mixed with bile and pancreatic juice until it meets the other (aptly named biliopancreatic) limb, 75 cm or more downstream, it is not efficiently absorbed.

11. **How much do patients usually lose after gastric bypass?**

Initially, about 70% of their excess weight. This takes place over the first 12 to 24 months. Patients (and doctors) need to understand that it is quite unusual to get all the way down to ideal weight. These operations are not intended to produce fitness models—rather—healthier patients with improved quality of life and improved longevity.

12. **Who are the best candidates for bariatric surgery?**

Most bariatric surgeons use Centers for Disease Control and Prevention (CDC) guidelines, which include BMI (>40, or >35 with weight-related comorbidities), and the ability to understand and comply with the perioperative routine. The latter is extremely important because the patient must relearn how to eat with his or her new anatomy. This operation is not without risk and has significant health and social consequences—imagine going out to dinner when you can eat only 10 teaspoons.

13. **What are the most serious complications of gastric bypass?**

Leak of the gastrojejunal anastomosis is the most feared complication, though it is second to pulmonary embolism as a cause of death in most series. The mortality rate is <1%, but not 0%. Wound complications (hernia, infection) are seen in about 10% of patients undergoing open surgery, and only about 1% in patients undergoing laparoscopic surgery.

14. **What is the most reliable sign of gastrojejunal leak?**

Tachycardia. A heart rate >110 should prompt concern for a leak. Some surgeons order routine contrast studies in all patients.

KEY POINTS

1. Morbid obesity is a serious medical condition that shortens life span.

2. Surgical weight loss promotes improved health and probably lengthens life span.

3. Although there are a number of possible surgical options, gastric bypass is the most tested.

4. Bariatric surgery requires an informed, compliant patient who understands there are significant risks.

BIBLIOGRAPHY

1. Adams TD, Gress RE, Smith SC et al.: Long-term mortality after gastric bypass surgery. N Engl J Med 357:753, 2007.

2. DeMaria EJ, Sugerman HJ, Kellum JM et al.: Results of 281 consecutive total laparoscopic Roux-en-Y gastric bypasses to treat morbid obesity. Ann Surg 235:640, 2002.

3. Hutter MM, Randall S, Khuri SF et al.: Laparoscopic versus open gastric bypass for morbid obesity: a multicenter, prospective, risk-adjusted analysis from the National Surgical Quality Improvement Program. Ann Surg 243:657, 2006.

4. Madan AK, Orth W, Ternovits CA et al.: Metabolic syndrome: yet another co-morbidity gastric bypass helps cure. Surg Obes Relat Dis 2:48, 2006.

IV. ENDOCRINE SURGERY

CHAPTER 57

HYPERPARATHYROIDISM

Christopher D. Raeburn, MD, and Robert C. McIntyre, Jr., MD

1. What is the prevalence of hyperparathyroidism (HPT)?

There are approximately 100,000 new cases of HPT annually in the United States. Women outnumber men by 2 to 1, and the risk increases with age. Primary HPT occurs in 1 in 500 women and in 1 in 2000 men older than 40. Approximately 10% of patients with primary HPT are referred for surgery.

2. What are the symptoms of hyperparathyroidism?

"Painful bones, renal stones, abdominal groans, psychic moans, and fatigue overtones." The classic symptoms and signs are:

Bones: arthralgia, osteoporosis, and pathologic fractures.

Stones: renal stones, renal insufficiency, polyuria, and polydipsia.

Abdominal groans: pancreatitis, peptic ulcer disease, and constipation.

Psychic moans: fatigue, weakness, and depression.

3. What is the most common cause of hypercalcemia in an outpatient as opposed to an inpatient?

HPT is the most common cause of hypercalcemia among outpatients and the second most common cause in the hospital setting. The most common cause of hypercalcemia in hospitalized patients is malignancy. Primary HPT and malignancy account for 90% of cases of hypercalcemia.

4. What is the differential diagnosis of hypercalcemia?

Endocrine:
   HPT.
   Hyperthyroidism.
   Addison's disease.
Malignancy:
   Bone metastasis.
   Paraneoplastic syndromes.
   Solid tumors (squamous or small cell lung carcinoma).
   Hematologic malignancy (myeloma, leukemia, lymphoma).
Increased intake:
   Milk alkali syndrome.
   Vitamin D intoxication.
Granulomatous disease:
   Sarcoidosis.
   Tuberculosis.
Miscellaneous:
   Familial hypocalciuric hypercalcemia (FHH).
   Thiazide.
   Lithium.

5. **What is the essential laboratory evaluation for HPT?**

   Elevated serum calcium (>10.3 mg/dl) should be assessed at least twice. Hypercalcemia must be associated with elevation of intact parathyroid hormone. Serum phosphate levels are low in nearly 80% of patients, and serum chloride is increased in 40% of patients. A chloride/phosphate ratio greater than 33 associated with hypercalcemia suggests primary HPT. Increased alkaline phosphatase levels occur only in the setting of advanced bone disease. Patients with elevated alkaline phosphatase associated with increased blood urea nitrogen (BUN) and creatinine are at increased risk of hungry bone syndrome after parathyroidectomy. A 24-hour urine collection for calcium and creatinine excretion excludes benign FHH. In patients with primary HPT, the 24-hour urine calcium is >150 mg/day versus <100 mg/day in those with FHH.

6. **Describe the embryology and anatomy of the parathyroid glands.**

   The upper parathyroid glands arise from the dorsal part of the fourth brachial pouch along with the lateral lobes of the thyroid. The lower parathyroid glands arise from the dorsal part of the third brachial pouch along with the thymus.

   The average weight of a normal parathyroid gland is 35 to 50 mg. The upper parathyroid gland lies on the posterior portion of the upper half of the thyroid, cephalad to the inferior thyroid artery, and posterior to the recurrent laryngeal nerve (RLN). The normal lower parathyroid gland is found on the lateral or posterior surface of the lower pole of the thyroid gland, caudal and anterior to the point that the inferior thyroid artery crosses the RLN.

   Four glands are present in 89% of patients, five in 8%, six in 3%, and less than four in 0%. The presence of as many as eight glands has been reported.

   The upper parathyroid glands' location is more constant. The most common ectopic sites of the upper glands are posterior to the esophagus or in the tracheoesophageal groove down into the posterior superior mediastinum. The lower parathyroid glands are more commonly ectopic and may be in the thyrothymic ligament, thymus, mediastinum (but outside the thymus), carotid sheath, or within the thyroid (3%).

7. **What are the indications for parathyroidectomy?**

   The 2002 NIH Workshop on Asymptomatic Hyperparathyroidism listed the indications as serum calcium >1.0 mg/dl above the upper limits of normal, 24-hour urinary calcium >400 mg, creatinine clearance reduced >30%, osteoporosis (bone mineral density t score <−2.5 at any site), age <50, and patients in whom surveillance is not possible or desired.

   Careful history indicates the majority of patients (>90%) have symptoms. The treatment of asymptomatic patients with minimal elevation (10.3 to 11.0 mg/dl) of serum calcium is controversial. However, at least four factors favor operation:

   - Patients with untreated primary HPT have an increased death rate caused by cardiovascular disease.
   - Patients with HPT have abnormal quality-of-life scores, and these scores improve to normal after operative success.
   - The cost of parathyroidectomy is equivalent to medical follow-up at 5 years.
   - Experienced endocrine surgeons have a high success rate (=95%) with low morbidity and mortality rates.

8. **Can a patient have hyperparathyroidism and a normal parathyroid hormone level?**

   Yes. A normal parathyroid response to elevated serum calcium is to decrease parathyroid hormone secretion. When serum calcium is high, the parathyroid hormone level should be at the low end of normal. A parathyroid hormone level at the high end of the normal in the setting of hypercalcemia is inappropriately elevated, and this is consistent with HPT. One should rule out FHH by doing a 24-hour urine calcium and creatinine.

9. **What is normocalcemic hyperparathyroidism?**

Occasionally, patients will be identified (often in the work up of osteoporosis) with an elevated parathyroid hormone level but normal serum calcium. The calcium is typically at the upper limits of the normal range. The majority of these patients will have elevated ionized calcium. If the calcium level is low, the diagnosis is secondary HPT which may be the result of vitamin D deficiency.

10. **Outline the traditional surgical strategy of an initial exploration for primary HPT.**

The traditional operation is a bilateral neck exploration to identify all four glands. A meticulously dry, blood-free operative field must be maintained. Tissue in the region of the recurrent laryngeal nerve (RLN) should not be clamped or divided until the nerve is definitively identified. If a solitary adenoma and three normal glands are found, the adenoma is removed, and one of the normal glands biopsied. Frozen-section examination confirms that the tissue is parathyroid but is unreliable to differentiate adenoma versus hyperplasia. Four-gland enlargement (hyperplasia) indicates either subtotal parathyroidectomy (leaving approximately 50 mg of well-vascularized parathyroid tissue in the neck) or total parathyroidectomy with autotransplantation of 50 mg of parathyroid tissue. If a remnant is left in the neck, it should be marked with a nonabsorbable suture or staple. In the setting of hyperplasia, a thymectomy eliminates the possibility of thymic supernumerary glands. If more than one enlarged gland is found in association with normal-appearing glands (double adenoma), all abnormal glands should be removed.

11. **What is the pathology of primary HPT?**

Primary HPT is caused by a single adenoma in 87% of cases; hyperplasia in 9%; double adenoma in 3%; and carcinoma in <1%. In familial HPT, multiple endocrine neoplasia (MEN) syndromes (I and II), and HPT as a result of end-stage renal disease, hyperplasia is the rule.

12. **What minimally invasive alternatives exist to the standard operative approach?**

Focused parathyroidectomy, minimally invasive radio-guided parathyroidectomy (MIRP), and endoscopic neck exploration are new techniques. A focused parathyroidectomy uses preoperative localization to guide a parathyroidectomy, avoiding a bilateral exploration. This approach is combined with intraoperative "rapid" parathyroid hormone assay. The parathyroid hormone is measured by a modified assay before operation and 10 minutes after adequate resection. A postresection level <50% of the preoperative level and within the normal range predicts success. The MIRP uses a sestamibi scan the morning of surgery and an intraoperative gamma probe to guide parathyroidectomy. The ratio of ex vivo radioactivity to background is measured to determine success and, thus, the end of the operation.

13. **What preoperative localization studies are available?**

The single best localization study is the sestamibi scan. Other noninvasive localization studies include ultrasound (US), computed tomography (CT), and magnetic resonance imaging (MRI). Invasive localization procedures include arteriography and venous sampling. The tests are most accurate with a single abnormal parathyroid gland. Localization procedures in cases of hyperplasia may be misleading.

Preoperative sestamibi scintigraphy or US are used to allow a minimally invasive parathyroidectomy.

Localization studies are mandatory before all reoperative parathyroidectomies for persistent or recurrent HPT and in patients with previous thyroid surgery.

14. **How is a sestamibi scan performed, and how accurate is it?**

Sestamibi is a radionuclide that is taken up by the heart, thyroid, salivary glands, and abnormal parathyroid tissue. A standard scan involves administering the sestamibi and performing planar imaging of the neck and upper chest at 30 minutes and 2 to 3 hours later. The radionuclide is typically seen in all of the aforementioned tissues on the early scan but typically "washes out" of the heart and thyroid quickly. For unclear reasons, the radionuclide is retained in the parathyroids longer so any remaining uptake seen on the delayed scan is specific for abnormal parathyroid tissue. The sensitivity and specificity of the sestamibi scan is about 85%.

An alternative approach is to give both Sestamibi and iodine or pertechnatate that is only taken up by the thyroid. The thyroid can be subtracted from the Sestamibi scan and reveal an adenoma. An alternative to planar imaging is single photon emission computed tomography (SPECT) which provides three-dimensional information presented as cross-sectional slices through the patient and can be reformatted as needed.

15. **What should one do if an adenoma is not found in the usual locations?**
Each normal gland should be biopsied for confirmation and marked. Normal parathyroid glands should not be removed. If three normal glands are identified, the surgeon should assess whether the missing gland is an upper or lower one. A missing upper gland often lies in the tracheoesophageal groove, posterior to the esophagus or in the posterior superior mediastinum. The common mistake is that the upper thyroid is not satisfactorily mobilized and dissection is not carried posterior enough. This exploration may require ligation of the superior thyroid artery and vein. The location of a missing lower gland is more variable. First, the thyrothymic ligament should be inspected. The thymus then can be resected through the neck incision. Next, the carotid sheath should be opened. Finally, the thyroid lobe on the side of the missing parathyroid should be palpated or examined by intraoperative US for nodules. If a nodule is found, a lobectomy is done and the tissue examined by frozen section; it may be an intrathyroidal parathyroid gland. A blind thyroid lobectomy is rarely helpful.

A sternotomy should never be done as part of an initial exploration. If the aforementioned maneuvers are unsuccessful in revealing a parathyroid adenoma, the surgeon should stop. A diagram of the location of the identified glands should be made for future reference. Persistent hypercalcemia indicates the need for localization procedures.

The undescended parathyroid is rare (<1%) and is located at or superior to the carotid bifurcation. This area cannot be explored through the standard incision and requires accurate preoperative localization studies.

16. **What is the outcome of surgery for primary hypocalcemia?**
The expected cure rate should be ≈95% for patients undergoing an initial exploration for primary HPT. Symptomatic improvement exceeds 95%. Quality-of-life scores return to normal at 6 months. After parathyroidectomy, 80% of symptomatic patients have improvement in bone density and renal function. Even in asymptomatic patients, urinary calcium and deoxypyridinoline levels decrease. Patients have fewer episodes of nephrolithiasis, gout, and peptic ulcer disease. Parathyroidectomy also appears to improve longevity in patients with primary HPT.

One recent series suggests that the cure rate is lower in a patient that has a negative preoperative sestamibi scans (99.3% versus 92.7%).

17. **What are the complications of parathyroidectomy?**
Permanent RLN injury occurs in <1% of patients; however, a temporary nerve paresis occurs in 3%. Temporary hypocalcemia occurs in 10% of patients, but permanent HPT occurs in only 2% of cases. An elevated preoperative alkaline phosphatase level and abnormal renal function may predict which patients are likely to have "hungry bone" syndrome.

18. **What are the signs and symptoms of hypocalcemia after surgery?**
Chvostek's sign is spasm of the facial muscles caused by tapping the facial nerve trunk. Trousseau's sign is carpal spasm elicited by occlusion of the brachial artery for 3 minutes with a blood pressure cuff.

The earliest symptom of hypocalcemia is perioral numbness or paresthesias typically in the hands or feet. Untreated, severe hypocalcemia can result in carpel-pedal spasm or tetany.

19. **How should patients with hypocalcemia be treated?**
Patients with tetany caused by hypoparathyroidism require emergency treatment with intravenous (IV) calcium to prevent laryngeal stridor and convulsions. One ampule of 10% calcium gluconate (90 mg elemental calcium per 10 ml) should be given in 100-ml saline over 15 minutes followed by an infusion of calcium (5 ampules of calcium gluconate in 500 ml of saline) at 50 ml/h. Maintaining calcium levels of 7.5 to 9.0 mg/dl is adequate. Oral calcium should be started as soon as possible in the form of calcium carbonate (Tums or Oscal) at 2 to 3 g/day in divided doses (3 to 4 times/day). Calcium citrate is preferred for patients with renal lithiasis because the citrate may be prophylactic against renal lithiasis. In most patients, vitamin D preparations increase intestinal absorption and can be given as calcitriol (Rocaltrol), 0.25 to 0.75 mg per day.

20. **Define persistent and recurrent HPT.**
Operative success is defined by long-term normocalcemia. Persistent HPT is defined as hypercalcemia within 6 months of surgery; recurrent HPT is defined as hypercalcemia after 6 months.

21. **What is the strategy for managing patients with persistent or recurrent HPT?**
First, the patient should be reevaluated to ensure that the hypercalcemia is caused by primary HPT and not some other cause. Patients should be evaluated for familial hypocalciuric hypercalcemia, which does not warrant reoperation. The severity of disease is evaluated to ensure that repeat operation is justified. Previous operative notes and pathology reports should be reviewed to assist in planning repeat therapy. Localization studies should be used extensively. Before reexploration, vocal cord function should be assessed in all patients.

Repeat cervical exploration is done through the previous incision. Because the strap muscles are usually adherent to the thyroid, a lateral approach through the plane between the sternocleidomastoid and strap muscles may be used instead of the usual medial approach. With positive localization studies or retrospective determination of the side of the missing adenoma, the dissection may be limited if an adenoma is found.

An alternative to repeat exploration in patients who are well suited is angiographic ablation of parathyroid tissue, which is especially useful for mediastinal adenomas because it avoids a median sternotomy. It is performed by delivering ionic contrast through an arterial catheter wedged into the feeding vessel.

When localization is successful, reoperation for persistent or recurrent HPT is curative in 85% to 90%. Reexploration when localization is unsuccessful has a 50% rate of failure.

22. **Define secondary and tertiary hyperparathyroidism.**
Overproduction of parathyroid hormone (PTH) caused in response to low blood calcium that is caused by another condition is called secondary HPT. The most common causes include vitamin D deficiency, chronic renal failure, calcium deficiency, and disorders of phosphate metabolism.

Tertiary HPT typically occurs after long-standing secondary HP and is characterized by autonomous secretion of PTH causing hypercalcemia. PTH secretion does not respond to calcium or vitamin D administration.

23. **What are the indications for parathyroidectomy in end-stage renal disease?**
The main indications for parathyroidectomy are:
- Severe hypercalcemia.
- Progressive and debilitating hyperparathyroid bone disease.
- Pruritus that does not respond to dialysis.
- Progressive extraskeletal calcification or calciphylaxis that is usually associated with hyperphosphatemia.
- Otherwise unexplained symptomatic myopathy.
- Renal transplant recipients with persistent HPT associated with hypercalcemia and renal insufficiency.

24. **What are the options for surgical treatment of secondary and tertiary HPT?**
Either subtotal parathyroidectomy or total parathyroidectomy with autotransplantation effectively corrects secondary and tertiary HPT.

Subtotal parathyroidectomy is done by excision of all identifiable parathyroid tissue except for 40 to 60 mg of one gland. Disadvantages of subtotal parathyroidectomy include risk of recurrent disease, which is complicated by greater morbidity if repeat neck exploration is required. Total parathyroidectomy with autotransplantation of small amounts of resected parathyroid tissue into the brachioradialis muscle in the forearm has the main advantage of the ease of removing recurrent hyperplastic glands without the added morbidity of neck reexploration.

25. **List the endocrinopathies in MEN I and II.**
MEN I (3 P's):
 Hy**p**er**p**arathyroidism.
 Pituitary adenoma.
 Pancreatic endocrine tumor.
MEN II (3 C's):
 Hyperparathyroidism (**c**alcium).
 Medullary thyroid cancer (**c**alcitonin).
 Pheochromocytoma (**c**atecholamines).

26. **What is the preferred operative approach for HPT in MEN patients?**
HPT develops in over 90% of patients with MEN I. Patients typically have multiple tumors, but they may be asymmetric in size. The preferred operation is subtotal parathyriodectomy with transcervical thymectomy (the most likely location of supernummary glands). Parathyroid tissue can be cryopreserved for subsequent autografting for hypoparathyroidism.

In MEN II, 20% to 30% of patients develop HPT, and multiple tumors are the norm. The HPT tends to be milder than in MEN I. All four glands need to be inspected with resection of only enlarged glands or subtotal parathyroidectomy. Intraoperative PTH levels may help guide resection.

27. **Who performed the first parathyroidectomy?**
In 1925, Felix Mendl performed the first successful parathyroidectomy at the Hochenegg Clinic in Vienna. His patient was Albert, a 34-year-old tram car conductor who could not work because of severe osteitis fibrosa cystica.

28. **Who was Captain Martell?**
An officer in the U.S. Merchant Marine, Captain Martell was the first patient in the United States to undergo surgery for primary HPT. Captain Martell had progressive HPT that reduced his height from 6 feet to a kyphotic 5 feet, 6 inches. After seven operations, the adenoma was finally removed from the mediastinum; however, the captain died in chronic renal failure.

BIBLIOGRAPHY

1. Ambrogini E, Cetani F, Cianferotti L et al.: Surgery or surveillance for mild asymptomatic primary hyperparathyroidism: a prospective, randomized clinical trial. J Clin Endocrinol Metab 92:3114-3121, 2007.

2. Eigelberger MS, Cheah WK, Ituarte PH et al.: The NIH criteria for parathyroidectomy in asymptomatic primary hyperparathyroidism: are they too limited? Ann Surg 239(4):528-535, 2004.

3. Gil-Cardenas A, Gamino R, Reza A et al.: Is intraoperative parathyroid hormone assay mandatory for the success of targeted parathyroidectomy? J Am Coll Surg 204(2):286-290, 2007.

4. Kebebew E, Hwang J, Reiff E et al.: Predictors of single-gland vs multigland parathyroid disease in primary hyperparathyroidism: a simple and accurate scoring model. Arch Surg 2006; 141:777-782.

5. Lambert LA, Shapiro SE, Lee JE et al.: Surgical treatment of hyperparathyroidism in patients with multiple endocrine neoplasia type 1. Arch Surg 140:374-382, 2005.

6. Lo CY, Lang BH, Chan WF et al.: A prospective evaluation of preoperative localization by technetium-99m sestamibi scintigraphy and ultrasonography in primary hyperparathyroidism. Am J Surg 193:155-159, 2007.

7. Nilsson IL, Aberg J, Rastad J et al.: Maintained normalization of cardiovascular dysfunction 5 years after parathyroidectomy in primary hyperparathyroidism. Surgery 2005; 137(6):632-638, 2005.

8. Pappu S, Donovan P, Cheng D et al.: Sestamibi scans are not all created equally. Arch Surg 140:383-386, 2005.

9. Phitayakorn R, McHenry CR. Incidence and location of ectopic abnormal parathyroid glands. Am J Surg 191: 418-423, 2006.

10. Richards ML, Wormuth J, Bingener J et al.: Parathyroidectomy in secondary hyperparathyroidism: is there an optimal operative management? Surgery 139:174-180, 2006.

CHAPTER 58

HYPERTHYROIDISM

Robert C. McIntyre, Jr., MD, and Christopher D. Raeburn, MD

1. **What are the signs and symptoms of hyperthyroidism?**
   General: Heat intolerance, perspiration, flushing, tremor, sleep disturbance, or hair loss.
   Psychological: Nervousness, emotional lability, anxiety, aggressiveness, or delusions.
   Cardiovascular: Palpitations, tachycardia, or supraventricular dysrhythmias.
   Respiratory: Breathlessness or hoarseness.
   Gastrointestinal: Increased appetite, weight loss, or increased frequency of bowel movements.
   Reproductive: Gynecomastia or irregular menses.
   Bone: Osteoporosis.
   Other: Ophthalmopathy or dermopathy.

2. **What are the three most common causes of hyperthyroidism?**
   Graves' disease.
   Toxic multinodular goiter (TMNG).
   Toxic nodule (Plummer's disease).

3. **How should hyperthyroidism be investigated?**
   A thyroid stimulating hormone (TSH) level is the best initial test. A low TSH with a high serum level of free thyroxine (T_4) or triiodothyronine (T_3) is diagnostic. A high TSH with an increase in free T_4 indicates the rare patient with a thyrotropin-producing pituitary tumor. Subclinical hyperthyroidism is a suppressed TSH with a high-normal T_4 or T_3.
   After the diagnosis of hyperthyroidism is made, the radioactive iodine uptake (RAIU) and scan can differentiate the many causes. A high uptake confirms hyperthyroidism resulting from overproduction of thyroid hormone. Uptake is usually measured at 4 to 6 hours then again at 24 hours. Uniform uptake on the scan suggests Grave's disease, patchy uptake is suggestive of a TMNG, and a unifocal area with suppression of the rest of the thyroid is diagnostic of a toxic solitary adenoma. Diffuse, low uptake suggests thyroiditis, which can cause a self-limited course of hyperthyroidism secondary to release of preformed thyroid hormone.

4. **How is the diagnosis of Grave's disease established?**
   Grave's disease can almost always be diagnosed on the basis of the clinical findings. The TSH will be low in association with an increased free T_4. If the free T_4 is normal, a free T_3 level is obtained to rule out T_3 toxicosis. Graves' is an autoimmune disease that results in the production of auto-antibodies that stimulate the TSH receptor (thyroid-stimulating immunoglobulins, TSI). Ophthalmopathy is unique to Grave's disease and is the result of thyroid autoantibodies that cross-react to the extraocular muscles. A RAIU shows uniform increased uptake.

5. **What are the three treatment options?**
   Antithyroid drugs (ATD), radioiodine, and surgery.

6. **Which drugs are useful for the treatment of hyperthyroidism? What are their mechanisms of action?**

   Methimazole (MMI) and propylthiouracil (PTU) are the mainstays of treatment. The goal of treatment is remission of Graves' disease during therapy or euthyroidism before treatment with radioiodine or surgery. Both drugs inhibit organification of iodine and coupling of iodothyronines. PTU also inhibits the peripheral monodeiodination of T_4 to the more physiologically active T_3. Therapy is usually maintained for 2 years. Patients must be monitored for side effects, which include rash, pruritus, hepatitis, cholestatic jaundice, lupus-like syndrome, and the rare but life-threatening complication of agranulocytosis.

   β-adrenergic antagonists ameliorate the signs and symptoms of disease. They should not be used alone except for short periods before radioiodine or surgical therapy. Iodine given as Lugol's solution (5% iodine and 10% potassium iodide in water, 0.3 ml/day) or potassium iodide (60 mg 3 times/day) inhibits the release of thyroid hormone. It is useful for short-term therapy in preparation for surgery, after radioiodine therapy to hasten the fall in hormone levels, and for treatment of thyroid storm. It causes a decrease in perfusion of the thyroid, which may reduce bleeding during thyroidectomy.

7. **What are the indications for and outcome of drug treatment?**

   ATD is reserved for mild hyperthyroidism and a small gland. Almost all patients will become euthyroid within 6 weeks of initiating therapy; however, recurrent hyperthyroidism occurs in 50% of patients when the drug is stopped. Long-term remission only occurs in 30% of patients. Relapse is most common in the first 6 months after cessation of treatment. Side effects of ATDs include agranulocytosis, hepatotoxicity, and rashes.

8. **What is the regimen of radioiodine treatment?**

   Radioiodine is the most common therapy. The usual dose of radioiodine is 10 to 15 mCi for Grave's disease. TMNG is treated with slightly higher doses of 25 to 30 mCi. Older patients and patients with significant comorbidity should receive ATDs before radioiodine to prevent I^{131} induced thyroid storm. Patients with significant eye disease and smokers should receive corticosteroids before radioiodine to prevent progression of ophthalmopathy.

   Pregnancy is an absolute contraindication. Women of childbearing age should be evaluated with a pregnancy test before treatment and should avoid pregnancy for 6 months after treatment.

9. **What is the outcome of radioiodine treatment?**

   Euthyroidism is not achieved for months after treatment. Once euthyroidism is achieved, recurrence of hyperthyroidism is rare. Hypothyroidism, the only serious side effect, is dose dependent. It occurs at a rate of 3% per year, affecting 50% of patients at 10 years, and nearly 100% at 25 years.

10. **What are the indications for thyroidectomy for hyperthyroidism?**

    1. Patients who are pregnant are difficult to treat medically.
    2. Patients with large goiter and low radioiodine uptake.
    3. Children.
    4. Noncompliant patients.
    5. Patients with nodules suspected to be cancer (cold).
    6. Patients with compression of the trachea or esophagus.
    7. Patients with cosmetic concerns.
    8. Patients with ophthalmopathy.
    9. Allergy or significant side effects to ATDs.
    10. Patients with significant comorbidity that need a rapid achievement of a euthyroid state.

11. **How should patients be prepared for surgery?**

Any patient with hyperthyroidism should be rendered euthyroid before surgery. Patients may be treated with antithyroid medication plus potassium iodine. β-adrenergic antagonists also may be used alone or in combination with the above regimen.

12. **What is the extent of thyroidectomy?**

The two surgical options for Graves' disease are subtotal thyroidectomy or near-total thyroidectomy. Near-total thyroidectomy is preferred for coexisiting malignancy and patients with severe ophthalmopathy. The goal of subtotal thyroidectomy is to preserve 4 to 8 g of well-vascularized thyroid tissue to avoid hypothyroidism. Because of the small risk of recurrence (10%), however, some surgeons prefer near-total thyroidectomy. In Plummer's disease, lobectomy or partial thyroidectomy for unilateral lesions and contralateral subtotal thyroidectomy for multiple lesions render the patient euthyroid.

13. **What is the incidence of hypothyroidism after surgery?**

All patients having a near-total thyroidectomy become hypothyroid and need T_4 replacement. Hypothyroidism occurs in 30% of patients following subtotal thyroidectomy.

14. **What is the appropriate treatment for toxic nodular goiter?**

Hyperthyroidism as a result of toxic nodular goiter is permanent and without spontaneous remission; ATDs are not appropriate long-term therapy. Radioiodine is the most common form of therapy. Larger doses (25 to 30 mCi) minimize the risk of persistent hyperthyroidism in such patients, who tend to be older and to have prominent cardiovascular symptoms of hyperthyroidism. Surgery is also quite effective, results in the most rapid achievement of euthyroidism and has a low recurrence rate.

15. **What is the appropriate treatment for hyperthyroidism resulting from thyroiditis?**

Subacute thyroiditis should be suspected if the patient has pain and tenderness in the thyroid region. A RAIU and scan show decreased uptake. The hyperthyroidism is usually mild and of short duration (weeks). Most patients do not need treatment but a β-adrenergic antagonist and salicylate or glucocorticoid are used for symptom control. Hypothyroidism may occur but usually is not permanent.

16. **What is the appropriate treatment for thyroid storm?**

Thyrotoxic crisis should be treated in the intensive care unit (ICU). General measures include hydration, antipyresis (acetaminophen), and nutrition. Specific measures include inhibition of T_4 synthesis and conversion to T_3 with PTU at a dose of 100 mg orally, via nasogastric (NG) tube or rectally every 6 hours. Iodides inhibit T_4 release (saturated solution of potassium iodide, SSKI 5 drops by mouth or NG tube every 6 hours). Steroids (dexamethasone, 2 mg every 6 hours) also inhibit T_4 release and conversion to T_3. β-adrenergic antagonists (propranolol or esmolol) may control cardiovascular manifestations. Other agents that lower thyroid hormone are iopanoic acid, lithium, and potassium perchlorate. The last management option is T_4 removal by plasmapherisis, hemoperfusion, or dialysis.

17. **What surgeon won the Nobel prize for his work with thyroid disease?**

Theodor Kocher won the Nobel Prize in Medicine in 1909 for his work on the physiology, pathology, and surgery of the thyroid gland. He was successful in reducing the high mortality rate of thyroidectomy in the late 1800s. In 1850 the mortality rate was 50%, but by 1898 the mortality rate at Kocher's clinic was 0.18%. His most significant achievement was in describing postoperative hypothyroidism as *cachexia strumipriva*.

WEBSITES

www.endocrinesurgery.org/

www.thyroid.org/

www.aace.com/

BIBLIOGRAPHY

1. Boger MS, Perrier ND: Advantages and disadvantages of surgical therapy and optimal extent of thyroidectomy for the treatment of hyperthyroidism. Surg Clin North Am 84(3):849-874, 2004.

2. Cooper DS: Antithyroid drugs. N Engl J Med 352(9):905-917, 2005.

3. Erbil Y, Giris M, Salmaslioglu A et al.: The effect of anti-thyroid drug treatment duration on thyroid gland microvessel density and intraoperative blood loss in patients with Graves' disease. Surgery 143(2):216-225, 2008.

4. Kang AS, Grant CS, Thompson GB et al.: Current treatment of nodular goiter with hyperthyroidism (Plummer's disease): surgery versus radioiodine. Surgery 132(6):916-923; discussion 923, 2002.

5. Lal G, Ituarte P, Kebebew E et al.: Should total thyroidectomy become the preferred procedure for surgical management of Graves' disease? Thyroid 15(6):569-574, 2005.

6. Palit TK, Miller CC 3rd, Miltenburg DM: The efficacy of thyroidectomy for Graves' disease: a meta-analysis. J Surg Res 90(2):161-165, 2000.

7. Schussler-Fiorenza CM, Bruns CM, Chen H: The surgical management of Graves' disease. J Surg Res 133(2):207-214, 2006.

8. Vidal-Trecan GM, Stahl JE, Eckman MH: Radioiodine or surgery for toxic thyroid adenoma: dissecting an important decision. A cost-effectiveness analysis. Thyroid 14(11):933-945, 2004.

9. Weetman AP: Graves' disease, N Engl J Med 343(17):1236-1248, 2000.

10. Witte J, Goretzki PE, Dotzenrath C et al.: Surgery for Graves' disease: total versus subtotal thyroidectomy—results of a prospective randomized trial. World J Surg 24(11):1303-1311, 2000.

CHAPTER 59

THYROID NODULES AND CANCER

Trevor L. Nydam, MD, and Robert C. McIntyre, Jr., MD

1. **What is the prevalence of thyroid nodules and cancer?**

   The prevalence of thyroid nodules increases throughout life. Nodules are 4 times more common in females than in males. The prevalence is dependent on the method of detection: by palpation 5%, by ultrasound (US) 35%, and by autopsy 50%. After exposure to radiation, nodules develop at approximately 2% annually, reaching a peak at 25 years. Each year in the United States, there are approximately 24,000 new cases of thyroid cancer. Up to 35% of thyroid glands examined at autopsy contain occult papillary cancer (<1.0 cm).

2. **What is the importance of the distinction between solitary and multiple thyroid nodules?**

   Traditionally, multiple thyroid nodules were considered benign, and solitary thyroid nodules were malignant. However, multiple series suggest that a dominant nodule in a multinodular gland carries the same risk of cancer as a solitary nodule (5%). US will often reveal multinodular disease in a gland with a known solitary nodule.

3. **What features of the history and physical examination indicate a higher risk of cancer?**

   Nodules occurring at the extremes of age are more likely to be cancerous, particularly in males. Rapid growth and local invasion raise the possibility of malignancy, but associated symptoms (e.g., hoarseness, dysphagia) are uncommon. A history of radiation exposure increases the frequency of both benign and malignant nodules. A family history of medullary or papillary thyroid cancer or Gardner's syndrome (i.e., familial polyposis) increases the risk of cancer.

   Cancer is more often found in patients with firm, solitary nodules. Fixation to adjacent structures, vocal cord paralysis, and enlarged lymph nodes also are associated with an increased risk of malignancy.

4. **What is the proper laboratory evaluation of a patient with a thyroid nodule?**

   The only biochemical test that is routinely needed is a serum thyroid-stimulating hormone (TSH) concentration to identify patients with unsuspected hyperthyroidism. In patients with suspected medullary thyroid carcinoma (MTC), serum calcitonin should be measured. Patients with MTC should have lymphocyte-derived DNA analysis for *ret* proto-oncogene mutation analysis. In patients with known multiple endocrine neoplasia (MEN) 2, serum calcium levels and 24-hour urine collection for assessment of catecholamines and their metabolic products should be done to evaluate for hyperparathyroidism (HPT) and pheochromocytoma before thyroidectomy.

5. **What imaging should be done in the evaluation of a thyroid nodule?**

   Patients with suppressed TSH (<0.5 μIU/mL) should undergo radioactive iodine uptake (RAIU) and scan to evaluate for hyperthyroidism resulting from Graves' disease, toxic multinodular goiter (TMNG), or an autonomous nodule. Patients with a normal or elevated TSH do not require scanning because this cannot reliably distinguish benign from malignant nodules.

   Thyroid US should be performed on all patients with nodules. It determines if there is a nodule that corresponds to a palpable abnormality, evaluates for other nodules, determines if a nodule is cystic, solid, or mixed, and is the best measure of the size of a nodule. Sonographic features are superior to size for determining risk of malignancy and include microcalcification, hypoechogenicity of a solid nodule, and intranodular hypervascularity. US improves the accuracy of fine-needle aspiration (FNA) biopsy, which should be performed on the nodule that is most concerning.

6. **What is the differential diagnosis of thyroid nodules?**
   Adenoma:
      Macrofollicular (colloid).
      Microfollicular.
      Embryonal.
      Hurthle cell.
   Carcinoma:
      Papillary.
      Follicular.
      Medullary.
      Anaplastic.
      Lymphoma.
      Metastatic.
   Cyst
   Nodular goiter with a dominant nodule
   Other:
      Inflammatory diseases (e.g., Hashimoto's thyroiditis).
      Developmental abnormalities.

7. **Which single test best predicts the need for surgical intervention?**
   The single best test to predict the need for surgery is fine-needle aspiration (FNA). If an adequate specimen is obtained, the three possible results are benign (70%), suspicious (15%), and malignant (5%). FNA is most reliable for the diagnosis of papillary carcinoma and in patients with medullary and anaplastic cancer. It is least reliable in distinguishing benign from malignant follicular and Hurthle cell neoplasms. The overall accuracy exceeds 95% in experienced hands. When FNA reveals cancer, it is 97% correct (3% false-positive rate); when it indicates a benign nodule, cancer is present in 4% of cases (4% false-negative rate). When the FNA is suspicious, 25% of nodules are malignant.

8. **Is levothyroxine treatment useful in the management thyroid nodules?**
   In regions of the world with low iodine uptake suppression of serum TSH to subnormal levels using levothyroxine may decrease benign nodule size. However, in iodine sufficient areas suppression treatment is not recommended.

9. **What are the types and distribution of thyroid cancer?**
      Papillary 80%.
      Follicular 15%.
      Medullary 5%.
      Anaplastic and lymphoma <1%.

10. **What are the axioms of thyroid surgery?**
    - A meticulously dry operative field must be maintained.
    - Tissue in the region of the recurrent laryngeal nerve (RLN) should not be cut or clamped until the nerve is definitively identified.
    - Every parathyroid gland should be treated as if it were the last functioning gland.
    - If malignancy is suspected, the entire operation should be done as if the lesion were cancer.

11. **Define the various types of thyroid procedures.**

   Subtotal thyroidectomy is intended to treat hyperthyroidism and leaves ~4 to 8 g of thyroid tissue to achieve an euthyroid state. A near-total thyroidectomy is used to treat carcinoma and leave less that 1 g of thyroid tissue at the ligament of Berry to avoid RLN injury. This operation has equivalent oncologic outcomes to total thyroidectomy that removes all visible thyroid tissue. However, near-total thyroidectomy may have a lower complication rate than total thyroidectomy.

12. **What is the minimal extent of thyroidectomy for a solitary thyroid nodule?**

   With the exception of small lesions in the thyroid isthmus, the minimal procedure for suspected malignancy should be lobectomy, including the isthmus (as a diagnostic biopsy). Enucleation or nodulectomy is to be avoided. Solitary autonomous nodules should be treated with lobectomy.

13. **What is the surgical therapy for thyroid carcinoma?**

   Thyroid carcinoma should be treated by near-total or total thyroidectomy except in young patients with small, well-differentiated tumors ($=1$ cm), no extrathyroidal invasion, or metastasis to lymph nodes or distant sites. In such cases, lobectomy with resection of the isthmus is adequate therapy. Near-total thyroidectomy eliminates multifocal cancer in the thyroid, allows postoperative radioiodine for the diagnosis and therapy of metastatic disease, decreases the risk of local-regional recurrence, and improves the accuracy of serum thyroglobulin as a marker for persistent or recurrent disease. For papillary carcinoma $\geq$1cm, total or near-total thyroidectomy improves overall survival. Enlarged cervical lymph nodes should be removed and examined by frozen section. If metastatic cancer is identified, a neck dissection is performed. "Berry picking" results in an increased rate of regional recurrence and should be avoided in favor of anatomic dissections.

   Because medullary thyroid cancer is not responsive to radioiodine or levothyroxine, a total thyroidectomy should be performed. A central neck dissection is mandatory to evaluate metastatic disease. If the central nodes are positive for cancer on frozen section, an ipsilateral modified neck dissection is performed. The contralateral neck may be observed.

   Surgery for anaplastic carcinoma is palliative and usually is limited to debulking and tracheostomy for relief of compressive symptoms.

14. **What is the incidence of metastatic disease to the lymph nodes?**

   At the time of the diagnosis of well-differentiated thyroid cancer (WDTC; papillary and follicular), 20% to 50% of patients will have microscopic metastasis if a prophylactic neck dissection is done. However, multiple studies fail to show a significant benefit to prophylactic neck dissection. Multiple authors advocate a central neck dissection at the time of the thyroidectomy in patients with WDTC because the thyroidectomy involves operating within the central neck. However, the risk of hypoparathyroidism and nerve injury may be higher than that of total thyroidectomy alone.

   In medullary thyroid cancer, 80% of patients will have positive nodes in the central and ipsilateral neck. Approximately 50% of patients will have nodal disease in the contralateral neck. Because MTC is radio-iodine and TSH insensitive, surgery is the only therapy and neck dissection is necessary.

15. **Can anything be done to identify patients with nodal disease before the initial operation?**

   US of the neck before thyroidectomy identifies nonpalpable node disease in 20% to 30% of patients and alters the operation performed based on physical examination. US is not sensitive in the central neck when the thyroid has not been removed. It is much more accurate in the lateral neck.

16. **Describe the arterial supply and venous drainage of the thyroid.**

   The blood supply to the thyroid gland comes from the superior and inferior thyroid arteries. Occasionally, a midline thyroid imma artery arises from the aortic arch. The superior thyroid artery is the first branch of the external carotid artery. The inferior thyroid artery arises from the thyrocervical trunk.

The three major veins are the superior, middle, and inferior thyroid veins. The superior and middle thyroid veins drain into the internal jugular vein, and the inferior vein drains into the innominate vein.

17. **Describe the anatomy of the recurrent laryngeal nerves.**
The right RLN arises from the vagus and loops around the right subclavian artery. The left vagus nerve gives off the left RLN and loops around the aorta at the ligamentum arteriosus. The RLNs run obliquely through the neck, usually in the tracheoesophageal groove. Low in the neck, the nerves are more lateral and course medially as they ascend. The right nerve runs more obliquely than the left. Occasionally, the RLN may branch before entering the larynx, usually on the left side. The motor fibers are usually in the most medial branch. In 1% of cases, the right RLN is not recurrent and enters the neck from a lateral and superior direction and is associated with an aberrant right subclavian artery.

18. **What defect results from injury to the RLN?**
Injury to a single RLN results in a paralyzed vocal cord, which causes a weak, hoarse voice. Patients may also have abnormal swallowing and problems with aspiration. Injury to both nerves causes paralysis of both cords and obstruction of airflow. This situation necessitates a tracheostomy. RLN injury occurs in 1% of thyroidectomies.

19. **Describe the anatomy of the superior laryngeal nerve and the defect that occurs with its injury.**
The superior laryngeal nerve gives off the external branch of the superior laryngeal nerve (EBSLN), which runs medial to the superior pole vessels to enter the cricothyroid muscle. This motor nerve (i.e., Amelita Galli-Curci nerve) increases tension of the vocal cords, allowing for high notes. The internal laryngeal nerve provides the sensory innervation to the posterior pharynx. It lies superior to the thyroid cartilage. Injury to the nerve leads to a weak, low voice that lacks resonance. Patients may also have problems with aspiration.

20. **Do patients have voice changes independent of injury to the nerves?**
In the absence of nerve injury, 80% to 85% of patients have a change in at least one voice parameter; however only 40% to 50% of patients report mild voice dysfunction. These early vocal symptoms resolve in most but may persist in approximately 15% of patients. This data is important to discuss with patient before operation.

21. **What is the other major complication of thyroidectomy?**
Temporary hypocalcemia occurs in 10% to 15% of patients, whereas permanent hypoparathyroidism occurs in 3% of patients who have had thyroidectomies.

22. **What are the postoperative therapies for well-differentiated thyroid carcinoma?**
Selected patients should be treated with postoperative radioiodine (I^{131}) for ablation of remnant tissue and distal disease. All patients with WDTC should be treated with levothyroxine (Synthroid) to suppress serum levels of TSH. This three-component therapy (i.e., surgery, I^{131}, and levothyroxine) results in the lowest recurrence rate.

23. **What are the indications for postoperative radioiodine (I^{131}) ablation?**
Recommended for all tumor, node, and metastasis (TNM) stage 2 to 4 disease and selected patients in stage 1 with risk factors. Risk factors include older age (>45 years old), male gender, tumor size, direct local invasion, nodal spread, and distant disease. Postoperative ablation and subsequent monitoring for persistent or recurrent disease requires TSH stimulation. Endogenous TSH stimulation is done with levothyroxine withdrawal. Exogenous TSH stimulation is done with recombinant human TSH (rhTSH).

24. **What is the appropriate degree of thyroid hormone suppression of TSH?**

    Retrospective studies suggest that high-risk patients should have TSH suppressed to <0.1 μIU/ml. Low-risk patients should be maintained at 0.1 to 0.5 μIU/ml (normal = 0.5 to 5.0 μIU/ml).

25. **What is the appropriate method of following patients after their initial course of treatment?**

    Patients with WDTC have a 30% risk of recurrence over 30 years of follow-up. Initially patients are followed at 6- to 12-month intervals depending on their risk stratification. A physical examination is done. TSH, Thyroglobulin (Tg), and thyroglobulin antibody levels should be checked with the patient on levothyroxine. An elevated Tg level with a suppressed TSH is worrisome for recurrence. If the Tg level is undetectable while on TSH suppression, a Tg level is done with TSH stimulation (endogenous or exogenous). An increase in the Tg level with TSH stimulation is also worrisome for recurrence. Fifteen percent to 20% of the population has Tg antibodies that interfere with the Tg assay and can cause either overmeasurement or undermeasurement. US of the neck has largely supplanted iodine scanning to detect recurrence.

26. **What is the appropriate management of patients with metastatic disease?**

    Local or regional disease in the neck is treated by reoperation. Compartment-oriented neck dissection is advocated for regional metastasis. Distant disease should be treated with radioiodine if the metastases take up iodine. Pulmonary micrometastasis should be treated at 6- to 12-month intervals as long as the disease continues to respond. Nonradioiodine avid disease is not benefited by routine treatment. In these patients, follow-up with TSH suppressive therapy is indicated. For selected patients, metastectomy or external beam radiation therapy (EBRT) may provide palliative benefit. Complete surgical resection of isolated bone metastasis should be considered. Alternatives, when metastases are not isolated, are radioiodine treatment or EBRT. Patients with advanced progressive disease that is not radioiodine avid can be entered into chemotherapy clinical trials. If clinical trials are not available, cytotoxic chemotherapy consists of a doxorubicin-based regimen.

WEBSITES

www.acssurgery.com

www.endocrinesurgery.org/

www.thyroid.org/

www.aace.com/

BIBLIOGRAPHY

1. Bilimoria KY, Bentrem DJ, Ko CY et al.: Extent of surgery affects survival for papillary thyroid cancer. Ann Surg 246:375-381, 2007.
2. Brandi ML, Gagel RF, Angeli A et al.: Guidelines for diagnosis and therapy of MEN type 1 and type 2. J Clin Endocrinol Metab 86:5658-5671, 2001.
3. Cooper DS, Doherty GM, Haugen BR et al.: Management guidelines for patients with thyroid nodules and differentiated thyroid cancer. Thyroid 16:109-142, 2006.
4. Haugen BR, Ridgway EC, McLaughlin BA et al.: Clinical comparison of whole-body radioiodine scan and serum thyroglobulin after stimulation with recombinant human thyrotropin. Thyroid 12:37-43, 2002.

5. Ito Y, Miyauchi A: Lateral and mediastinal lymph node dissection in differentiated thyroid carcinoma: indications, benefits, and risks. World J Surg 31:905-915, 2007.

6. Jonklaas J, Sarlis NJ, Litofsky D et al.: Outcomes of patients with differentiated thyroid carcinoma following initial therapy. Thyroid 16:1229-1242, 2006.

7. Leboulleux S, Girard E, Rose M et al.: Ultrasound criteria of malignancy for cervical lymph nodes in patients followed up for differentiated thyroid cancer. J Clin Endocrinol Metab 92:3590-3594, 2007.

8. Lim CY, Yun JS, Lee J et al.: Percutaneous ethanol injection therapy for locally recurrent papillary thyroid carcinoma. Thyroid 17:347-350, 2007.

9. Mazzaferri EL, Robbins RJ, Spencer CA et al.: A consensus report of the role of serum thyroglobulin as a monitoring method for low-risk patients with papillary thyroid carcinoma. J Clin Endocrinol Metab 88:1433-1441, 2003.

10. Mittendorf EA, Wang X, Perrier ND et al.: Followup of patients with papillary thyroid cancer: in search of the optimal algorithm. J Am Coll Surg 205:239-247, 2007.

11. Pacini F, Molinaro E, Castagna MG et al.: Recombinant human thyrotropin-stimulated serum thyroglobulin combined with neck ultrasonography has the highest sensitivity in monitoring differentiated thyroid carcinoma. J Clin Endocrinol Metab 88:3668-3673, 2003.

12. Sawka AM, Thephamongkhol K, Brouwers M et al.: Clinical review 170: A systematic review and metaanalysis of the effectiveness of radioactive iodine remnant ablation for well-differentiated thyroid cancer. J Clin Endocrinol Metab 89:3668-3676, 2004.

13. Stojadinovic A, Shaha AR, Orlikoff RF et al.: Prospective functional voice assessment in patients undergoing thyroid surgery. Ann Surg 236(6):823-832, 2002.

14. Stulak JM, Grant CS, Farley DR et al.: Value of preoperative ultrasonography in the surgical management of initial and reoperative papillary thyroid cancer. Arch Surg 141:489-494, 2006.

CHAPTER 60

SURGICAL HYPERTENSION

Thomas A. Whitehill, MD, and Joel Baumgartner, MD

1. **What are the surgically correctable causes of hypertension?**
   Renovascular hypertension, pheochromocytoma, Cushing's syndrome, primary hyperaldosteronism (Conn's syndrome), coarctation of the aorta, and unilateral renal parenchymal disease. Surgical hypertension accounts for 5% of all hypertensive patients.

2. **Which form of surgical hypertension is most common?**
   Renovascular hypertension is most common. Although the overall frequency of renovascular hypertension among patients with elevated diastolic blood pressure (DBP) is about 3%, moderate or severe diastolic hypertension may be caused by renal artery occlusive disease in as many as 25% of cases. Pheochromocytoma, hyperaldosteronism, Cushing's disease, and coarctation of the aorta each are found in only 0.1% of all patients who are hypertensive.

3. **What are the most common causes of renovascular hypertension?**
   Atherosclerosis causes 70% of cases; it affects men twice as often as women. The second most common cause is fibromuscular dysplasia (25%). Of the many pathologic subtypes, the most common is medial fibrodysplasia (85%); it invariably affects women. Last is developmental renal artery stenosis (10%), which is often associated with neurofibromatosis and abdominal aortic coarctation.

4. **What clinical criteria support the pursuit of investigative studies for suspected renovascular hypertension?**
   Although no clinical characteristics are pathognomonic of renovascular hypertension, the following findings strongly suggest the presence of an underlying renal artery stenotic lesion:
   - Hypertension in very young individuals or in women younger than 50 years of age.
   - Rapid onset of severe hypertension after age 50 years.
   - Hypertension refractory to three-drug regimens.
   - Initial presentation with DBP >115 mm Hg or sudden worsening of presumed preexisting hypertension.
   - Accelerated or malignant hypertension.
   - Deterioration of renal function after the initiation of antihypertensive agents, especially angiotensin-converting enzyme (ACE) inhibitors.
   - Systolic or diastolic upper abdominal or flank bruits.

5. **What is the renin-angiotensin-aldosterone system?**
   Renin is released from the juxtaglomerular apparatus of the kidney in response to changes in renal cortical afferent arteriolar perfusion pressure. Renin acts locally and in the systemic circulation on renin substrate (angiotensinogen), a nonvasoactive α_2 globulin is produced in the liver to form angiotensin I. Angiotensin I undergoes enzymatic cleavage by ACE in the pulmonary circulation to produce angiotensin II, a potent vasopressor responsible for the vasoconstrictive element of renovascular hypertension. Angiotensin II increases adrenal gland production of aldosterone with subsequent retention of sodium and water; this process establishes the volume element of renovascular hypertension.

6. **How do ACE inhibitors work?**

   Direct inhibition of ACE decreases concentrations of angiotensin II, which leads to decreased vasopressor activity and decreased aldosterone secretion. Removal of angiotensin II negative feedback on renin secretion leads to increased plasma renin activity.

7. **Should patients with renovascular hypertension be treated medically or surgically?**

   Although large, prospective randomized studies comparing drug and interventional therapy have not been published, surgical treatment and percutaneous transluminal renal angioplasty (PTRA) have been favored over drug therapy by most physicians. The key is early recognition of the problem.

8. **When should patients with renovascular hypertension be treated with PTRA?**

   Clear indications for PTRA include nonorificial atherosclerotic lesions and medial fibrodysplastic lesions limited to the main renal artery.

9. **What findings on history and physical examination should lead to a suspicion of pheochromocytoma?**

   Pheochromocytomas are tumors primarily of the adrenal medulla and extraadrenal paraganglia cells. Approximately 90% of them are found within the adrenal gland, and the remaining 10% are scattered along the abdominal paravertebral sympathetic chain or in ganglia located remotely (e.g., urinary bladder, pelvic nerves). Tumors are classified as functioning when they produce catecholamines, always autonomously and usually in great excess. The predictable clinical effects of increased endogenous cathecholamine outpouring is sustained hypertension with episodes of increased blood pressure, tachycardia, headache, palpitations, or flushing. Rarely, patients maintain periods of normotension with infrequent and unpredictable paroxysmal episodes of hypertension.

10. **How is pheochromocytoma diagnosed?**

    Diagnosis is best confirmed by 24-hour urine collection for excreted catecholamines, metanephrines, and vanillylmandelic acid. The best single test to confirm the diagnosis of pheochromocytoma is still debated; some believe that the metanephrine level is the most precise (85%). Plasma catecholamines are also a specific test, but given the variability of results in individual patients and in many assays, the current approach should continue to emphasize the use of urinary catecholamines. Eighty percent of patients with pheochromocytoma have at least one urinary metabolite greater than twice the normal value. The diagnosis of pheochromocytoma should be followed by studies to localize the tumor.

11. **What is the best test to localize a pheochromocytoma?**

    Computed tomography (CT) scanning, magnetic resonance imaging (MRI), and I^{131}-metaiodobenzylguanidine (MIBG) scanning are three available imaging modalities. Because 97% of pheochromocytomas are intraabdominal and almost always >2 cm, an abdominal CT scan (thin cuts through the adrenal bed from the diaphragm to the aortic bifurcation) rarely misses a lesion and provides good anatomic detail. MRI has been increasingly used because 90% of pheochromocytomas are characteristically bright on T_2-weighted images. MIBG is best used in patients who are suspected to have extraadrenal, multifocal, or recurrent pheochromocytoma. It is less sensitive than CT and MRI. MIBG is best reserved for patients at higher risk for multiple or extraadrenal tumors and malignant pheochromocytoma.

12. **Describe the immediate antihypertensive treatment in patients with pheochromocytoma.**

Hypertension from pheochromocytoma is caused by activation of vascular smooth muscle α_1-receptors, which results in vasoconstriction. Thus, the best acute treatment is intravenous (IV) administration of an α_1-antagonist or α-blocker; options include phenoxybenzamine, prazosin, or terazosin. Second-line agents include calcium channel blockers and ACE inhibitors. Antiarrhythmic β-blockade should be avoided initially because these agents cause both unopposed peripheral α_1-receptor stimulation and decreased cardiac output (CO; secondary to high vascular resistance). Congestive heart failure may be precipitated by β-blocking the heart before lowering the blood pressure.

13. **How is primary hyperaldosteronism (Conn's syndrome) diagnosed?**

Conn's syndrome, which results from autonomous mineralocorticoid hypersecretion, is characterized by hypertension, hypokalemia, hypernatremia, metabolic alkalosis, and periodic muscle weakness and paralysis, often caused by an aldosterone-secreting adenoma. The syndrome is now identified by the combined findings of hypokalemia, suppressed plasma renin activity despite sodium restriction, and high urinary and plasma aldosterone levels after sodium repletion in hypertensive patients.

14. **Why does Cushing's syndrome or Cushing's disease cause hypertension?**

Both cause hypercortisolism or excessive amounts of glucocorticoids. In the cardiovascular system, glucocorticoids produce increased cardiac chronotropic and inotropic effects, along with an increased peripheral vascular resistance. Receptors in the distal renal tubules respond to glucocorticoids by increasing tubular resorption of sodium. These receptors belong to a different class from receptors that mediate the more potent actions of aldosterone.

15. **What findings suggest aortic coarctation?**

Lower blood pressure in the legs than in the arms and diminished or absent femoral pulses. Rib notching may be evident on chest radiograph in patients with long-standing, hemodynamically significant coarctation. Bruits may be heard over the chest or abdominal wall. Adults may even develop congestive heart failure and renal failure.

16. **How does aortic coarctation cause hypertension?**

No single cause has been identified. Mechanical obstruction to ventricular ejection is one component that leads to upper extremity hypertension. Hypoperfusion of the kidneys with resulting activation of the RAAS probably contributes. Abnormal aortic compliance, variable capacity of collateral vessels, and abnormal setting of baroreceptors also have been implicated.

KEY POINTS: SURGICAL HYPERTENSION

1. The causes of surgically correctable hypertension include renovascular hypertension, pheochromocytoma, Cushing's syndrome, Conn's syndrome, coarctation of the aorta, and unilateral renal parenchymal disease.

2. The most common cause of renovascular hypertension is atherosclerosis.

3. The diagnosis of pheochromocytoma is confirmed by 24-hour urine collection for excreted catecholamines, metanephrines, and vanillylmandelic acid.

4. Conn's syndrome is characterized by hypertension, hypokalemia, hypernatremia, metabolic alkalosis, and periodic muscle weakness and paralysis.

BIBLIOGRAPHY

1. Bloch MJ, Basile J: Diagnosis and management of renovascular disease and renovascular hypertension. J Clin Hypertens (Greenwich) 9:381, 2007.

2. Coen G, Calabria S, Lai S et al.: Atherosclerotic ischemic renal disease: diagnosis and prevalence in an hypertensive and/or uremic elderly population. BMC Nephrol 4:2, 2003.

3. Hansen KJ, Deitch JS, Oskin TC et al.: Renal artery repair: consequences of operative failures. Ann Surg 277:678-690, 1998.

4. Kebebew E, Duh Q-Y: Benign and malignant pheochromocytoma: diagnosis, treatment and follow-up. Surg Oncol Clin North Am 7:765, 1998.

5. Mittendorf EA, Evans DB, Lee JE et al.: Pheochromocytoma: advances in genetics, diagnosis, localization, and treatment. Hematol Oncol Clin North Am 21:509, 2007.

6. Lairmore TC, Ball DW, Baylin SB et al.: Management of pheochromocytomas in patients with multiple endocrine neoplasia type 2 syndromes. Ann Surg 217:595, 1993.

7. Rossi GP, Pessina AC, Heagerty AM: Primary aldosteronism: an update on screening, diagnosis and treatment. J Hypertens 26:613, 2008.

8. Nicholson T: Magnetic resonance angiography for the diagnosis of renal artery stenosis. Clin Radiol 58:257, 2003.

9. Oskin TC, Hansen KJ, Deitch JS et al.: Chronic renal artery occlusion: nephrectomy versus revascularization. J Vasc Surg 29:140, 1999.

10. Palmaz JC: The current status of vascular intervention in ischemic nephropathy. J Vasc Interv Radiol 9:439, 1998.

11. Stanley JC: Surgical treatment of renovascular hypertension. Am J Surg 174:102, 1997.

12. Wong JM, Hansen KJ, Oskin TC et al.: Surgery after failed percutaneous renal artery angioplasty. J Vasc Surg 30:468, 1999.

CHAPTER 61

ADRENAL LAPAROSCOPIC ADRENALECTOMY INCIDENTALOMA

Janeen R. Jordan, MD, and Robert C. McIntyre, Jr., MD

1. **What are the anatomy and secretory products of the adrenal gland?**

   There are two adrenal glands, each located in the retroperitoneum superior to the kidneys. The blood supply consists of three arteries: the superior adrenal artery that is a branch of the inferior phrenic artery; the middle adrenal artery that is a branch of the abdominal aorta; and the inferior adrenal artery that is a branch of the renal artery. The main central vein on the right usually exits the upper one third of the gland and drains directly to the vena cava. The left central vein is longer and drains to the left renal vein. In addition to the central veins, a series of small veins parallels the arteries.

   The cortex has three distinct zones: the zona glomerulosa adjacent to the outer capsule where aldosterone is produced; the zona fasciculata that produces glucocorticoids (cortisol) and some sex steroids; and the zona reticularis that is adjacent to the medulla and produces cortisol, androgens and estrogens.

   - **G**lomerulsa   Salt (aldosterone)
   - **F**asiculata   Sugar (Cortisol)
   - **R**eticularis   Sex (androgens and estrogens)

   The medulla is derived from neural crest cells, acts as a sympathetic ganglion, and secretes catecholamines, specifically, norepinephrine, epinephrine, and dopamine.

2. **What questions need to be considered when an adrenal tumor is identified?**

   Is the tumor functional?
   Is the tumor benign or malignant?
   Is the tumor primary or metastatic?
   Is the tumor cortical or medullary?

3. **What is the incidence of incidental adrenal tumors?**

   An incidental adrenal tumor (incidentaloma) is a clinically inapparent adrenal tumor discovered by imaging done for another indication. These tumors are found in 1.4% to 9% of patients in autopsy series and in 0.4% to 4% of patients undergoing computed tomography (CT) scan of the abdomen. The incidence increases with age, obesity, and hypertension.

4. **What is the differential diagnosis of an incidental adrenal tumor?**

   The differential diagnosis of an adrenal incidentaloma with the reported distribution from multiple series are as follows:

   Adrenal cortex
   - Nonfunctioning adenoma 36% to 94%.
   - Cortisol-producing adenoma (CPA) 2% to 15%.
   - Aldosterone-producing adenoma (APA) 0% to 2%.
   - Adrenalcortical cancer 0% to 25%.

   Adrenal medulla
   - Pheochromocytoma 0% to 11%.

Metastasis
- No past history of cancer 0% to 21%.
- Past history of cancer 32% to 73%.

Other
- Cysts 4% to 22%.
- Myelipomas 7% to 15%.
- Hematoma 0% to 4%.
- Ganglioneuroma 0% to 6%.
- Granulomas 0% to 5%.

5. **What is the function of aldosterone?**

Aldosterone is the principle mineralocorticoid. It increases sodium (Na) and water resorption by the kidney in exchange for potassium or hydrogen. Aldosterone release is stimulated by angiotensin II, which is derived from the renin-mediated conversion of angiotensinogen to angiotensin I that is converted to angiotensin II by angiotensin-converting enzyme (ACE). Renin release from the kidney is stimulated by hypovolemia, β-adrenergic stimulation, and prostaglandins. Hyponatremia and hyperkalemia directly stimulate aldosterone secretion. Aldosterone secretion is also stimulated by adrenocorticotropic hormone (ACTH). Because ACTH has diurnal variation, aldosterone and cortisol levels vary depending on the time of the day.

6. **What is primary hyperaldosteronism?**

Primary hyperaldosteronism (hyperaldo), also known as Conn's disease, is a clinical syndrome characterized by hypertension and hypokalemia (although, 20% of patients may have normal serum potassium levels). Any patient with early onset hypertension that is difficult to control or is associated with hypokalemia should be screened. Between 0.05% and 2.0% of hypertension is caused by hyperaldosteronism. Primary hyperaldo is caused by APA (65% of cases) or primary adrenal hyperplasia. Other less common clinical entities comprising primary hyperaldo include idiopathic, adrenal carcinoma, and glucocorticoid-remediable aldosteronism.

7. **How do you screen for hyperaldosteronism?**

The diagnosis is made in the presence of an inappropriately elevated plasma aldosterone (PA) level with a suppressed plasma renin activity (PRA). Patients must be off diuretics, β-blockers, and ACE inhibitors for 2 weeks. They should consume at least 150 mEq of Na per day and are given potassium supplements. Upright blood samples are collected and a PA/PRA ratio >20 is suggestive. A 24-hour urine aldosterone level 20 mg/day is also suggestive.

  To confirm the diagnosis, a saline load test is often done. A patient is given 2 L of saline over 4 hours. Basal and 4-hour PA, PRA, and 18-Hydroxycorticosterone are obtained. Saline should suppress aldosterone levels but patients with primary hyperaldo will have undetectable PRA with PA levels >15 ng/dl before and after loading.

8. **How do you image the patient with primary hyperaldosteronism?**

Abdominal CT scan will identify lesions >5 mm. Magnetic resonance imaging (MRI) is just as accurate but does not give additional information and is more expensive. Anatomic imaging is unable to differentiate APA from hyperplasia. For that reason patients should undergo adrenal vein sampling (AVS) that can influence management in up to 25% of patients. The ratio of aldosterone on the affected side to the unaffected gland is greater than 10:1. Cortisol is also measured to confirm the samples are in fact from the adrenal veins. The test is often done with and without ACTH stimulation.

9. **What is the treatment of primary hyperaldosteronism?**

Patients with APA should undergo unilateral adrenalectomy. If AVS reveals hyperplasia, Spironolactone (50 to 200 mg twice a day) is the agent of choice. Amiloride is an alternative, and some success is reported with calcium channel blockers and ACE inhibitors.

10. **What is the outcome of unilateral adrenalectomy for APA?**

Seventy percent to 85% of patients will either be cured of hypertension or will have significant improvement and need less drug therapy. Hypokalemia is cured in >90% of cases. Factors that suggest a favorable outcome include young age, shorter duration of hypertension, less severe hypertension, higher creatinine clearance.

11. **What are the common clinical features of pheochromocytoma?**

Pheochromocytomas are tumors of the adrenal medulla that produce catecholamines including norepinephrine, epinephrine, and dopamine. The five P's of the paroxysm are:
- Pressure (high blood pressure).
- Pain (headaches).
- Perspiration (profuse).
- Palpitations.
- Pallor.

12. **What is the "rule of 10" in relation to pheochromocytoma?**

The seven 10's of pheochromocytoma are:
- 10% are malignant.
- 10% are extra adrenal.
- 10% are multiple or bilateral.
- 10% arise in childhood.
- 10% are familial.
- 10% incidentally discovered.
- 10% recur following resection.

13. **What neuroendocrine disorders are associated with pheochromocytomas?**
- Multiple endocrine neoplasia (MEN) IIA: associated with mutation of the RET proto-oncogene. Associated with hyperparathyroidism (HPT) and medullary thyroid cancer. (3 C's: catecholamines, calcium, calcitonin).
- MEN IIB: also associated with mutation of the RET proto-oncogene. Associated with neurogangliomas and medullary thyroid cancer.
- Von Hippel Lindau (VHL) disease: caused by mutations of the VHL tumor suppressor gene on chromosome 3. Pheochromocytomas are accompanied with angiomatosis, hemangioblastomas, renal cell carcinoma or tumors, or cysts of the pancreas.

14. **What is the workup for a pheochromocytoma?**

Screening is done in patients with "spells," resistant hypertension, familial disorders (MEN II, VHL, familial pheochromocytoma), and incidentalomas. The most sensitive screening studies are 24-hour urine metanephrines and catecholamines. Total metanephrines are typically >1000 μg, Normetanephrine >400 μg, and catecholamines are >2 times the normal. The sensitivity is 98% in sporadic cases and 90% including syndromic patients. Specificity is 98%. Recent enthusiasm for fractionated plasma-free metanephrines is a result of the high sensitivity of 97% to 100%, but this test has a lower specificity (85% to 89%) and should only be done in high-risk patients (inconclusive urine studies, vascular adrenal mass, family history, MEN II, VHL).

Imaging should not be done until the biochemical test confirms the diagnosis. 90% are in the adrenals, 98% are in the abdomen, and they are usually not hard to localize. MRI is preferred over CT. If a unilateral adrenal pheochromocytoma is found then ^{123}I-methaiodobenzylguanidine (MIBG) is not necessary. However, if a paraganglioma is found then MIBG is done to evaluate for additional tumors and malignant disease. In patients with negative abdominal imaging consider CT of the head, neck, and chest.

15. **How should a patient with a pheochromocytoma be prepared for surgery?**
α-adrenergic blockade should be started at least 7 to 10 days before operation to control blood pressure and expand the contracted blood volume. Phenoxybenzamine is the preferred agent starting 10 mg every day, twice a day and increasing by 10 to 20 mg in divided doses every 2 to 3 days until control of blood pressure and spells. Patients should be warned about orthostasis. β-blockade should never be started before α-blockade and is indicated for tachycardia associated with α-blockade. Intraoperative hypotension can be controlled with nitroprusside, phentolamine, or nicardipine.

16. **What is Cushing's Syndrome?**
Cushing's Syndrome is a collection of clinical manifestations caused by excess cortisol. Features include:
- Obesity, especially truncal, moon facies, and buffalo hump.
- Thin skin, striae, hirsutism.
- Muscle weakness and wasting.
- Hypertension.
- Menstrual irregularity.
- Osteoporosis.
- Pancreatitis.
- Increased infection risk.
- Depression.

17. **How is Cushing's syndrome different from Cushing's disease?**
Cushing's disease is a result of a pituitary tumor releasing ACTH that stimulates the release of cortisol from the adrenal gland. Cushing's syndrome is the clinical manifestation of the excess cortisol despite the etiology.

18. **What are the causes of Cushing's syndrome?**
Exogenous steroid administration.
Pituitary Cushing's syndrome.
Ectopic ACTH production.
Adrenal CPA.
Adrenal carcinomas.
Adrenal micronodular and macronodular hyperplasia, adrenal hyperplasia.

19. **How can the causes of Cushing's syndrome be classified, and which is most common?**
Overall exogenous Cushing's syndrome is most common. Otherwise, Cushing's syndrome can be classified as ACTH dependent (80%) and ACTH independent (20%):

ACTH Dependent (80%)	ACTH Independent (20%)
Pituitary adenoma (85%)	Adrenal adenoma (>50%)
Ectopic ACTH (15%)	Adrenal carcinoma (<50%)
Adrenal hyperplasia	
Exogenous (common)	

20. **What is the diagnosis modality and treatment for Cushing's syndrome?**
The single best screening test is a 24-hour urinary-free cortisol. Another widely used test is the dexamethasone suppression test. A basal cortisol and ACTH level is done. The diagnosis is suggested with a high cortisol. The patient is given 1 mg dexamethasone at 11 PM and the cortisol is measured at 8 AM. Patients with Cushing's syndrome will have a cortisol >5 mg/dl, and it will not suppress. The dexamethasone suppression test will aid in determining the localization of the tumor. If low-dose dexamethasone is given, cortisol levels will *not* suppress if the tumor is in the adrenal gland. If there is no suppression, the study is repeated with

high-dose dexamethasone (8 mg) that will suppress ACTH secretion from pituitary tumors. Next, ACTH is measured in the plasma. If ACTH is high the tumor is likely extra adrenal. If plasma ACTH is low, this suggests an adrenal cause. Therefore, low plasma ACTH + suppression with *high* dose dexamethasone = adrenal origin.

21. **What is the outcome of resection of adrenal cortisol-producing adenomas?**
    Adrenalectomy results in excellent improvement in the symptoms of Cushing's syndrome and improves patient quality of life. Hypertension and diabetes will resolve in 65% to 80% of patients. The physical changes of Cushing's syndrome will resolve in 85%. These improvements take 6 to 12 months to occur. Exogenous steroids will be necessary for 3 to 36 months after unilateral adrenalectomy. Cosyntropin stimulation studies are done every 3 to 6 months to determine when steroids can be discontinued.

22. **What is the functional evaluation of an incidentaloma?**
    A careful history and physical examination may suggest a particular tumor type and biochemical studies to be performed. Initial tests should include low dose dexamethasone suppression test, 24-hour urine for metanephrines and catecholamines (especially in hypertensive patients), and serum potassium and plasma aldosterone level.

23. **What are the rules of resection for incidentalomas?**
    Incidentalomas with the following characteristics should be resected:
    - All functioning tumors.
    - Tumors >5 cm.
    - Any size tumor with imaging features concerning for malignancy.
    - Tumors that grow with serial imaging.

24. **What imaging features of incidentalomas are suggestive of malignancy?**
    Most adrenal carcinomas are large (>4 cm). Carcinomas may have an irregular shape with unclear margins and be heterogeneous. Necrosis, hemorrhage, or calcification is common. They are usually solitary unilateral tumors with an attenuation of >10 Hounsfield Units (HU) on unenhanced CT scan. They tend to be vascular and have contrast washout <50% at 10 minutes on enhanced CT scan. By MRI, they are hyperintense compared to the liver on T_2 images.

25. **Which tumors or disorders commonly appear as bilateral adrenal masses?**
    Metastatic tumors, hyperplasia (congenital adrenal hyperplasia), and adenomas.

26. **How should adrenal cortical carcinoma be treated, and what is the primary determinant of outcome?**
    In the absence of distant disease open resection aiming at a R0 (R zero) resection is the treatment of choice. In patients not amenable to surgery, mitotane (alone or in combination with cytotoxic drugs) remains the treatment of choice. Commonly used cytotoxic agents include etoposide, doxorubicin, cisplatin, and streptozotocin. Postoperative disease-free survival at 5 years is 30%. Local, peritoneal, or distant recurrence occurs in 70%.

27. **What is Addison's disease?**
    Addison's disease is adrenal insufficiency in which the adrenal gland produces insufficient amount of glucocorticoids and sometimes mineralocorticoids. Clinically, patients present with hyperpigmentation, low blood pressure with hyperkalemia, hypercalcemia, hypoglycemia, and hyponatremia. Addison's disease may be the result of primary adrenal insufficiency, polyendocrine deficiency syndrome, tuberculosis, and amyloidosis. Secondary adrenal insufficiency is the result of reduced pituitary ACTH release. Secondary adrenal insufficiency is usually as a result of panhypopituitarism most commonly from space-occupying lesions in the sella. It is treated by replacement of glucocorticoids and mineralocorticoids (hydrocortisone and fludrocortisone).

28. **What is Addisonian crisis, and how is it treated?**
Addisonian crisis is severe adrenal insufficiency resulting from untreated or undiagnosed Addison's disease. It may also occur as a result of trauma (bilateral adrenal hemorrhage), infection or with the sudden cessation of exogenous glucocorticoids. It presents with dehydration, hypotension, altered mental status, hypoglycemia, and possibly convulsions. It is a medical emergency that can be fatal. The diagnosis is made by cosyntropin stimulation testing. In this test, blood cortisol is measured before and after a synthetic form of ACTH is given by injection. Measurement of cortisol in blood is repeated 30 to 60 minutes after an intravenous (IV) ACTH injection. IV replacement of cortisol, glucose and saline are required for treatment.

29. **What are the relative potencies of steroids?**

	Glucocorticoid	Mineralocorticoid	Duration
Hydrocortisone	1.0	1.0	Short
Cortisone	0.7	0.7	Short
Prednisone	4.0	0.7	Short
Methylprednisolone	5.0	0.5	Short
Dexamethasone	30.0	0.0	Long
Fludrocortisone	10.0	400.0	Long

30. **Which U.S. President had Addison's disease?**
John F. Kennedy was officially diagnosed with Addison's disease in 1947. However, he may have been diagnosed much earlier than has been commonly thought. At that time Addison's disease was classically described as being caused by tuberculosis which Kennedy never had. When Lyndon B. Johnson's campaign made reference to Kennedy's Addison's disease using it as an argument against his nomination for president, Kennedy's campaign countered that he never had the disease.

BIBLIOGRAPHY

1. Allolio B, Fassnacht M: Adrenocortical carcinoma: clinical update. J Clin Endocrinol Metab 91:2027-2037; 2006.

2. Annane D, Maxime V, Ibrahim F et al.: Diagnosis of adrenal insufficiency in severe sepsis and septic shock. Am J Respir Crit Care Med 174(12):1319-1326, 2006.

3. Barnett CC Jr, Varma DG, El-Naggar AK et al.: Limitations of size as a criterion in the evaluation of adrenal tumors. Surgery 128(6):973-982; discussion 982-983, 2000.

4. Brunt LM, Moley JF: Adrenal incidentaloma. World J Surg 25(7):905-913, 2001.

5. Goldstein RE, O'Neill JA Jr, Holcomb GW 3rd et al.: Clinical experience over 48 years with pheochromocytoma. Ann Surg 229(6):755-764; discussion 764-766, 1999.

6. Gonzalez RJ, Tamm EP, Ng C et al.: Response to mitotane predicts outcome in patients with recurrent adrenal cortical carcinoma. Surgery 142(6):867-875; discussion 867-875, 2007.

7. Grumbach MM, Biller BM, Braunstein GD et al.: Management of the clinically inapparent adrenal mass ("incidentaloma"). Ann Intern Med 138(5):424-429, 2003.

8. Kudva YC, Sawka AM, Young WF Jr: Clinical review 164: the laboratory diagnosis of adrenal pheochromocytoma: the Mayo Clinic experience. J Clin Endocrinol Metab 88(10):4533-4539, 2003.

9. Porterfield JR, Thompson GB, Young WF Jr et al.: Surgery for Cushing's syndrome: an historical review and recent ten-year experience. World J Surg 32:659-677, 2008.

10. Quayle FJ, Spitler JA, Pierce RA et al.: Needle biopsy of incidentally discovered adrenal masses is rarely informative and potentially hazardous. Surgery 142(4):497-502; discussion 502-504, 2007.

11. Sawka AM, Young WF, Thompson GB et al.: Primary aldosteronism: factors associated with normalization of blood pressure after surgery. Ann Intern Med 135(4):258-261, 2001.

12. Sprung CL, Annane D, Keh D et al.: Hydrocortisone therapy for patients with septic shock. N Engl J Med 358(2):111-124, 2008.

13. Tan YY, Ogilvie JB, Triponez F et al.: Selective use of adrenal venous sampling in the lateralization of aldosterone-producing adenomas. World J Surg 30(5):879-885; discussion 886-887, 2006.

14. Terzolo M, Angeli A, Fassnacht M et al.: Adjuvant mitotane treatment for adrenocortical carcinoma. N Engl J Med 356(23):2372-2380, 2007.

15. Young WF Jr: Clinical practice. The incidentally discovered adrenal mass. N Engl J Med 356(6):601-610, 2007.

BREAST MASSES

Ann Marie Kulungowski, MD, and Christina A. Finlayson, MD

1. What are the three parts of breast screening that assist in the early diagnosis of breast cancer?

Breast self-examination (BSE) should begin at age 20 and be performed monthly. The breast is usually easiest to examine on the days immediately following the menstrual cycle. BSE can be frustrating to patients, particularly when they have fibrocystic change because they are not certain what they are feeling or supposed to feel. The technique of BSE should be taught early and reinforced regularly. If a palpable tumor develops, women who regularly perform BSE present with tumors 1 cm or smaller more frequently than women who do not perform BSE. Improvement in survival from breast cancer has not been demonstrated, however. Some women should not practice BSE because of the psychological trauma they suffer from repetitive false-positive findings. Those women need to rely on their physician to do a breast examination once or twice a year.

Clinical or physician breast examination (CBE) also should begin at age 20 and be performed annually for women at average risk for breast cancer. Although tumors between 0.5 cm and 1.0 cm occasionally can be detected by an experienced physician, tumors between 1.0 and 1.5 cm can be detected 60% of the time. As the tumor grows, 96% of tumors larger than 2.0 cm can be identified on physician physical examination. Clinical breast examination should be part of the primary care physician's health maintenance and screening program.

Screening mammography has had the most substantial impact on the early diagnosis of, and subsequent decrease in mortality from, breast cancer.

2. When should routine mammography begin?

All major U.S. medical organizations currently recommend that women who are at average risk for the development of breast cancer should begin mammography screening at age 40. Mammography should be performed annually. This screening regimen will result in a 30% or greater decrease in death from breast cancer. Women with a family history of early breast cancer should begin screening mammography 10 years before the age that the youngest first-degree family member was diagnosed with breast cancer.

3. Does a normal or negative mammogram guarantee that no cancer is present?

No. Mammography has a false-negative rate of at least 15%. For a breast cancer to be detected on mammography, it must have tissue characteristics that are different from the surrounding tissue. Some tumors, particularly lobular carcinoma, invade the surrounding breast tissue in a way that does not alter the characteristics of the breast tissue. Such tumors are often not visible on mammogram.

4. What is the role of screening magnetic resonance imaging as an adjunct to mammography?

American Cancer Society guidelines published in 2007 recommend screening magnetic resonance imaging (MRI) for women with a greater than 20% lifetime risk of developing breast cancer. This includes women who have a strong family history of breast or ovarian cancer and women who have received chest radiation for Hodgkin's disease as teenagers or young adults. Annual screening MRI should be added for women who have a BRCA mutation, women who have not been tested for BRCA mutations but have a first-degree relative with a BRCA mutation, or women who have a lifetime risk of greater than 20% determined by BRCAPRO or other statistical models that predict risk. Annual MRI screening is also recommended for women with Li-Fraumeni, Cowden, or Bannayan-Riley-Ruvalcaba syndromes and their first-degree relatives.

Currently there is insufficient evidence to recommend for or against screening in MRI in women with a lifetime risk 15% to 20%, lobular carcinoma in situ or atypical lobular or ductal hyperplasia with an associated family history, heterogeneously dense breasts by mammography, or women with a history of breast cancer, including ductal carcinoma in situ (DCIS). MRI screening is not recommended for any women with less than a 15% lifetime risk of breast cancer.

MRI is quite sensitive for identifying breast cancer but is criticized for having a lower specificity that leads to additional imaging and biopsies to further characterize lesions that prove to be false-positives. As with all diagnostic studies, the need for additional evaluation must be weighed against the benefit of finding an occult breast cancer. The ability to detect cancer by MRI is strongly influenced by the quality of the image and the radiologist's familiarity with reading breast MRI. Breast MRI should only be done in facilities that have the capability to evaluate any abnormalities that are found including the ability to perform MRI-guided biopsy. MRI should be used in conjunction with mammography and is not an independent screening modality for breast cancer.

5. **What is the role of ultrasound in the diagnosis of breast cancer?**
   To date, ultrasound (US) has been used as an adjunct to further evaluate abnormalities found on mammography and physical examination but is not used as a screening tool. US can distinguish benign simple cysts from solid masses or complex cysts. It is particularly valuable in young women in which the density of the breast tissue limits the value of mammography. If a patient with a complaint of a palpable mass that has benign characteristics on physician physical examination has a negative targeted US, the negative predictive value for cancer is 99.8%.

6. **What is the difference between a screening and a diagnostic mammogram?**
   Screening mammography is done in asymptomatic women to look for clinically occult breast cancer. Two views of each breast are obtained. When a woman has a breast complaint, such as a mass or an abnormal screening mammogram, diagnostic mammography is performed. A diagnostic mammogram pays particular attention to the area of clinical concern. Additional views taken at multiple angles or compression views taken with increased magnification of the abnormality help to distinguish between benign and malignant changes.

7. **How are mammographic abnormalities characterized?**
   The American College of Radiography has developed a standard interpretation score to decrease ambiguity in mammographic reporting:
   Bi-Rads
   0 Requires further evaluation.
   1 Negative (normal examination without any findings).
   2 Benign (normal examination with a definitely benign finding).
   3 Probably benign (<3% chance of malignancy).
   4 Suspicious (30% chance of malignancy).
   5 Highly suspicious or malignant.
   - **Category 0** is a temporary designation that requires further diagnostic imaging by either US or compression (magnification) views of the abnormality. After further evaluation, such mammograms are reclassified into one of the other categories.

- **Categories 1 and 2** require no further evaluation; the usual mammographic schedule is not altered.
- For **category 3**, a short-interval (6-month) diagnostic mammogram of the affected breast is recommended. Alternatively, a biopsy may be performed.
- **Categories 4 and 5** require a biopsy.

8. **Which biopsy techniques aid in the diagnosis of mammographic abnormalities?**

Several image-guided biopsy techniques maximize diagnostic yield while minimizing patient discomfort and loss of normal tissue:

Tru-cut core biopsy is performed with a 14- to 18-gauge coring needle. Several tissue samples (at least seven) are obtained.

Mammotome biopsy is performed with an 11-gauge vacuum-assisted biopsy needle. Mammotome can remove an entire lesion or area of calcification. A marking clip can be left in the breast at the site of the abnormality. Core biopsy and mammotome can be performed with local anesthesia alone.

The **advanced breast biopsy instrument** (ABBI) removes up to a 2-cm core of breast tissue. It usually requires local anesthesia and mild sedation and usually is performed in the operating room (OR).

Needle localization breast biopsy is a surgical procedure requiring the radiologist to place a thin wire into the breast at the site of the abnormality. In the OR, the wire and the breast tissue surrounding the wire are removed. This procedure can be done with local anesthesia with or without sedation.

Although **fine needle aspiration** (FNA) is excellent for evaluation of palpable abnormalities, its sensitivity and specificity for image-guided biopsy are not acceptable.

With the exception of FNA, each of these techniques has an equivalent success rate in identifying the pathology associated with the mammographic abnormality. A 5% false-negative rate is associated with each of these techniques.

9. **What are the characteristics of a dominant breast mass?**

Identification of a dominant mass, especially in premenopausal women, can be challenging. Typically, a dominant mass can be palpated in three dimensions, and its density is distinct from surrounding breast tissue. Symptoms of equal importance are nodule, lump, thickening, and asymmetry. Breast cancer cannot be excluded by physical examination alone. "Failure to be impressed by physical examination findings" is the most common reason cited for a delay in the diagnosis of breast cancer.

10. **What are the four most frequently encountered palpable breast masses?**

Most dominant masses are benign. Examples include cysts, fibroadenomas, and fibrocystic masses. Carcinoma, although not the most common form of breast mass, is the reason that all persistent, dominant masses require a diagnosis. Other less common causes of palpable breast masses are lipomas, granulomas, fat necrosis, epidermal inclusion cysts, and lactational adenomas.

11. **What are the differential characteristics of the most common palpable masses?**

A **cyst** is a regular, mobile mass that may be tender. It may be quite firm or fluctuant. A **fibroadenoma** is usually smooth, firm, elongated (longer than it is wide), and mobile with discrete borders. **Fibrocystic changes** often are described as "lumpy-bumpy" breast tissue. There may be a discrete focal area of fibrosis that is more dominant than the background irregular tissue.

Carcinoma is an irregular, hard, painless mass. In advanced stages it may become fixed to the chest wall or be associated with overlying skin changes. Although this is the classic presentation, carcinoma may present in a form similar to benign lesions. Lobular carcinoma often appears as a soft mass or area of thickening. Because physical examination alone is unreliable in definitively excluding breast cancer, a biopsy must be obtained for all persistent, dominant solid masses.

12. **A 32-year-old woman presents with the complaint of a breast lump. Which questions about the patient's history are important in the evaluation of the mass?**

The size of the mass, whether it has changed in size, how long it has been present, whether it is painful, skin changes, nipple discharge, or changes in relation to the menstrual cycle may be helpful. Evaluation of any breast condition includes an assessment of risk factors for breast cancer, including personal or family history of breast, ovarian, or other cancers; age at menarche; age at first full-term pregnancy; age at menopause, if applicable; birth control or hormone replacement use; and history of previous breast biopsy.

13. **The mass identified in question 10 is discrete, not tender, easily palpable, and has gradually increased in size. What is the most appropriate next step?**

Breast imaging can be useful in further defining the characteristics of a breast mass. US of a discrete mass can determine if it is cystic or solid. There are specific US criteria for defining a simple cyst. A simple cyst can be aspirated or observed. A complex cyst must be further evaluated by aspiration (to see if it completely resolves) or by excisional biopsy. With a complex cyst, FNA or core biopsy has a higher risk of sampling error of the solid component. A solid mass requires a tissue diagnosis.

14. **How is a cyst aspiration performed?**

A 22-gauge needle is inserted into the cyst, and fluid is withdrawn. Generally, a 10-ml syringe is adequate, although occasionally cysts contain larger amounts of fluid. If the cyst is quite deep and difficult to fix between the physician's fingers, the aspiration can be performed under US guidance. Aspiration of a cyst is both diagnostic and therapeutic. After aspiration, the mass should resolve completely. If a mass persists or recurs after two aspirations, it should be excised. Cyst fluid may be clear or cloudy yellow, green, gray, or brown. A purely blood aspirate or an aspirate of what appears to be old blood should be sent for cytology, and excision of the lesion should be performed.

15. **What techniques are available for diagnosis of a palpable, solid breast mass?**

FNA, core biopsy, incisional biopsy, and excisional biopsy have a role in diagnosing palpable breast masses. Which technique is used depends on the nature of the lesions and available technical support.

FNA recovers cells from the mass and requires a dedicated cytopathologist for accurate interpretation. Several benign and malignant lesions can be characterized accurately by FNA, but FNA cannot discriminate between invasive and in situ carcinoma. To be used effectively, it must be correlated with physical examination and breast imaging.

Core biopsy is also a sampling technique that removes 14- to 18-gauge pieces of tissue for histologic evaluation by the pathologist. Because it is a sampling, there is a risk of missing the lesion and obtaining a false-negative result. Again, correlation with physical examination and imaging is important to avoid failure to diagnose a breast cancer.

Incisional biopsy is rarely used today. It has a role when a highly suspicious lesion that is a candidate for neoadjuvant treatment fails to be definitively diagnosed on core biopsy.

Excisional biopsy completely removes the target lesion. It provides the most tissue for pathologic evaluation and, in benign disease, is both diagnostic and therapeutic.

16. **What is the role for breast imaging in the evaluation of a palpable breast mass?**

Breast imaging helps to define the lesion and screens the remainder of the breast for secondary lesions. In general, breast imaging is done before biopsy because the artifact from the biopsy can interfere with the interpretation of the study.

In women younger than 30, in whom the risk of malignancy is low, mammography should be reserved for the most suspicious lesions. For women over 30, evaluation of a mass suspicious for malignancy includes mammography to characterize the mass and evaluate the remainder of the breast. US can reliably differentiate between cystic and solid masses. It is quite unusual (less than 2%) that US will fail to identify a clinically significant breast mass. A cyst aspiration or biopsy can be performed accordingly.

17. What is the "triple-negative test" or "diagnostic triad"?

There are three components to diagnosing a palpable breast abnormality: physical examination, breast imaging, and biopsy. Benign lesions do not have to be removed, but the difficulty is in differentiating between a benign and a malignant lesion. When the characteristics of a mass on physical examination indicate low suspicion for malignancy, the mammogram is benign, and FNA recovers benign cells, the likelihood that the lesion is benign is 98%. Treatment options include excision for definitive diagnosis or observation. If observation is elected, the abnormality should be reexamined within 3 months to confirm that it is stable. If any component of the diagnostic triad is worrisome, definitive diagnosis, usually with excisional biopsy, is necessary.

BIBLIOGRAPHY

1. Elmore JG, Armstrong K, Lehman CD et al.: Screening for breast cancer. JAMA 293:1245-1256, 2005.

2. Geller BM, Barlow WE, Ballard-Barbash R et al.: Use of the American College of Radiology BI-RADS to report on the mammographic evaluation of women with signs and symptoms of breast disease. Radiology 222:536-542, 2002.

3. Hendrick RE: Mortality reduction from screening mammography. Breast Dis 13:303-307, 2003.

4. Mendelson, EB: Problem-solving ultrasound. Radiol Clin N Am 42:909-918, 2004.

5. Pruthi S, Brandt KR, Degnim AC et al.: A multidisciplinary approach to the management of breast cancer, part 1: prevention and diagnosis. Mayo Clin Proc 82:999-1012, 2007.

6. Saslow D, Boetes C, Burke W et al.: American Cancer Society guidelines for breast screening with MRI as an adjunct to mammography. CA Cancer J Clin 57:75-89, 2007.

7. Yang W, Dempsey P: Diagnostic breast ultrasound: current status and future directions. Radiol Clin N Am 45:845-861, 2007.

CHAPTER 63

PRIMARY THERAPY FOR BREAST CANCER

Kristine E. Calhoun, MD, and Benjamin O. Anderson, MD

1. **How is breast cancer diagnosed?**

   A breast cancer diagnosis requires tissue confirmation by needle sampling or surgical biopsy. Historically, **excisional biopsy** was the gold standard, but needle sampling has become the preferred initial diagnostic method using **core needle biopsy** or, if an expert breast cytologist is available to interpret the specimen, **fine needle aspiration** (FNA). Needle sampling (1) allows complete operative planning, including decisions about lumpectomy or the use of sentinel node mapping and (2) does not distort the breast shape or architecture for future clinical breast examination (CBE) and breast imaging.

2. **What are the limitations of needle sampling?**

   Both FNA and core-needle biopsy can have false-negative results caused by sampling error. If the needle sampling diagnosis is negative for cancer and these findings correlate with the clinical presentation and breast imaging findings (mammogram and ultrasound [US]), all of which suggest a benign breast process **(concordance)**, the patient may have clinical follow-up examination without further intervention. However, if the needle sampling results do not match the findings from clinical examination or breast imaging **(discordance)**, additional tissue sampling, such as excisional biopsy, needs to be performed.

3. **How do fine needle aspiration and core needle biopsy differ?**

   FNA cytology is technically simple to perform, can be read immediately, and costs only pennies. However, FNA cytology requires an expert cytologist for correct interpretation and cannot be used to distinguish noninvasive (in situ) from invasive cancer. By contrast, core needle biopsy (using standard 14-gauge or large bore 8-gauge vacuum-assisted sampling) obtains true histology specimens that functionally resemble miniature surgical biopsies but do not distort the breast tissue or leave large scars after healing. Core needle biopsy can distinguish invasive from noninvasive cancer, ductal from lobular histology, and high-grade from low-grade disease. Special sections of core needle biopsy specimens can be prepared for immunohistochemistry (IHC) staining to determine estrogen receptor (ER), progesterone receptor (PR) status and Her-2/neuoncogene overexpression. A pathologist skilled in reading standard surgical breast slides should also be comfortable reading breast core-needle slides, but may not be comfortable interpreting a breast FNA. Because of its versatility and the relative paucity of breast cytology expertise, core needle biopsy has largely become the standard in the United States.

4. **Why should the breast be imaged before performing a surgical breast biopsy?**

   Breast cancer typically starts as clinically occult disease that gradually becomes palpable as the cancer evolves and grows in the breast. Even experienced surgeons can be surprised to find that seemingly small palpable cancers can be much more extensive in the breast than anticipated based on CBE alone. Preoperative imaging helps surgeons optimize surgical outcomes by avoiding these surprises.

The mammogram is the surgeon's road map, illustrating the distribution of fatty and dense tissues within the breast and simultaneously identifying additional lesions in the same or opposite breast. Breast US is good for visualizing a specific lesion or palpable mass within the breast and can be used to guide needle sampling. Breast magnetic resonance imaging (MRI) is currently used by many cancer centers to assess extent of disease beyond what is seen on standard imaging once cancer is already diagnosed.

5. **Does a delay between biopsy and definitive treatment adversely affect cure?**
No, if the delay is only for days or weeks. In general, breast cancers evolve slowly, treatment should be initiated within 3 to 4 weeks of initial diagnosis. Delays of longer than 3 to 6 months should be avoided. There is more urgency with pregnancy-associated breast cancer, in which tumor growth can be much more rapid. It is not appropriate to delay the treatment of a breast cancer until the end of pregnancy, particularly when some chemotherapeutic agents (e.g., doxorubicin [Adriamycin]) can be safely given during pregnancy.

6. **How is breast cancer staged?**
See Table 63-1.

TABLE 63-1. STAGING OF BREAST CANCER

TNM	Histology	Tumor Size	Nodal Metastases	Distant Metastases
0	Noninvasive	Any	—	—
I	Invasive	≤2 cm (T1)	No (N0)	No
IIA	Invasive	≤2 cm (T1)	Yes, 1–3 (N1)	No
		2–5 cm (T2)	No (N0)	No
IIB	Invasive	2–5 cm (T2)	Yes, 1–3 (N1)	No
		>5 cm (T3)	No (N0)	No
IIIA	Invasive	<2 cm (T1)	Yes, 4–9 (N2)	No
		2–5 cm (T2)	Yes, 4–9 (N2)	No
		>5 cm (T3)	Yes, 1–3 (N1)	No
		>5 cm (T3)	Yes, 4–9 (N2)	No
IIIB	Invasive	Involved muscle or skin (T4)	No/Yes (N0, N1, N2)	No
IIIC	Invasive	Any size (Any T)	Yes, 10+ (N3)	No
IV	Invasive	Any size	Yes or no	Yes

7. **Why is staging of breast cancer important?**
Breast cancer stage correlates with likelihood of relapse and fatality. Tumor, node, and metastasis (TMN) staging summarizes data about tumor size, axillary node metastases, and distant metastases. Stage 0 cancers are noninvasive cancers (e.g., ductal carcinoma in situ [DCIS]); stage I breast cancers are small node-negative invasive cancers; stage II cancers are intermediate-sized cancers with or without axillary nodal metastases; stage III cancers are locally advanced cancers, usually with axillary nodal metastases; and stage IV cancers are those that have already metastasized to distant sites.

8. **What is the overall survival rate after definitive multimodality treatment?**
   Stage 0 (DCIS): Nearly 100% 10-year overall disease-specific survival rate.
   Stage I: 90% 10-year overall disease-specific survival rate.
   Stage II: 75% 10-year overall disease-specific survival rate.
   Stage III: 40% 10-year overall disease-specific survival rate.
   A gradual incremental improvement in breast cancer survival over recent years has been attributed to earlier detection and improved systemic therapy. Cytotoxic chemotherapy (e.g., CMF, Adriamycin, paclitaxel [Taxol]) for hormone-receptor negative cancers, hormonal therapy (e.g., tamoxifen, aromatase inhibitors) for hormone-receptor positive cancers, and biologic therapy (e.g., herceptin for Her-2/neuoncogene overexpressing cancers) have improved disease-free and overall survival in breast cancer patients, even those with advanced disease.

9. **What is the difference between noninvasive (in situ) and invasive breast cancers?**
   Noninvasive (in situ) cancers are lesions in which the malignant cells remain confined to the duct or lobule in which they originated. In situ cancers have minimal chance of spreading to nodes or distant sites. Invasive cancers have traversed the basement membrane of their originating duct or lobule and concomitantly may have developed metastatic potential. In situ cancers have cells that are largely biologically incompetent and are unable to establish growth in distant tissues, so even if cells from these early cancers "escape" from the duct or are pushed into surrounding tissues during needle sampling, they remain unable to create metastatic disease. Thus, the primary reason for treating in situ cancer is to stop it from transforming into invasive cancer that does have the potential to spread to distant sites. Complete lymph node dissection is not warranted for in situ lesions. Sentinel node mapping, however, may be used in conjunction with surgical treatment of DCIS, when the patient is going to undergo mastectomy or if invasive cancer is also suspected.

10. **Where does invasive breast cancer spread (other than to lymph nodes)? Which diagnostic tests are useful for identifying such metastases?**
    Breast cancer can spread to the bones, lung, liver, peritoneal surfaces, and brain. **Bone scans** are quite sensitive but less specific for bone metastases. Standard radiographs help distinguish metastases from benign inflammatory conditions. Lung metastases are identified by **chest radiographs** or **computed tomography (CT) scan.** Liver metastases can be identified using **liver function tests** (LFTs), but these tests are neither specific nor sensitive, with 25% of breast cancer patients with documented liver metastases having normal LFT results. Liver imaging tests (abdominal CT, US, or MRI) are more expensive but more reliable. Brain metastases are imaged by **head CT** or **MRI scanning,** but only in the symptomatic patient.

11. **Which tests should be obtained before surgery to screen for metastases?**
    All patients with symptoms suggesting metastatic disease (bone pain, pulmonary symptoms, jaundice, seizures, or focal neurologic symptoms) should be fully evaluated after invasive breast cancer has been diagnosed.
    A standard minimal preoperative workup for invasive disease consists of a **chest radiograph** and **LFTs.** In reality, the utility of these tests among early-stage cancers is low. Routine chest radiography identifies unsuspected lung metastases in <1% of patients. Chest radiography often is justified for preoperative planning and is useful as a baseline test for future comparison. The measurement of circulating tumor markers (CEA, CA-125, etc.) is of little or no value in most circumstances and should be discouraged.

12. **What are the alternatives for primary surgical treatment of invasive breast cancer?**
    1. Mastectomy
       A. Modified radical mastectomy (MRM): Modified radical mastectomy (removal of the breast and the level 1, level 2 axillary lymph nodes), has replaced radical mastectomy

(removal of breast, lymph nodes, and pectoralis muscle) as the standard of care for patients with node positive disease who undergo mastectomy. The pectoralis minor muscle can be removed with minimal morbidity in a modified radical mastectomy to facilitate dissection of the highest (level III) lymph nodes (if involved), although most surgeons are not trained in this technique today.

B. Total, or simple, mastectomy: This variation of mastectomy involves removal of the whole breast, but eliminates routine axillary node dissection. It is often coupled with sentinel node biopsy in those with clinically node negative breast cancers, because once the breast is removed, sentinel node biopsy is no longer possible.

2. **Partial mastectomy (lumpectomy or quadrantectomy):** Breast conservation therapy requires the removal of the tumor with a margin of normal breast tissue (negative margins) and is followed by postoperative breast irradiation. Trials with 20-year follow-up have shown that survival is equivalent for patients treated with lumpectomy and radiation, total mastectomy, and radical mastectomy. Mastectomy is preferred when negative margins cannot be achieved. Lumpectomy can be coupled with sentinel node biopsy if the patient is clinically node negative or with axillary node dissection if the patient has documented nodal disease.

13. **What is the National Surgical Adjuvant Breast and Bowel Program?**
The National Surgical Adjuvant Breast and Bowel Program (NSABP) is a U.S.-based trialist group that performed many of the classic randomized trials that have shaped our modern approach to breast cancer therapy. The NSABP helped demonstrate that breast cancer can be a systemic problem at the time of diagnosis and that smaller operations can be equivalent to larger ones for curative potential. Most recently, the NSABP has reported that tamoxifen can decrease the chances that a woman with a high risk of developing breast cancer will do so.

14. **What is the significance of the NSABP B-06 trial?**
NSABP B-06 was a multicenter study that randomized nearly 2000 women with stage I and II tumors (<4 cm) to one of three treatment arms: segmental mastectomy (SM; a.k.a., lumpectomy) alone, SM with radiation, and total mastectomy (TM). All patients underwent axillary dissection, and patients with positive nodes received adjuvant chemotherapy. There was **no difference in overall survival rates** between the groups, but radiation therapy decreased local recurrence in patients treated with lumpectomy. There were **no differences in disease-free survival or overall survival rates** among any of the three treatment groups, indicating that breast conservation therapy is effective for achieving both local and distant disease control.

15. **What is the difference among quadrantectomy, lumpectomy, and partial mastectomy?**
The differences are minimal because they all refer to removing part of the breast, just in varying amounts, for the purposes of treating breast cancer. The original quadrantectomy promoted by the Italians in the 1980s included excision of the entire involved breast quadrant, along with the overlying skin. Standard lumpectomies remove less tissue and may or may not involve skin removal, but they still demand negative surgical margins for both invasive cancer and DCIS. In these cancer operations, the surgeon is intending to achieve "negative" or "free" margins, meaning that cancer is not found tracking microscopically up to the edge of the removed tissues. This stands in contrast to "surgical biopsy," in which the surgeon is trying to remove as little tissue as possible to make a histologic diagnosis of a questionable lesion, and there is no intention to remove excess tissue or achieve negative margin status.

16. **Are some patients poor candidates for breast conservation therapy?**
Contraindications (relative or absolute) to breast conservation include (1) cancers that cannot be excised with negative margins without mastectomy, (2) cancers that are too large

relative to the breast to obtain acceptable cosmetic results, (3) multicentric cancers, and (4) patients who do not desire or who have a specific contraindication to adjuvant radiation therapy (e.g., scleroderma).

17. What is oncoplastic surgery?

This is a collection of procedures that use combined oncologic and reconstructive principles in performing a partial mastectomy. Large, full-thickness segments of breast are excised, usually in conjunction with the overlying skin. Using mastopexy techniques, the gland is remodeled on the chest wall to preserve the breast's natural shape and appearance without creating an unsightly tissue divot under the skin.

18. After mastectomy, which patients may undergo immediate breast reconstruction (i.e., during the same operation)?

Patient selection for immediate reconstruction can be controversial. Most agree that those with noninvasive (in situ) or early invasive (stage I and selected stage II) breast cancers may be offered immediate reconstruction using a myocutaneous flap, a temporary tissue expander that is replaced by an implant, or a combination of the both. It is disadvantageous to perform immediate reconstruction in patients with locally advanced (stage III) breast cancers because these patients may ultimately require postmastectomy chest wall irradiation. Radiation adversely affects the cosmetic outcome in reconstructed tissue flaps, may lead to tissue flap loss, and can promote capsular contracture around implants.

19. When is chest wall radiation therapy indicated after mastectomy?

The majority of mastectomy patients do not require radiation therapy. Exceptions are those with large, T3 (>5 cm) primary invasive cancers, positive or close mastectomy margins, or four or more positive axillary nodes, all of which are associated with an increased risk of locoregional recurrence. The possible benefit of radiation with one to three positive axillary nodes is currently being studied.

20. What is sentinel lymph node mapping for breast cancer?

The historic gold standard for staging the axilla in patients with invasive breast cancer was a level 1 + level 2 axillary lymph node dissection, which provides important staging information, but was often associated with morbidity, the most notable of which is lymphedema of the arm. Sentinel lymph node mapping, where a radioactive tracer (technetium labeled sulfur colloid), blue dye (lymphazurin), or combination of both are injected into the breast to identify the first upstream axillary node(s) to which a primary breast cancer drains, was introduced in the 1990s and is currently the standard of care for axillary staging. If the sentinel lymph nodes are negative for cancer, it is not necessary to node dissection to perform a completion.

21. Are there risks of axillary staging by sentinel lymph node mapping?

Sentinel node mapping appears most appropriate for breast cancers with clinically node negative axillae. The technique may be less reliable with large (T3) cancers and nodes extensively replaced with cancer. Thus, the primary risk of sentinel node mapping is that it may understage a patient by suggesting that the cancer is node negative when, in fact, nodal metastases are present in other "nonsentinel" lymph nodes (i.e., a false-negative result). As a result, the patient may be treated with less aggressive chemotherapy than is appropriate to minimize cancer mortality. The risk of a false-negative sentinel node biopsy is less than 5% for surgeons trained in the procedure.

22. Which tests should be obtained after surgery to screen for metastases or as baseline studies for future comparison?

The usefulness of metastatic screening tests correlates with the locoregional tumor and nodal (TN) staging determined at surgery. Patients with more advanced cancers are at higher risk for developing cancer recurrence with metastases, making additional diagnostic studies valuable. **Bone scan, CT scan (chest, abdomen, pelvis)**, and **PET scan** are used among higher risk patients and occasionally reveal previously unappreciated metastatic disease. Some physicians also use **circulating tumor markers** such as CEA CA-27, 29 to follow treatment results and monitor for evidence of cancer recurrence, although the value of these studies is debatable.

Conversely, baseline studies are best avoided in asymptomatic patients with early cancers because the chance of a false-positive test is higher than the chances of finding clinically occult distant metastases. For example, with stage I breast cancer, the likelihood of a false-positive result on bone scans vastly exceeds the likelihood of a true-positive result. Similarly, **brain imaging (CT or MRI)** should be reserved for those patients with neurologic symptoms because of low yield in asymptomatic patients.

23. What is "neoadjuvant" therapy for breast cancer?

Locally advanced but operable (stage IIIA, B, C, and some stage II) cancers have a higher likelihood of recurrence after surgery. Neoadjuvant therapy (before surgery), also referred to as primary chemotherapy, is used to decrease the local tumor burden and begin treatment of presumed micrometastatic disease at the earliest possible time. It does not appear that the timing of chemotherapy relative to surgery influences survival time from diagnosis, although this is being studied. Neoadjuvant chemotherapy may downstage some cancers that are otherwise marginal for breast conserving therapy into successful lumpectomy candidates.

24. What is "inoperable" breast cancer?

Inoperable breast cancer has advanced beyond the boundaries of surgical resection. The spread may be regional (involving large amounts of the chest wall skin) or distant (distant metastases, stage IV). Ipsilateral supraclavicular lymph node metastases are a poor prognostic indicator, but are currently staged as stage III, not stage IV, disease. Primary therapy for such advanced cancers is systemic treatment (chemotherapy or hormonal therapy) rather than surgery. Surgery combined with radiation therapy becomes an adjuvant therapy for local control of disease after a good response to systemic treatment, and increasing numbers of reports actually argue for resection of the primary lesion even in stage IV disease.

25. How is DCIS treated?

As the earliest form of breast cancer requiring treatment, DCIS has the widest range of treatment choices. Also called intraductal carcinoma, DCIS can be safely treated by breast conservation therapy (lumpectomy plus adjuvant radiation), provided that the disease is excised with negative margins. If negative margins cannot be achieved, then mastectomy is recommended for disease control. Although axillary dissection for staging is not indicated, sentinel lymph node biopsy may be offered if mastectomy is the operation of choice. Because it lacks metastatic potential, DCIS does not require systemic drug treatment. Tamoxifen may play a role in breast cancer prevention, and it lowered local recurrence after lumpectomy and radiation in the NSABP B-24 trial.

26. Can some cases of DCIS be treated by lumpectomy without radiotherapy?

Using carefully collected retrospective data, Silverstein and colleagues developed a prognostic index (scoring system) for DCIS based on histologic grade, tumor size, and margin width. Their data suggest that small (<1 cm) non-high-grade DCIS lesions excised with wide surgical margins do not require radiation therapy in addition to lumpectomy. However, eliminating radiation treatment after lumpectomy for DCIS remains controversial. Several phase III randomized studies have shown the benefits of local control with radiation therapy. In addition, one recent group demonstrated a 12% local recurrence rate at 5 years following only local excision, leading the authors to conclude that the elimination of radiation resulted in unacceptably high recurrence rates.

27. **How does DCIS management differ from that for lobular carcinoma in situ (LCIS)?**

DCIS is considered a preinvasive, or noninvasive, malignancy. It is treated surgically with lumpectomy or mastectomy, with or without radiation therapy, similar to how invasive breast cancer is managed. The overall goal is negative margin resection. By contrast, lobular carcinoma in situ (LCIS) is viewed as a "risk factor" lesion for the development of subsequent breast cancer and is generally not thought to be "cancer" per se. If diagnosed on a core needle biopsy, a subsequent excisional biopsy is recommended to rule out the concurrent existence of either DCIS or an invasive cancer. If LCIS is identified on a surgical specimen, negative margin resection is not required.

28. **Why are patients with LCIS not treated surgically?**

LCIS does not invariably degenerate into invasive cancer, although women with biopsy proven LCIS have up to a 25% chance of developing breast cancer during their lifetimes. The cancer may be ductal or lobular and may develop in either breast. LCIS is, therefore, considered to be a marker for high breast cancer risk, warranting careful surveillance with serial mammography, physical examination, and MRI. Because future breast cancer risk is the same for both breasts, bilateral mastectomy would be the only logical surgical procedure for this condition. Such aggressive therapy is not warranted in the majority of patients, although it may be considered in high risk individuals on a case by case basis.

29. **Can drugs be used to prevent breast cancer among women at high risk?**

In the NSABP P-01 Tamoxifen Prevention Trial, women at heightened risk for the development of breast cancer (>1.66% 5-year risk) developed fewer breast cancers when given tamoxifen versus placebo. For women with LCIS, the 5-year breast cancer incidence was 6.8% in the placebo group and 2.5% in the tamoxifen group, representing a 56% absolute reduction in breast cancers. However, the number of breast cancers that were prevented rivaled the number of tamoxifen-associated complications, including endometrial cancers and thrombotic events. No survival benefit to tamoxifen prophylaxis has yet been observed. At this time, women with LCIS and no major medical contraindications may be offered tamoxifen as an option for cancer prevention, although they may reasonably decline when presented with the complete data.

KEY POINTS: PRIMARY THERAPY FOR BREAST CANCER ✔

1. Historically, excisional biopsy was the gold standard for the diagnosis of breast cancer.

2. Now, the preferred initial diagnostic method is core needle biopsy or FNA.

3. The surgical alternatives for treatment of primary invasive breast cancer are modified radical mastectomy, total mastectomy, or partial mastectomy.

4. The NSABP B-06 trial found no difference in overall survival in women with stage I and II breast cancer who underwent either SM, SM with radiation, and TM, but radiation decreased local recurrence in the lumpectomized breast.

WEBSITE

www.acssurgery.com

BIBLIOGRAPHY

1. Anderson BO, Calhoun KE, Rosen EL: Evolving concepts in the management of lobular neoplasia. J Natl Compr Canc Netw 4(5):511-522, 2006.

2. Buzdar AU: Preoperative chemotherapy treatment of breast cancer—a review. Cancer 110:2394-2407, 2007.

3. Calhoun KE, Anderson BO: Prophylactic mastectomy and the clinical management of high-risk breast cancer patients. Community Oncol 3(6):379-382, 2006.

4. Chen CY, Calhoun KE, Masetti R et al.: Oncoplastic breast conserving surgery: a renaissance of anatomically-based surgical treatment. Minerva Chir 61:421-434, 2006.

5. Fisher B, Anderson S, Bryant J et al.: Twenty-year follow-up of a randomized trial comparing total mastectomy, lumpectomy, and lumpectomy plus irradiation for the treatment of invasive breast cancer. N Engl J Med 347:1233-1241, 2002.

6. Fisher B, Costantino JP, Wickerham DL et al.: Tamoxifen for prevention of breast cancer: current status of the National Surgical Adjuvant Breast and Bowel Project P-1 Study. J Natl Cancer Inst 97:1652-1662, 2005.

7. Lehman CD, Gatsonis C, Kuhl CK et al.: MRI evaluation of the contralateral breast in women with recently diagnosed breast cancer. N Engl J Med 356:1295-1303, 2007.

8. Lyman GH, Giuliano AE, Somerfield MR et al.: American Society of Clinical Oncology guideline recommendations for sentinel lymph node biopsy in early-stage breast cancer. J Clin Oncol 23:7703-7720, 2005.

9. Morrow M, Strom EA, Bassett LW et al.: Standard for breast conservation therapy in the management of invasive breast carcinoma. Ca Cancer J Clin 52:277-300, 2002.

10. Saslow D, Boetes C, Burke W et al.: American Cancer Society guidelines for breast screening with MRI as an adjunct to mammography. CA Cancer J Clin 57:75-89, 2007.

11. Silverstein MJ: The University of Southern California/Van Nuys prognostic index for ductal carcinoma in situ of the breast. Am J Surg 186(4):337-343, 2003.

12. Truong PT, Olivotto IA, Kader HA et al.: Selecting breast cancer patients with T1-2 tumors and one to three positive axillary nodes at high postmastectomy locoregional recurrence risk for adjuvant radiotherapy. Int J Radiat Oncol Biol Phys 61:1337-1347, 2005.

13. Wong JS, Kaelin CM, Troyan SL et al.: Prospective study of wide excision alone for ductal carcinoma in situ of the breast. J Clin Oncol 24:1031-1036, 2006.

14. Veronesi U, Cascinelli N, Mariani L et al.: Twenty-year follow-up of a randomized study comparing breast-conserving surgery with radical mastectomy for early breast cancer. N Engl J Med 34:1232, 2002.

15. Yen TW, Kuerer HM, Ottesen RA et al.: Impact of randomized clinical trial results in the national comprehensive cancer network on the use of tamoxifen after breast surgery for ductal carcinoma in situ. J Clin Oncol 25:3251-3258, 2007.

VI. OTHER CANCERS

CHAPTER 64

WHAT IS CANCER?

Karyn Stitzenberg, MD, MPH, and John A. Ridge, MD, PhD

1. What is a neoplasm?

A neoplasm (tumor) is a new growth in which cells grow progressively under conditions that do not prompt the growth of normal cells. A malignant neoplasm (cancer) is composed of cells that invade other tissues and spread.

2. What kinds of cancers are there?

Malignant tumors of epithelial (surface tissue) cells are **carcinomas.** Malignant tumors of mesenchymal (connective tissue) cells are **sarcomas.** Carcinomas and sarcomas are **solid** tumors. Hematologic malignancies, such as leukemia, are **liquid** tumors of mesenchymal origin.

3. What about skin cancers?

Melanoma behaves similarly to other solid tumors. In contrast, most basal cell and squamous skin cancers are life threatening only if neglected. They occur in tremendous numbers and are seldom fatal with proper treatment. Although the general principles of cancer management apply to non-melanoma skin cancers, they usually are not considered in the same class with other solid tumors.

4. Why is cancer bad for you?

There is no simple answer. The replacement of normal tissue by tumor eventually causes organ dysfunction. If a tumor outgrows its blood supply and becomes necrotic, local inflammation ensues. Often obstruction (with compromise of the lumen) of the gastrointestinal (GI) tract, bile ducts, or airway develops as the tumor grows. Occasionally the cancer bleeds (but life-threatening bleeding is rare). Nerve invasion or inflammation typically causes pain, which may be excruciating. Cancers also may elaborate humoral factors (e.g., gastrin) that cause symptoms.

5. Are all cancers life threatening?

Cancer is a fatal disease. It is uncommon for a patient with an untreated cancer to die of something else. Still, currently more than 50% of patients with cancer in the United States are cured.

6. How do cancers start?

No one knows, but cells begin to grow under circumstances when they should not. They stop responding to antigrowth signals, promote their own blood supplies, are seemingly able to replicate endlessly, and do not undergo programmed cell death (apoptosis).

7. Is this process the same for all cancers?

No, the order in which these changes take place seems to vary among types of cancer and even between individual tumors with the same histologic type. Occasionally, a single mutation alone causes cancer, but many genetic alterations are usually involved.

8. How is cancer diagnosed?

Cancer is diagnosed histopathologically. Pathologists have a variety of criteria for diagnosing cancer. They look for disordered growth, changes in the cell nucleus, changes in the structure of the cell, and invasion of the abnormal cells into nearby or distant tissues, adjacent blood vessels and lymphatics.

9. **What is immunohistochemistry?**

Pathologists use labeled antibodies directed against certain cell proteins to help them identify the type of cell. For example, if an antibody directed against the estrogen receptor stains the cancer cells in a lymph node, it is likely that cancer has spread from the breast.

10. **What is a metastasis?**

A metastasis is a group of cancer cells that have spread from the original tumor location to another nonadjacent organ. The cells in the metastasis are similar to those of the original tumor. Metastases develop from cancer cells traveling in the bloodstream or lymphatics. However, most cancer cells in the bloodstream and lymphatics are not capable of creating metastases. Only rarely do bloodstream cells actually develop into distant tumor implants. This process is known as the invasion-metastasis cascade. There are many steps in the cascade. Cancer cells must come to rest in tissues conducive to their growth and acquire traits that allow them to colonize and develop a blood supply in the new environment.

11. **Do all cancers spread?**

About 25% of patients with solid tumors have detectable metastases at the time of diagnosis. Fewer than 50% of the remainder develop metastases during the course of treatment. At diagnosis, a cancer is usually at least 1 cm in diameter (and often much larger), containing millions of cells. It is surprising that metastases have not occurred in all patients at the time of diagnosis.

12. **Does this process have an effect on how surgeons treat patients with cancer?**

Operations to treat benign conditions are designed to remove as little tissue as possible while creating a new and desirable physiologic or anatomic state. Cancer operations, on the other hand, are designed to remove as much tissue as possible while leaving the patient with acceptable function. Cancer operations typically remove the primary tumor and the lymph nodes draining the primary site. Surgical resection is the single most effective treatment for solid tumors.

13. **Why are lymph nodes removed during cancer operations?**

More than 100 years ago, William S. Halsted (if you do not know the answer to any historical question posed on rounds, you should always guess "Halsted") appreciated that tumor recurrence on the chest wall after mastectomy was related to tumor in remaining lymph nodes. Halsted believed that cancer of the breast spread in an orderly fashion (or perhaps even contiguously) from the primary tumor to regional lymph nodes and eventually to distant sites. He popularized en bloc dissection of the breast with axillary lymph nodes for treatment of breast cancer. Conceptually, this approach was adopted for surgical treatment of most solid tumors.

14. **What is a sentinel lymph node?**

Sentinel lymph nodes are the first stop for tumor cells metastasizing through lymphatics from the primary tumor. Often there is more than one sentinel node, even for a small tumor. If no tumor is present in a sentinel lymph node(s), it is unlikely that tumor is present in any of the other nodes. Sentinel lymph node mapping has been used for cancers of many organs (including the skin, breast, colon, thyroid, and head and neck). Careful evaluation of sentinel lymph nodes has proven reliable in the staging of melanoma and breast cancer. With a tumor-free sentinel node, patients with melanoma and breast cancer can now be spared far more morbid lymphadenectomies (lymph node dissections).

15. **Do solid tumors spread in an orderly way?**

Not necessarily. Another view of breast cancer behavior became popular by the 1970s. Bernard Fisher postulated that cancer is widespread at its inception. He stated that "breast cancer is a systemic disease . . . and that variations in effective local regional treatment are unlikely to effect survival substantially."

16. **How do these different models of cancer affect treatment?**
    Surgeons who believe that tumors spread in an orderly way tend to perform complete lymph node dissections in concert with resection of the primary tumor. They generally believe that lymphadenectomy will cure some patients who have lymph node involvement without distant metastases and that local or regional recurrence is a preventable cause of death. Surgeons who believe that lymph node metastases are simply markers for systemic disease are usually far less aggressive in performing lymph node dissections, because in their view, removal of lymph nodes that contain tumor will not cure patients who probably already have metastatic disease.

17. **Do we know which model is correct?**
    Both are probably inadequate. Even when they have lymph node involvement, some solid tumors (e.g., squamous cancer of the head and neck, colon cancer) often have no distant metastases. Their spread seems to be an orderly process. Other solid tumors (e.g., small cell lung cancer and prostate cancer) often metastasize widely even when they are small. For such cancers, lymph node involvement is a reliable sign of widespread cancer. Sarcomas seldom metastasize to the lymph nodes, but patients may develop distant metastases limited to the lungs alone. Remarkably, such patients sometimes are cured by resection of the distant lung lesions.

18. **How else can solid tumors be treated with curative intent?**
    Instead of surgical removal of the primary tumor and appropriate lymph nodes, the entire area may be treated with curative radiation. Some types of cancer are more responsive to radiation than others. The side effects of curative radiation treatment are formidable. Similar to those of surgery, they must be explained to the patient. When radiation kills cancer, it injures adjacent normal tissues. The damage to normal tissues continues over the course of the patient's life. Although radiotherapists are getting better at directing their beams, the tolerance of nearby tissues to radiation remains the limiting factor in treatment of cancers with radiation alone. For the same reason, radiation can usually only be used once for any given treatment area.

19. **What is adjuvant therapy?**
    Adjuvant means "assisting or aiding," but we use this term to mean assisting after surgical or radiotherapeutic control of the primary tumor. Adjuvant chemotherapy is of documented benefit in the treatment of breast cancer, colorectal cancer, stomach cancer, pancreatic cancer, and ovarian and testicular tumors. Adjuvant radiation therapy is effective in reducing the risk of tumor recurrence around a surgical site. Adjuvant radiation therapy is often used in treating patients with rectal, breast, head and neck, and stomach cancers and sarcomas. Conceptually, both surgery and radiation are local and regional therapies. Although chemotherapy is obviously a systemic treatment, it may help sensitize tumors to radiation.

20. **What is neoadjuvant therapy?**
    The term neoadjuvant does not really mean anything, but it is often used to describe chemotherapy or radiation therapy administered before the treatment truly intended to be curative. It might be more accurately described as "induction" treatment.

21. **What cancer treatments are available in addition to surgery, radiation therapy, and cytotoxic chemotherapy?**
    Hormonal manipulation has been used for decades to slow the growth of some tumors. Stimulation of the patient's immune system to combat cancer is potentially promising. This approach may involve vaccines, training of T cells, or enhancement of the immune response. New types of anticancer agents include drugs that interfere with tumor angiogenesis, antibodies and other drugs that interfere with growth factor receptors, other sorts of drugs that alter intracellular signaling, and drugs that restore cell cycle control. The limitation of all of these

approaches resides in our inability to specify a target unique to cancer cells. Hence, while damaging tumor cells, treatments also damage the rest of the body with potentially fatal toxicity.

22. **What is targeted therapy?**
The term *targeted therapy* refers to drugs or other agents that interact with specific molecules, or "targets," on the cancer cell, interfering with the tumor's ability to grow, divide, and communicate with other cells. Most targeted agents consist of a monoclonal antibody that interacts with a molecular target on the cancer cell. Targeted therapies are directed toward molecules unique to cancer cells, allowing them to attack tumors without attacking normal cells. Examples of molecular targets include certain types of tyrosine kinases and growth factor receptors.

23. **Does the body fight cancer on its own?**
Certainly. Some scientists believe that early cancers are regularly extirpated by the immune system (as we "catch" cancer every day) and that clinical cancers reflect a breakdown in immune surveillance. Immunocompromised patients with transplants or acquired immunodeficiency syndrome (AIDS) have less effective immune surveillance. These patients develop cancers with frightening frequency. In fact, rejection and sepsis are no longer the most common causes of death among kidney transplant patients; cancer is. "Spontaneous remissions" of melanoma and renal cell carcinoma do occur and are presumably immunologically mediated.

24. **What is a tumor-infiltrating lymphocyte?**
Tumor-infiltrating lymphocytes (TILs) are lymphoid cells (T cells) that infiltrate solid tumors and appear naturally reactive to autologous tumor antigens. Compared with circulating lymphocytes, TILs more aggressively target cancer. These TILs are believed to play a significant role in the body's immune response to cancer. In general, the presence of circulating TILs is a good prognostic sign. The field of adoptive immunotherapy is focused on harnessing the power of TILs to treat cancer.

25. **What are palliative treatments?**
Palliative means "affording relief by not curing."

26. **What are some examples of palliative procedures?**
Resection of the primary tumor in the face of distant metastases may be performed to treat bleeding or obstruction. Procedures to bypass intestinal or biliary obstruction in patients with unresectable cancer are common. Tracheotomies are created for patients who are unable to breathe because of upper airway obstruction. Feeding tubes may permit enteral nutrition in patients who cannot eat. Removal of isolated brain metastases often improves the patient's quality of life. Many patients with functioning endocrine tumors benefit from reduction in tumor mass.

27. **What is cytoreductive surgery?**
Cytoreductive ("debulking") procedures are designed to decrease tumor burden. Simply reducing tumor bulk is seldom sufficient to prolong survival. For cytoreductive surgery to be beneficial, the nonsurgical (adjuvant) therapy must be highly effective, such as radiation for glioblastoma or chemotherapy for ovarian cancer.

CONTROVERSY

28. **Is axillary lymph node treatment for breast cancer of therapeutic value, or does it merely help select patients who should receive chemotherapy?**
Those who believe that axillary lymph node dissection confers only information about tumor behavior rather than a therapeutic benefit usually cite the National Surgical Adjuvant Breast and

Bowel Program (NSABP) B-04 trial. There was no statistically significant difference in survival curves between patients whose axillae were treated initially and patients who received delayed treatment to the axilla. In addition to other problems, however, the study lacked the power to prove the point. To have a 90% chance of detecting a 7% survival difference between the treatment groups the NSABP should have enrolled 2000 patients (not just 550) in each arm. Hence, a substantial survival advantage resulting from axillary dissection might not have been recognized. The study was not designed to prove that the two approaches were equivalent, and it has been overinterpreted. It takes a much larger trial to prove equivalence than to show a difference. Indeed, subsequent randomized trials in the management of breast cancer and observational studies demonstrate an independent survival advantage conferred by treatment of the axilla. This experience with breast cancer reinforces the importance of actually understanding clinical trials.

BIBLIOGRAPHY

1. Bland KI, Scott-Conner CEH, Menck H et al.: Axillary dissection in breast-conserving surgery for state I and II breast cancer: A National Cancer Data Base study of patterns of omission and implications for survival. J Am Coll Surg 188:586-596, 1999.

2. Cabanes PA, Salmon RJ, Vilcoq JR et al.: Value of axillary dissection in addition to lumpectomy and radiotherapy in early breast cancer. Lancet 339:1245-1248, 1992.

3. Fisher B, Jeong J-H, Anderson S et al.: Twenty-five year follow-up of randomized clinical trial comparing radical mastectomy, total mastectomy, and total mastectomy followed by irradiation. N Engl J Med 312:674-681, 1985.

4. Hanahan D, Weinberg RA: The hallmarks of cancer. Cell 100:57-70, 2000.

5. Harris JR, Osteen RT: Patients with early breast cancer benefit from effective axillary treatment. Breast Cancer Res Treat 5:17-21, 1985.

6. Hellman S: Natural history of small breast cancers. J Clin Oncol 12:2229-2234, 1994.

7. Morton DL, Thompson JF, Cochran AJ et al.: Sentinel-node biopsy or nodal observation in melanoma. N Engl J Med 355:1307-1317, 2006.

8. Rosenberg SA: Progress in human tumor immunology and immunotherapy. Nature 411:380-384, 2001.

9. Scheel C, Onder T, Karnoub A et al.: Adaptation versus selection: the origins of metastatic behavior. Cancer Res 67:11476-11479, 2007.

10. Veronesi U, Paganelli G, Viale G et al.: Sentinel-lymph-node biopsy as a staging procedure in breast cancer: update of a randomized controlled study. Lancet Oncol. 7:983-990, 2006.

11. Whelan TJ, Julian J, Wright J: Does locoregional radiation therapy improve survival in breast cancer? A meta-analysis. J Clin Oncol 18:1220-1229, 2000.

CHAPTER 65

MELANOMA

Martin D. McCarter, MD

1. What is melanoma?

The term *melanoma* implies a malignant tumor; *malignant melanoma* is redundant. The most malignant of all skin cancers, melanoma usually forms from a preexisting nevus or mole but may develop de novo.

2. What is the incidence of melanoma?

It is the sixth most common cancer in the United States, and currently is the cancer with the most rapid rise in incidence in the United States. The lifetime risk in the year 2000 was 1 in 75 versus 1 in 150 in 1985. Over 59,000 new cases of melanoma are reported each year with more than 8000 deaths from the disease.

3. What are the types of moles? Which are most prone to malignant change?

Intradermal: the most benign form.
Junctional: the junctional component may be the site of melanoma formation.
Compound: intradermal and junctional together; intermediate activity.
Spitz: once called juvenile melanoma, it is actually a spindle cell epithelioid nevus that is quite benign.
Dysplastic: the most likely to turn malignant (especially in dysplastic nevus syndrome).

4. What are the risk factors in melanoma formation?

- Large number of moles (>50 moles >2 mm in diameter).
- Changing nevi.
- History of melanoma.
- Family history of melanoma.
- Light, poorly tanning skin; blonde or reddish-brown hair.
- History of episodic, acute, severe sunburns.
- Dysplastic nevus syndrome, or familial atypical multiple mole melanoma syndrome (FAMMM).

5. Which skin lesions often mimic a primary melanoma?

- Spitz nevus (spindle cell epithelioid nevus).
- Mycosis fungoides.
- Atypical benign nevus.
- Extramammary Paget's disease.
- Halo nevus.
- Bowen's disease.
- Recurrent benign nevus after inadequate excision.
- Dark sebaceous keratoses.
- Metastatic melanoma to skin.
- Kaposi's sarcoma.
- Pigmented basal cell carcinoma.

6. **What is the familial melanoma syndrome?**

   The inherited FAMMM syndrome has been defined as the occurrence of melanoma in one or more first- or second-degree relatives and the presence of >50 moles of variable size, some of which are atypical histologically. The risk of melanoma in this syndrome runs as high as 100% in the person's lifetime. People with FAMMM frequently have a mutation in p16 mapped to chromosome 9.

7. **What are common sites of melanoma development?**

   The most common sites are the posterior trunk in men and lower extremities in women. All sun-exposed areas are possible sites. Uncommon sites for melanoma formation are the soles of the feet, palms, and genitalia. Unusual noncutaneous sites for melanoma formation are the eye, anus, and gastrointestinal (GI) tract.

8. **Where is the incidence of melanoma the highest in the world?**

   Melanoma is most common in Australia, especially the northern part of the continent, where light-skinned descendants of the original settlers are exposed to tropical sun.

9. **What are the warning signs of melanoma?**

   Skin lesions that display:
   - **A** = **A**symmetry.
   - **B** = Irregular **b**order.
   - **C** = **C**olor: variable; spotted; often very black with irregular tan areas; red or pink spots; ulcerated when advanced (bleeds easily).
   - **D** = **D**iameter (>5 to 6 mm).
   - **E** = **E**nlargement or **E**levation.

10. **What are the types of melanoma and their incidence?**

    Superficial spreading: 75% of all cases; most common.
    Nodular: 15% of cases; most malignant; well circumscribed; deeply invasive.
    Lentigo maligna melanoma: 5% of cases; relatively good prognosis.
    Acral lentiginous: 5% of cases; most common type in people of color; appears on the soles, palms, subungual sites.

11. **Which moles should be considered for removal?**

    Growing and darkening nevi should be excised, especially in sun-sensitive patients. Itching is a sign of early malignant change. Ulceration is a late sign. Because melanoma may be familial in origin, children of patients with melanoma should be carefully screened for very dark nevi.

12. **How should suspicious nevi be biopsied?**

    Total excision of the lesion with a narrow (1-mm) margin of normal skin plus primary repair should be done. Partial incisional biopsy is acceptable if the lesion is large or if total excision would require reconstructive surgery. Punch biopsy, incisional biopsy, or saucerization are all appropriate as long as a **full-thickness** specimen is obtained. Thorough pathologic study is essential.

13. **Do melanomas spontaneously regress or even disappear?**

    Remarkably, some melanomas can regress or even disappear. Approximately 10% of melanoma patients with metastasis present with metastasis from an unknown primary site.

14. **What are the Breslow and Clark classifications of melanoma invasion?**

    Clark selected five levels of melanoma thickness in the skin:
    - Level I: intradermal melanoma that does not metastasize; may be better termed atypical melanotic hyperplasia: a benign lesion.

- Level II: melanoma that penetrates the basement membrane into the papillary dermis.
- Level III: melanoma that fills the papillary dermis and encroaches on the reticular dermis in a pushing fashion.
- Level IV: melanoma that invades the reticular dermis.
- Level V: melanoma that works its way into the subcutaneous fat.

The **Breslow method** requires an optical micrometer fitted to the ocular position of a standard microscope. This technique is a more exact determination of tumor invasion. Lesions are classified as follows:

= 1.0 mm
1.01 to 2.0 mm
2.01 to 4.0 mm
= 4.0 mm

Lesions <1 mm include melanoma in situ and thin invasive tumors. The cure rate in the latter is over 95% with excision. Tumors of 1.0 to 4.0 mm are called intermediate but involve risk of metastasis. Lesions >4.0 mm are high-risk lesions with a poor cure rate.

All melanomas should be checked by both methods because some tumors may show a low Breslow measurement with a deeper Clark level, indicating a great risk of recurrence and spread. Measurement of thickness is important, and the tumor should be measured from the total height of the lesion vertically at the point of maximal thickness. In addition, if ulceration is present, the measurement should be from the bottom of the ulcer crater down to the deepest margin of the lesion (see Fig. 65-1).

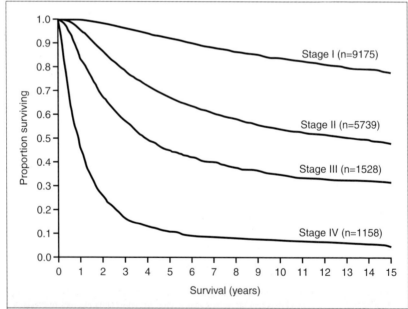

Figure 65-1. Estimated survival by melanoma stage (Balch CM, Buzaid AC, Soong SJ et al.: Final version of the American Joint Committee on Cancer staging system for cutaneous melanoma, J Clin Oncol 19(16): 3635-3648, 2001. Reprinted with permission from the American Society of Clinical Oncology.)

15. **What is the tumor, node, metastasis staging system for melanoma?**
    The tumor, node, metastasis (TNM) staging system is the most comprehensive classification of melanoma. Using established risk factors for advanced disease, it stratifies patients based on the thickness of the melanoma, ulceration, micrometastases or nodal metastases, and distant metastatic disease. Last revised in 2001, it more accurately predicts overall prognosis. See Table 65-1.

TABLE 65-1. TUMOR, NODE, AND METASTASIS CLASSIFICATION OF MELANOMA		
T Classification	**Thickness**	**Ulceration Status**
T1	≤1 mm	a = without ulceration and level II/III b = with ulceration or level IV/V
T2	1.01–2.0 mm	a = without ulceration b = with ulceration
T3	2.01–4.0 mm	a = without ulceration b = with ulceration
T4	>4.0 mm	a = without ulceration b = with ulceration
N Classification	**Number of Metastatic Nodes**	**Nodal Metastatic Mass**
N1	1 node	a = micrometastasis (microscopically discovered) b = macrometastasis (clinically evident)
N2	2–3 nodes	a = micrometastasis b = macrometastasis c = in transit mets/satellite without metastatic nodes
N3	4 or more nodes, or matted nodes, or in stansit/satellite mets with metastatic nodes	
M Classification	**Site**	**Serum Lactate Dehydrogenase**
M1a	Distant skin, subcutaneous, or nodes	Normal
M1b	Lung metastatsis	Normal
M1c	All other visceral metastasis Any distant metastasis	Normal Elevated

Used with the permission of the American Joint Committee on Cancer (AJCC), Chicago, Illinois. The original source for this material is the AJCC Cancer Staging Manual, Sixth Edition (2002) published by Springer Science and Business Media LLC, www.springerlink.com.

16. **What are the chances of nodal and systemic spread of the various degrees of melanoma invasion?**
See Table 65-2.

TABLE 65-2. ESTIMATED RISK OF SENTINEL LYMPH NODE METASTASIS BASED ON TUMOR THICKNESS	
Tumor Thickness	Relative Risk of Sentinel Lymph Node Metastasis
≤1.0 mm	<5%
1.01–2.0 mm	10%–20%
2.01–4.0 mm	25%–35%
≥4 mm	35%–55%

17. **What are the characteristics of a subungual melanoma?**
Subungual lesions are often mistaken for a chronic inflammatory process; therefore, most patients present quite late. They are usually older than patients with other forms of cutaneous melanoma. The great toe is the most common site of origin. Amputation at or proximal to the metatarsal phalangeal joint and regional sentinel lymph node biopsy is advised. The primary lesions are usually deeply invasive, and the lymph nodes are positive for cancer in the majority of cases, either at the time of the original diagnosis or at subsequent follow-up.

18. **Describe the technique of sentinel lymph node biopsy.**
The sentinel lymph node (SLN) biopsy is based on the theory that lymph from a solid neoplasm initially drains to a central, sentinel node. These sentinel nodes are the first nodes at risk for metastatic disease. The nodes can be biopsied and examined with serial sectioning and immunohistochemical staining. The SLN identification technique requires the cooperation of a surgeon, radiologist, and pathologist. Lymphoscintigraphy with the injection of radioactive technetium sulfur colloid (99mTeSC) is performed around the site of the primary melanoma. This identifies the regional nodal basins at risk. In the operating room for intradermal injection of blue contrast dye (lymphazurin 1%) around the primary site. A handheld gamma detector identifies the hot spot, and a small incision is made over this area for removal of the SLN. A combination of blue contrast dye and radiocolloid provides the highest yield of sentinel node identification.

KEY POINTS: MELANOMA

1. The term *melanoma* implies a malignant tumor.

2. Melanoma is the sixth most common cancer in the United States and the fastest rising cancer in men.

3. The warning signs of melanoma are skin lesions that display asymmetry, irregular borders, color changes, diameter >5 to 6 mm, and enlargement or elevation (ABCDE).

4. The surgeon's role is to provide local control with adequate margins (1 or 2 cm) and assess prognosis (sentinel lymph node biopsy).

19. **How is sentinel lymph node biopsy changing the treatment of melanoma?**
The presence of metastasis in the SLN is an independent predictor of overall survival. SLN biopsy also selectively, with minimal morbidity, identifies patients who are at high risk for recurrence. Although an absolute benefit for regional node dissection or adjuvant therapy have not been proven, these are often offered to provide local control of the disease and prognostic information.

20. **Does elective lymph node dissection improve cure rates in patients with melanoma?**
No.

21. **What is the accuracy of sentinel lymph node biopsy for melanoma?**
In general the procedure is 95% accurate in predicting the presence of additional nodal metastasis in the region sampled. There is a 5% false-negative rate. Of those with a completion lymph node dissection, approximately 20% will have additional positive nodes. One advantage of the SLN technique is enhanced pathologic analysis with multiple fine cuts of only a few select nodes.

22. **What features of melanoma are unfavorable for prognosis and metastatic risk?**
Tumor thickness (Breslow), anatomic invasion of dermis (Clark), nodal status, angiolymphatic invasion, regression, microsatellitosis, neurotropism, mitotic index ($>6/mm^2$), trunk versus extremities, ulceration, and male gender are unfavorable.

23. **If indicated, which types of node dissection should be performed?**
If there is no evidence of gross involvement of nodes except for the histologically positive SLN, a functional (i.e., a function preserving, not radical) type dissection is preferred because it preserves vital nerves and vessels.

24. **What margin is appropriate for treating a primary melanoma?**
Surgical science is alive and well! Through a series of prospective randomized trials, the following guidelines have been established:

Tumor Thickness	Recommended Clinical Margin
≤ 1.0 mm	1.0 cm
1.01 to 2.0 mm	1 to 2 cm
2.01 to 4.0 mm	2.0 cm
≥ 4 mm	2.0 cm

25. **Are there other treatments that improve survival in melanoma patients?**
Not yet. Any number of adjuvant treatments, vaccines, rabbits feet and combinations (biochemotherapy) have been employed. Response rate as high as 40% have been achieved but do not translate into improved survival. Dacarbazine (DTIC) is the chemotherapy approved by the Food and Drug Administration (FDA) for advanced melanoma.

26. **What about immunotherapy?**
Interleukine-2 and Interferon-gamma are approved treatments for melanoma but are only active in 5% to 10% of patients. Many vaccines have been tried as well with no improvement in overall survival.

27. **Can radiotherapy be helpful in melanoma treatment?**
Radiotherapy is quite helpful as palliative treatment of metastatic disease.

28. **When should amputation be used in the management of locally advanced melanoma?**
Rarely. With the development of isolation perfusion, the indications for major limb amputation are rare. Amputation does not impact on survival and as such should be used only for local control of disease that cannot be managed in a limb preserving manner. Partial digital amputation is the recommended therapy for subungual melanoma to achieve local control.

29. **What is isolation limb perfusion? How is it used in melanoma?**
Although studies have not shown that isolation perfusion conveys a survival advantage in primary melanoma, this technique is often used in setting of multiple or recurrent intransit metastases of an extremity. Melphalan (commonly used) or other chemotherapy preparations (e.g., interferon, tumor necrosis factor [TNF]) are circulated through an isolated extremity using a pump oxygenator at mild hyperthermic temperatures. Successful isolation perfusion preserves a functional extremity, has a superior response rate, and incurs less morbidity than systemic therapy.

30. **What is the treatment of a patient with metastatic nodes confined to a single area when the primary site is unknown?**
If careful workup reveals no other foci of melanoma, regional lymph node dissection should be carried out.

31. **Now you've done it. That patient with a lymph node dissection has developed lymphedema. How do you manage it?**
Early recognition and treatment are the key. It occurs 10% to 20% of patients. Physical therapy and custom made compressive garments may help reduce the severity of the edema.

32. **What should you do in the follow-up care of patients undergoing curative surgery for melanoma?**
Besides frequent physical examinations, chest radiographs and liver function tests (LFTs) are important.

33. **Is there a role for surgery in patients with stage IV (metastatic) melanoma?**
Absolutely. In selected patients (generally a long disease-free interval, single site of disease), up to 30% who undergo a resection will be alive at 5 years (compared to les than 5% who do not undergo resection).

WEBSITES

www.nccn.org/

www.cancer.org

BIBLIOGRAPHY

1. Balch CM, Buzaid AC, Soong SJ et al.: Final version of the American Joint Committee on Cancer staging system for cutaneous melanoma. J Clin Oncol 19(16): 3635-3648, 2001.
2. Balch CM, Houghton AN, Sober AJ et al.: *Cutaneous melanoma*, 4th ed., St. Louis, 2003, Quality Medical Publishing.
3. Blazer DG 3rd, Sondak VK, Sabel MS: Surgical therapy of cutaneous melanoma. Semin Oncol 34(3):270-280, 2007.
4. Jakub JW, Reintgen DS, Shivers S et al.: Regional node dissection for melanoma: techniques and indication. Surg Oncol Clin N Am 16(1):247-261, 2007.
5. Morton DL, Thompson JF, Cochran AJ et al.: Sentinel-node biopsy or nodal observation in melanoma. N Engl J Med 355(13):1307-1317, 2006.
6. Noorda EM, Vrouenraets BC, Nieweg OE et al.: Isolated limb perfusion in regional melanoma. Surg Oncol Clin N Am 15(2):373-384, 2006.

7. Rousseau DL Jr, Ross MI, Johnson MM et al.: Revised American Joint Committee on Cancer staging criteria accurately predict sentinel lymph node positivity in clinically node-negative melanoma patients. Ann Surg Oncol 10(5):569-574, 2003.

8. Spanknebel K, Temple L, Hiotis S et al.: Randomized clinical trials in melanoma, Surg Oncol Clin N Am 11(1):23-52, 2002.

9. Thompson JF, Scolyer RA, Uren RF: Surgical management of primary cutaneous melanoma: excision margins and the role of sentinel lymph node examination. Surg Oncol Clin N Am 15(2):301-318, 2006.

10. Young SE, Martinez SR, Essner R: The role of surgery in treatment of stage IV melanoma. J Surg Oncol 94(4):344-351, 2006.

CHAPTER 66

PAROTID TUMORS

Michael L. Lepore, MD, FACS

1. **Describe the location and characteristics of the parotid gland.**

   The paired parotid glands are the largest of the three major salivary glands arising as invagination of oral ectoderm into the surrounding mesenchymal tissue. The distinguishing histologic feature of the parotid gland is that its acinar cells are made up mainly of serous secreting cells. The parotid gland compartment is roughly triangular in shape, bounded superiorly by the zygomatic arch, posteriorly by the external auditory canal, and inferiorly by the styloid process, the styloid muscle, and the jugular and internal carotid vessels; anteriorly it is bounded by the masseter muscle. The tail of the parotid gland may extend inferior-posterior to the level of the sternocleidomastoid muscle and mastoid process.

2. **What is the relationship of the facial nerve to the parotid gland?**

   The nerve runs through the parotid gland, dividing the parotid gland into a superficial and deep lobe. The nerve lies laterally to the styloid process and to the posterior belly of the digastric muscle and medial to the mastoid tip. As the nerve exits the stylomastoid foramen, it gives off three motor branches: one to the stylohyoid muscle, one to the posterior belly of the digastric muscle, and lastly to the three postauricular muscles. The nerve will then turn laterally to enter the posterior aspect of the parotid gland. After entering the gland, it divides at the pes anserinus into a temporofacial and cervicofacial division. The temporofacial division divides into the temporal, zygomatic, and buccal branches. The cervicofacial division divides into the marginal mandibular and cervical branches. The deep lobe lies between the temporofacial and cervicofacial divisions.

3. **What branch of the facial nerve follows the parotid duct along its course, and what is its significance?**

   The buccal branch of the facial nerve travels superiorly along the entire course of Stenson's duct. In difficult parotidectomies when the facial nerve cannot be located at the stylomastoid foramen, the relationship of the facial nerve to the Stenson's duct is one method that the nerve can be identified peripherally. Following this nerve distally will lead directly to the temporofacial division.

4. **What is the salivary gland unit?**

   The salivary gland unit is composed of either serous or mucous acini cells. The secretions from these cells drain into an intercalated duct that connects to a striated duct that in turn drains into an excretory duct. Surrounding the acini and intercalated ducts are myoepithelial cells. These myoepithelial cells contract to force saliva into the ductal system.

5. **What is the significance of the salivary gland unit in tumor development?**

   There are currently two theories of tumor development based on the salivary gland unit.
   a. Bicellular theory: tumors arise from stem cells. The excretory duct reserve cell will give rise to squamous cell and mucoepidermoid carcinomas. The intercalated duct reserve cell gives rise to the pleomorphic adenoma, oncocytomas, adenoid cystic carcinomas, adenocarcinomas, and acinic cell carcinomas.

b. Multicellular theory: each tumor type is associated with a specific differentiated cell of origin within the salivary gland unit. Therefore, excretory duct cells give rise to squamous cell carcinomas; intercalated duct cells give rise to pleomorphic adenomas; striated ducts give rise to oncocytomas; and acinar cells give rise to acinic cell carcinomas.

6. **What are the four most common benign tumors of the salivary gland origin and their characteristics?**

   a. The pleomorphic adenoma (mixed tumor) accounts for approximately 80% of all benign parotid tumors. They are slow growing and are not well encapsulated. The recurrence rate is 1% to 5% with appropriate excision. Malignant degeneration may occur in approximately 2% to 10% of cases.

   b. Warthin tumor (papillary cystadenoma lymphomatosum or adenolymphoma). This tumor occurs later in life. It is the second most common tumor representing approximately 5% of all benign tumors. There is a male predominance. Approximately 12% of Warthin's tumors occur bilaterally.

   c. Oncytoma occurs in the sixth decade of life and is composed of large oxyphilic cells. Oncocytes found in these tumors and Warthin tumors are responsible for concentration of technetium 99m pertechnetate.

   d. Monomorphic adenoma includes the following: basal cell adenoma, clear cell adenoma, and glycogen-rich adenoma. The most common of the three is the basal cell adenoma. These tumors are well circumscribed and encapsulated.

7. **What is the treatment of benign tumors of the parotid gland?**

   The treatment is a superficial parotidectomy with preservation of the facial nerve. Before the gland is removed it should be properly oriented and tagged for the pathologist. If there is a close margin then patient should be observed for recurrence particularly in the case of pleomorphic adenomas.

8. **What is the role of intraoperative facial nerve monitoring in parotid gland surgery?**

   Facial nerve monitoring is a useful means of identifying the facial nerve particularly during difficult parotid gland surgical cases. Multiple peripheral probes are placed normally at four locations: at the region of the temporal branch that innervates the frontalis muscle; at the region of the zygomatic branch that innervates the orbicularis oculi muscle; at the region of the buccal branch that innervates the orbicularis oris muscle; and at the region of marginal mandibular nerve that innervates the muscle of the depressor muscle of the lower lip. When the major divisions of the facial nerve are stimulated distally facial movement will be evident.

9. **What is the significance of a "dumbbell tumor"?**

   Occasionally, deep lobe parotid tumor may present on examination as a mass in the lateral pharyngeal wall. This is primarily the result of a weakness in the stylomandibular membrane.

10. **Of all the three paired major salivary glands, which gland has the highest incidence of salivary gland neoplasms?**

    The parotid gland has the highest incidence of salivary gland neoplasms. Approximately 80% of all neoplasms located in this gland are benign. A good rule of thumb to remember with respect to malignant tumors is the 25/50/75 rule. As the salivary gland gets smaller, the incidence of malignancies increases. Thus in the parotid gland the incidence of malignancies is 25%, in the submandibular gland it is 50%, and in the sublingual gland it is 75%.

11. **What is the work-up for a mass in the parotid space?**

    The work-up is based on the clinical history and physical findings on examination of the patient. Classically, patients with a tumor involving the parotid gland will complain of a painless mass that is slow growing in the preauricular region (80%), or at the angle of the mandible (tail of the parotid gland). If the mass is painful (30%), or branches of the facial nerve are not functioning (7% to 20%), then one should have a high index of suspicion for a parotid malignancy. Approximately 80% of patients with facial nerve paralysis have nodal metastasis at the time of diagnosis. A careful examination of the oral cavity, scalp, and flexible endoscopy should be performed to rule out other tumors that may have metastasized to the gland. Examination of the neck should look for adenopathy denoting metastatic disease or lymphoma. Fine needle aspiration (FNA) may be easily performed in the clinical setting. Contrast computed tomography (CT) scan and magnetic resonance imaging (MRI) scanning are helpful in determining the location and extent of the mass; however, benign pathology can give similar findings: poorly defined borders and enhancement.

12. **Why is the significance of facial nerve weakness or paralysis in association with parotid gland enlargement?**
Involvement of the facial nerve in the presence of a parotid mass is usually an indication that a malignant process is present. The degree of paralysis should be noted clinically and photos taken for documentation.

13. **Describe the five most common malignant parotid tumors and their characteristics?**
   a. Mucoepidermoid carcinoma is the most common malignant tumor of the parotid gland accounting for 30% of all parotid malignancies. It is classified as to low grade or high grade malignancies. The low grade form has a higher ratio of mucous cells to epidermoid cells and behaves like benign tumors. In the case of high grade tumors, there is a higher portion of epidermoid cells and may resemble squamous cell carcinomas. The later have a high propensity for metastasis.
   b. Adenocarcinoma represents approximately 15% of parotid gland tumors. The neoplasms present as firm or hard masses attached to the surrounding tissue. Adenocarcinomas lack keratin, and therefore are easily differentiated from mucoepidermoid carcinomas.
   c. Adenoid cystic carcinoma (cylindromas) accounts for 6% of all salivary gland neoplasms. It is the most common malignancy of the submandibular and minor salivary glands. Adenoid cystic carcinomas are unpredictable and may remain quiescent for a long time. These tumors grow along perineural planes and have a high incidence of distant metastasis particularly to the lungs. There are three histologic types of the cribriform, solid, cylindromatous, and tubular. The solid form has the worst prognosis and the cribriform is considered to be the most benign of the group.
   d. Malignant mixed tumors (carcinoma expleomorphic adenoma) are believed to develop from a preexisting pleomorphic adenoma. It appears to represent 2% to 5% of parotid malignancies.
   e. Lymphoma of the parotid gland most commonly occur in elderly males. The entire parotid gland and regional lymph nodes are enlarged. FNA with flow cytometry may assist in diagnosing this condition because the treatment consists of chemotherapy followed by radiation therapy.

14. **What is the current classification of malignant parotid gland tumors?**
Parotid tumors are classified according to the American Joint Committee on Cancer (AJCC).
Primary tumor
TX Tumor extent unknown or cannot be assessed
T0 No evidence of a primary tumor
T1 Tumor <2 cm in greatest diameter
T2 Tumor >2 cm but <4 cm in greatest diameter
T3 Tumor >4 cm or tumor having extraparenchymal extension
T4a Tumor invades skin, mandible, ear canal, or facial nerve

T4b Tumor invades skull base or pterygoid plates or encases the carotid artery

All categories are subdivided into a) no local extension, b) local extension

Lymph nodes

N0 No regional lymph node metastasis

N1 Metastasis to a single ipsilateral node <3 cm

N2a Metastasis to a single ipsilateral node >3 cm but <6 cm

N2b Metastasis in multiple ipsilateral lymph nodes, none more than 6 cm in greatest dimension

N2c Metastasis in bilateral or contralateral lymph nodes, none more than 6 cm in greatest dimension

N3 Metastasis in a lymph node >6 cm in greatest dimension

Metastasis

M0 No distant metastasis

M1 Distant metastasis

15. How are parotid tumors managed?

Although the treatment options may vary from case to case and location (superficial or deep lobe), parotid tumors can be categorized into the following groups:

Group 1: T1 or T2N0 low grade malignancies (acinic cell carcinoma and low grade mucoepidermoid carcinomas).

A superficial parotidectomy is performed with preservation of the facial nerve.

Group 2: T1 or T2N0 high grade malignancies (high grade mucoepidermoid carcinomas, adenocarcinomas, and malignant mixed tumors).

a. Total parotidectomy is performed if the deep lobe is involved.

b. If the facial nerve is not involved it should be preserved. If involved it should be resected and immediately graft with a sural nerve graft.

c. Lymph node dissection is performed.

d. Patient should receive postoperative radiation therapy.

Group 3: T3N0 or and N1 high grade cancers and recurrent cancers.

a. The treatment of choice is aggressive radical surgical resection to include the deep lobe if involved.

b. If branches of the facial nerve are involved then they should be removed and grafted at the time of surgery. If the tumor involves the stylomastoid foramen then a mastoidectomy needs to be performed and the nerve followed in the fallopian canal until negative margins are obtained.

c. A modified neck dissection is performed in all T3N0 categories and a radical neck dissection in T3N+ categories. The patient should receive postoperative radiation therapy.

Group 4: T4 category.

a. In this group a radical parotidectomy is performed to include the surrounding tissue involved (buccal fat, skin, ear canal, mastoid bone).

b. The facial nerve is usually involved and sacrificed.

c. Primary reconstruction of all involved areas is performed at the time of surgery. The patient will need postoperative radiation therapy.

16. What are the most common malignant parotid tumors in children?

Well-differentiated mucoepidermoid carcinoma.

17. What are the potential complications of parotid gland surgery?

Skin flap

Bleeding (hematoma)

Infection

Salivary gland fistula

Temporary facial paresis in 10% of patients (usually the result of a stretched nerve) and permanent facial paresis in <2% of patients.

Frey's syndrome (flushing and sweating of the skin overlying the surgical site). This is the result of postoperative uninterrupted preganglionic parasympathetic nerve branches to the parotid into the more superficial sweat glands of the skin.

18. **What is the role of fine needle aspiration biopsy in the diagnosis of parotid gland enlargement?**
FNA is a useful diagnostic adjunct in the evaluation of masses in the head and neck. FNA is highly dependent on the experience of the pathologist. Therefore, its role in the evaluation of salivary gland tumors is some what controversial. It has a sensitivity of >90% and a specificity of >95%. It has a positive predictive value of approximately 84% and a negative predictive value of approximately 77%. It is an excellent method of differentiating between a benign (lymphadenopathy) and a malignant process.

19. **What parotid gland malignancy has a high incidence of perineural invasion?**
Adenoid cystic carcinoma is commonly associated with a high incidence of perineural invasion.

20. **Why should you be careful when dealing with cystic lesions of the parotid gland?**
Cystic lesions of the parotid gland were once thought to be rare lesions. However in the last 20 years, the incidence of cystic lesions has increased particularly in the population affected by human immunodeficiency virus (HIV). When a mass is noted in the parotid gland in a patient who is HIV positive one must think of a lymphoepithelial cyst that is frequently associated with patients who are HIV positive.

21. **Are intraoperative frozen sections reliable to differentiate between benign and malignant parotid tumors, and would you resect the facial nerve on the basis of a frozen section?**
At times, it is difficult for a pathologist to make a conclusive diagnosis based on frozen sections, consequently he or she will have a tendency to defer the diagnosis until an adequate work-up is performed. Therefore, most surgeons will hesitate before performing a major destructive procedure until the final pathologic diagnosis is received in writing. The surgeon will normally perform a superficial lobe parotidectomy and at a second operation obtain clear surgical margins, which may include resecting and grafting of the facial nerve.

22. **Is there a role for chemotherapy in the treatment of parotid gland malignancies?**
Parotid gland tumors normally respond poorly to chemotherapy. Adjuvant chemotherapy is currently indicated only for palliation. Platinum-based agents are most commonly used because they induce apoptosis and cell death. On the other hand, doxorubicin-based agents promote cell arrest.

23. **Is there a role of immuno-histochemical staining in parotid gland tumor identification?**
Newer investigations into the microcellular processes of salivary gland neoplasms can be performed on biopsied or sectioned tissue to assist in the diagnostic work up. Staining for silver nucleolar organizer region can help to differentiate benign or inflammatory lesions from malignant ones. Cytoplasmic immunostainings for pRb or p130 (tumor suppressor gene family) directly correlated with increased tumor grade in salivary gland malignancies. The loss of immunostaining for p63 in myoepithelial cells can be used to look for malignant cells to distinguish pleomorphic adenomas from carcinoma expleomorphic adenomas. Immunostaining for mucin expression can help differentiate acinic cell carcinoma from mucoepidermoid carcinomas. Acinic cell carcinomas express MUC3 but not MUC5AC, on the other hand, mucoepidermoid carcinomas uniquely express MUC5AC but not MUC3.

24. **Is there a role of immuno-histochemistry in predicting survival in parotid gland malignancies?**

    a. Immuno-histochemical staining for mucin expression in mucoepidermoid carcinomas demonstrated an increased MUC1 expression in these tumors correlated with increased tumor progression and a worse prognosis, however, an increase in MUC4 expression demonstrated decreased progression and better survival.

    b. Proteins were also evaluated such as heparinase and endo-β-D-glucuronidase. When these substances were expressed, they negatively correlated with survival particularly in mucoepidermoid carcinomas, adenocarcinoma, squamous cell, and acinic cell carcinomas.

    c. Ki-67, a nuclear antigen that measures proliferative capacity, was studied in parotid tumors. When high levels of Ki-67 were found in the tumors, poor survival was noted.

KEY POINTS

1. The most common benign tumor of the parotid gland is a pleomorphic adenoma.

2. The most common malignant tumor of the parotid gland is a mucoepidermoid carcinoma.

3. Adenoid cystic carcinoma has the highest incidence of perineural invasion.

4. FNA biopsy is a useful diagnostic tool that may assist the surgeon in the preoperative evaluation.

5. The presence of facial nerve paralysis is a good indication of an underlying malignant process.

BIBLIOGRAPHY

1. Arabi Mianroodi AA, Sigston EA, Vallance NA : Frozen section for parotid surgery: should it become routine? ANZ J Surg 76:736-739, 2006.

2. Balakrishnan K, Castling B, McMahon J et al.: Fine needle aspiration cytology in the management of a parotid mass: a two centre retrospective study. Surgeon 3:67-72, 2005.

3. Brennan JA, Moore EJ, Shuler KJ: Prospective analysis of the efficacy of continuous intraoperative nerve monitoring during thyroidectomy, parathyroidectomy and parotidectomy. Otolaryngol Head Neck Surg 1:537-554.

4. Carlson GW: The salivary glands: embryology, anatomy, and surgical applications. Surg Clin North Am 80: 261-273, 2000.

5. English GM, editor: *Otolaryngology*, vol 5 Philadelphia, 2000, J. B. Lippincott.

6. Huang RD, Pearlman S, Friedman WH et al.: Benign cystic vs. solid lesions of the parotid gland in HIV patients. Head Neck 13:522-526, 1991.

7. Koyuncu M, Sesen T, Akan H et al.: Comparison of computed tomography and magnetic resonance imaging in the diagnosis of parotid tumors. Otolaryngol Head Neck Surg 129:726-732, 2003.

8. Lee JH, Lee JH, Kim A et al.: Unique expression of MUC3, MUC5AC and cytokeratins in salivary gland carcinomas. Pathol Int 55:386-390, 2005.

9. Medina JE: Neck dissection in the treatment of cancer of major salivary glands. Otolaryngol Clin North Am 31:815-822, 1998.

10. Rabinov JD: Imaging of salivary gland pathology. Radiol Clin North Am 38:1047-1057, 2000.

11. Spiro RH: Diagnosis and pitfalls in the treatment of parotid tumors. Semin Surg Oncol 7:20-24, 1991.

12. Zbaren P, Schar C, Hotz MA et al.: Value of fine-needle aspiration cytology of parotid gland masses. Laryngoscope 111:1989-1992, 2001.

CHAPTER 67

NECK MASSES

Nathan W. Pearlman, MD

1. **A 34 year-old man presents with an ipsilateral 2- to 3-cm mass just below the angle of the mandible. What is the differential diagnosis?**

   Nonspecific lymph node enlargement
   Branchial cleft cyst
   Intraoral infection
   Salivary gland tumor
   Viral or bacterial infectious process
   Lymphoma
   Carotid body tumor
   Metastatic carcinoma
   Tuberculosis
   Prominent normal anatomy

2. **Normal anatomy?**

   Yes. In some patients, a neck "mass" is nothing more than a normal submaxillary gland or omohyoid muscle that has become prominent as a result of a slight enlargement or loss of surrounding fat. The key finding is a similar, but perhaps somewhat smaller mass in the same location on the other side.

3. **Does this patient seem awfully young for metastatic cancer?**

   Not really. Metastatic thyroid cancer frequently presents as an enlarged neck node in patients between the ages of 20 and 40. Although nasopharynx cancer and tongue cancer are uncommon in this age group, they are not rare.

4. **Is there any way to narrow this list of possibilities?**

   - Nonspecific lymphadenopathy: relatively asymptomatic, or only mildly painful, recent onset, nodes are mobile and <3 cm, overlying skin is normal.
   - Infectious mononucleosis: large, confluent, painful nodes, recent onset (with or without low grade fever), bilateral, soft texture, and normal overlying skin.
   - Bacterial infection: enlarged, indurated painful nodes, unilateral, and overlying skin erythematous.
   - Carotid body tumors: tender or painless, unilateral or bilateral, long standing, rubbery consistency, cannot be separate from the carotid pulse.
   - Branchial cleft cysts: unilateral, soft, nontender, long standing, and transilluminate.
   - Lymphoma: nodes nontender, >3 cm, unilateral or bilateral, relatively soft, recent onset. Signs of systemic illness (recurring fevers, weight loss, etc.) may or may not be present.
   - Salivary gland tumor (submaxillary, parotid): rubbery, nontender, relatively immobile. Remember, when examining the patient, the tail of the parotid extends down to the angle of the mandible.
   - Metastatic carcinoma: nodes hard, nontender, often >3 to 4 cm, usually present for at least several weeks.
   - Tuberculosis: mimics all of these conditions.

5. **Why not just remove the mass or lymph node to see what it is?**

Excisional biopsy should never be the initial diagnostic maneuver unless absolutely necessary. If lymphoma or an unusual infection is present, but not suspected, the node may be mishandled when sent to pathology or microbiology. If metastatic cancer is the problem, scarring created by the biopsy will make any subsequent neck dissection more difficult than necessary. A better choice for initial diagnosis is fine needle aspiration (FNA), which is 95% accurate and avoids the problems of open biopsy.

6. **A complete head and neck examination shows nothing abnormal, but fine needle aspiration of the mass reveals squamous cancer in a lymph node. What should be done next?**

Examination of the mouth, pharynx, larynx, esophagus, and tracheobronchial tree (triple endoscopy) under anesthesia. If nothing is seen, proceed to blind biopsy of the nasopharynx, base of tongue, and pyriform sinuses.

7. **Is this a bit much?**

No. The squamous cancer came from somewhere in the region and the most likely spot is somewhere in the upper aerodigestive tract (mouth, pharynx, etc.). In approximately 15% of cases, the primary tumor is detected only by examination under anesthesia, and in another 10% of patients a second, synchronous, primary tumor of the aerodigestive tract will be found.

8. **Why carry out a head and neck examination in the office if I am going to proceed to triple endoscopy anyway?**

Examination of the patient while awake provides information about tongue and laryngeal function that cannot be obtained while asleep and helps in treatment planning. In addition, examination under anesthesia may be a blind search because of collapse of the tongue and pharynx, unless directed by findings noted while awake.

9. **Should I get a CT or MRI scan?**

Yes. Both modalities provide information that may be difficult to obtain by physical examination, such as involvement of tissues at the base of the skull. However, these tests do not replace the measures already outlined.

10. **All that is done, and I still cannot find a primary tumor. What now?**

Two options exist. One can proceed to a functional or modified ipsilateral neck dissection, preserving as much function as possible; then use postoperative irradiation to treat the neck and likely site of the primary tumor. Alternatively, one may use primary irradiation alone, with surgery reserved for persistence, or recurrence, of disease in the neck.

11. **What if the primary tumor never shows up? Does this influence survival?**

No. Prognosis is determined by the presence of metastatic disease, in this case in the neck nodes.

12. **If the mass or enlarged node is in the posterior triangle of the neck, is the work-up still the same?**

Yes. Although most oral or pharyngeal tumors spread first to nodes in the anterior triangle, it is not uncommon for nasopharyngeal or hypopharyngeal tumors, thyroid cancers, and lymphomas to present as enlarged posterior triangle nodes.

13. **What if fine needle aspiration of the nodes shows only lymphocytes or shows adenocarcinoma?**

The presence of only lymphocytes most likely represents inflammation or lymphoma; however, if the "node sits just below the ear lobe, it may be a Warthin's tumor (cystadenoma lymphomatosum) of the parotid gland. Adenocarcinoma found on FNA usually indicates metastases from thyroid cancer, or a primary site below the clavicles; however, it could also represent spread from a salivary gland cancer.

If the FNA obtains only lymphocytes, it may now be reasonable to excise the node for better histologic staging; but, as noted previously, excision should not be the first step.

14. **Lumps in the neck are common, and relatively few patients have cancer. Is this type of work-up overkill and too expensive?**

No. Most patients with a lump in the neck have a benign process that will get better on its own without surgery. Thus, initial observation for several weeks is really the *most* cost-effective approach. Then, if you or the patient still wants to know "what it is," FNA is cheaper, less morbid, and usually just as informative as open biopsy.

On the other hand, if neck lumps are routinely excised without a differential diagnosis, the physician will be constantly surprised by the findings. If the node is benign, the patient had needless surgery. If cancer, or infection is present, the work-up previously outlined will still need to be undertaken—and then in a field dirtied by the biopsy. This is not cost effective; but, rather a waste of time and resources.

BIBLIOGRAPHY

1. Attie JN, Setzon M, Klein I. Thyroid cancer presenting as an enlarged cervical lymph nodes. Am J Surg 166:428-430, 1993.
2. King AD, Ahuja AT, Yeung DKW et al.: Malignant cervical lymphadenopathy: diagnostic accuracy of diffusion-weighted MR imaging. Radiology 245:806-813, 2007.
3. Lee NK, Byers RM, Abbruzzese JL et al.: Metastatic adenocarcinoma to the neck from an unknown primary source. Am J Surg 162:306-309, 1991.
4. Nasuti JF, Yu G, Boudousquie A et al.: Diagnostic value of lymph node fine needle aspiration cytology: an institutional experience of 387 cases observed over a 5-year period. Cytopathology 11:18-31, 2000.
5. Rice DH, Sprio RH: Metastatic carcinoma of the neck, primary unknown. In *Current Concepts in Head and Neck Cancer*, Atlanta, 1989, American Cancer Society.
6. Tarantino DR, McHenry CR, Strickland T et al.: The role of the fine-needle aspiration biopsy and flow cytometry in the evaluation of persistent neck adenopathy. Am J Surg 176:413-417, 1998.
7. Troost EG, Vogel WV, Merkx MA et al.: 18-FLT PET does not discriminate between reactive and metastatic lymph nodes in primary head and neck cancer patients. J Nucl Med 48:726-735, 2007.

WHAT IS ATHEROSCLEROSIS?

Nancy C. Andersen, MD, and Craig H. Selzman, MD

CHAPTER 68

1. Do you have to be old to have atherosclerosis?

No. The initial (or type I) lesion, consisting of lipid deposits in the intima, has been well characterized in infants and children.

2. What is a fatty streak?

Fatty streaks or type II lesions are visible as yellow-colored streaks, patches, or spots on the intimal surface of arteries. Microscopically, they are characterized by the intracellular accumulation of lipid.

3. What is a foam cell?

A foam cell is any cell that has ingested lipids, thus giving the histologic appearance of a sudsy vacuole. In general, a foam cell refers to a lipid-laden macrophage; however, other cells that uptake lipids, particularly vascular smooth muscle cells, also may be considered foam cells.

4. Describe the progression of atherosclerosis.

Although the sequence of events is not always consistent, fatty streaks progress to type III or intermediate lesions. This growth is characterized by extracellular pools of lipid, which are generally clinically occult. However, when the pools coalesce to create a core of extracellular lipid (type IV lesion or atheroma), the blood vessel architecture has been altered sufficiently to become clinically overt. With smooth muscle cell (SMC) proliferation and collagen deposition, the atheroma becomes a fibroatheroma (type V). The fibroatheroma is characterized by thrombogenic surface defects that provoke intramural hemorrhage or intraluminal thrombus (type V lesion), resulting in vessel occlusion, which, in the case of a coronary artery, results in myocardial infarction (MI).

5. Of 100 medical student volunteers, how many have significant atherosclerosis?

In 1953, Enos reported autopsy findings from 300 U.S. male battle casualties in Korea (average age, 22 years). He noted that 77% of the hearts had some gross evidence of coronary atherosclerosis. About 39% of the men had luminal narrowing, estimated at 10% to 90%, and 3% had plaques causing complete occlusion of one or more coronary vessels. However, a subsequent study evaluating 105 combat casualties in Vietnam demonstrated that only 45% exhibited atherosclerosis, and fewer than 5% were considered severe. Finally, a recent study looking at 105 trauma victims corroborated the Korean War study by demonstrating a 78% incidence of atherosclerosis, with left main or significant two- and three-vessel involvement in 20%.

6. What are the classic risk factors for atherosclerotic cardiovascular disease?

The classic risk factors include tobacco use, hyperlipidemia, hypertension, diabetes mellitus, and family history of cardiovascular disease. More recent evidence suggests the importance of obesity, emotional stress (weaker), and physical inactivity (that's you).

7. **How do such diverse risk factors produce similar disease?**

That is the million-dollar question. Do parallel pathways lead to a final atherosclerotic lesion, or do the apparently dissimilar risk factors activate signals that converge to a few dominant events, promoting the development of atherosclerosis? Certainly, this question has broad therapeutic implications. It would be a lot easier to inhibit a single proximal point in this process rather than to treat multiple divergent, more distal cellular pathologic events.

8. **What is the response to injury?**

The premise that atherogenesis represents an exaggerated inflammatory, fibroproliferative response to injury has evolved into an attractive unifying hypothesis of vascular disease and repair. Mechanical, metabolic, and toxic insults may injure the vessel wall. The common denominator is endothelial injury. Disruption of the endothelium not only results in endothelial cell dysfunction but also allows adhesion and transmigration of circulating monocytes, platelets, and T lymphocytes. Within the developing lesion, the activated cells release potent growth-regulatory molecules that may act in both a paracrine and autocrine manner. Under the influence of cytokines and growth factors, vascular smooth muscle cells (VSMCs) adapt to a synthetic phenotype and begin proliferation and migration across the internal elastic lamina into the intimal layer. Stimulated VSMCs allow the deposition of extracellular matrix, thus converting the initial lesion to a fibrous plaque.

9. **What is C-reactive protein? Is it just another random, nonclinically relevant marker of inflammation?**

C-reactive protein (CRP) is one of many acute phase proteins elaborated from hepatocytes on inflammatory stimulation. Originally isolated from the serum of patients with pneumonia, it has a high binding affinity for pneumococcal C-polysaccharide. Although CRP is best known as an active peptide by neutralizing foreign antigens, controlling tissue damage, and promoting tissue repair, it is increasingly considered a sensitive marker of inflammation. Unlike other markers of inflammation, CRP levels are stable over long periods of time, have no diurnal variation, can be measured inexpensively with available high-sensitivity assays, and have shown specificity in predicting risk of cardiovascular events. Indeed, elevation of CRP levels might be more predictive of cardiac events than elevation of low-density lipoprotein (LDL) levels. These observations may influence therapy because nonhyperlipidemic patients with elevated CRP levels might benefit from aggressive statin (3-hydroxyl-3-methylglutaryl [HMG]-reductase inhibitors) therapy.

10. **Does vascular injury mean only direct physical injury, as with an angioplasty catheter?**

No. Injury is a catch-all word that includes physical injury, such as angioplasty, hypertension, and shear forces (atherosclerotic lesions typically occur at bifurcations), and other diverse insults, including viruses, bacteria, nicotine, homocysteine, and oxidized LDLs.

11. **Are lipids important?**

The lipid hypothesis of atherosclerosis suggests that the cellular changes in atherosclerosis are reactive events in response to lipid infiltration. Indeed, antilipid therapy is one of the few strategies that has induced regression of atherosclerosis in randomized, prospective clinical trials. Strong evidence also derives from patients with genetic hyperlipidemias; homozygotes rarely live beyond age 26 years.

12. **What is the metabolic syndrome?**

Often referred to as syndrome X, metabolic syndrome is a phenomenon in older, sedentary people who have hyperinsulinemia associated with elevated blood sugar, high blood pressure, and increased triglycerides with decreased high-density lipoprotein (HDL) cholesterol levels. The prevalence in the United States is estimated to be nearly 25% of the population. Clinically, such patients develop premature cardiovascular disease. Insulin resistance with elevated insulin levels, with or without overt diabetes, fuels important aspects of atherogenesis, including dyslipidemias, endothelial dysfunction, hypertension, and SMC proliferation. For the trivia fans and not to be confused with your in-laws, a similar condition has been observed in overweight horses known as equine metabolic syndrome.

13. **What is leptin? What is its association with atherosclerosis?**
Leptin is a hormone secreted by adipocytes that maintains homeostasis between energy stores and energy expenditure through regulation of appetite and food intake. Alterations in the signaling pathway of leptin, whether through leptin resistance or leptin depletion, can result in excessive food intake and obesity. Leptin is also proatherogenic. It signals proliferation of monocytes, promotes oxidative stress in the endothelial cell, and prompts hypertrophy and proliferation of vascular smooth muscle cells.

14. **Why would vitamin E be (even theoretically) protective against cardiovascular disease?**
Antioxidant therapy with vitamins C and E and beta-carotene is intuitively sound. In vitro, these agents afford resistance of LDL to oxidation and reduce elaboration of vessel-injuring reactive oxygen species. Reactive oxygen metabolites (as much as 5% of oxygen), such as superoxide and hydrogen peroxide, directly injure vascular cells, impair endothelial vasomotor function, promote platelet aggregation and leukocyte adhesion, and stimulate vascular SMC proliferation. Although descriptive, case-control, and prospective cohort studies have found inverse associations between the frequency of coronary artery disease (CAD) and dietary intake of antioxidant vitamins, randomized therapeutic trials thus far have exhibited no benefit of doing so.

15. **What is homocysteine?**
This amino acid intermediate in the metabolism of methionine is an essential amino acid in the synthesis of both animal and plant proteins. Excessive homocysteine in the vessel wall reacts with low density proteins (LDPs) to create damaging reactive oxygen species. Epidemiologic evidence correlates elevated levels of homocysteine and decreased levels of folate with cardiovascular disease.

16. **How does homocysteine rank as a risk factor for atherosclerosis?**
It is estimated that 10% of the risk of CAD in the general population is attributable to homocysteine. An increase in 5 μmol/L in plasma homocysteine concentration (normal, 5 to 15 μmol/L) raises the risk of coronary disease by as much as an increase of 20 mg/dl in the cholesterol concentration.

17. **Should everyone take folate supplements?**
Folic acid, vitamins B_{12} and B_6, and pyridoxine are important cofactors for the enzymatic processing of homocysteine. Indeed, the reduction in mortality from cardiovascular causes since 1960 has been correlated with the increase in vitamin B_6 supplementation in the food supply. Although these supplements may decrease homocysteine levels, the expected decrease in cardiovascular events has not yet been documented in prospective, randomized clinical trials. In fact, the results of the HOPE-2 study concluded that in patients with vascular disease or diabetes over 55 years old, dietary supplementation with folic acid, B_6 and B_{12} for 5 years did not reduce the risk of major cardiovascular events.

18. **What microorganisms have been implicated in atherosclerosis?**
Bacteria include *Chlamydia pneumoniae, Helicobacter pylori*, streptococci, and *Bacillus typhosus*. Viruses include influenza, herpes virus, adenovirus, and cytomegalovirus.

19. **Are individuals with sexually transmitted diseases at greater risk for cardiovascular disease?**

    The initial epidemiologic description linking *Chlamydia* species to atherosclerosis was reported by venerologists in South America in the 1940s. *C. pneumoniae*, a ubiquitous respiratory organism, is the predominant species subsequently identified in cardiovascular lesions. More than 50% of the population has antichlamydial antibodies (ACAs) by age 50 years; yet this 50% of the population does not have this sexually transmitted disease (STD).

20. **Is there an *H. pylori* peptic ulcer equivalent in atherosclerosis? Should we all take a macrolide a day?**

    The jury is still out. It is unlikely that eradication of *Chlamydia* species will have the same profound effect on disease as eradication of *H. pylori*. However, *C. pneumoniae* may be another factor, exacerbating the response to injury. Evidence suggests that antibiotic therapy decreases the number of cardiovascular events in patients with elevated ACA titers.

21. **If you have multiple cavities, should you electively schedule your coronary artery bypass surgery?**

    In several cohort studies, chronic periodontis was associated with a 15% greater risk of developing coronary heart disease. Closer evaluation suggests that this link is actually much weaker. The major problem of existing studies is the high incidence of tobacco abuse in patients with dental disease. Interestingly, when you maximize oral hygiene by full dental extraction, edentulous people had a similar risk of heart disease with those with chronic periodontis.

22. **What is the role of the endothelium?**

    A healthy blood vessel wall is lined by a monolayer of phenomenally metabolically active endothelial cells. The surface area of the endothelium is approximately 5000 m^2 but comprises only 1% of the total body weight. While acting as a physical barrier to protect the underlying vessel and allowing formed blood elements to flow freely, thus preventing thrombosis, this seemingly bucolic layer is a central control center of vascular physiology. The endothelium is a key docking point for monocytes, neutrophils, and lymphocytes by virtue of its ability to express sticky, cell-specific adhesion molecules. The endothelium is a source for cytokines and peptide growth factors that act in both autocrine and paracrine fashion to promote atherogenesis.

23. **What are some of the products of endothelial cells that govern vasomotor tone?**

    Factors that favor vascular relaxation include nitric oxide and prostacyclin. Conversely, factors favoring vascular constriction include thromboxane, leukotrienes, free radicals, endothelins, and cytokines (e.g., tumor necrosis factor [TNF] and interleukin-1).

24. **What is the importance of vascular thrombosis?**

    Thrombosis is central to the pathogenesis of acute arterial insufficiency and acute coronary or cerebrovascular syndromes, including unstable angina, non-Q-wave MI, acute (ST-elevation) MI, and vessel occlusion after vascular intervention (angioplasty).

25. **Describe the three main phases of platelet involvement with thrombus formation.**

    The three main phases of platelet involvement in thrombus formation are platelet adhesion, activation, and aggregation. With exposure of the subendothelial space after vascular injury, platelets adhere to exposed basement membrane proteins such as proteoglycans, collagen, fibulin and laminin and molecules secreted locally, such as von Willebrand Factor (vWF), through their membrane glycoprotein receptors. Platelet activation occurs following adhesion, enhancing the ability of nearby platelets to attach to the developing thrombus. This process is energy dependent, requiring adenosine triphosphate (ATP). The predominant stimulators of activation include collagen, vWF, epinephrine, and thromboxane A2. Lastly platelet aggregation occurs, in which platelets collect in an amplified manner leading to final thrombus formation. This step is mediated by the glycoprotein IIb/IIIa receptor and its interaction with vWF, fibronectin, and fibrinogen. This process takes only minutes. Pharmacologic blockade of the glycoprotein IIb/IIIa receptor is actively used by our cardiology colleagues for treatment of acute coronary syndromes.

26. **What is the mechanism of plaque rupture?**
The structural support for an atherosclerotic plaque is the fibrous cap, an organized layer of SMCs and connective tissue. This cap serves as a subendothelial barrier between the vessel lumen and the atherosclerotic necrotic core, filled with lipid droplets, inflammatory cells, and calcium salts. When the fibrous cap is thin, it can be damaged by inflammatory cytokines and proteases released by macrophages, T-cells, and mast cells. Once destroyed, the contents of the necrotic core are exposed, prompting thrombosis and near or total artery occlusion. This process occurs in up to 70% of coronary artery thrombosis.

27. **What are some of the clinical complications of atherosclerotic plaque formation?**
Aneurysmal dilatation, arterial stenosis and occlusion, arterial wall rupture, and thromboembolic events leading to MI and stroke.

28. **If atherosclerosis is an inflammatory disease, should we all be taking an aspirin a day?**
Maybe. Strategies aimed at limiting the inflammatory cascade offer promise as antiatherosclerosis therapy. Examples in daily use include aspirin, fibrinolytics, HMG-reductase inhibitors, and estrogens. Others in the preclinical arena include gene therapy, anticytokine therapy, and antigrowth factor therapy. Certainly, primary prevention is important in limiting the initial injury stimulus. However, the smoldering inflammation involved with atherosclerosis may best be attacked by modifying the vascular cells' response to these insults.

BIBLIOGRAPHY

1. Ayada K, Yokota K, Kabayashi K et al.: Chronic infections and atherosclerosis. Ann NY Acad Sci 1108:594-602, 2007.
2. Davi G, Patrono C: Platelet activation and atherothrombosis. N Engl J Med 357:2482-2494, 2007.
3. Enos WF, Holmes RH, Beyer J: Coronary disease among United States soldiers killed in action in Korea. JAMA 152:1090-1093, 1953.
4. Fruchart JC, Nierman MC, Stroes ESG: New risk factors for atherosclerosis and patient risk assessment. Circulation 109:III-15-III-19, 2004.
5. Hansson GK: Inflammation, atherosclerosis, and coronary artery disease. N Engl J Med 352:1685-1695, 2005.
6. Selzman CH, Miller SA, Harken AH: Therapeutic implications of inflammation in atherosclerotic cardiovascular disease. Ann Thorac Surg 71:2066-2074, 2001.
7. The Heart Outcomes Prevention Evaluation (HOPE) 2 Investigators: Homocysteine lowering with folic acid and B vitamins in vascular disease. N Engl J Med 354:1567-1577, 2006.
8. Zimmerman MA, Selzman CH, Raeburn CD et al.: Diagnostic implications of C-reactive protein in atherosclerosis. Arch Surg 138:220-224, 2003.

CHAPTER 69

ARTERIAL INSUFFICIENCY

Carlos A. Rueda, MD, and Mark R. Nehler, MD

1. **Describe claudication and its physiology.**
   Intermittent claudication consists of reproducible lower extremity muscular pain induced by exercise and relieved by short periods of rest. It is caused by arterial obstruction to affected muscular beds, which restricts the normal exercise-induced increase in blood flow, producing transient muscle ischemia. Studies have shown that more than half of patients with intermittent claudication have never complained of this symptom to their physicians, assuming that difficulty with walking is a normal consequence of aging. Finally, only one third or less of patients with peripheral arterial disease (PAD) have typical claudication; others have atypical leg pain or are asymptomatic because medical comorbidities limit ambulation.

2. **List the different nonoperative therapies for intermittent claudication.**
   Risk factor modification, exercise, and pharmacologic therapies. Smoking cessation reliably doubles walking distances, and the need for eventual amputation in patients with lower extremity arterial occlusive disease decreases after smoking cessation. Exercise (defined as walking until onset of leg pain, resting, and then resuming walking) for 30 to 60 minutes, 3 days per week for 6 months has also been demonstrated in multiple randomized trials to increase walking distance by more than 100%. Currently, the only Food and Drug Administration (FDA)-approved drugs for the treatment of claudication are pentoxifylline (minimally effective) and cilostazol (appears more effective). Pharmacological therapy should also target dyslipidemia, hypertension, and glycemic control. In addition, life-long antiplatelet therapy is essential.

3. **Define critical limb ischemia.**
   Critical limb ischemia potentially threatens the viability of the limb. Symptoms include rest pain (Fontaine stage III [e.g., foot pain at rest]) typically occurring at night when the patient is supine and the gravity contribution to foot arterial pressure is no longer present. This pain is relieved with foot dependency or short periods of ambulation. Poor tissue circulation does not heal minor skin breakdown caused by incidental trauma. These ischemic ulcers (Fontaine stage IV) are frequently painful and can progress to gangrene. Critical limb ischemia implies chronicity and should be distinguished from acute limb ischemia, which is due to sudden (defined as 2 weeks or less) reduction in limb perfusion.

4. **What is the ankle brachial index (ABI)?**
   ABI is the highest ankle pressure (anterior tibial or posterior tibial artery) divided by the higher of the two brachial pressures. The normal ABI is slightly >1 (1.10). An ABI of 1.0 to 0.5 is typical of patients with claudication. Patients with rest pain have an ABI <0.5, and patients with tissue necrosis often have an ABI much lower.

5. **Describe the natural history of claudication.**
   Multiple natural history studies have documented the benign nature of claudication. The cumulative 10-year amputation rate is 10%. One third of patients experience symptom deterioration, and half of these patients require some sort of revascularization. Continued smoking and diabetes are major risk factors for progression.

6. **Describe the natural history of critical limb ischemia.**
Critical limb ischemia often requires revascularization or primary amputation. Percutaneous interventions are increasingly used as the primary therapy with surgical procedures or amputation used if they fail. Noninterventional treatment groups from several pharmacologic trials for critical limb ischemia noted improvement of symptoms over time in 40% of patients. Because patients with critical limb ischemia have a threefold higher risk of cardiovascular mortality than those with intermittent claudication, 50% of patients with critical limb ischemia succumb to cardiac disease within 5 years. Finally, a subgroup of patients with critical limb ischemia cannot be effectively treated with surgical or endovascular revascularization. Meticulous wound management can help patients with uncomplicated chronic nonhealing ulcers without revascularization. In randomized trials 15% to 20% of placebo patients heal at 6 months, but recurrence rates are high. Other therapies, including angiogenesis, are in clinical trial stage.

7. **What are segmental limb pressures? How are they used?**
Just as the ABI is recorded at the ankle, cuffs at the high thigh, above knee, and below knee level can record pressures. Noting the location of decreases in arterial pressure can determine the level of the vascular obstruction. Typically, a reduction in pressure of 20 mm Hg or greater between segments is considered significant and will help determine the level of obstruction.

8. **Describe the natural history of graft occlusions.**
Although bypass grafts can dramatically improve lower extremity circulation, they have a limited life expectancy. When these grafts fail, the limb involved is frequently in worse circulatory trouble than before the bypass. This is because of division of major arterial collateral pathways during the operation and thrombus propagation or embolization to occlude distal arteries at the time of graft occlusion.

9. **What is the prognosis of young patients with vascular disease?**
Significant atherosclerosis in young patients (age <40 years) is infrequent. These patients are almost exclusively heavy smokers with a high incidence of hypercoaguable states (defective fibrinolysis, anticardiolipin antibodies, homocysteinemia, or deficiencies in natural anticoagulants). Those with limb-threatening conditions frequently progress to limb loss despite attempts at revascularization. Reconstructive procedures have limited longevity and require frequent revision in this population.

10. **Describe the anatomic distribution of vascular disease in diabetes.**
Patients with diabetes are unique. They have a predilection for calcification of the arterial wall, rendering diagnostic studies (ankle pressure, ABI) unreliable because of false elevation. The digital arteries are usually spared, and the great toe pressure can be used to approximate the ankle pressure. The inflow arteries (i.e., aorta, iliacs, common femorals) are usually spared. Intermittent disease is often present in the superficial femoral and popliteal arteries. Significant occlusive disease most commonly affects the profunda femoris, posterior and anterior tibials, and pedal arteries, with relative sparing of the peroneal artery.

11. **What are the implications of renal failure on outcomes?**
Patients with end-stage renal failure who have critical limb ischemia are at the end of life, with 3 year survival rates <30%, similar to patients with metastatic cancer. In addition, the healing potential for partial foot amputations after successful revascularization is limited. Reconstructions in these patients are technically difficult because of calcified distal targets. The combination of these problems has caused many vascular surgeons to discourage vascular reconstructions in these patients.

12. Discuss the concept of inflow versus outflow.

The limb is thought of as a separate circulation network when planning revascularization procedures. Adequate leg circulation requires blood to enter the leg from the heart (inflow) and reach the foot from the thigh (outflow). In the normal limb, the inflow to the leg is via the aorta and iliacs and common and deep femoral arteries. The normal outflow to the foot is the popliteal and three tibial arteries (anterior, posterior, and peroneal). For bypasses to work, they need adequate inflow (i.e., blood coming into them) and outflow (i.e., a vascular bed to supply). Treatment of inflow and outflow is often accomplished through hybrid procedures that require the use of both endovascular and surgical procedures to treat all critical lesions in one patient. For example, an iliac stenosis may be treated with percutaneous transluminal angioplasty and a popliteal occlusion with surgical bypass.

13. What are the choices for autogenous conduits?

The success of infrainguinal bypass is highly dependent on the conduit (what the graft is made of). The best choices for conduit in order of preference would be a single segment greater saphenous vein, spliced pieces of saphenous vein, spliced lesser saphenous veins, arm veins, spliced arm veins, and prosthetic material with a distal vein cuff. Cryopreserved cadaver veins are expensive and are generally of limited durability. Prosthetic grafts are best used for above-the-knee popliteal targets because they bend at the knee joint and the size mismatch at more distal arteries decrease their longevity in these positions markedly. However, heparin-bonded polytetrafluoroethylene (PTFE) grafts have been used with comparable patency rates to autologous vein grafts for the treatment of occlusive vascular disease in the lower extremities. This material shows promise for patients with limited autogenous conduit options.

14. What are the indications for arteriography?

Arteriography is only performed to plan future operations or interventions. Diagnostic arteriography without intervention is rarely used in lower extremity occlusive disease. Arteriography is expensive and carries a finite risk of bleeding, arterial injury with thrombosis, and renal failure from contrast agent toxicity (combined 3%).

15. What are the patency rates of inflow procedures?

The durability of vascular reconstructions is measured by patency. Patency has three types, all measured via a life table method, which accounts for the moderate number of deaths (primarily cardiac origin) occurring in vascular patients over time. Patency can be **primary** (the graft has remained functioning without any intervention), **assisted primary** (the graft has never thrombosed but has required some intervention to keep it functioning), or **secondary patency** (the graft has thrombosed, but an intervention has reopened it and it is again functioning). The four most common procedures to improve inflow are iliac angioplasty, aortofemoral bypass, femorofemoral bypass, and axillofemoral bypass. The most durable is the aortofemoral bypass, which has a 10-year primary patency of 80%. Five-year primary patency rates for iliac angioplasty, axillofemoral, and femorofemoral bypass are 65%, 70%, and 70%, respectively.

16. What are the patency rates of infrainguinal bypass procedures?

Infrainguinal bypasses include grafts to the above-knee popliteal, below-knee popliteal, the tibials, and the pedal arteries. Five-year primary patency rates for above-knee popliteal grafts with saphenous vein and prosthetic are 80% and 65%, respectively. Five-year primary patency rates for below-knee saphenous vein popliteal grafts are 75%. Five-year primary patency rates for tibial bypasses are 65%. Five-year primary patency rate for pedal bypass is 50%. Heparin bonded PTFE grafts have achieved comparable results to autologous saphenous vein in low-risk patients in small series and are a potential alternative for patients who do not have a suitable vein.

17. Name the primary cause of perioperative mortality.

The majority (>90%) of all peripheral vascular disease patients have underlying coronary artery disease (CAD). Because of the ambulatory limitations of their peripheral vascular disease, most of these patients have no overt coronary symptoms. The most common cause of perioperative mortality in vascular surgery is myocardial infarction (MI). The decision to work-up and revascularize (surgically or with angioplasty and stenting) CAD in these patients before the vascular operation is an area of ongoing controversy.

18. Name the primary cause of perioperative morbidity.

Wound complications occur in about 25% of patients undergoing lower extremity bypass for critical limb ischemia. Postoperative lymphedema, ischemic neuropathy, and prolonged (often measured in months rather than weeks) wound healing are all important issues for these patients.

19. What are the causes of graft failure?

About 20% to 50% of patients undergoing infrainguinal bypass surgery will experience graft failure. Early failure (within 30 days) is caused by technical problems with the operation (graft kinking or twisting, narrowing of the anastomosis, bleeding, infection, intimal flaps, or embolization). Graft failure at months 2 through 18 is most often caused by fibrointimal hyperplasia at distal anastomoses or venous valve sites within the graft. Late graft failure (>18 months) is most frequently caused by recurrent atherosclerosis. Hypercoagulable states are an unusual cause of graft failure.

20. What therapeutic options are available for graft failure?

If a vein graft fails immediately postoperatively, the correct approach is to explore the distal anastomosis and to fix the presumed technical problem. If a graft fails weeks to months after implantation, the correct course is somewhat controversial. Exploring the graft to mechanically remove thrombus and repair any stenoses has a poor success rate and is not recommended. Using thrombolytic therapy to open the graft and then repair any underlying stenoses seems attractive, but the longevity of grafts treated in this manner has been poor, with <50% remaining patent at 1 year. Replacing the vein graft with a new bypass provides the most durable alternative providing it is technically possible and the patient is an operative candidate. The main challenges in replacing the vein graft are finding appropriate inflow and outflow vessels and appropriate bypass graft conduit. Inflow grafts that occlude are usually managed with operative thrombectomy and revision of the distal anastomotic stenosis.

21. What method of graft surveillance should be used?

Because of the limited options for occluded vein bypass grafts, ultrasound (US) studies are used to detect stenoses within the graft before occlusion. Various criteria have been championed to accurately detect >50% narrowing within the graft or native inflow and outflow arteries. Examinations of the graft are conducted at 1, 3, 6, 9, and 12 months postoperative and yearly thereafter. Natural history data indicate that grafts with >50% stenoses left untreated have high intermediate-term failure rates. Recurrent symptoms and changes in the ABI are too insensitive to detect these lesions.

22. What therapeutic options are available for graft stenoses?

The majority of vein graft stenoses are caused by fibrointimal hyperplasia of sclerotic portions of the graft or valve sites. These lesions are a firm rubber consistency and less amenable to long-term success with percutaneous angioplasty although focal lesions are usually initially treated in this manner. Open techniques (resection and interposition vein grafting or vein patch angioplasty) are more durable but also cause more patient morbidity. In summary, the results of intervention on failing grafts is superior to the results of intervention on those that have already failed.

23. **What is the role of iliac angioplasty and stenting?**
Iliac artery atherosclerotic lesions that respond best to balloon angioplasty are of short length (<3 cm) and are confined to the common iliac artery. Patients without diabetes fare better than patients with diabetes. Current reports of initial success is >90%, which has improved with the usage of stents to treat iatrogenic arterial dissections (splitting the arterial wall at the intima or media layers). Newer endovascular techniques combining angioplasty and stents have long-term patency rates (6 to 8 years) of more than 80% in well-selected patients. Most patients with aortoiliac disease without complete long segment occlusions are initially managed with endovascular techniques.

24. **How is viability determined in cases of acute ischemia?**
The five P's of acute ischemia are **p**ain, **p**allor, **p**ulselessness, **p**aresthesia, and **p**aralysis. Early findings with acute ischemia include absent pulse, pain, and pallor. Paresthesia and paralysis are later findings. Classical teaching states irreversible muscle ischemia after 6 hours. However, in clinical practice, there are many overlaps. Perhaps the most sensitive finding that indicates limb nonviability is muscle rigor in the calf. The vast majority of ischemic limbs can be managed with initial heparin therapy followed by angiography and surgery or thrombolysis the next day(s).

25. **How is thrombus distinguished from embolus in acute ischemia?**
The diagnosis of acute thrombotic versus embolic lower extremity arterial occlusion is complicated. Findings suggestive of embolus include no history of vascular disease, normal contralateral leg circulation, no history of cardiac arrhythmia or recent MI, and no known cardiac thrombus. Patients with embolus frequently have rather profound leg ischemia because of the proximal nature of the occlusion (aortic or femoral bifurcation) and the absence of any developed collaterals. Occasionally, arteriography is required to differentiate between the two.

26. **When is thrombolysis indicated?**
Thrombolytic therapy requires a patient without contraindications (bleeding risks) and a thrombus that can be crossed with a guidewire. The lytic medication (urokinase, streptokinase, or tissue plasminogen activator) needs to be placed directly within the thrombus. Acute native arterial occlusions should not have evidence of patent outflow arteries (e.g., a thrombosed popliteal artery aneurysm). Arterial embolus in an extremity that is not severely ischemic and can tolerate the time course of successful thrombolysis (frequently multiple hours of intraarterial infusion and repeat trips to the angiography suite for angiograms to help determine optimal catheter repositioning for complete thrombus lysis). Percutaneous thrombectomy benefits include completing the thrombectomy in less time, avoiding delayed reperfusion injury, and decreasing the risk of bleeding from the use of thrombolytics. The use of thrombolytic therapy for graft occlusions is more controversial because of the relatively poor long-term durability of these grafts after flow is restored.

27. **What is compartment syndrome?**
Reperfusion after acute ischemia can lead to profound tissue swelling in the involved extremity. Edema of the involved muscle can increase the pressure within the fascia bound muscle compartments (i.e., anterior, lateral, deep posterior, and superficial posterior) to a level that exceeds the capillary perfusion pressure (>30 mm Hg). Muscle death is then inevitable unless the pressure is relieved by opening the compartments surgically, a procedure known as fasciotomy. Patients complain of intense pain and swelling, with associated paresthesia. Pedal pulses can remain palpable.

28. **What is the role of endovascular therapy in infrainguinal occlusive disease?**
Endovascular therapy is increasingly being used to treat infrainguinal occlussive disease in patients with claudication and critical limb ischemia. This includes angioplasty and stenting for

stenoses and recanalization for long segment occlusions. In addition, atherectomy devices have been used for treating stenoses in the femoral, popliteal, and tibial arteries. Early results are favorable and these techniques are currently being used as frequently or even more frequently than surgical bypass. The long-term durability is relatively unknown at present.

KEY POINTS: ARTERIAL INSUFFICIENCY

1. ABI is the highest ankle pressure divided by the higher of the two brachial pressures.

2. Critical limb ischemia potentially threatens the viability of the limb.

3. Patients with end-stage renal failure that have critical limb ischemia are at the end of life, with 3-year survival rates <30%.

4. If a vein graft fails immediately postoperatively, the correct approach is to explore the distal anastomosis and to fix the presumed technical problem.

WEBSITES

www.acssurgery.com

www.vascular web.org

BIBLIOGRAPHY

1. Amonkar SJ, Cleanthis M, Nice C et al.: Outcomes of intra-arterial thrombolysis for acute limb ischemia. Angiology 58(6):734-742, 2007.

2. Gerhard-Herman M, Gardin JM, Jaff M et al.: Guidelines for noninvasive vascular laboratory testing: a report from the American Society of Echocardiography and the Society for Vascular Medicine and Biology. Vasc Med 11(3):183-200, 2006.

3. Hiatt WR, Krantz MJ: Masterclass series in peripheral arterial disease. Antiplatelet therapy for peripheral arterial disease and claudication. Vasc Med 11(1):55-60, 2006.

4. Klein WM, van der GY, Seegers J et al.: Dutch iliac stent trial: long-term results in patients randomized for primary or selective stent placement. Radiology 238(2):734-744, 2006.

5. Landis GS, FariesPL: New techniques and developments to treat long infrainguinal arterial occlusions: use of reentry devices, subintimal angioplasty, and endografts. Perspect Vasc Surg Endovasc Ther 19(3):285-290, 2007.

6. Lau H, Cheng SW, Hui J: Eighteen-year experience with femoro-femoral bypass. Aust N Z J Surg 70:275-278, 2000.

7. Nehler MR, Hiatt WR: Exercise therapy for claudication. Ann Vasc Surg 13:109-114, 1999.

8. Novo S, Coppola G, Milio G: Critical limb ischemia: definition and natural history. Curr Drug Targets Cardiovasc Haematol Disord 4(3):219-225, 2004.

9. Taylor SM, Kalbaugh CA, Blackhurst DW et al.: Postoperative outcomes according to preoperative medical and functional status after infrainguinal revascularization for critical limb ischemia in patients 80 years and older. Am Surg 71(8):640-645, 2005.

10. Wind J, Koelemay MJ: Exercise therapy and the additional effect of supervision on exercise therapy in patients with intermittent claudication. Systematic review of randomised controlled trials. Eur J Vasc Endovasc Surg 34(1):1-9, 2007.

CHAPTER 70

CAROTID DISEASE

Jennifer M. Worth, MD, and Bernard Timothy Baxter, MD

1. **What primary diseases affect the carotid arteries?**
   Atherosclerosis is by far the most common disease affecting the carotid arteries accounting for 90% of lesions in the Western world. The carotid artery also can be affected by kinking secondary to arterial elongation, fibromuscular dysplasia, extrinsic compression (e.g., neoplasm), radiation-induced changes, trauma (causing bleeding, occlusion, or dissection) and inflammatory arteriopathies (e.g., Temporal arteritis, Takayasu's arteritis).

2. **What are the histological features of atherosclerotic plaques?**
   Plaques are likely formed according to the response to injury hypothesis. Plaques begin in the intima and media through a complex series of events. Initially smooth muscle cells (SMCs) are recruited and connective tissue proteins are produced in excess. Incorporation of low-density lipoprotein (LDL) cholesterol, monocytes, and platelets leads to formation of the mature plaque consisting of a lipid core and a fibrotic cap covering the core. Hemorrhage into the plaque (intraplaque hemorrhage) may cause sudden growth acutely increasing the degree of stenosis or causing occlusion.

3. **What are the clinical sequelae of atherosclerotic disease?**
   Thrombosis and embolization are the most common complications of atherosclerotic plaques. Thrombosis and embolization typically occur when the outer fibrous layer of the plaque is degraded by enzymes from inflammatory cells exposing the lipid core. This core is highly thrombogenic and friable predisposing to thrombosis and embolization of lipids and platelet aggregates. Atherosclerosis may also be a factor in development of carotid artery aneurysms, although this is controversial because they may occur without atherosclerosis.

4. **What are the most common symptoms of carotid artery disease?**
   - Transient ischemic attack (TIA)
   - Cerebrovascular accident (CVA)
   - Amaurosis fugax

5. **Define TIA, CVA, and amaurosis fugax.**
   These clinical terms describe a spectrum of cerebral ischemic syndromes. A **TIA** is a neurologic deficit that lasts <24 hours but typically last only minutes. Clinically, a **CVA,** or acute stroke, is defined by a persistent neurologic deficit lasting >24 hours. **Amaurosis fugax** is an episode of transient (minutes to hours) monocular blindness, often likened to a window shade being pulled across the eye. It is caused by an acute decrease in blood flow secondary to embolization through the ophthalmic artery to the retina. When this occurs, blood flow to the periphery of the retina is lost first with the ischemia (loss of vision) working its way toward the center of the retina, hence the sensation of shade being pulled down.

6. **What are Hollenhorst plaques?**
   Hollenhorst was an ophthalmologist who first described refractile plaques of cholesterol in the retinal vessels. They are usually seen at branch points in the vessel and are the result of

arterial to arterial emboli. The most common source is a carotid bifurcation plaque, but they may originate from disease in the common carotid or the ascending aorta.

7. **What mechanisms produce neurologic deficits?**
   - Embolization from proximal atherosclerotic arteries (ascending aorta, aortic arch, carotid arteries), the heart, or in the case of a right to left cardiac shunt, the venous system (paradoxical emboli)
   - Reduced cerebral blood flow from shock
   - Atherosclerotic occlusive disease progressing to thrombosis
   - Intracranial hemorrhage

8. **What is the natural history of a TIA?**
   The natural history of a TIA is defined by the pathology of the ipsilateral carotid artery. In patients with severe stenosis (>70%), the risk of ipsilateral stroke within 24 months is 26%. For those with moderate disease (50% to 69%), the risk is 22% at 5 years. With minimal stenosis (<30%), the risk is 1% at 3 years (see Required Reading in Chapter 1).

9. **What is the effect of medication on TIAs and stroke?**
   Acetylsalicylic acid (aspirin) is a cyclooxygenase inhibitor that decreases platelet stickiness and inflammation. It lowers the incidence of stoke in women. Although it has not been shown to lower stroke incidence as a single endpoint in men, it has been shown to lower the incidence of myocardial infarction (MI) and stroke when these endpoints are combined. Other antiplatelet agents (clopidogrel, dipyridamole) may be added when patients are symptomatic on aspirin, but there is no prospective data to demonstrate that any combination is superior to aspirin alone.
   Statin therapy is approved and recommended for stroke prevention in patients with TIAs, stroke, or significant carotid stenosis.

10. **What does a carotid bruit signify?**
    A carotid bruit is a general marker for atherosclerosis that lacks specificity; it indicates an increased risk of both cardiac and cerebral vascular events. Absence of a bruit does not indicate absence of disease.

11. **Does the sound of a bruit correlate with the degree of stenosis?**
    No. As a stenosis progresses, the bruit may actually diminish or disappear as flow decreases.

12. **What preliminary test should be ordered to evaluate a cervical bruit or carotid stenosis based on clinical findings such as TIA or CVA?**
    Duplex ultrasound (US) is accurate and inexpensive. To confirm carotid disease or look for other sites of disease when carotid duplex does not correlate with symptoms, magnetic resonance angiography or computed tomography angiography (CTA) are now used to assess the arch vessels and intracranial circulation. Because cerebral angiography is invasive and associated with additional risk including a small risk of stroke, it is reserved for cases where specific, additional anatomic information is required.

13. **When is intervention indicated for symptomatic carotid artery disease?**
    Intervention is strongly indicated for symptomatic carotid artery disease associated with >70% stenosis. The absolute risk reduction of stroke is 17% at 2 years. There is a smaller benefit in patients with symptomatic stenoses of 50% to 69% (6.5% risk reduction at 5 years). Symptomatic patients with stenosis of <50% do not benefit from intervention.

KEY POINTS: CAROTID DISEASE

1. The symptoms of carotid disease include TIA, CVA, and amaurosis fugax.

2. A carotid bruit is a general marker for atherosclerosis including both coronary artery and cerebrovascular disease.

3. Intervention is strongly indicated for symptomatic carotid artery disease associated with >70% stenosis.

14. **Should a patient with asymptomatic stenosis undergo surgery?**
The absolute reduction in risk of stroke is 6% over a 5-year period in asymptomatic patients with >60% stenosis who undergo carotid endarterectomy (CEA) plus aspirin versus patients treated with aspirin alone (5.1% versus 11%). Thus, CEA should be performed for asymptomatic carotid disease when the patient is expected to live at least 3 years and when the CEA can be performed with a combined stroke and mortality rate of <3%.

15. **What are the complications of carotid endarterectomy?**
TIA or stroke (approximately 2%)
Hematoma
Cranial nerve injury
Hypertension
Hypotension

16. **Which cranial nerves may be injured during CEA? What are the clinical signs of injury?**
The **marginal mandibular branch of the facial nerve** (cranial nerve [CN] VII): injury may cause droop of the ipsilateral corner of the mouth
Glossopharyngeal nerve (CN IX): difficulty in swallowing both solids and liquids
Recurrent laryngeal branch of the vagus nerve (CN X): hoarseness, loss of effective cough
Superior laryngeal nerve (branch of the vagus, CN X): voice fatigue, loss of high-pitch phonation
Hypoglossal nerve (CN XII): deviation of the tongue to the ipsilateral side, difficulty with speech and chewing

17. **What is the danger of wound hematoma after surgery?**
The main danger is airway compromise, which may necessitate emergent decompression by opening of the wound. Whether drains placed in the wound bed prevent hematoma formation is not clear.

18. **When do neurologic events occur during CEA?**
 - Dissection: dislodgement of material from the arterial wall with embolization
 - Clamping: ischemic infarct
 - Postoperatively: intimal flap, reperfusion

19. **What is a shunt? When is it used?**
A shunt is a small plastic tube that diverts blood flow around the surgically opened carotid artery while endarterectomy is performed. A shunt is used to ensure adequate cerebral blood flow and to avoid intraoperative cerebral ischemia. Many surgeons routinely use shunts, but others use them selectively, if at all. The decision to use a shunt is based on known absence of collateral circulation or intraoperative assessment, including temporary clamping of the

carotid under local anesthesia, measurement of stump pressure, intraoperative electroencephalography, or transcranial Doppler. None of these methods is 100% accurate.

20. **What is stump pressure?**
Stump pressure is the back pressure of the internal carotid artery after clamping. It is used to assess the adequacy of cerebral perfusion. The "safe" pressure varies from physician to physician, but mean pressure should be at least 40 mm Hg.

21. **Does stenosis recur after carotid endarterectomy?**
Yes. The reported incidence has been quite variable and ranges from <2% to as much as 36%. During the first 24 months after operation, restenosis is thought to be secondary to myointimal hyperplasia. Beyond this time, it is caused by progression of disease (atherosclerosis). The incidence is lower when the arteriotomy is closed with a vein patch angioplasty.

22. **What is the most common complication associated with reoperation endarterectomy?**
CN injury (reported incidence ≈2% to 20%). Most injuries are transient, however.

23. **In which layer of the artery is the carotid endarterectomy performed?**
The outer layers of the tunica media.

24. **What anatomic landmark is useful in identifying the level of the carotid artery bifurcation?**
The common facial vein.

25. **How many branches of the internal carotid artery are located in the neck?**
None.

26. **When the internal carotid artery is occluded, which branches of the external carotid artery form collaterals and reestablish circulation in the circle of Willis?**
The periorbital branches of the external carotid artery form communications with the ophthalmic artery, a branch of the internal carotid.

27. **What are the functions of the carotid sinus and the carotid body?**
Both are located at the carotid bifurcation and are innervated by the glossopharyngeal and vagus nerves, respectively. The function of the carotid sinus is regulation of blood pressure. Hypertension stimulates efferent impulses to the vasomotor center in the medulla, inhibiting sympathetic tone and increasing vagal tone. The carotid body regulates respiratory drive and acid-base status via chemoreceptors. It also induces bradycardia when manipulated (this is your target during carotid massage for cardiac dysrhythmias).

28. **When was the first successful surgical procedure of the extracranial carotid artery performed? Who is credited with it?**
In 1954 by Eastcott.

CONTROVERSY

29. **What is the role of carotid artery stenting?**
Although CEA remains the standard of care for carotid artery disease, percutaneous angioplasty with stenting (CAS) has been investigated as an alternative. The underlying rationale is to decrease morbidity, hospital costs, and anesthetic risks in addition to improving long-term patency. Currently, "high-risk" symptomatic patients are considered for carotid stenting.

Multiple reports have been published in the last 10 years looking at the use of stents in carotid artery disease. These studies have clearly established that some type of cerebral protection device is required to reduce the risk of embolization. The most commonly used devices are filters placed distal to the stenosis to capture debris released during angioplasty and stenting. Recent randomized trials suggest that CAS is not equivalent to CEA, but the studies have been limited by heterogeneous (symptomatic and asymptomatic) patient populations. Proponents of CAS cite problems with these studies that may have favored surgery and note the continued improvements in technology. There are a number of important randomized trials enrolling patients at this time including the CREST (carotid revascularization endarterectomy versus stent) trial sponsored by National Institutes of Health (NIH) that will randomize 1400 symptomatic patients and 1100 asymptomatic patients.

WEBSITE

www.acssurgery.com

BIBLIOGRAPHY

1. Barnett HJM, Taylor DW, Eliasziw M et al.: Benefit of carotid endarterectomy in patients with symptomatic moderate or severe stenosis. N Engl J Med 339:1415-1425, 1998.

2. Executive Committee for the Asymptomatic Carotid Atherosclerosis Study: endarterectomy for asymptomatic carotid artery stenosis. JAMA 273:1421-1429, 1995.

3. Halliday A, Mansfield A, Marro J et al.: Prevention of disabling and fatal strokes by successful carotid endarterectomy in patients without recent neurological symptoms: randomised controlled trial. MRC Asymptomatic Carotid Surgery Trial (ACST) Collaborative Group. Lancet 363:1491, 2004.

4. Illig KA, Narins CR: Patient selection for carotid stenting versus endarterectomy: a systematic review. J Vasc Surg 44:661-672, 2006.

5. Luebke T, Aleksic M, Brunkwall J: Meta-analysis of randomized trials comparing carotid endarterectomy and endovascular treatment. Eur J Vasc Endovasc Surg 34:470-479, 2007.

6. Mas JL, Chantellier G, Beyssen B et al.: Endarterectomy versus stenting in patients with symptomatic severe carotid stenosis. N Engl J Med 355:1660-1671, 2006.

7. Moore WS, Kempszinski RF, Nelson JJ et al.: Recurrent carotid stenosis: results of the asymptomatic carotid atherosclerosis study. Stroke 29:2018-2025, 1998.

8. North American Symptomatic Carotid Endarterectomy Trial Collaborators: Beneficial effect of carotid endarterectomy in symptomatic patients with high-grade stenosis. N Engl J Med 325:445-453, 1991.

9. Paraskevas KI, Hamilton G, Mikhailidis DP: Statins: an essential component in the management of carotid artery disease. J Vasc Surg 46:373-386, 2007.

10. SPACE Collaborative Group: 30 day results from the SPACE trial of stent-protected angioplasty versus carotid endarterectomy in symptomatic patients: a randomised non-inferiority trial. Lancet 368:1239-1247, 2006.

CHAPTER 71

ABDOMINAL AORTIC ANEURYSM

Carlos A. Rueda, MD, and Mark R. Nehler, MD

1. **What is an abdominal aortic aneurysm (AAA)?**
   Aorta 50% increase in normal aortic diameter. Normal infrarenal aortic diameter is 2.0 cm for men. A definition of AAA as an aorta = 3.0 cm in diameter is appropriate.

2. **What is the incidence of AAA?**
   - Three percent in unselected adult patients screened with ultrasound (US)
   - Five percent in patients with known coronary artery disease (CAD)
   - Ten percent in patients with known peripheral vascular disease

3. **What is the etiology of AAA?**
   Elastin is the primary load-bearing element of the aorta. In the normal human aorta, there is a gradual reduction in the amount of elastin present in the distal compared with the proximal aorta. Elastin fragmentation and degeneration are observed histologically in AAA walls. These observations help explain the predilection of AAAs in the infrarenal aorta. Absence of vasa vasorum in the infrarenal aorta has led to the suggestion of a nutritive deficiency. The degradation of aortic media in aneurysmal disease implies a disrupted balance between proteolytic enzymes and their inhibitors.

4. **Do AAAs have a genetic component?**
   Multiple reports describe a familial subgroup of AAAs. Therefore, screening of AAA patients' first-degree relatives who are 50 years old and older makes sense. Two prospective studies demonstrated that approximately 30% of these relatives also harbor an AAA. The proposed genetic defect has been linked to abnormal type III collagen.

5. **Are patients with AAA prone to aneurysms in other vascular beds?**
   Yes. Forty percent of patients with a popliteal artery aneurysm harbor an AAA. Seventy-five percent of patients with a femoral artery aneurysm also have an AAA. Patients with thoracic aneurysms have a 20% chance of having a simultaneous AAA. Five percent of patients develop aortic aneurysms proximal to their graft at ≈5 years after infrarenal AAA repair.

6. **Can AAAs reliably be detected on physical examination?**
   No. The aortic bifurcation is at the level of the umbilicus. Therefore, the pulsatile mass of an AAA is located in the epigastrium. Thus, only relatively large AAAs can be detected in thin patients.

7. **Can AAAs be detected by radiography?**
   Plain abdominal or lumbar spine radiographs can detect occult AAA in about 20% of cases. A thin rim of calcification identifies the aneurysmal aortic wall. The majority of AAAs contain insufficient calcium to be visualized by radiography.

8. **Which imaging method is the best for screening patients for AAA?**
   Abdominal US permits measurement accuracy within 0.3 cm and data in both cross-sectional and longitudinal dimensions.

9. **What is the best single imaging modality to plan AAA repair?**
   The contrast-enhanced computed tomography (CT) scan is the best one. Diameter measurements are accurate within 0.2 cm. Venous anomalies (i.e., retroaortic or circumaortic left renal vein, inferior vena cava [IVC] duplication, and left-sided IVC) that dramatically alter the operative approach are well visualized on CT. Although CT is excellent at detecting aneurysmal rupture or leak (92% accuracy and 100% specificity), it is less useful for predicting suprarenal aneurysm involvement (sensitivity, 83%; specificity, 90%; positive predictive value, 48%).

10. **What is the manifestation of a symptomatic AAA?**
    Acute low back pain is the most common presenting symptom (82%), but only one third of AAAs are diagnosed before rupture. A hypotensive elderly man with acute onset of low back pain has a leaking AAA until proven otherwise.

11. **What is the appropriate management of a patient suspected of a ruptured AAA?**
    Just before emergent surgical exploration, patients who are hemodynamically unstable with a pulsatile abdominal mass should have an electrocardiogram (ECG) to rule out myocardial infarction (MI).

12. **Should all patients presenting with AAA rupture undergo repair?**
    Patients in profound shock or cardiac arrest at the time of presentation have little chance of survival. Extreme age, dementia, metastatic cancer, and other severe end-stage medical problems should force you to reassess this allocation of medical resources.

13. **Do all patients with ruptured AAAs make it to surgery?**
    Approximately half of patients with a ruptured AAA die before reaching the hospital. One fourth of those who make it to the hospital die before they can be brought to the operating room (OR). Therefore, only 25% of patients make it to surgery.

14. **How is a ruptured AAA treated operatively?**
    The patient should not be anesthetized until completely prepped and draped and ready for immediate incision because the blood pressure may decrease dramatically on induction of anesthesia. Rapid proximal aortic control is the key to successful outcome of operations for ruptured AAA. This can be at the diaphragm (in an unstable patient, with free intraperitoneal bleeding or a retroperitoneal hematoma that extends proximal to the left renal vein) or at the infrarenal aortic segment (in a stable patient with a lower retroperitoneal hematoma). Intraluminal balloon occlusion of the aorta is an option with free intraperitoneal rupture. As soon as control is obtained, the patient is resuscitated and clamps are moved to the more standard infrarenal location. Distal control can also be obtained with balloons or packs to prevent iliac venous injury.

15. **How should patients with symptomatic nonruptured AAAs be managed?**
    Symptomatic AAAs are rapidly expanding and at high risk for rupture. Therefore, most vascular surgeons agree that symptomatic but intact AAAs should be repaired expeditiously (as early as is conveniently possible).

16. **Are there any alternatives to open surgical repair for ruptured AAA?**
    Endovascular prosthetic grafts have been successfully placed in high-risk patients with symptomatic AAAs or contained ruptures both in the aortic and aortoiliac position.

17. **What are the rupture rates of AAAs?**
    A 5-cm diameter AAA has an annual rupture risk of <1%. The risk of AAA rupture increases with size. Annual rupture risk is 10% for a 6-cm AAA and 30% for AAAs >7 cm.

18. **How fast do AAAs enlarge?**

    The average expansion rate of all AAAs is 0.4 cm/year. However, 20% of all AAAs demonstrate no change in size over time. Conversely, 20% expand at a rate >0.5 cm/year. Rapid expansion (0.5 cm/6 months) is considered to be predictive of rupture and an indication for repair.

19. **When are angiograms helpful in the diagnostic workup for AAA?**

    Traditionally, angiography has been indicated in patients when there is concern regarding the extent of the proximal neck, concomitant visceral occlusive disease, renal artery anomalies, a prior colectomy with need to visualize the visceral circulation, or lower extremity occlusive or aneurysmal disease. More recently, thin slice (3 mm or less) CT angiograms are used to plan for the endovascular repair of an AAA (EVAR). Standard angiography is rarely used preoperatively as it is now part of the endovascular therapy.

20. **What is the difference between extraperitoneal and transabdominal approach?**

    Elective aortic graft placement can be carried out equally well via a transperitoneal or extraperitoneal approach. The former provides better pelvic exposure. The extraperitoneal approach provides superior exposure of the suprarenal aorta and facilitates postoperative pulmonary management.

21. **What are endografts? Are they durable?**

    It is estimated that 50% to 60% of AAAs are repaired with an endovascular graft. Endovascular grafts are graft-covered stents that are placed via the femoral artery by interventional (i.e., radiographic) methods to exclude the aneurysm without the need for an abdominal incision or cross-clamping the aorta. Multiple different series of successful endovascular AAA repair have been reported. Successful endograft placement has been reported in a wide variety of high-risk operative candidates. Many vascular surgeons and interventionalists are making aortic endograft placement their preferred treatment for patients with AAAs. The major drawbacks are late leaks or rupture from the graft, the cost of the procedure, and the need for long-term patient follow-up.

22. **What are the advantages and disadvantages of an endovascular repair of an AAA (EVAR)?**

    Recent studies suggest that EVAR has short-term reduced operative mortality over open AAA repair in anatomically suitable and relatively healthy patients. However, this reduced operative mortality disappeared in patients considered unfit for major surgery. In addition, EVAR requires ongoing surveillance and longer follow-up than open AAA repair. Some evidence suggests that EVAR is more expensive and leads to a greater number of complications and re-interventions. Open AAA repair may be preferred for younger, healthier patients and for whom long-term durability and follow-up is of concern. In contrast, older, sicker patients with increased operative risks and shorter life expectancy may be best treated with EVAR.

23. **What are the complications of EVAR? How are they treated?**

    There can be continued arterial perfusion of the aneurysm sac after EVAR. This is termed *endoleak*, and it occurs in 15% to 20% of EVAR. Type I endoleak results from antegrade flow at the stent graft attachment site. These are treated with proximal or distal extension grafts at the time of discovery. Type II endoleak results from retrograde flow in a collateral side branch of the aneurysm such as the lumbar arteries or inferior mesenteric artery. Because most of these endoleaks are self-limiting, observation is appropriate when the AAA is not increasing in size. However, type II endoleaks can be treated with percutaneous coil embolization or open repair if the AAA increases in size. Type III endoleak results from antegrade flow at the junction point between graft components. These are repaired with a secondary endograft. Type IV endoleak results from graft wall porosity and can be treated with secondary stenting or with observation. Aortic CT scans are conducted at regular intervals post-EVAR to identify late type II endoleaks that can lead to delayed AAA rupture.

24. **Describe the evaluation needed for a patient receiving EVAR.**
    A history and physical examination with a careful focus on the cardiopulmonary system is essential along with appropriate laboratory data. A CTA with fine cuts and three-dimensional reconstructions can help measure the diameter and evaluate the neck length, angulation, and thrombus. It will also provide valuable data on vessel diameter (iliac and femoral arteries), calcification, and tortuosity to determine the suitability of the patient and the type of device that will best seal the aneurysm. In general the proximal aortic neck diameter below the lowest renal artery should be between 20 and 28 mm and at least 15 mm or more in length.

25. **What are the technical aspects of EVAR?**
    Longitudinal incisions in the groin expose the femoral arteries, although many centers are doing it percutaneously. Subsequent proximal and distal control of the common, superficial, and profunda femoral arteries will allow the introduction of sheaths, wires, and the endovascular device to repair the AAA. The patient receives systemic heparinization before arterial puncture. An aortogram confirms the anatomical landmarks needed for graft deployment and the distance from the renal arteries to the common iliac artery bifurcation to accurately select the graft length. The location of the renal arteries must be noted and the C-arm not moved until deployment of the graft is completed. In some cases, after deployment of the aortic graft sealing is accomplished with gentle balloon angioplasty. A contralateral limb within the iliac artery is deployed and overlaps the main graft to achieve a good seal and avoid a type III endoleak. A repeat angiogram confirms placement and identifies type I and type III endoleaks. After extraction of the wires and sheaths the femoral arterotomies are closed with non-absorbable suture and the incisions closed in two layers or percutaneous closure devices are used.

26. **At what size should asymptomatic AAAs be repaired electively?**
    They should be repaired electively when the AAA reaches 5.5 cm in diameter. The only benefit for repair of an asymptomatic AAA is to prevent subsequent rupture and death. Therefore, all candidates for elective repair must expect to live at least 5 years.

27. **What are the technical aspects of AAA surgery?**
    The two important decisions are the location of arterial clamps and the type of graft to place. The majority of cases can be managed by placing the arterial clamp below the renal arteries. This avoids prolonged ischemia to the kidneys. The aneurysm is opened after clamping proximally and distally. Lumbar artery orifices are oversewn to prevent bleeding from collateral arteries. The inferior mesenteric artery is often occluded, but when it is patent and not vigorously backbleeding, it may require reimplantation.

28. **What are the major noncardiac complications of AAA repair?**
    Renal failure (elevation in creatinine) and intestinal ischemia (bloody diarrhea).

KEY POINTS

1. An AAA is defined as a ≥ 50% increase in normal aortic diameter.
2. Forty percent of patients with a popliteal artery aneurysm harbor an AAA.
3. CT is the single best imaging modality to plan an AAA repair.
4. AAA should be repaired electively when the size reaches 5.5 cm in diameter.
5. Neck length, angulation, and thrombus of the AAA determines if EVAR is feasible.

WEBSITES

www.acssurgery.com

www.vascularweb.org

BIBLIOGRAPHY

1. Harkin DW, Dillon M, Blair PH et al.: Endovascular ruptured abdominal aortic aneurysm repair (EVRAR): a systematic review. Eur J Vasc Endovasc Surg 34(6):673-681, 2007.

2. Tambyraja A, Murie J, Chalmers R: Predictors of outcome after abdominal aortic aneurysm rupture: Edinburgh Ruptured Aneurysm Score. World J Surg 31(11):2243-2247, 2007.

3. Endovascular aneurysm repair versus open repair in patients with abdominal aortic aneurysm (EVAR trial 1): randomised controlled trial. Lancet 365(9478):2179-2186, 2005.

4. Greenhalgh RM, Brown LC, Kwong GP et al.: Comparison of endovascular aneurysm repair with open repair in patients with abdominal aortic aneurysm (EVAR trial 1), 30-day operative mortality results: randomised controlled trial. Lancet 364(9437):843-848, 2004.

5. Endovascular aneurysm repair and outcome in patients unfit for open repair of abdominal aortic aneurysm (EVAR trial 2): randomised controlled trial. Lancet 365(9478):2187-2192, 2005.

6. Faries PL, Cadot H, Agarwal G et al.: Management of endoleak after endovascular aneurysm repair: cuffs, coils, and conversion. J Vasc Surg 37(6):1155-1161, 2003.

7. Lecroy C, Passman MA, Taylor S et al.: Should endovascular repair be used for small abdominal aortic aneurysms? Vasc Endovascular Surg 42:113-119; discussion, 120-121, 2008.

8. Powell JT, Brown LC, Forbes JF et al.: Final 12-year follow-up of surgery versus surveillance in the UK Small Aneurysm Trial. Br J Surg 94(6):702-708, 2007.

9. Alonso-Perez M, Segura RJ, Sanchez J et al.: Factors increasing the mortality rate for patients with ruptured abdominal aortic aneurysms. Ann Vasc Surg 15(6):601-607, 2001.

10. Lederle FA, Johnson GR, Wilson SE et al.: Rupture rate of large abdominal aortic aneurysms in patients refusing or unfit for elective repair. JAMA 287:2968-2972, 2002.

11. Lederle FA, Wilson SE, Johnson GR et al.: Immediate repair compared with surveillance of small abdominal aortic aneurysms. N Engl J Med 346:1437-1444, 2002.

CHAPTER 72

VENOUS DISEASE

Franklin L. Wright, MD, and Thomas A. Whitehill, MD

1. Where does deep venous thrombosis (DVT) originate?
More than 95% of DVTs develop in the deep veins of the lower extremities; the majority originate in the valve sinuses of the calf veins.

2. What is the usual source of a pulmonary embolus?
Calf vein thrombosis may propagate proximally into the deep venous system to involve the popliteal, femoral, or iliac veins (or a combination of veins). These proximal DVTs are the culprits in >90% of pulmonary emboli (PE).

3. What is Virchow's triad?
(1) Hypercoagulability, (2) disruption of an intact venous intimal lining, and (3) stasis of venous blood flow. In most patients with DVT, at least two of these three components are operative.

4. What are the major hypercoagulable syndromes (thrombophilia)?
Factor V Leiden mutation, antithrombin III deficiency, protein C deficiency, protein S deficiency, dysfibrinogenemia, lupus anticoagulant, antiphospholipid syndrome, elevated factor VIII, prothrombin 20210A mutation, and abnormalities of fibrinolysis are the major examples. The most common is the factor V Leiden mutation (i.e., activated protein C resistance).

5. What causes venous intimal injury?
Venous intimal changes may be secondary to vein wall trauma, infection, inflammation, indwelling catheters, or surgery. Venodilation during anesthesia and surgery may produce microscopic intimal tears and stasis. The injured venous intima initiates the release of thromboplastic substances that can activate the coagulation cascade.

6. What causes stasis of venous blood flow?
Venostasis is common in surgical patients; it occurs during anesthesia, after certain types of trauma, and with perioperative immobility.

7. What are the usual clinical risk factors for DVT?
Risk factors include malignancy (especially pancreatic, genitourinary, stomach, lung, colon, brain, ovary, kidney, and breast cancer), age older than 40 years, obesity, history of venous thrombosis or PE, family history, major surgical procedures, inflammatory bowel disease (IBD), pregnancy, hormone therapy, limited mobility, paralysis, hypercoagulable state, and trauma.

8. What signs and symptoms suggest DVT? How can DVT be accurately diagnosed?
The signs and symptoms are calf or thigh pain, tenderness, increased skin temperature, swelling, or superficial venous dilatation. None of these signs is specific for DVT. Even the well-known Homan's sign (i.e., calf pain with dorsiflexion of the foot) is unreliable; its accuracy is only 50%. Doppler ultrasound (US) examination (duplex scanning) detects DVT proximal to the calf veins with >95% accuracy; unfortunately, it is not as sensitive in detecting calf vein DVT. Ascending venography is still the reference standard.

9. **Is there any value to D-dimer testing?**

   Measurement of D-dimer cross-linked fibrin degradation products (FDPs), formed by the action of plasmin on cross-linked fibrin, has been proposed as an alternative to initial noninvasive testing. A sensitivity of 96.8% and a specificity of 35.2% have been reported for the enzyme-linked immunosorbent assay (ELISA) test, making it theoretically possible to limit noninvasive testing to those with positive D-dimer testing. Unfortunately, the ELISA test is time consuming and impractical as a screening test. More rapid (1 hour) ELISA assays are now available. Prospective evaluation of the safety of withholding anticoagulation therapy in patients who are D-dimer negative has been limited. False-positive results are a problem in patients with malignancy, infection, pregnancy, trauma, hemorrhage, or recent surgery.

10. **What methods of perioperative DVT prophylaxis should be used? In which surgical patients?**

    Perioperative DVT prophylaxis is strongly recommended in all high-risk patients who are older than 40 years and undergoing major general or orthopedic procedures. In general surgical patients, well-applied prophylactic measures decrease the relative risk of DVT by 67%. The best prophylaxis for DVT includes preoperative and postoperative walking. Intermittent pneumatic compression stockings and some form of anticoagulant prophylactic therapy (low-dose unfractionated heparin [LDUH] or low molecular weight heparin [LMWH]) are recommended as the patient's risk profile increases; anticoagulant prophylaxis is frequently underapplied given the high prevalence of risk factors among hospitalized patients.

11. **How does heparin work?**

    Heparin binds to antithrombin III (ATIII), rendering it more active. Low-dose heparin (5000 U administered subcutaneously every 8 to 12 hours until the patient is fully ambulatory) activates ATIII, inhibits platelet aggregation, and decreases the availability of thrombin.

12. **What is LMWH?**

    LMWH is a fragment of heparin produced by chemical breakdown. It exerts its anticoagulation effect by binding with ATIII and inhibiting several coagulation enzymes, principally factor Xa. It has a longer half-life than standard preparation heparin and can be administered once daily. LMWH gives a more predictable anticoagulant response at high doses and thus can be administered without monitoring (it is not necessary to follow the partial thromboplastin time).

13. **Should the placement of an inferior vena cava (IVC) filter ever be considered?**

    In patients with a documented, recurrent PE while taking adequate anticoagulation therapy or with an absolute contraindication to anticoagulation, an inferior vena cava (IVC) filter can be placed to prevent embolization or propagation of clot to the lungs. IVC filters are associated with a subsequent significant increase in the rate of DVT. Despite renewed interest in IVC filters as a result of advances in retrievable devices, insufficient evidence exists to expand these indications.

14. **How long should anti-coagulation be continued post-DVT?**

    Patients with a transient/reversible cause (e.g., trauma, surgery) of an initial DVT may be anticoagulated for 3 months (LMWH or vitamin-K antagonist [i.e., warfarin]). Treatment should extend for 6 to 12 months for an initial DVT of unknown origin. Risk factors for recurrent DVT include personal or strong family history of DVT, thrombophilic state (e.g., cancer, hypercoagulable syndrome), persistently elevated D-dimer after therapy, or residual clot on follow-up duplex Doppler US. In the presence of one of these risk factors the physician must weigh the risks and benefits of lifelong anticoagulation in consultation with the patient.

15. **What are the characteristics of chronic venous insufficiency and postphlebitic or postthrombotic syndrome?**

    The primary characteristic is venous valvular incompetence or persistent venous obstruction with distal ambulatory venous hypertension. After DVT, involved venous segments eventually recanalize to some degree. However, their delicate valves remain scarred or trapped by residual organized thrombus. The loss of valvular function disables the venomotor pump. The vein walls become thicker and less compliant, increasing resistance to proximal blood flow. These factors result in distal venous hypertension. Protein-rich fluids, fibrin, and red blood cells are extravasated and deposited through large pores in the distended microcirculation during periods of venous hypertension. This process leads to inflammation, scarring, fibrosis of the subcutaneous tissues, and discoloration by hemosiderin deposition ("brawny" edema). The resultant inflammatory reaction, scarring, and interstitial edema create a further barrier to capillary flow and diffusion of oxygen; adequate nutrition to the skin is inhibited. These changes may lead to tissue atrophy and ulceration (i.e., venous stasis ulcer).

16. **Do all patients with DVT develop postphlebitic or postthrombotic syndrome?**

    No. Approximately one third to one half of patients with a DVT will develop a clinically relevant postphlebitic syndrome, generally in the first 2 years post-DVT. Recent epidemiologic studies suggest that the incidence of venous ulceration is about 5%. Of interest, 50% of patients with venous ulcers have no history of DVT (probably because of previous asymptomatic calf vein DVT).

17. **How are patients with postphlebitic syndrome treated?**

    With proper patient education and compliance, postphlebitic stasis sequelae can be controlled by nonoperative means in well over 90% of patients, particularly if no residual venous outflow obstruction complicates valvular incompetence. Nonoperative treatment consists of graded elastic compression stockings (or Unna boots) to retard swelling and periodic leg elevation during the day. Patients must be taught to elevate their legs above the heart ("toes above your nose") at regular intervals (e.g., 10 to 15 minutes every 2 hours). Compliance is critical.

18. **Distinguish between phlegmasia alba dolens and phlegmasia cerulea dolens.**

    Iliofemoral venous thrombosis is characterized by unilateral pain and edema of an entire lower extremity, discoloration, and groin tenderness. A total of 75% of the cases of iliofemoral venous thrombosis occur on the left side, presumably because of compression of the left common iliac vein by the overlying right common iliac artery (May-Thurner syndrome). In **phlegmasia alba dolens** (literally, painful white swelling), the leg becomes pale and white. Arterial pulses remain normal. Progressive thrombosis may occur with propagation proximally or distally and into neighboring tributaries. The entire leg becomes both edematous and mottled or cyanotic. This stage is called **phlegmasia cerulea dolens** (literally, painful purple swelling). When venous outflow is seriously impeded, arterial inflow may be reduced secondarily by as much as 30%. Limb loss is a serious concern; aggressive management (i.e., venous thrombectomy, catheter-directed lytic therapy, or both) is necessary.

19. **What is venous claudication?**

    When venous recanalization fails to occur after iliofemoral venous thrombosis, venous collaterals develop to bypass the obstruction to venous outflow. These collaterals usually suffice while the patient is at rest. However, leg exercise induces increased arterial inflow, which may exceed the capacity of the venous collateral bed and result in progressive venous hypertension. The pressure buildup in the venous system results in calf pain commonly described as tight, heavy, or bursting (venous claudication). Relief is obtained with rest and elevation but is not as prompt as with arterial claudication.

20. **How can one distinguish primary varicose veins from secondary varicose veins?**
    Primary varicose veins result from uncomplicated saphenofemoral venous valvular
    incompetence and have a greater saphenous distribution, positive tourniquet test result, no
    stasis sequelae (dermatitis or ulceration), and no morning ankle edema (lymphedema).
    Secondary varicose veins are most commonly a consequence of deep and perforator venous
    incompetence secondary to postphlebitic syndrome.

21. **Why do people develop primary varicose veins?**
    The most common cause is congenital absence of venous valves proximal to the saphenofemoral
    junction. There are normally no valves in the vena cava or common iliac veins and only
    an occasional valve in the external iliac veins. Thus, the sentinel valve in the common femoral
    vein just above the saphenofemoral junction is of critical importance. However, anatomic studies
    reveal that this valve is absent on one or the other side in 30% of patients.

22. **How, when, and in whom should varicose veins be treated?**
    Varicose veins that cause discomfort or serious cosmetic embarrassment require treatment.
    Better results are obtained with early treatment before continuous retrograde pressure and flow
    down the superficial system and into communicating perforating veins (whenever the patient
    is standing) cause secondary, irreversible perforator incompetence. High saphenous vein
    ligation at an early stage can arrest progression of this gravitational process. The distal
    varicosities can be managed by selective surgical stripping, sclerotherapy, or both.

KEY POINTS: VENOUS DISEASE

1. More than 95% of DVTs develop in the deep veins of the lower extremities; the majority
   originate in the valve sinuses of the calf veins.

2. Virchow's triad consists of hypercoagulability, disruption of an intact venous intimal lining,
   and stasis of venous blood flow.

3. The best prophylaxis for DVT includes preoperative and postoperative walking, however,
   prophylactic anticoagulation should be considered for the many surgical patients who have
   significant risk factors for DVT.

WEBSITE

www.acssurgery.com

BIBLIOGRAPHY

1. Clarke-Pearson DL, Dodge RK, Synan I et al.: Venous thromboembolism prophylaxis: patients at high risk to fail
   intermittent pneumatic compression. Obstet Gynecol 101:157, 2003.

2. Franks PJ, Sharp EJ, Moffatt CJ: Risk factors for leg ulcer recurrence: a randomized trial of two types of
   compression stockings. Age Ageing 24:490, 1995.

3. Gallix BP, Achard-Lichere C, Dauzat M et al.: Flow-independent magnetic resonance venography of the calf.
   J Magn Reson Imaging 17:421, 2003.

4. Geerts WH, Pineo GF, Heit JA et al.: Prevention of venous thromboembolism. Chest 126:338S-400S, 2004.

5. Ginsberg JS: Management of venous thromboembolism. N Engl J Med 335:1816, 1996.

6. Janssen MC, Wollersheim H, Verbruggen B et al.: Rapid D-dimer assays to exclude deep venous thrombosis and pulmonary embolism: current status and new developments. Semin Thromb Hemost 24:393, 1998.

7. Kahn SR: Frequency and determinants of the postthrombotic syndrome after venous thromboembolism. Curr Opin Pulm Med 12:299, 2006.

8. Meissner MH, Wakefield TW, Ascher E et al.: Acute venous disease: venous thrombosis and venous trauma. J Vasc Surg 46S: 25S, 2008.

9. Philbrick JT, Heim S: The d-dimer test for deep venous thrombosis: gold standards and bias in negative predictive value. Clin Chem 49:570, 2003.

10. Sorensen HT, Mellemkjaer L, Steffensen FH et al.: The risk of a diagnosis of cancer after primary deep venous thrombosis or pulmonary embolism. N Engl J Med 338:1169, 1998.

11. Young T, Tang H, Aukes J et al.: Vena caval filters for the prevention of pulmonary embolism. Cochrane Database Syst Rev 4: CD006212, 2007.

CHAPTER 73

NONINVASIVE VASCULAR DIAGNOSTIC LABORATORY

Darrell N. Jones, PhD, Jason Q. Alexander, MD, and Tony T. Nguyen, DO

1. **What is the role of the vascular diagnostic laboratory (VDL) in the assessment and treatment of patients with suspected vascular disease?**

   Although traditional evaluation by an experienced physician remains the foundation of vascular diagnosis, clinical assessment has its limitations. For example, only one third of cervical bruits are associated with significant carotid artery disease; conversely, as many as two thirds of patients with severe carotid disease present without a cervical bruit. Half of patients with extensive deep venous thrombosis (DVT) of the lower extremity lack signs and symptoms referable to the lower extremities, and more than half of patients presenting with clinical signs of DVT are venographically normal. As many as 40% of patients with diabetes have no large-vessel peripheral arterial occlusive disease. The vascular diagnostic laboratory (VDL) provides objective, quantitative, and functional status data to delineate the severity of extracranial cerebrovascular disease, peripheral arterial occlusive disease, and acute and chronic venous disease.

2. **What differentiates the VDL from diagnostic radiology and ultrasound?**

   The VDL provides functional information rather than or in addition to the morphologic data provided by radiology tests and general ultrasound (US) images. This information is particularly important for peripheral arterial occlusive disease, chronic venous insufficiency, and postoperative surveillance of vascular interventions. Anatomic information about the site of stenosis or occlusion is of limited value without knowledge of the functional significance when assessing peripheral arterial disease. Treatment options for patients with chronic venous insufficiency is dependent on function of the deep and superficial venous systems rather than ultrasonographic evidence of blockages. Early identification of narrowings in the postoperative period may allow early intervention to extend durability of repair.

CEREBROVASCULAR DISEASE

3. **Which noninvasive tests should be used to diagnose extracranial carotid artery disease?**

   Duplex ultrasound (US) has a sensitivity of 97% in detecting carotid artery disease and an accuracy of 95% in correctly classifying carotid stenoses as >50% reduction in diameter. Although catheter-based angiography is the gold standard for evaluation of carotid artery occlusive disease, this procedure is associated with a 1.2% stroke rate. Computed tomography angiography (CTA) and magnetic resonance angiography (MRA) also demonstrate high sensitivity and specificity for carotid occlusive disease, but to obtain these results requires the administration of contrast agents (usually either renagraffin or gadolinium) that carry a risk of nephropathy or systemic fibrosis. These risks are not associated with duplex ultrasonography.

4. **What is duplex ultrasound?**

Duplex US uses both image and velocity data (hence the name duplex) in a nearly simultaneous presentation of US echo images (often referred to as "gray scale" or B-mode US and blood velocity waveforms obtained by Doppler US. The Doppler signals are obtained from a single small region of the blood vessel. Average velocities can be estimated for multiple such regions over a large area of the vessel. By assigning colors to the velocities, blood flow can be visually represented. Such a presentation, called colorflow duplex US, aids the duplex examination but cannot replace the information obtained from the Doppler velocity waveform.

5. **Why is blood velocity important in assessing the degree of carotid artery stenosis?**

It is often difficult to measure accurately the arterial lumen on a B-mode US image because the acoustic properties (and hence the image) of noncalcified plaque, thrombus, and even blood may be similar. Arterial narrowing forces blood through a narrower channel, which increases the blood velocity. This velocity can characterize the degree of arterial narrowing. Current practice classifies the degree of internal carotid stenosis based exclusively on the Doppler velocity data.

6. **What are the velocity criteria and categorical ranges of carotid artery stenosis?**

The criteria developed at the University of Washington (Table 73-1) are the most widely accepted. Note that progressive carotid stenosis increases the flow velocity signal as the volume of blood is squeezed through a smaller and smaller orifice. Unfortunately, there is no universally excepted criteria for estimation of carotid stenosis based on velocity measurements. Ultrasonography is not only dependent on each individual ultrasonographer but also the type of machine. Ultimately, ultrasonography can only estimate stenoses ranges resulting from the aforementioned variables and variation in different patients (e.g., patients with improved ejection fraction [EF] will have elevated velocities compared with patients having lesser EF but similar narrowings). Thus any noninvasive VDL must continually evaluate the criteria that they employ and compare to gold standard measurements (catheter-based angiography) to verify their criteria.

TABLE 73-1. UNIVERSITY OF WASHINGTON CRITERIA

Stenosis	Criteria
0%	Peak systolic velocity <125 cm/sec and no velocity disturbance
1%–15%	Peak systolic velocity <125 cm/sec with turbulence during systolic deceleration
16%–49%	Peak systolic velocity <125 cm/sec with turbulence in the entire cardiac cycle
50%–79%	Peak systolic velocity >125 cm/sec and diastolic velocity <140 cm/sec
80%–99%	Diastolic velocity >140 cm/sec
100%	Absent flow velocity signal

7. **Is duplex ultrasonography capable of determining whether the internal carotid is occluded?**

As the stenosis in a vessel becomes tighter, the velocity of blood flow increases. At a critical point, however, the diameter of the stenosis becomes so narrow that blood can no longer traverse at a high speed and will actually slow down. When the stenosis approaches occlusion the velocity of the blood flow will slow down to the point that it is no longer in the range of the US machine. The duplex study may then interpret an internal carotid artery as occluded when in fact there is "trickle flow" or a "string sign." This is an important differentiation but internal carotid artery occlusion rarely requires intervention, but a critical stenosis associated with trickle flow or a string sign carries a significant risk of stroke.

8. **How accurate is duplex ultrasound of the internal carotid if the contralateral internal carotid is occluded?**
When the contralateral internal carotid artery is occluded the body will often adjust to maintain the same anterior cerebral perfusion by increasing flow in the internal carotid of interest. This increased flow leads to elevated velocities determined by Doppler. Because these velocities are used to estimate stenosis, the Doppler may artificially predict a tighter stenosis than is in fact present.

VENOUS DISEASE

9. **What noninvasive test is used to diagnose acute DVT?**
Duplex US has replaced venous occlusion plethysmography as the accepted standard. Colorflow duplex is useful because it helps to identify small veins from the muscle and fascial layers. The US assessment involves the following steps:
   1. Examine the vein for echogenic thrombus.
   2. Compress the vein, using pressure on the US probe, looking for complete collapse. Inability to compress the vein suggests thrombosis. Partial compression suggests partial thrombosis.
   3. A Doppler signal from the vein that is phasic with respiration suggests no proximal occlusive thrombus. A signal that is spontaneously present but nonphasic suggests flow around an occlusion via small collateral veins. Absence of a Doppler signal in the vein suggests absence of flow.

10. **Can duplex ultrasound be used for surveillance in patients at high risk for DVT?**
Diagnosis of DVT in asymptomatic patients presents a dilemma. The sensitivity of duplex US is reduced from the reported 95% to <80% for above-knee detection of DVT in asymptomatic patients. Calf DVT detection is much worse, with sensitivities as low as 20% in many reported series. However, serial contrast venography, although more specific, is not a practical surveillance strategy.

11. **Which veins are anatomically deep veins, and which veins are superficial veins?**
Differentiating between superficial and deep veins is important as superficial venous thrombosis carries almost no risk of pulmonary embolism (PE) unless first propagating into the deep system. The deep system is identified beneath muscular fascial layers in the body. For greater simplicity, it is often easiest to remember that *if* a vein runs with a named artery it is considered a deep vein. Thus, the vein that runs with the superficial femoral artery (formerly called the superficial femoral vein), the femoral vein, is a deep vein. There are a few exceptions to this rule but are largely limited to muscular calf veins, the gastrocnemius and soleal veins.

12. **What noninvasive tests are useful for evaluation of venous incompetence?**
Doppler US can detect venous reflux in the deep veins of the legs and in the greater and lesser saphenous veins. With experience, the test can be done using a simple Doppler (continuous wave versus pulsed Doppler), but duplex US is often used to facilitate identification of the vein segments and valves and to position a pulsed Doppler sample reliably. When a venous valve is incompetent, flow in the vein perpetuates peripherally if pressure is applied in the more central portion of the limb. Differentiating between competent and incompetent venous valves in the superficial and deep system impacts options for therapy.

PERIPHERAL ARTERIAL OCCLUSIVE DISEASE

13. **What is the primary test for diagnosis of lower extremity ischemia?**
    The ankle brachial index (ABI) or systolic pressure ratio is normally greater than or equal to
    1.0. Typically, Doppler US is used (instead of a stethoscope) as the flow sensor distal to
    the pressure cuff, but plethysmographic instruments also may be used. Doppler signals are
    usually monitored at the posterior tibial artery or dorsalis pedis artery. The ABI is the ratio of
    the highest systolic blood pressure (SBP) measured at either the dorsalis pedis artery or
    posterior tibial artery compared to the highest SBP measurement at the brachium of either arm.
    Unfortunately, calcified vessels can prevent compression by pressure cuffs thus suggesting
    artificially high SBP. This is most notable in patients who are diabetic who may demonstrate ABI
    greater than 1.0 despite hemodynamically significant lower extremity stenotic disease.

14. **What is gained by measuring pressures at limb levels other than the ankle?**
    Segmental limb pressure (SLP) measurements, performed at the upper thigh, lower thigh, calf,
    and ankle, localize the arterial segment(s) involved in peripheral arterial occlusive disease.

15. **What tests are used for assessing peripheral artery disease in patients who
    are diabetic who may have incompressible arteries caused by medial calcification?**
    Pulse volume recording (PVR) is a pneumoplethysmographic technique that tracks the limb
    volume changes over the cardiac cycle. It measures the segmental pressure changes with
    pneumatic cuffs as a function of the limb volume changes. The relative PVR amplitudes identify
    the presence of peripheral artery disease and localize the arterial segment involved. The PVR
    is unaffected by medial calcification. Great toe pressure also may be used to diagnose and assess
    disease severity in diabetic patients because medial calcification rarely affects the digital arteries.

16. **How should the patient with suspected intermittent claudication be evaluated?**
    The patient first should be evaluated by obtaining ABIs or SLPs at rest. The patient with ischemia
    at rest does not normally need further evaluation. The patient with mild arterial insufficiency
    at rest or even normal resting pressures should perform an exercise stress test (treadmill
    walking using either fixed or variable load protocols) followed by ABIs. The distance that the
    patient is able to walk allows assessment of functional disability, and the postexercise reduction
    in ankle pressure, or lack thereof, allows assessment of whether the disability is caused by
    arterial insufficiency rather than musculoskeletal or neurologic pain.

DUPLEX ULTRASOUND SURVEILLANCE OF VASCULAR THERAPY

17. **What is the importance of duplex ultrasound surveillance of autogenous lower
    extremity bypass grafts?**
    Duplex surveillance of infrainguinal autogenous bypass grafts is critical to the postoperative
    care in the vascular patient. Occluded autogenous grafts usually do not respond to attempts to
    regain patency and often require entirely new bypasses. Multiple studies have demonstrated
    that physical examination (e.g., loss or diminished distal pulse) or return of ischemic symptoms
    fail to identify new stenoses before occlusion. Early identification of stenosis within or at the
    periphery of grafts may be treated by minimally invasive open or endovascular techniques
    before occlusion occurs. Duplex US can easily identify stenoses both within the graft and at the
    anastomoses by demonstrating significant velocity shifts at these points.

18. **Does duplex ultrasound have any role in surveillance of infrainguinal
    revascularization?**
    Infrainguinal revascularization can be simply categorized as autogenous vein or graft bypass and
    above or below knee bypass. Numerous studies have verified that the patency rate differs

depending on which type of conduit is used and the location of the distal anastomosis: vein graft above the knee being best and below knee prosthetic graft being worst in terms of graft failure. It has been documented that early detection of graft failure resulting from significant stenosis and subsequent intervention have a better outcome compared to salvage of an occluded graft. Vein grafts are more likely to develop a progressive stenosis leading to occlusion compared to prosthetic graft, which generally do not stenose before occlusion. Duplex US, therefore, has a role in graft surveillance of vein graft to improve patency. Although prosthetic grafts do not routinely demonstrate intragraft stenosis, they may exhibit progression of atherosclerotic disease of hemodynamically significant narrowing at the anastomoses. If these narrowings are identified and treated it may be possible to extend prosthetic graft patency as well. Furthermore, current literature tends to support surveillance US for following endovascular stenting and angioplasty in attempts to identify early restenosis to expedite reintervention.

19. **What is the role for surveillance duplex ultrasound following carotid endarterectomy (CEA)?**
The rationale for surveillance duplex US following carotid endarterectomy (CEA) is twofold. Most vascular surgeons will evaluate the repair of the ipsilateral carotid on a 6-month to annual basis. The incidence of recurrent stenosis is rare but early identification may allow more immediate or minimally invasive intervention before a patient becomes symptomatic. Of potentially greater significance during surveillance duplex US examination is evaluation of the contralateral carotid artery. Up to one quarter of patients undergoing CEA will demonstrate progression from nonhemodynamically significant disease to significant atherosclerotic disease in the contraleteral internal carotid artery over the next 10 years.

CONTROVERSIES

20. **Can carotid endarterectomy be performed on the basis of duplex study alone?**
The argument for elimination of arteriography in selected cases is persuasive because the carotid arteriogram alone has a morbidity rate >1%. This rate may represent 25% of the usual total morbidity associated with CDEA. However, to realize the benefit of surgery based on duplex US, the duplex study must have a high positive predictive value (PPV). Fortunately, the PPV is high for severe lesions that meet suitably strict criteria (e.g., peak systolic velocities >290 cm/sec and end-diastolic velocities >80 cm/sec).

21. **Does duplex ultrasound have any role in the preoperative evaluation of peripheral vascular disease?**
Contrast arteriography (CA) is still the gold standard imaging modality in the work-up of limb ischemia. However, duplex US is gaining popularity as the preferred modality of choice to image the arterial vasculature to evaluate for potential revascularization. Duplex has several advantages over contrast arteriography that makes it appealing. It can identify areas of thickened or calcified vessels that are still patent and therefore, would be falsely identify as a potential distal target on contrast imaging or MRA. Volume flow measurements by duplex allows a more objective assessment of hemodynamically significant lesion as compared to a subjective assessment by CA. Other benefits of duplex are the ability to assess the underlying disease of the vessel to determine whether a lesion is a chronic occlusion or an acute embolus with little underlying disease, aneurysms with partial thrombus and no luminal dilation, which would appear normal on CA, and the presence of ulcerated or irregular plaques, which would be a source of embolization. The feasibility and portability of the duplex as a bedside study allows for a more cost-effective and time efficient study and thus, reducing hospital cost and stays. The ability to concurrently evaluate the venous system for potential conduit is also attractive.

22. **What is the potential adverse affects of magnetic resonance angiography in patients with renal insufficiency?**

    Nephrogenic systemic fibrosis (NSF), first recognized in 1997, is a disease affecting renal failure or dialysis patients. It is characterized by a scleroderma-like dermatosis with thickening of the skin resulting in indurated plaque lesions. It commonly involves extremities causing contractures but can also have visceral involvement, which increases morbidity and mortality. Although the actual pathogenesis is currently unknown, there are many associated risk factors including gadolinium-containing contrast media. Because MRA carries the risk of NSF and CTA carries a risk of contrast nephropathy, duplex US may be the diagnostic modality of choice in patients with renal insufficiency.

23. **What are the disadvantages of duplex ultrasound?**

    Duplex US do have limitations. Factors that limits its visualizations are severely calcified vessels, severe lymphedema, dermatitis, ulcer wounds, or hyperkeratosis, and rest pain or noncompliant patients. Extremely low-flow states with peak systolic velocity (PSV) <20 cm/sec can make duplex interpretations unreliable, as is the case with critically stenotic internal carotid artery (ICA) disease that may be incorrectly interpreted as occluded.

24. **Should D-dimer blood tests be required before patients are evaluated by ultrasound for DVT?**

    D-dimer is a degradation product of cross-linked fibrin. Blood plasma levels of D-dimer are often elevated in patients with DVT. However, DVT is not the only cause of elevated D-dimers and cannot be used instead of US to diagnose the presence of DVT. Conversely, in selected patient subgroups, a low D-dimer level has a high negative predictive value and can prevent unnecessary US testing. The test should be restricted to nonsurgical patients, patients who are not anticoagulated, patients in the outpatient setting, and patients in whom there is a low clinical suspicion of DVT such as a painful limb without swelling or bilateral ankle swelling.

25. **Is there a therapeutic component to the noninvasive vascular diagnostic laboratory?**

    Duplex US is now being used to localize and guide treatment of many iatrogenic pseudoaneurysms. When a patient develops a pseudoaneurysm after arterial cannulation with a long and narrow neck, treatment can be instituted employing compression at the neck using the US probe. If the flow can be obstructed using the probe (usually requiring 20 to 30 minutes of pressure), the pseudoaneurysm will often thrombose. Additionally, US can be used to guide thrombin injection into the pseudoaneurysms themselves. Injection is performed only in pseudoaneurysms with long, narrow necks. Cannulation of the aneurysm with a needle is confirmed with US. Colorflow is applied to the aneurysm during thrombin injection to confirm thrombosis. This method, while carrying a small risk of distal embolization, eliminates the discomfort to the patient of extended ultrasound compression.

26. **What is the role of duplex ultrasound in the treatment and management of abdominal aortic aneurysms (AAA)?**

    Conventional US is quite good at identifying abdominal aortic aneurysm (AAA) but suffers when attempting to determine aneurysm size. This is more significant in large patients or aneurysms containing an abundance of thrombus. Computed tomography (CT) scan remains the test of choice for anatomic delineation of AAA, especially when evaluating for the appropriateness of endovascular AAA repair (EVAR). Duplex US may be valuable in determining success of repair during surveillance after EVAR. Although this application remains controversial, post-EVAR duplex US can identify leaks and evaluate aneurysm sac growth while avoiding the contrast load incumbent to post-EVAR CT scan surveillance.

KEY POINTS: NONINVASIVE VASCULAR DIAGNOSTIC LABORATORY

1. Duplex US has a sensitivity of 97% in detecting carotid artery disease and an accuracy of 95% in correctly classifying carotid stenoses as >50% reduction in diameter.

2. The primary test for diagnosis of lower extremity ischemia is the ABI.

3. The noninvasive test used to diagnose acute DVT is duplex US.

4. Duplex US surveillance of lower extremity revascularization and CEA has become a critical component of the noninvasive VDL.

5. The role of duplex US is rapidly expanding in conjunction with the expansion of minimally invasive vascular therapies. This role includes not only diagnosis but surveillance and therapy.

WEBSITE

www.acssurgery.com

BIBLIOGRAPHY

1. Ascher E, Marks NA, Hingorani AP et al.: Duplex-guided endovascular treatment for occlusive and stenotic lesions of the femoral-popliteal arterial segment: a comparative study in the first 253 cases. J Vasc Surg 44:1230-1237, 2006.

2. Baker WF: Diagnosis of deep venous thrombosis and pulmonary embolism. Med Clin North Am 82:459-476, 1998.

3. Ballotta E, Da Giau, Meneghetti G et al.: Progression of atherosclerosis in asymptomatic carotid arteries after contralateral endarterectomy: a 10-year prospective study. J Vasc Surg 45:516-522, 2007.

4. Carter A, Murphy MO, Halka AT et al.: The natural history of stenoses within lower limb arterial bypass grafts using a graft surveillance program. Ann Vasc Surg 21:695-703, 2007.

5. Clorius S, Technau K, Watter T et al.: Nephrogenic systemic fibrosis following exposure to gadolinium-containing contrast agent. Clin Nephrol 68:249-252, 2007.

6. Gerlock AJ, Giyanani VL, Krebs C: *Applications of noninvasive vascular techniques*, Philadelphia, 1988, W.B. Saunders.

7. Hanson JM, Atri M, Power N: Ultrasound-guided thrombin injection groin pseudoaneurysm: Doppler features and technical tips. Br J Radiology 81:154-163, 2008.

8. Hingorani AP, Ascher E, Marks N: Duplex arteriography for lower extremity revascularization. Perspect Vasc Surg Endovasc Ther 19:6-20, 2007.

9. Luedde M, Krumsdorf U, Zehelein J et al.: Treatment of iatrogenic femoral pseudoaneurysm by ultrasound-guided compression therapy and thrombin injection. Angiology 58:435-439, 2007.

10. Moneta GL, Edwards JM, Papanicolaou G et al.: Screening for asymptomatic internal carotid artery stenosis: duplex criteria for discriminating 60% to 99% stenosis. J Vasc Surg 21:989-997, 1995.

11. Mueller-Hulsbeck S, Order BM, Jahnke T: Interventions in infrainguinal bypass grafts. Cardiovasc Intervent Radiol 29:17-28, 2006.

12. Olsen DM, Rodriguez JA, Vranic M et al.: A prospective study of ultrasound scan-guided thrombin injection of femoral pseudoaneurysm: a trend toward minimal medication. J Vasc Surg 36:779-782, 2002.

13. Roth SM, Bandyk DF: Duplex imaging of lower extremity bypasses, angioplasties, and stents. Semin Vasc Surg 12:275-284, 1999.

14. Sato DT, Goff CD, Gregory RT et al.: Endoleak after aortic stent graft repair: diagnosis by color duplex ultrasound scan versus computed tomography scan. J Vasc Surg 28:657-663, 1998.

15. Shirit D, Levi H, Huerta M et al.: Appropriate indications for venous duplex scanning based on D-dimer assay. Ann Vasc Surg 16:304-308, 2002.

16. Wolf YG, Johnson BL, Hill BB et al.: Duplex ultrasound scanning versus computed tomographic angiography for postoperative evaluation of endovascular abdominal aortic aneurysm repair. J Vasc Surg 32:1142-1148, 2000.

17. Zierler RE, Sumner DS: Physiologic assessment of peripheral arterial occlusive disease. In Rutherford RB, editor: *Vascular surgery*, 5th ed., Philadelphia, 2000, W.B. Saunders.

CHAPTER 74

CORONARY ARTERY DISEASE

Joseph C. Cleveland, Jr., MD

1. What is angina, and what causes it?

Angina pectoris reflects myocardial ischemia. Patients often describe the sensation as pressure, choking, or tightness. Angina is typically produced by an imbalance between myocardial oxygen supply and myocardial oxygen demand. The classic presentation is a man (male/female ratio of 4:1) out shoveling snow on a cold night after a big meal after having a fight with his wife.

2. How is angina treated?

The treatment options for angina include medical therapy or myocardial revascularization. Medical treatment is directed toward decreasing myocardial oxygen demand. Strategies include nitrates (nitroglycerin, isosorbide), which dilate coronary arteries minimally but also decrease blood pressure (afterload) and therefore myocardial oxygen demand; **β-receptor antagonists,** which decrease heart rate, contractility, and afterload; and **calcium channel antagonists,** which decrease afterload and may prevent coronary vasoconstriction. **Aspirin** (antiplatelet therapy) is also important. Newer antiplatelet agents such as clopidogrel (Plavix) and eptifibatide (Integrilin) are promoted in the management of acute coronary syndromes. Plavix, however, is a potent, efficacious agent, and operation (i.e., coronary artery bypass grafting [CABG]) within 1 week of Plavix exposure increases the risk of postoperative bleeding by threefold.

If medical therapy is unsuccessful in alleviating angina, myocardial revascularization with either percutaneous coronary intervention (PCI), with or without placement of a stent, or CABG may be appropriate.

3. What are the indications for coronary artery bypass graft?

1. **Left main coronary artery stenosis:** Stenosis >50% involving the left main coronary artery is a robust predictor of poor long-term outcome in patients who are medically treated. A substantial portion of the myocardium is supplied by this artery. Even if the patient is asymptomatic, survival is markedly improved with CABG. Left main coronary disease is a class I indication for CABG according to the American Heart Association/American College of Cardiology (AHA/ACC) guidelines for CABG surgery.
2. **Three-vessel coronary artery disease (70% stenosis) with depressed left ventricular (LV) function (i.e., <0.50) or two-vessel coronary artery disease (CAD) with proximal left anterior descending (LAD) involvement:** In randomized trials, patients with three-vessel disease and depressed LV function showed a survival benefit with CABG compared with medical therapy.
3. CABG also confers survival benefit in patients with **two-vessel CAD with a tight proximal LAD stenosis and an ejection fraction (EF) <0.50 or demonstrable ischemia on noninvasive testing.** An important caveat, however, in managing patients with depressed LV function is that operative mortality increases when the EF falls below 30%.
4. **Angina despite aggressive medical therapy:** Patients who have lifestyle limitations because of CAD are appropriate candidates for CABG, provided surgery can be performed with acceptable risk. Data from the Coronary Artery Surgery Study (CASS) suggest that patients treated with surgery have less angina, fewer activity limitations, and an objective increase in exercise tolerance compared with medically treated patients.

4. What is done during a "traditional" CABG procedure?

CABG is an arterial bypass procedure that can be done both on bypass and off bypass. The left internal mammary artery (LIMA) is harvested as a pedicled graft, with other conduits including the greater saphenous vein or radial artery procured as well. Cardiopulmonary bypass (CPB) is established by cannulating the ascending aorta and the right atrium, and the heart is arrested with cold blood cardioplegia. Segments of the greater saphenous vein are then reversed and sewn with the proximal (inflow) portion of the bypass graft originating from the ascending aorta and the distal (outflow) portion of the bypass graft anastomosed to the coronary artery distal to the obstructing lesion. The LIMA is typically sewn to the LAD. When the anastomoses are finished, the patient is weaned from CPB, and the chest is closed. Typically, one to six bypass grafts are constructed (hence the terms *triple* or *quadruple bypass*).

5. What is an off-pump CABG (OPCAB)?

CABG can be performed without CPB and arrest of the heart. When done with the heart beating through a median sternotomy, CABG is then called an off-pump coronary artery bypass (OPCAB). The heart is positioned with commercially available stabilization devices, and the vessel to be bypassed is immobilized and snared to provide temporary occlusion. The venous or arterial conduit is then sewn to the immobilized coronary artery, and the occlusion of the vessel is released.

6. Why would one choose an OPCAB instead of a traditional CABG?

CABG with CPB remains the gold standard with 85% of CABG procedures reported to the Society of Thoracic Surgeons National Adult Cardiac Database still being performed with CPB. However, CPD is associated with several adverse clinical consequences such as acute lung dysfunction, stroke, renal failure, liver failure, bleeding, and the promotion of a proinflammatory state. It is thought, although not yet well delineated, that performing CABG without CPB may reduce these complications. Patients with comorbidities of lung disease, cerebrovascular disease, renal disease, or severe peripheral vascular disease may have improved outcomes when CABG is performed without the use of CPB. The trade-off for avoidance of CPB may unfortunately include compromised graft patency, as most reports promoting OPCAB do not include graft patency data, and early reports of OPCAB described more early graft occlusions with this technique.

7. Does CABG improve myocardial function?

Yes. Hibernating myocardium is improved by CABG. Myocardial hibernation refers to the reversible myocardial contractile function associated with a decrease in coronary flow in the setting of preserved myocardial viability. Some patients with global systolic dysfunction exhibit dramatic improvement in myocardial contractility after CABG.

8. Is CABG helpful in patients with congestive heart failure?

Possibly. CABG improves CHF symptoms that are related to ischemic myocardial dysfunction. Conversely, if heart failure is secondary to long-standing irreversibly infarcted muscle (i.e., scar), CABG does not prove beneficial. The critical preoperative evaluation must assess the viability of dysfunctional myocardium. A rest-redistribution thallium scan can determine the segments of myocardium that are still viable, however, cardiac magnetic resonance imaging (MRI) is supplanting radionuclide imaging as a better test to detect hibernating myocardium.

9. Is CABG valuable in preventing ventricular arrhythmias?

No. Most ventricular arrhythmias in patients with CAD originate from the border of irritable myocardium that surrounds infarcted muscle. Implantation of an automated implantable cardiac defibrillator (AICD) is indicated for patients with life-threatening ventricular tachyarrhythmias.

10. What is the difference between PCI and CABG?

Several randomized, controlled clinical trials have compared PCI with CABG. Although collectively they analyzed data from several thousand patients, the vast majority (>80%) of patients who originally met inclusion criteria were excluded from participation for a variety of reasons. It is important to understand that although randomized controlled trials are the gold standard for comparison between two therapies, a significant criticism of these CABG versus PCI trials includes the relatively low risk of the populations studied, which may not be reflective of real world patients who undergo either CABG or PCI (see Controversies).

Several important features emerged from these trials. Overall mortality and adverse cardiac event (myocardial infarction [MI]) rates were no different for CABG and PCI. One study, the Bypass Angioplasty Revascularization Investigation (BARI) study showed a clinically relevant higher survival in type 2 diabetics undergoing CAB than those diabetics who had PCI. This differential survival persisted for 10 years of follow-up.

The major difference between the two treatment strategies was freedom from angina and reintervention. Overall, 40% of patients treated with percutaneous transluminal coronary angioplasty (PTCA) required repeat PTCA or CABG, whereas roughly 5% of patients treated with CABG required reintervention. The patients who underwent CABG also experienced fewer episodes of angina compared with the patients treated with PTCA.

The more recent trials comparing drug eluting stents (DES) versus CABG do establish a much lower rate of restenosis with DES—roughly 8% to 10%. However, DES have been associated with catastrophic thrombosis—occurring suddenly and without antecedent clinical signs—months to even years after placement. The thrombosis of these stents is much more likely to cause sudden death, or a substantial MI than restenosis seen by bare metal stents (BMS). Because of this propensity toward thrombosis with DES, patients are committed to dual antiplatelet therapy (both acetylsdisylic acid [ASA] and clopidogrel) for a minimum of 1 year, and many patients with DES in place are now being continued on dual antiplatelet therapy indefinitely.

The unavoidable conclusion is that the recommendation of PCI or CABG should be individualized for each patient. The two therapies should not be viewed as exclusionary or competitive; some patients may benefit from a combination of PCI and CABG. CABG results in a more durable revascularization, although with the inherent risk of perioperative complications.

KEY POINTS: CORONARY ARTERY DISEASE

1. Hibernating myocardium is improved by CABG.
2. CABG is not helpful in preventing ventricular arrhythmias.
3. The rule of thumb for vessel patency is 90% patency at 10 years for the internal mammary graft, 50% patency at 10 years for saphenous vein grafts, and 80% patency at 1 year for PCI of stenotic vessel with a BMS.

11. What is the rule of thumb for vessel patency?

Internal mammary graft:	90% patency at 10 years
Saphenous vein graft:	50% patency at 10 years
PCI with BMS of stenotic vessel:	80% patency at 1 year

12. What operative and technical problems are associated with CABG?

The operative complications broadly include technical problems with the bypass graft anastomosis, sternal complications, and incisional complications associated with the saphenous vein harvest incision. Technical problems with the coronary artery anastomosis usually lead to MI.

Sternal complications predictably result in sepsis and multiple organ failure (MOF). Incisions for saphenous vein harvest also may result in problems with edema, infection, and pain postoperatively.

13. What are the risks of CABG? Which comorbid factors increase the operative risk for CABG? Why are large databases useful for the reporting of data?

Estimating operative risk is a critical component of counseling patients before surgical revascularization. The Society of Thoracic Surgeons (STS) and the Veterans' Administration have developed and promoted two large national databases. The STS database now includes outcomes on over 2 million patients and represents the largest cardiothoracic outcomes and quality improvement program in the world. Factors that increase the risk of CABG include depressed left ventricular ejection fraction (LVEF), previous cardiac surgery, priority of operation (emergency versus elective), New York Heart Association Classification, age, peripheral vascular disease, chronic obstructive pulmonary disease (COPD), and decompensated heart failure at the time of surgery. These comorbidities figure prominently in outcome. Quite simply, raw mortality data for CABG can be misleading. Different surgeons can perform identical operations but have different raw mortality rates if one surgeon operates on young triathletes with CAD and the other surgeon operates on old couch potatoes who smoke two packs of cigarettes per day. Through assessment of these comorbid factors, a fairer representation of predicted to observed outcome can be determined. In this manner, using observed to expected outcomes with risk-adjusted models represents a more honest comparison of CABG mortality rates. As both the public and payers of health care demand transparency in outcomes, the STS database serves as a model for all other specialties to appropriately collect and risk-adjust data for quality improvement.

14. What steps are taken if a patient cannot be weaned from CPB?

The surgeon is in fact treating shock. As in hypovolemic shock (e.g., a bullet transecting the aorta), the basic principles include the following:

- Volume resuscitation until left-sided and right-sided filling pressures are optimized.
- When filling pressures are adequate, initiation of inotropic support.
- Push inotropic support to toxicity (usually ventricular tachyarrhythmias) and insert an intraaortic balloon pump (IABP). The ultimate extension of CPB includes the placement of an LV or right ventricular assist device (or both). These devices can support the circulation while allowing for myocardial recovery.

CONTROVERSIES

15. Is there an advantage to surgical revascularization with all arterial conduits?

Probably, however, the data are much less strong than the data supporting the clear advantage of a LIMA to LAD bypass over a vein graft to LAD bypass. The logical extension of the observation that an internal mammary artery has superior patency to a saphenous vein has sparked an interest in total arterial revascularization. Instead of using saphenous veins as bypass conduits, some surgeons also use the right internal mammary artery, the gastroepiploic artery, and the radial artery as bypass conduits instead of vein. Convincing data suggest a survival benefit and freedom from angina when the LIM artery is used as a conduit. The data supporting total arterial revascularization are much less clear.

16. What are the options for a patient with continued angina who is deemed not suitable for CABG?

For patients on optimized medical treatment who are not surgical candidates (because of prohibitive comorbidities or poor quality coronary artery targets for bypass), an alternative is a procedure called transmyocardial revascularization (TMR). TMR uses a laser to burn small holes from the endocardium to the epicardium. Although it was originally believed that the laser brought blood from the endocardial capillary network to the myocardium, it has been repeatedly observed that laser-created channels are filled with thrombus within 24 hours and subsequently occluded. Therefore, it is postulated that the laser energy invokes an inflammatory response with a resultant increase in angiogenic factors (vascular endothelial growth factor, tumor growth factor β, and fibroblast growth factor). Although promising experimental data and clinical trials support TMR as therapeutic, one wonders if a placebo effect is not operative in promoting anginal relief.

17. **What therapy should I offer to a 65-year-old male with diabetes mellitus, stable lifestyle limiting angina, multivessel coronary artery disease (no proximal left anterior descending involvement), and normal ventricular function (ejection fraction = 65%)?**
This type of patient explores the debate and interface between three options: (1) continued medical therapy, (2) multivessel PCI, and (3) CABG. A persuasive argument can be made for each therapy, although as surgeons, we would offer this patient a CABG. The key to appropriate decision making for this patient includes a multidisciplinary team of physicians, including cardiologists, and cardiac surgeons to fully inform the patient of his options and the expected benefits, outcomes, and long-term issues with each line of therapy. The decision to undergo multivessel PCI while this patient is on the catheterization table because "the problem can be fixed at this moment without a big operation" leaves this patient without a fair chance to be adequately counseled and informed of his options. In discussion with this patient, highlight that although CABG represents the most invasive therapy for his CAD, it offers him the most durable long-term treatment of his disease with a small upfront risk of mortality or morbidity and a relatively short (weeks to month) recovery period.

WEBSITE

www.acssurgery.com

BIBLIOGRAPHY

1. Cleveland JC Jr, Shroyer ALW, Chen AY et al.: Off-pump coronary artery bypass grafting decreases risk-adjusted mortality and morbidity. Ann Thorac Surg 72:1282-1288, 2001.

2. Eagle KA, Guyton RA, Davidoff R et al.: ACC/AHA 2004 guideline update for coronary artery bypass graft surgery: a report of the American College of Cardiology/American Heart Association Task Force on Participation Guidelines (Committee to update the 1999 Guidelines for Coronary Artery Bypass Surgery). American Heart Association Web Site. Available at: www.americanheart.org/presenter.jhtml?identifier=9181.

3. Gundry SR, Romano MA, Shattuck OH et al.: Seven-year follow-up of coronary artery bypasses performed with and without cardiopulmonary bypass. J Thorac Cardiovasc Surg 115:1273-1277, 1998.

4. Hannan EL, Racz MJ, Walford G et al.: Long-term outcomes of coronary-artery bypass grafting versus stent implantation. N Engl J Med 352:2174-2183, 2005.

5. Horvath KA, Aranki SF, Cohn LH et al.: Sustained angina relief 5 years after transmyocardial laser revascularization with a CO2 laser. Circulation 104(suppl I):I81-I84, 2001.

6. Taggart DP: Coronary artery bypass grafting is still the best treatment for multivessel and left main disease, but patients need to know. Ann Thorac Surg 82:1966-1975, 2006.

7. The final 10-year follow-up: results from the BARI randomized trial. J Am Coll Cardiology 49:1600-1606, 2007.

CHAPTER 75

MITRAL STENOSIS

T. Brett Reece, MD, and David A. Fullerton, MD

1. **What causes mitral stenosis?**
   Rheumatic fever.

2. **Which gender most commonly gets mitral stenosis?**
   Women, by a ratio of 2:1.

3. **What are the physical findings of mitral stenosis?**
   On auscultation, an opening snap and a diastolic murmur are heard best at the apex.

4. **How is the diagnosis confirmed?**
   By echocardiography, preferably transesophageal echocardiography (TEE).

5. **What is the Gorlin formula?**
   A formula used to calculate the area of a heart valve. In simplified terms:

   Mitral valve area = cardiac output (CO) ÷ √mean pressure gradient across the valve

6. **What is the normal size of the mitral valve?**
   The normal cross-sectional area is 4 to 6 cm^2.
   Mild mitral stenosis is <2 cm^2.
   Severe mitral stenosis is <1 cm^2.

7. **How is the mitral valve area determined by echocardiogram?**
   By measuring the blood flow velocity across the valve (the velocity increases with stenosis) and measuring the time required for the flow velocity to decline (referred to as the pressure half-time).

   Mitral valve area = 220 ÷ pressure half-time

8. **What is the pathophysiology of mitral stenosis?**
   Increased left atrial pressure is necessary to push blood through a stenotic mitral valve from the left atrium into the left ventricle. Increased left atrial pressure is transmitted retrograde into the pulmonary veins and pulmonary capillaries and ultimately into the pulmonary arteries. It gives the patient a sensation of dyspnea. A left atrial pressure of approximately 25 mm Hg increases pulmonary capillary pressure enough to produce pulmonary edema.
   Example: to maintain adequate left ventricular filling across a 1.5-cm^2 valve, a pressure gradient of 20 mm Hg is required. With a normal left ventricular end-diastolic pressure of 5 mm Hg, a 20-mm Hg gradient produces a left atrial pressure of 25 mm Hg. Left atrial pressure rises even further as flow across the valve increases (increased CO). This high left atrial pressure backs up and floods the lungs (pulmonary edema).

9. **What is the main symptom of mitral stenosis?**
   Dyspnea on exertion (DOE).

10. **What hemodynamic conditions precipitate symptoms in patients with mitral stenosis?**

   Tachycardia: Because blood flows through the mitral valve during diastole, a shorter diastole (tachycardia) means less time for blood to move through the stenotic mitral valve, which decreases stroke volume.

   Loss of atrial kick: As left atrial pressure increases, the left atrium stretches bigger and the normally organized atrial impulse becomes chaotic (i.e., atrial fibrillation). Increased pressure is required to move blood through the stenotic valve. Loss of presystolic atrial contraction may decrease left ventricular filling by as much as 30%.

11. **What complications may result from mitral stenosis?**
   1. Hemoptysis from severe pulmonary venous congestion.
   2. Thromboembolism in patients in atrial fibrillation.
   3. Endocarditis.
   4. Pulmonary hypertension and right-sided heart failure.

12. **Why does mitral stenosis cause pulmonary hypertension?**
   - Retrograde transmission of increased left atrial pressure.
   - Reflex pulmonary vasoconstriction initiated by left atrial distention.
   - Hypertrophy of the pulmonary arteries, leading to remodeling of the pulmonary vasculature.

13. **What is the medical therapy of mitral stenosis?**
   - β-blockers slow the ventricular rate to about 60 beats per minute.
   - Digoxin slows the ventricular rate (by slowing atrioventricular nodal conduction) in patients with atrial fibrillation.
   - Furosemide (Lasix) to reduce pulmonary edema.
   - Warfarin (Coumadin) is used if the patient is in atrial fibrillation.

14. **What is the natural history of mitral stenosis?**
   The survival with moderate mitral stenosis is approximately 50% at 10 years.

   Survival in asymptomatic patients is 80% at 10 years, but plummets to 0% to 15% once symptoms develop. Moreover, mean survival in these patients with pulmonary hypertension is <3 years.

15. **What are the indications for mechanical intervention in mitral stenosis?**
   - Symptomatic patients with moderate-to-severe mitral stenosis (valve area <1.5 cm^2 or transvalvular gradient of 5 to 10 mm Hg).
   - Asymptomatic patients with a mitral valve area <1 cm^2, transvalvular gradient of >10 mm Hg, or pulmonary artery systolic pressure >50 mm Hg.

16. **What is the procedure of choice for mitral stenosis?**
   If the patient has mobile valve leaflets, no calcium in the valve leaflets, and minimal concurrent mitral regurgitation, then balloon valvuloplasty with a catheter may be an option.

17. **Which patients may be appropriate for balloon valvuloplasty?**
   Again, this can be a tough call, but patients may be candidates if they are without calcification of the mitral annulus or leaflets, have little or no mitral regurgitation, and have little or no fusion of the mitral chordae tendineae. Left atrial thrombus is also a contraindication for the procedure.

18. **What are the results of balloon valvuloplasty?**
   - Mortality rate <1%.
   - Initial success can be as high as 95% in properly selected patients.

- Valve area may increase to 2 cm^2.
- <90% event-free (you and your patient do not want "events") survival at 7 years, again in properly selected patients.

19. **Which operations may be done for mitral stenosis?**
   - **Mitral commissurotomy:** The mortality rate is <2%, and recurrence of mitral stenosis is 2% per year. This operation is rarely done today.
   - **Mitral valve replacement:** The mortality rate is 6%.

BONUS QUESTION

20. **What is the Lutembacher syndrome?**
   Mitral stenosis associated with an atrial septal defect. This results in a left-to-right shunt and overworks the right ventricle.

KEY POINTS: MITRAL STENOSIS

1. Mitral stenosis is caused by rheumatic fever.

2. Physical findings include auscultation of an opening snap and a diastolic murmur, heard best at the apex.

3. Symptoms usually become manifest with tachycardia from exercise or atrial fibrillation.

4. Balloon mitral valvuloplasty is the procedure of choice for mitral stenosis. Mitral commissurotomy and mitral valve replacement are the two operations that may be done for mitral valve stenosis.

WEBSITE

www.acssurgery.com

BIBLIOGRAPHY

1. Bonow RO, Carabello B, Chatterjee K et al.: ACC/AHA 2006 guidelines for the management of patients with valvular heart disease. Circulation 114:e84-e231, 2006.

2. Fawzy ME, Shoukri M, Al Buraiki et al.: Seventeen years clinical and echocardiographic follow up of mitral balloon valvuloplasty in 520 patients, and predictors of long-term outcome. J Heart Valve Dis 16:454-460, 2007.

3. Hammermeister K, Sethi GK, Henderson WG et al.: Outcomes 15 years after valve replacement with mechanical versus bioprosthetic valve: Final report of the VA randomized trial. J Am Coll Cardiol 36:1152-1158, 2000.

4. Lung B, Garbarz E, Michand P et al.: Late results of percutaneous mitral commissurotomy in a series of 1024 patients. Analysis of late clinical deterioration: frequency, anatomic finding and predictive factors. Circulation 99:3270-3278, 1999.

5. Palacios IF, Sanchez PL, Harrell KC et al.: Which patients benefit form percutaneous mitral balloon valvuloplasty? Prevalvuloplasty and post valvuloplasty variables that predict long-term outcome. Circulation 106:1183-1188, 2002.

CHAPTER 76

MITRAL REGURGITATION

T. Brett Reece, MD, and David A. Fullerton, MD

1. **List the causes of mitral regurgitation.**
   Rheumatic fever
   Senile mitral annular calcification
   Endocarditis
   Papillary muscle dysfunction from ischemia
   Ruptured chordae tendineae
   Annular dilatation from left ventricular dilation

2. **What is the pathophysiology of mitral regurgitation?**
   The left ventricle ejects blood via two routes: (1) antegrade, through the aortic valve or (2) retrograde, through the mitral valve. The amount of each stroke volume ejected retrograde into the left atrium is the **regurgitant fraction**. To compensate for the regurgitant fraction, the left ventricle must increase its total stroke volume. This ultimately produces volume overload of the left ventricle and leads to ventricular dysfunction.

3. **What are the symptoms of mitral regurgitation?**
   Dyspnea on exertion and loss of exercise tolerance are the symptoms of heart failure.

4. **What determines left atrial pressure in mitral regurgitation?**
   The compliance of the left atrium.

5. **Why does acute mitral regurgitation cause severe symptoms?**
   With acute mitral regurgitation, the normal left atrium is noncompliant. Hence, left atrial pressure increases rapidly, flooding the lungs (i.e., congestive heart failure [CHF]) and causing severe symptoms. Conversely, chronic mitral regurgitation is associated with progressive dilation of the left atrium. With increased left atrial compliance, the left atrial pressure may not increase.

6. **What hemodynamic conditions exacerbate mitral regurgitation?**
   Increased left ventricular afterload: Increased systemic arterial blood pressure increases the impedance against which the left ventricular must pump to eject blood antegrade. The regurgitant fraction is therefore increased (more blood goes backwards through the mitral valve).

7. **What is the murmur of mitral regurgitation?**
   A holosystolic murmur is best heard at the apex with radiation to the left axilla.

8. **How is the diagnosis confirmed?**
   By color Doppler echocardiography, especially transesophageal echocardiography (TEE; the left atrium lies right on the esophagus). The regurgitant jet may be accurately visualized and quantified. Echocardiography also allows determination of the anatomic abnormality of the mitral valve apparatus that is responsible for the regurgitation. Furthermore, the defined anatomy defines the likelihood of valve repair.

9. **What is the medical therapy for mitral regurgitation?**
   - Afterload reduction with angiotensin-converting enzyme (ACE) inhibitors.
   - Diuretics (furosemide) for lower left ventricular preload.
   - Digoxin provides ventricular rate control for patients in atrial fibrillation.
   - Warfarin (Coumadin) is used for patients in atrial fibrillation.

10. **What are the indications for surgery in patients with mitral regurgitation?**
    - Severe mitral regurgitation, especially with a ruptured chordae tendineae.
    - Symptoms despite medical therapy.
    - Progressive mitral regurgitation by echocardiography.
    - Deteriorating left ventricular systolic function. Because mitral regurgitation lowers the total impedance of left ventricular ejection (much of each stroke volume escapes via the low resistance mitral valvular "back door"), the left ventricular ejection fraction (LVEF) should be greater than normal in the presence of mitral regurgitation. An LVEF <55% in the presence of mitral regurgitation suggests left ventricular dysfunction.
    - Pulmonary artery pressure increases with exercise.

11. **How is mitral regurgitation corrected?**
    Mitral valve repair. Mitral valve repair is the preferred surgical procedure. This preserves the mitral apparatus, maintaining the continuity between the left ventricular muscle and the mitral annulus via the chordae tendineae. Loss of this continuity by resection of the apparatus places the left ventricle at a mechanical disadvantage that over time leads to left ventricular dilatation and dysfunction.
    Mitral valve replacement. An inability to repair the regurgitant valve mandates replacement. If replacement is necessary, efforts should be made to preserve the posterior leaflet of the mitral valve. In most series, mitral valve replacement is required in <30% of cases.

12. **Why is it preferable to repair rather than replace the mitral valve?**
    - Lower operative mortality.
    - Less risk of thromboembolism.
    - Less risk of endocarditis.
    - Less need (if any) for chronic anticoagulation.
    - Better long-term left ventricular function.
    - Avoids valve-related complications.

13. **How is the mitral valve repaired?**
    The redundant portion(s) of the valve leaflet(s) is resected, the leaflet is reapproximated, and the mitral annulus is plicated and reinforced with a prosthetic annuloplasty ring. The annuloplasty ring is sewn around the perimeter of the annulus on the left atrial side of the valve. In so doing, the mitral leaflets are supported by competent chordae tendineae, and the circumference of the mitral annulus is decreased. Competency of the repaired valve is assessed intraoperatively using TEE.

14. **What is the operative mortality of mitral valve repair versus mitral valve replacement?**
    Repair: 2%; replacement: 6%.

15. **How durable are mitral valve repairs?**
    The risk of requiring another mitral valve operation is approximately 2% per year.

16. **What is the role of minimally invasive surgery in patients with mitral regurgitation?**
    Minimally invasive approaches can be applied to many patients undergoing mitral valve surgery. "Minimally invasive" may refer to many things ranging from a limited incision, to a limited

sternotomy, to a thoracotomy, or even with use of robotics. All these approaches can be used with repair or replacement. Theoretical advantages of the minimally invasive approaches include a possible decrease in postoperative bleeding and postoperative pain. Finally, minimally invasive approaches have been safely performed in patients with previous sternotomy undergoing subsequent cardiac procedures. The robotic approach may be particularly useful in facilitating repair of the mitral valve for myxomatous degeneration.

BONUS QUESTION

17. **What is systolic anterior motion (SAM) of mitral valve?**
    SAM is a complication of mitral valve repair. After mitral valve repair, the anterior leaflet of the mitral valve may billow into the left ventricular outflow tract during systole, creating two problems: (1) dynamic left ventricular outflow tract obstruction and (2) mitral regurgitation (anterior displacement of the anterior leaflet causes it to be foreshortened). SAM should be suspected if cardiac output (CO) is low after mitral valve repair and may be diagnosed by echocardiography. It is exacerbated by an increased contractile state of the myocardium, so inotropic agents should be avoided. Patients with SAM are treated by volume-loading and β-blocking agents. If these measures fail, the valve should be replaced.

KEY POINTS: MITRAL REGURGITATION

1. The symptoms are dyspnea on exertion and loss of exercise tolerance.

2. The murmur of mitral regurgitation is a holosystolic murmur heard best at the apex with radiation to the left axilla.

3. Mitral valve regurgitation is corrected with mitral valve repair or mitral valve replacement.

4. Mitral valve repair is preferable to replacement because of lower operative mortality rates, less risk of thromboembolism, less risk of endocarditis, better long-term left ventricular function, and less need (if any) for chronic anticoagulation.

5. Repair also avoids prosthetic valve-related complications.

WEBSITE

www.acssurgery.com

BIBLIOGRAPHY

1. Bonow RO, Carabello B, Chatterjee K et al.: ACC/AHA 2006 guidelines for the management of patients with valvular heart disease. Circulation 114:e84-e231, 2006.

2. Carabello BA: The ten most commonly asked questions about mitral regurgitation. Cardiol Rev 10:321-322, 2002.

3. Enruquez-Sarano M, Nkomo V, Mohty D et al.: Mitral regurgitation: natural history in operated and nonoperated patients. Adv Cardiol 39:122-129, 2002.

4. Galloway AC, Grossi EA, Bizekis CS et al.: Evolving techniques for mitral valve reconstruction. Ann Thorac Surg 236:288-293, 2002.
5. Irvine T, Li XK, Shan DJ et al.: Assessment of mitral regurgitation. Heart 88(suppl 4):iv11-iv19, 2002.
6. Soltesz EG, Cohn LH: Minimally invasive valve surgery. Cardiol Review 15:109-115, 2007.

CHAPTER 77

AORTIC VALVULAR DISEASE

Cyrus J. Parsa, MD

1. **What are the most common causes of aortic stenosis?**
   Age-related degenerative calcific aortic stenosis is the most common cause in adults. Aortic stenosis is more common in men than women.

2. **What is the most common anatomic anomaly in aortic stenosis?**
   Bicuspid aortic valve (normal valve is tricuspid) occurs in 2% of the general population. More than 50% of patients with aortic stenosis older than age 15 have a bicuspid aortic valve.

3. **What are the most common symptoms of aortic stenosis in adults? Infants?**
   Most patients with aortic stenosis are asymptomatic. In adults, the development of angina, syncope, or dyspnea on exertion (congestive heart failure [CHF]) portends a poor prognosis unless valve replacement is performed. CHF is the most common presentation of aortic stenosis in infants.

4. **What is the expected survival of patients with aortic stenosis?**
   Asymptomatic patients with aortic stenosis have a near-normal life expectancy. Once symptomatic, estimated survival if expectant management is pursued is 2 years (CHF), 3 years (syncope), and 4 years (angina). After symptoms occur, the composite 3-year mortality of patients who do not undergo valve surgery is 75%. Hence, it is important to catch patients before they are symptomatic.

5. **What is the most feared complication of aortic stenosis?**
   Sudden death.

6. **What physical findings suggest aortic stenosis?**
   Systolic crescendo-decrescendo (diamond-shaped) murmur, diminished peripheral pulses, or delayed pulse upstroke (call it *pulsus parvus et tardus* if you want to shine on medicine rounds).

7. **What are the typical findings of aortic stenosis on chest radiographs and electrocardiogram (ECG)?**
   Both chest radiographs and ECG may show normal results even with severe aortic stenosis; thus, these are not good screening tests. On chest radiograph, calcification of the aortic valve and an enlarged cardiac silhouette may be seen. ECG is fairly sensitive in detecting left ventricular hypertrophy (LVH) and may also reveal conduction defects such as P-R interval prolongation (these occur secondary to extension of valvular calcification into the adjacent conduction tissue).

8. **How is the diagnosis of aortic stenosis confirmed?**
   Echocardiography with Doppler ultrasound (US) is nearly 100% accurate in diagnosing hemodynamically significant aortic stenosis. The measured variable is actually velocity (v) across the valve. Velocity is converted to gradient using the Bernoulli equation where gradient $= 4v^2$. This data is then used to derive or estimate the aortic valve area (AVA).

9. **When is cardiac catheterization indicated in patients with aortic stenosis confirmed by echocardiography?**

   Class I recommendations from the most recent American College of Cardiology/American Heart Association (ACC/AHA) Task Force Guidelines indicate: (1) coronary angiography for patients undergoing aortic valve replacement (AVR) at risk for coronary artery disease (CAD) because approximately 50% of patients with aortic stenosis will have some degree of associated CAD. Patients requiring AVR who have surgically treatable CAD should have coronary artery bypass graft (CABG) performed at the time of the valve surgery. (2) Cardiac catheterization for hemodynamic measurements when the severity of symptomatic aortic stenosis (AS) is inconclusive on noninvasive testing or the clinical findings and noninvasive tests do not correlate, and (3) Coronary angiography is recommended in patients with AS in whom pulmonary autograft (Ross procedure) is planned and the origins of both coronary arteries were not clearly delineated by noninvasive studies.

10. **When is an operation indicated for aortic stenosis?**

    Asymptomatic patients with aortic stenosis rarely require surgery; however, essentially all patients with symptomatic aortic stenosis should undergo aortic valve replacement. ACC/AHA class I guidelines support AVR for symptomatic patients with severe AS, patients with severe AS who are undergoing cardiac surgery for other reasons (e.g., CAD, other valve problems, or aortic surgery), and patients with severe AS with ejection fraction (EF) <50%. Class IIa recommendations are that an AVR can be performed for moderate AS in patients undergoing cardiac surgery for other reasons because the natural history of AS is that of a progressive disease that will probably warrant surgical repair within the next few years anyway. The average increase in gradient is 7 to 10 mm Hg per year; however, there is significant variation across patients.

11. **What should be given to all patients with AS undergoing elective clean-contaminated or contaminated surgery?**

    Antibiotic prophylaxis is indicated in all patients with AS for prevention of infective endocarditis and in patients with a rheumatic etiology of AS to prevent recurrent rheumatic fever.

12. **What hematologic disorder occurs in patient with severe aortic stenosis?**

    Impaired platelet function and decreased levels of von Willebrand factor (vWf) occur in patients with severe AS. This acquired vWf deficiency is associated with epistaxis or ecchymoses in 20% patients.

13. **Can aortic valvotomy be used to treat aortic stenosis?**

    Although valvotomy effectively palliates patients with congenital aortic stenosis, it is rarely curative. Most children with the condition will require AVR later in life. AVR, not valvotomy, is the procedure of choice in adults.

14. **What is the Ross procedure?**

    The patient's own pulmonary valve and proximal pulmonary artery are harvested (autograft) and used to replace the native, diseased aortic valve. A pulmonary allograft or homograft (harvested and frozen from a human cadaver) is then used to reconstruct the right ventricular outflow tract.

15. **What type of valvular prosthesis should be used in children requiring aortic valve replacement?**

    In children younger than 15 years (and young adults between the ages of 15 and 40 years), rapid calcification occurs in porcine valves placed in the aortic position. Thus, mechanical valves (or the Ross procedure; see question 14) should be used.

16. **What type of valvular prosthesis should be used in adults requiring aortic valve replacement?**

Whether to use a mechanical or a bioprosthetic valve depends on the patient's age, risk of lifelong anticoagulation, and ultimately patient preference. Although by no means unanimous, most cardiac surgeons would recommend a mechanical prosthesis for patients under the age of 60 years old. Mechanical aortic valves afford excellent long-term relief of hemodynamically significant aortic stenosis but require lifelong anticoagulation. Bioprosthetic valves in the aortic position do not require anticoagulation; however, 30% of these valves exhibit structural deterioration at 10 to 15 years. Freedom from reoperation for patients with bioprosthetic aortic valves is >90% at 10 years, but <70% at 15 years. A mechanical valve prosthesis is recommended to patients having redo valve surgery because reoperative risks are substantial for a third valve operation.

17. **What are the most common causes of aortic insufficiency?**

Infective valvular endocarditis, aortic dissection, connective tissue disease (e.g., Marfan and Ehlers-Danlos syndromes), aortitis (syphlitic or giant cell), iatrogenic (after aortic balloon valvotomy), aortic cusp prolapse associated with ventricular septal defects, and prosthetic (mechanical) valve dysfunction.

18. **What physical findings suggest aortic insufficiency?**

A rapid rise and fall of the arterial pulse (refer to this as a *water-hammer pulse* or, better yet, a *Corrigan's pulse* to dazzle your chief medicine resident). The diastolic pressure can be low in severe cases with a widened pulse pressure. These patients will exhibit a diastolic murmur as opposed to AS patients who exhibit a systolic ejection murmur.

19. **What is a Quincke's pulse?**

Capillary pulsations secondary to aortic insufficiency that can be detected by transmitting a light through the patient's fingertip or by pressing a glass slide on his or her lip.

20. **How is the diagnosis of aortic insufficiency confirmed?**

As with aortic stenosis, echocardiography or Doppler US are the tests of choice. Cardiac magnetic resonance imaging (MRI) is a recent advance that may be a useful diagnostic adjunct in these patients.

KEY POINTS: AORTIC VALVULAR DISEASE

1. The most common causes of aortic stenosis are congenital anomalies and calcific (degenerative) disease.

2. The most feared complication of aortic stenosis is sudden death.

3. Aortic stenosis is associated with a systolic ejection murmur, whereas aortic insufficiency is associated with a diastolic murmur.

4. Surgical intervention is indicated for all symptomatic patients with aortic stenosis and aortic insufficiency. The ACC/AHA guidelines provide class I recommendations for surgical indications in both groups.

5. Minimally invasive valve surgery is feasible and well used.

6. Patients with aortic stenosis should receive antibiotic prophylaxis before noncardiac surgeries.

7. Percutaneous AVR is in its infancy; only elderly patients with significant comorbidities can be enrolled in studies at centers that deploy these valves.

21. **When is an operation indicated for aortic insufficiency?**

    This depends on the cause of the aortic insufficiency and whether it is acute or chronic. Aortic insufficiency caused by an ascending aortic dissection is a surgical emergency. Aortic insufficiency secondary to infective endocarditis may or may not require aortic valve replacement (see question 22). Patients with chronic (mild to moderate) aortic insufficiency that does not progress enjoy a near-normal life expectancy. Patients with severe aortic insufficiency require valve surgery before they develop irreversible left ventricular dysfunction. ACC/AHA class I recommendations indicate AVR is indicated: for severe symptomatic patients irrespective of left ventricular (LV) function; for asymptomatic patients with chronic, severe aortic insufficiency with evidence of decreased LV function (EF = 50%); for patients with chronic, severe aortic insufficiency who are undergoing cardiac surgery for other reasons (see question 10). Class IIa recommendations indicate that AVR is indicated for asymptomatic, severe aortic insufficiency, with preserved LV function (EF >50%) if LV dimensions increase or enlarge (end-systolic LV diameter = 55 mm or end-diastolic LV diameter = 75 mm).

22. **What are the indications for aortic valve replacement in patients with infective endocarditis?**

    Progressive CHF, recurrent septic emboli, infection uncontrolled by antibiotics (often fungal, gram-negative rods or Staphylococcus aureus) and a prolongation of the P-R interval. Although hard to believe, the junction of the left and noncoronary aortic valvular cusps is immediately adjacent to the atrioventricular (A-V) node. Thus, a perivalvular abscess can slow A-V conduction.

23. **What is the operative mortality of aortic valve replacement?**

    Thirty-day mortality is 4.3% according to the Society of Thoracic Surgeons database (see referenced Web sites). In low-risk patients, the mortality can approach 1%; however, the mortality increases to 8% if AVR is combined with CABG. Multiple valve replacement and CABG increases perioperative mortality to 18.8%.

24. **What are the complications of aortic valve replacement?**

    - Bleeding requiring reexploration (2%).
    - Heart block (2%), again, caused by the proximity to the A-V node.
    - Stroke (1%) caused by air or calcium left in the heart after closure of the aortotomy.
    - Low cardiac output (= 5%) in patients with preoperative LV failure.

25. **What are the long-term results of aortic valve replacement?**

    Patients who survive the immediate perioperative period improve both symptomatically and functionally, and age-corrected survival returns to near normal (75% at 10 years). Aortic valve replacement partially reverses LVH and dilatation.

26. **What are the minimally invasive surgical options for AVR?**

    The approaches in order of use or popularity include: upper hemisternotomy approach, right anterior thoracotomy via the second interspace, right parasternal approach (complicated by postoperative lung herniation), and transverse sternotomy (less popular).

27. **What are the potential benefits of minimally invasive AVR?**

    Purported benefits of these approaches are superior cosmesis, decreased postoperative pain, and faster postoperative recovery with identical mortality to that of a full median sternotomy approach. A potential additional benefit is that these approaches limit dissection of unnecessary areas of the mediastinum, preserving intact pericardium that makes a potential redo operation technically less challenging.

28. **Can balloon aortic valvotomy be used for adult calcific aortic stenosis?**

Initially, it was hoped that BAV could replace surgery and provide long-term palliation in older patients who are at higher surgical risk because of decreased ventricular function. BAV can increase the AVA from 0.6 cm^2 to 0.9 cm^2 but is associated with a high incidence of recidivism over the subsequent months; in other words, the benefit is short-lived. Unfortunately, this group fare the poorest after balloon valvotomy; <50% are alive at 1 year after BAV.

29. **What are the indications for balloon valvotomy?**

Balloon valvotomy is effective in infants and young children with congenital aortic stenosis and a tiny aortic annulus. The intermediate results are similar to surgical valvotomy. In adults, balloon valvotomy should be used primarily as a bridge to aortic valve replacement or transplantation in patients who are critically ill. Temporary improvement in ventricular function suggests that the patient will benefit from AVR. Balloon valvotomy may also relieve the symptoms of women with severe aortic stenosis in the second trimester of pregnancy.

30. **Is percutaneous aortic valve replacement feasible?**

This modality is truly in its infancy. Trials are currently underway in the United States looking at this modality for patients with prohibitive mortality for conventional AVR. The largest current trials (REVIVE and RECAST) indicate feasibility, but are complicated by paravalvular leaks and an increase in cerebrovascular accidents. Options include: balloon aortic valvuloplasty, valved stents, balloon-expandable valves, and self-expanding valves. One of the biggest hurdles with this therapy is the large-caliber catheter requirements for deployment (particularly in patients with calcified, stenotic, artherosclerotic vessels). This has fostered attempts at a transapical approach via a small left thoracotomy. This approach is currently under study protocol in the United States.

CONTROVERSIES

31. **Should the Ross procedure ever be performed?**

For: The Ross procedure provides excellent, long-term (sometimes lifelong) hemodynamic relief of aortic stenosis and avoids the need for mechanical valves, thus avoiding the need for anticoagulation. An additional benefit is the regenerative capacity of the aortic autograft; it may actually increase in size as the patient grows.

Against: The Ross procedure is a technically demanding operation and has a significant learning curve with high associated morbidity. The procedure destroys a normal pulmonary valve, thus potentially giving the patient two (instead of one) valve diseases.

32. **Should a tissue valve be used in young adults between ages 15 and 30 years?**

For: Anticoagulation is not necessary for tissue valves placed in the aortic position; thus, the risk of significant bleeding complications in active patients is avoided. For women in the childbearing years, the advantages are real.

Against: Early valve dysfunction secondary to valve calcification occurs more aggressively in younger patients; thus, valve replacement may be necessary before 10 years.

33. **Should minimally invasive approaches to aortic valve replacement be attempted?**

For: AVR can be performed via a ministernotomy. This approach avoids a complete sternotomy and may improve cosmesis and decrease blood loss.

Against: AVR via conventional sternotomy is surprisingly well tolerated and has excellent long-term results. Comparative studies have identified no difference in quality of life between minimally invasive and conventional aortic valve replacement. Furthermore, long-term results of the minimally invasive approach are not yet available.

WEBSITES

www.acssurgery.com

www.ctsnet.org/

www.sts.org/sections/stsnationaldatabase/riskcalculator/

BIBLIOGRAPHY

1. Akins CW, Hilgenberg AD, Vlahakes GJ et al.: Results of bioprosthetic versus mechanical aortic valve replacement performed with concomitant coronary artery bypass grafting. Ann Thorac Surg 74:1098-1106, 2002.

2. Al-Halees Z, Pieters F, Qadoura F et al.: The Ross procedure is the procedure of choice for congenital aortic valve disease. J Thorac Cardiovasc Surg 123:437-441, 2002.

3. Bonacchi M, Prifti E, Giunti G et al.: Does ministernotomy improve postoperative outcome in aortic valve operation? A prospective randomized study. Ann Thorac Surg 73:460-465, 2002.

4. Bonow RO, Carabello BA, Chatterjee K et al.: ACC/AHA 2006 guidelines for the management of patients with valvular heart disease: a report of the American College of Cardiology/American Heart Association Task Force on Practice Guidelines (Writing Committee to Develop Guidelines for the Management of Patients With Valvular Heart Disease). American College of Cardiology Web site. Available at: www.acc.org/qualityandscience/clinical/guidelines/valvular/index.pdf.

5. Borer JS: Aortic valve replacement for the asymptomatic patient with aortic regurgitation: a new piece of the strategic puzzle. Circulation 106:2637-2639, 2002.

6. Carrol JD. Editorial: the evolving treatment of aortic stenosis: do new procedures provide new treatment options for the highest risk patients? Circulation 114:533-535, 2006.

7. Chaliki HP, Mohty D, Avierinos JF et al.: Outcomes after aortic valve replacement in patients with severe aortic regurgitation and markedly reduced left ventricular function. Circulation 106:2687-2693, 2002.

8. Detter C, Fischlein T, Feldmeier C et al.: Aortic valvotomy for congenital valvular aortic stenosis: a 37-year experience. Ann Thorac Surg 71:1564-1571, 2001.

9. Lamb HJ, Beyerbacht HP, de Roos A et al.: Left ventricular remodeling early after aortic valve replacement: differential effects on diastolic function in aortic valve stenosis and aortic regurgitation. J Am Coll Cardiol 40:2182-2188, 2002.

10. Lichtenstein SV, Cheung A, Ye J et al.: Transapical transcatheter aortic valve implantation in humans: initial clinical experience. Circulation 114:591-596, 2006.

11. Mihaljevic T, Cohn LH, Unic D et al.: One thousand minimally invasive valve operations: early and late results. Ann Surg 240:529-534, 2004.

12. McCrindle BW, Blackstone EH, Williams WG et al.: Are outcomes of surgical versus transcatheter balloon valvotomy equivalent in neonatal critical aortic stenosis? Circulation 104(suppl I):I152-II58, 2001.

13. Paparella D, David TE, Armstrong S et al.: Mid-term results of the Ross procedure. J Card Surg 16:338-343, 2001.

14. Rankin JS, Hammill MS, Ferguson TB et al.: Determinants of operative mortality in valvular heart surgery. J Thorac Cardiovasc Surg 131:547-557, 2006.

15. Russo CF, Mazzetti S, Garatti A et al.: Aortic complications after bicuspid aortic valve replacement: long-term results. Ann Thorac Surg 74:S1773-S1776, 2002.

16. Walther T, Simon P, Dewey T et al.: Transapical minimally invasive aortic valve implantation. Circulation 116: I-240-I-245, 2007.

17. Webb JG, Chandavimol M, Thompson C et al.: Percutaneous aortic valve implantation retrograde from the femoral artery. Circulation 113:842-850, 2006.

18. Webb JG, Pasupati S, Humphries K et al.: Percutaneous transarterial aortic valve replacement in selected high-risk patients with aortic stenosis. Circulation 116:755-763, 2007.

19. Yener N, Oktar GL, Erer D et al.: Bicuspid aortic valve. Ann Thorac Cardiovasc Surg 8:264-267, 2002.

THORACIC SURGERY FOR NON-NEOPLASTIC DISEASE

Laurence H. Brinckerhoff, MD

CHAPTER 78

PLEURAL EFFUSION

1. What is a pleural effusion?

Pleural fluid is generated in normal adults at a rate of 5 to 10 L per 24 hours in the combined hemithoraces, but normal adults have only 20 ml of pleural fluid present at any time. Pleural effusions develop when there is either increased production or decreased resorption. Pathologic conditions leading to effusions include increased capillary permeability (inflammation, tumor), increased hydrostatic pressure (e.g., in congestive heart failure [CHF]), decreased lymphatic drainage (tumor, radiation fibrosis), decreased oncotic pressure (hypoalbuminemia), or combinations of these.

2. How does one determine the cause of a pleural effusion?

History and physical examination, chest radiograph (upright and decubitus), and thoracentesis are used. Thoracentesis should be used to evaluate the pleural fluid. Bloody fluid is typical of trauma, pulmonary embolism (PE), or malignancy. Milky fluid can be evidence of a chylothorax (triglyceride >110), and purulent fluid evidence of an empyema. Fluid should be checked for cell count; cytology; acid-base balance (pH); Gram stain; culture; and glucose, protein, lactate dehydrogenase (LDH), amylase, and triglyceride level. Exudates have a protein ratio >0.5 and an LDH ratio >0.6. The most common cause of transudate is CHF; the most common cause of exudate is malignancy. Glucose <60 mg/dl is seen in parapneumonic effusions, rheumatoid effusion, tuberculous pleuritis, and malignancy.

3. What is the management of a pleural effusion?

Treatment for effusions differs based on the types, transudative or exudative. Thoracentesis or a tube thoracostomy should be used to evacuate the effusion and determine the type. If the effusion is transudative, one should correct the underlying problem (e.g., CHF). If the effusion is exudative, one needs to consider operative intervention (e.g., pleurodesis or decortication). A decortication is the removal of an infective rinde from the lung surface allowing for full expansion of the lung tissue thus filling an infected pleural space. A pleurodesis is used to treat a malignant effusion. A pleurodesis (stick the parietal and visceral pleurae together) can be performed with sclerosants (talc) or mechanical abrasion. Pleural symphysis (stuck pleura) results in decreased surface area for production, eliminates the pleural space for accumulation, and prevents lung collapse and compression. Chest tubes are generally removed when output is <150 ml per 24 hours.

4. What does an air-fluid level on an initial chest radiograph indicate?

An air-fluid level before any drainage procedure may represent a bronchopleural fistula. These fistulas may resolve with chest tube drainage or require open thoracotomy for definitive repair.

EMPYEMA

5. **What is an empyema, and what causes it?**
   An empyema is a purulent (infected) effusion. Fluid or blood in the pleural space can be directly inoculated with bacteria during surgery or trauma (33%) or by contamination from contiguous sites (50%) such as bronchopulmonary infection (most common). Most empyemas are parapneumonic, and the most commonly involved organisms are *Staphylococcus aureus*, enteric gram-negative bacilli, and anaerobes. Many times, infections are polymicrobial. Often there is no growth of an empyema culture because of effective antibiotic therapy or inadequate culture techniques, particularly with anaerobes.

6. **What are the three stages of empyema development?**
   They are the **exudative** stage (low viscosity fluid), **fibrinopurulent** stage (transitional phase with heavy fibrinous deposits and turbid fluid), and **organizing** stage (capillary ingrowth with lung trapping by collagen). This process usually evolves over 6 weeks.

7. **How is an empyema diagnosed?**
   Characteristic clinical and radiographic findings are used. Computed tomography (CT) scan is helpful in defining loculations. Thoracentesis may reveal frank pus. Gram stain may show many white blood cells (WBCs) and organisms. Biochemical analysis varies, but it is generally an exudate with a low pH (<7), high LDH (>1000 IU/L), and low glucose (<50 mg/dl).

8. **How should an empyema be treated?**
   Antibiotic therapy directed by Gram stain and culture. If early in the disease process, tube thoracostomy may be curative. Instillation of fibrinolytic enzymes (e.g., streptokinase or tissue plasminogen activator [tPA]) may be helpful if the empyema is early and loculated. An infected loculated (lots of discontinuous cystic pockets) effusion <14 days old should undergo video-assisted thoracoscopic surgery (VATS) decortication (i.e., resection of the thickened, adherent peel). The probability of conversion to open thoracotomy increases with the age of the effusion or empyema.

9. **What is a decortication?**
   The cortex is the outside wall or peel of the empyema (like an orange). Thus, decortication is the surgical release of the lung and removal of the abscess cavity walls. Successful decortication allows the lung to expand and fill the entire pleural space; if complete expansion does not occur, then the effusion may recur, and continued lung trapping is likely. There are two indications for decortication: ongoing signs of infection (fever, sepsis high WBC) after drainage and a significant rinde on the lung resulting in a trapped lung.

10. **What are the complications of an empyema if left untreated?**
    The most common is pulmonary fibrosis with lung trapping and resultant dyspnea. Others include contraction and deformity of the chest wall, spontaneous drainage through the chest wall (empyema necessitans), bronchopleural fistula, osteomyelitis, pericarditis, mediastinal or subphrenic abscess, sepsis, and death. None of these outcomes is particularly appealing, so in the absence of overwhelming contraindications, all empyemas warrant therapy.

INFECTIONS AND TUBERCULOSIS

11. **What is a lung abscess, and how is it treated?**
    A lung abscess is a localized site of infection located within the lung tissue with associated tissue necrosis. There are many potential lung infections that can produce lung abscesses, but anaerobic infections remain the most frequent types of pathogens. Unlike abscesses in other

area of the body, most lung abscesses do not require drainage and can be treated with systemic antibiotic therapy. Surgery is only considered when medical therapy has failed.

12. What are the clinical manifestations of pulmonary tuberculosis?

They can be almost anything or nothing (it has been stated that if you know tuberculosis, you know all of medicine), but the most common symptoms and signs are chronic fever; weight loss; night sweats; and cough, sometimes with hemoptysis. Chest radiograph typically shows upper lobe infiltrates, with or without cavitation, and can be misdiagnosed as a neoplastic process. Patients who are human immunodeficiency virus (HIV) positive and who are immunocompromised usually have mediastinal adenopathy, pleural effusions, and a miliary pattern.

13. How is the diagnosis of pulmonary tuberculosis made?

Positive acid-fast bacilli (AFB; "red snappers") smear in sputum sample; sensitivity improves with bronchoalveolar lavage (BAL) specimens. Culture growth will identify specific organism (i.e., atypicals) and drug sensitivity (watch out for multidrug resistance [MDR]).

14. What is the current medical treatment for active tuberculosis?

Initial therapy consists of a 6-month regimen with isoniazid, rifampin, and pyrazinamide for the first 2 months, and then isoniazid and rifampin for another 4 months. With this schedule, 95% of patients have tuberculosis-negative sputum at the end of therapy. Partial responders should receive therapy for longer than 6 months, and those with MDR-TB may receive ethambutol or streptomycin.

15. What are the indications for surgery in patients with tuberculosis?

Surgery is indicated for complications of the disease. The most common surgical indication in the United States is MDR-TB with destroyed lung and persistent cavitary disease. This lung tissue is resistant to drug penetration and can also "spill" organisms into healthy lung tissue. Other indications include hemoptysis, exclusion of lung cancer, bronchial stenosis, bronchopleural fistula, middle lobe syndrome, or mycobacterium other than tubercle bacilli (MOTT).

16. What is MOTT, and what is the role of surgery with this disease?

Atypical mycobacterial infections, nontuberculosis mycobacterial infections, and infection with mycobacteria other than tuberculosis are synonyms. The most common of these organisms is the *Mycobacterium avium* complex (MAC). Others include *M. chelonae* and abscesses, *M. kansaii, M. fortuitum,* and *M. xenopi.* MAC typically produces fibrocavitary disease of the upper lobes or the middle lobe or lingula of thin, white women. Surgery is indicated for localized disease, and in combination with drug therapy, it results in sputum conversion in ≈95% of patients with relapse rates of <5%. Other indications for surgery are the same as for regular tuberculosis.

KEY POINTS: THORACIC SURGERY FOR NON-NEOPLASTIC DISEASE

1. An empyema is a purulent (infected) effusion. The primary treatment is drainage.

2. The three stages of empyema are the exudative stage (low viscosity fluid), fibrinopurulent stage (transitional phase with heavy fibrinous deposits and turbid fluid), and organizing stage (capillary ingrowth with lung trapping by collagen).

3. Surgery is indicated for complications of tuberculosis, with the most common indication in the United States being MDR-TB with destroyed lung and persistent cavitary disease.

WEBSITE

www.acssurgery.com

BIBLIOGRAPHY

1. American Thoracic Society: Diagnosis and treatment of disease caused by nontuberculous mycobacteria. Am J Respir Crit Care Med 156(suppl 2 pt 2):S1-S25, 1997.

2. Colice GL, Curtis A, Deslauriers J et al.: Medical and surgical treatment of parapneumonic effusions: an evidence-based guideline. Chest 118:1158-1171, 2000.

3. Davis B, Systrom DM: Lung abscess: pathogenesis, diagnosis and treatment [Review]. Curr Clin Top Infect Dis 18:252-273, 1998.

4. de Hoyos A, Sundaresan S: Thoracic empyema. Surg Clin North Am 82:643-671, 2002.

5. Molnar TF: Current surgical treatment of thoracic empyema in adults [Review]. Eur J of Cardiothorac Surg 32 (3):422-430, 2007.

6. Pomerantz M, Brown J: Surgery of pulmonary mycobacterial disease. In Kaiser LR, Kron IL, Spray TL, editors: *Mastery of cardiothoracic surgery*, Philadelphia, 1998, Lippincott-Raven, 1998.

7. Takeda S, Maeda H, Hayakawa M et al.: Current surgical intervention for pulmonary tuberculosis. Ann Thorac Surg 79(3):959-963, 2005.

8. Wiedeman HP, Rice TW: Lung abscess and empyema. Semin Thorac Cardiovasc Surg 7:119-128, 1995.

CHAPTER 79

LUNG CANCER

Jamie M. Brown, MD

1. How common is lung cancer?

The incidence of lung cancer is approximately 180,000 new cases annually or 54.2 per 100,000 patients. More than 162,000 patients die annually, so the overall survival rate is 10%. This number has not improved over the past 35 years despite some treatment advances because of:

1. Teenage smoking and smoking in general.
2. Increased incidence in nonsmokers.
3. Presentation of lung cancer in advanced stage in most patients.

2. What risk factors are thought to be important in the development of lung cancer?

Ninety percent of patients have a smoking history
Chemicals (aromatic hydrocarbons, vinyl chloride)
Radiation (radon gas and uranium)
Asbestos
Metals (chromium, nickel, lead, and arsenic)
Environmental factors (air pollution, coal tar, petroleum products)

3. Do genes and heredity play a role in lung cancer?

Yes. A family history of lung cancer probably increases the risk of getting lung cancer. Furthermore, a large array of important biomarkers that influence prognosis have been identified in lung cancer cells and lung cancer tissue.

Past:

- Light microscopic evidence of vascular invasion
- Lymphatic invasion
- Cellular pleomorphism and mitotic figures

Present:

- Proto-oncogenes, growth factors, growth factor receptors
- Insulin-like growth factor (IGF)
- Epidermal growth factor receptor (EGFR)
- K-*ras* mutation (cell growth regulation)
- C-*myc* overexpression (cell growth)
- *bcl*-2 underexpression (loss of apoptosis regulation)
- Loss of tumor suppressor genes
- p53
- Retinoblastoma (RB gene)
- Chromosomal allele loss
- Fragile histidine triad gene (FHit)
- Retinoic acid receptor a (RARa)
- Overactivation of angiogenesis
- Platelet-derived growth factor (PDGF)
- Vascular endothelial-derived growth factor (VEGF)

Future:
- Gene therapy directed at those listed in present
- Antiangiogenesis therapy
- Immunopotentiation
- Adoptive immunotherapy: isolation, expansion, and reinfusion of tumor-infiltrating lymphocytes
- Nonspecific immunostimulation
- Tumor vaccines
- No single marker yet has a clear meaning with respect to prognosis in a given patient.

4. **What are the major histologic types of lung cancer?**

The most important distinction is between small cell and non-small cell carcinoma because of fundamental differences in tumor biology and clinical behavior (Table 79-1). Patients with small cell lung cancer are classified as having either limited or extensive disease. **Limited** means that all known disease is confined to one hemithorax and regional lymph nodes, including mediastinal, contralateral hilar, and ipsilateral supraclavicular nodes. **Extensive** describes disease beyond these limits, including brain, bone marrow, and intraabdominal metastases.

With small cell or neuroendocrine carcinoma, the small cell type is usually extensive at presentation, and 5-year survival is 5%. Neuroendocrine carcinoma, which is well differentiated, is known as *atypical carcinoid* and has a good prognosis but is not "benign."

TABLE 79-1. MAJOR HISTOLOGIC TYPES OF LUNG CANCER

Type	Incidence	Comments
Non–small cell carcinomas	80%	
Adenocarcinoma	40%	Has increased in nonsmokers
Squamous cell carcinoma	40%	Referred to as epidermoid, is associated histologically with keratin pearls, and is promoted by smoking and other inhaled irritants
Large-cell carcinoma	15%	
Bronchoalveolar carcinoma	5%	Single nodule, multiple nodules, or nonresolving infiltrate on chest radiography
Small cell carcinoma	20%	Very poor prognosis

5. **Is lung cancer screening effective?**

Old dogma: No.

Current thinking: Maybe. The thinking is as follows: lung cancer accounts for more cancer deaths than other cancers. Eighty-five percent of patients present with advanced uncurable lung cancer. We have not changed survival for lung cancer. Early-stage cancers that are asymptomatic can be found by chest radiograph and helical computed tomography (CT). Unfortunately CT also detects many false positives. Also, public health policy does not endorse screening for lung cancer.

6. **How do patients with lung cancer present?**

Cough	70%
Weight loss	10%
Bone pain	30%
Paraneoplastic syndrome	10%
Asymptomatic	10%

7. **What is a paraneoplastic syndrome?**
Paraneoplastic syndromes of lung cancer may be **metabolic** (e.g., hypercalcemia, Cushing's syndrome), **neurologic** (e.g., peripheral neuropathy; polymyositis; or Lambert-Eaton syndrome, which is similar to myasthenia gravis), **skeletal** (e.g., clubbing, hypertrophic osteoarthropathy), **hematologic** (e.g., anemia, thrombocytosis, disseminated intravascular coagulation [DIC]), or **cutaneous** (e.g., hyperkeratosis, acanthosis nigricans, dermatomyositis). Of interest, the presence of a paraneoplastic syndrome does not influence the ultimate curability of the lung cancer.

8. **Does the staging system for lung cancer have prognostic and therapeutic importance?**
Yes. The patient's survival is related to the stage at presentation (Table 79-2).

TABLE 79-2. STAGING OF LUNG CANCER

Stage	Subset	Description
I	Ia	Intraparenchymal tumor with or without extension to the visceral pleura, 2 cm from the carina, and no lymph node metastases spread
	Ib	Tumor >3 cm or through parietal pleura, no positive nodes
II	IIa	Primary tumor is similar to that of stage I with extension to interbronchial lymph nodes (N_1)
	IIb	Tumor invades chest wall without nodal involvement (T_3N_0)
III	IIIa	Extension of tumor into hilar or mediastinal lymph nodes (N_2) or chest wall with N_1 nodes
	IIIb	All elements of IIIa plus extension of tumor to mediastinal structures (heart or great vessels) or contralateral hilar, paratracheal, or supraclavicular lymph nodes (N_3)
IV		Malignant pleural effusion or metastatic disease (M_1)

9. **Describe the work-up of a patient with a mass on chest radiograph.**
The work-up should be directed toward diagnosis, staging, and risk assessment.
1. Diagnosis
   - CT and positron emission tomography (PET): defines size, mets, nodes, and malignancy risk
   - Sputum cytology: low diagnostic yield
   - Bronchoscopy: low diagnostic yield if tumor not visible
   - CT-guided fine needle aspiration aspiration (FNA)
   - Thoracoscopy and biopsy: wedge excision

2. Staging
   - CT scan (chest): tumor, mediastinal lymph node assessment
   - PET: 90% sensitive and 80% specific for nodes, mets
   - Bronchoscopy: endobronchial invasion
   - Thoracoscopy: lymph node sampling
   - Mediastinoscopy: sample N2 and N3 nodes
3. Risk assessment
   - Pulmonary
   Spirometry: ventilation/perfusion (V/Q) screening; if borderline, must leave patient with approximately 800 ml forced expiratory volume (FEV_1) after resection
   Arterial blood gas (ABG) analysis
   - Cardiac
   Electrocardiogram (ECG)
   History of myocardial infarction (MI), prior intervention
   - Cardiopulmonary
   Able to walk a flight of stairs; if yes, will tolerate lobectomy
   Maximal oxygen (O_2) consumption <15 milliliters per kilogram per minute

10. **How are patients with lung cancer treated?**
    The most effective treatment for lung cancer is surgical resection. Unfortunately, 75% of patients present with advanced disease and are not candidates for resection. Fortunately, preoperative chemotherapy with a cisplatinum-containing regimen has increased the number of patients with stage III who are candidates for resection. This recent innovative therapy may translate into improved survival rates. For stage III lung cancer, several clinical trials have shown an advantage to preoperative chemotherapy and radiation treatment called neoadjuvant therapy. Even lower-stage disease or tumors at high risk of recurrence may benefit from newer chemotherapeutic regimens.

KEY POINTS: LUNG CANCER

1. The overall survival rate for patients with lung cancer is 10%.
2. Ninety percent of patients have a smoking history.
3. The most effective treatment for lung cancer is surgical resection.

11. **Do chemotherapy radiation therapy have a place in the therapy of lung cancer?**
    Radiation therapy is effective palliative but not curative therapy for lung cancer. Specifically, patients who present with a superior vena cava syndrome or a blocked bronchus with distal pneumonia frequently can be "opened up" with radiation therapy. Radiation is also excellent for the palliation of pathologic bone pain. Some—but not all—clinical trials have shown some benefit from preoperative chemoradiation treatment in advanced-stage lung cancer. There is evidence to suggest that patients with stage Ib, IIa, or b lung cancer benefit from induction chemotherapy. The treatment of stage III disease based on the presence of mediastinal lymph nodes is still controversial, despite much attention and many trials over the last 10 years. For now most patients with stage III disease have only a 20% survival at best. Most should be offered induction preoperative chemotherapy.

12. **What is the survival rate of patients treated for non-small cell lung cancer at 5 years?**

Stage I: Ia	65% (up to 84 % with no nodes or N1)
Ib	55%
Stage II: IIa	55%
IIb	40%
Stage III: IIIa	20%
IIIb	10%
Stage IV:	2%

Note that for chest wall invasion with no lymph nodes, survival is 50% at 5 years, although this is still called stage IIb. Also, if stage Ia (small tumor, no positive nodes) cancer is not resected, survival decreases from 70% to 7%.

13. **What is mediastinoscopy?**
Mediastinoscopy is a staging procedure in which the paratracheal, subcarinal, and proximal peribronchial lymph nodes are sampled from a small incision made in the suprasternal notch.

14. **What are the indications for mediastinoscopy?**
Mediastinal staging is indicated in patients with either apparent or documented lung cancer who have:
- Known lung cancer with mediastinal lymph nodes >1 cm accessible by cervical mediastinal exploration, as assessed by CT scan.
- Adenocarcinoma of the lung and multiple mediastinal lymph nodes <1 cm.
- Central or large (>5 cm) lung cancers with mediastinal lymph nodes <1 cm.
- Lung cancer and are at high risk of thoracotomy and lung resection.
- Highly suggestive PET scan for mediastinal nodal mets.

If the mediastinoscopy has negative results, the surgeon should proceed with thoracotomy, biopsy, and curative lung resection.

15. **Is malignant pleural effusion or recurrent nerve involvement with tumor an absolute contraindication to surgical resection for lung cancer?**
A malignant pleural effusion defines the tumor—T as T4 and the clival stage is at least IIIB. Most such patients will have metastatic disease after evaluation. Rarely, and small malignant pleural effusion will occur in the presence of a pleurally based but resectable primary tumor. Conversely, both King George V and Arthur Godfrey had successful surgical resections in the face of recurrent nerve involvement with tumor.

WEBSITE

www.acssurgery.com

BIBLIOGRAPHY

1. Arriagada R, Bergman B, Dunaunt A et al.: Cisplatin based adjuvant chemotherapy in patients with completely resectednon-small-cell carcinoma. N Engl J Med 350:351-360, 2004.
2. Ginsberg RJ, Ruckdeschel JC, editors: *Lung cancer: past, present, and future. Part I. Chest surgery clinics of North America*, vol. 10, Philadelphia, 2000, W.B. Saunders.

3. Mountain EF: Revision in the international system for staging lung cancer. Chest 111:1710, 1997.

4. Pass HI: Adjunctive and alternate treatment of bronchogenic lung cancer. Chest Surg Clin North Am 1:1-20, 1991.

5. Saunders CA, Dussek JE, O'Doherty MJ et al.: Evaluation of fluorine 18-fluorodeoxyglucose: whole body positron emission tomography imaging in staging lung cancer. Ann Thorac Surg 67:790-797, 1999.

6. Sonett JR, Krasna MJ, Suntharalingam M et al.: Safe pulmonary resection after chemotherapy and high-dose thoracic radiation. Ann Thorac Surg 68:316-320, 1999.

7. Strauss GM: Prognostic markers in resectable non-small-cell lung cancer. Hematol Oncol Clin North Am 11:409-434, 1997.

8. Toloza EM, Harpole L, Detterbeck F et al.: Invasive staging of non small cell lung cancer. Chest 123:157S-166S, 2003.

CHAPTER 80

SOLITARY PULMONARY NODULE

Jamie M. Brown, MD, and Marvin Pomerantz, MD

1. What is a solitary pulmonary nodule?

A solitary pulmonary nodule or "coin lesion" is found on chest radiograph, or computed tomography (CT), and is <3 centimeters. It is surrounded completely by lung parenchyma.

2. What causes a solitary pulmonary nodule?

The most common causes of a pulmonary nodule are either neoplastic (carcinoma, 60% to 70% of resected nodules) or infectious (granuloma). Pulmonary nodules may also represent lung abscess, pulmonary infarction, arteriovenous malformations, resolving pneumonia, pulmonary sequestration, and hamartoma. As a general rule of thumb, likelihood of malignancy is proportionate to the nodule's size, the patient's age, and history of smoking. Thus, whereas lung cancer is rare (although it does occur) in 30-year-old individuals, in 50-year-old smokers, the chance that a solitary pulmonary nodule represents malignancy is 50% to 60%. In a 70-year-old person with a smoking history and a 2.9-cm pulmonary nodule the malignancy risk is 75%.

3. How does a solitary pulmonary nodule present?

Typically, a solitary nodule presents incidentally as a finding on routine chest radiograph. In several large series, more than 75% of lesions were surprise findings on routine chest radiograph. Fewer than 25% of patients had symptoms referable to the lung. Solitary nodules are now seen on other sensitive imaging tests such as helical CT.

4. How frequently does a solitary pulmonary nodule represent metastatic disease?

Fewer than 10% of solitary nodules represent metastatic disease. Accordingly, an extensive work-up for a primary site of cancer other than the lung is not indicated.

5. Can a tissue sample be obtained by fluoroscopic or CT-guided needle biopsy?

Yes, but the results do not change the treatment. If the needle biopsy tissue indicates cancer, the nodule must be removed. If the needle biopsy is negative for cancer, the nodule must still be removed. Positron emission tomography (PET) is 90% sensitive in identifying malignant tumors. Nodule characteristics on CT scanning combined with PET may be 90% accurate in ruling out malignancy.

6. Are radiographic findings important?

Only relatively. The resolution of CT scanners allows the best identification of characteristics that suggest cancer:
1. Indistinct or irregular spiculated borders of the nodule.
2. The larger the nodule, the more likely it is to be malignant.
3. Calcification in the nodule generally is associated with benign disease (the opposite of breast cancer). Specifically, whereas central, diffuse, or laminated calcifications are typical of a granuloma, calcifications with more dense and irregular "popcorn" patterns are associated with hamartomas. Unfortunately, eccentric foci of calcium or small flecks of calcium may be found in malignant lesions.

4. Nodules can be studied using a CT scanner by measuring their change in relative radiodensity after injection of contrast. This is called Hounsefield attenuation and improves the accuracy of predicting the presence of malignancy.

KEY POINTS: SOLITARY PULMONARY NODULE

1. A solitary pulmonary nodule or "coin lesion" is <3 cm and is discrete on chest radiograph.

2. The most common causes of a pulmonary nodule are either neoplastic or infectious.

3. If the lesion proves to be cancer, anatomic lobectomy is the procedure of choice.

7. **What social or clinical findings suggest that a nodule is malignant rather than benign?**
Unfortunately, none of the findings is sufficiently sensitive or specific to influence the work-up. Both increasing age and a long smoking history predispose patients to lung cancer. Winston Churchill should have had lung cancer, but he did not. Thus, the fact that the patient is the president of the spelunking club (histoplasmosis), has a sister who raises pigeons (cryptococcosis), grew up in the Ohio River Valley (histoplasmosis), works as sexton for a dog cemetery (blastomycosis), or just took a hiking trip through the San Joaquin Valley (coccidioidomycosis) is interesting associated history but does not affect the work-up of a solitary pulmonary nodule.

8. **What is the most valuable bit of historic data?**
The patient's age and smoking history. Beyond the obvious, the most valuable data piece is an old chest radiograph. If the nodule is new, it is more likely to be malignant, whereas if the nodule has not changed in the past 2 years, it is less likely to be malignant. Unfortunately, even this observation is not absolute.

9. **If a patient presents with a treated prior malignancy and a new solitary pulmonary nodule, is it safe to assume that the new nodule represents metastatic disease?**
No. Even in patients with known prior malignancies, <50% of new pulmonary nodules are metastatic. Thus, the work-up should proceed exactly as for any other patient with a new solitary pulmonary nodule.

10. **How should a solitary pulmonary nodule be evaluated?**
A complete travel and occupational history is interesting but does not affect the evaluation. Because of the peripheral location of most nodules, bronchoscopy has a diagnostic yield of <50%. Even in the best hands, sputum cytology has a low yield. CT scanning is recommended because it can define to a degree the nodule (size, calcification, density, etc.), identify other potentially metastatic nodules, and delineate the status of mediastinal lymph nodes. As indicated previously, percutaneous needle biopsy has a diagnostic yield of approximately 80% but rarely alters the subsequent management. PET scanning may suggest cancer with accuracy. More importantly, PET scanning may suggest the presence of extramediastinal or covert mediastinal disease with more sensitivity than CT scanning.
The mainstay of management in patients who can tolerate surgery is resection of the nodule, usually by lobectomy if cancer is suspected, for diagnosis by either a minimally invasive thoracoscopy approach or a limited thoracotomy. Decisions to observe pulmonary nodules should be made selectively (e.g., old patient poor candidate for surgery) and with a careful follow-up plan.

11. **If the lesion proves to be cancer, what is the appropriate surgical therapy?**
    Like all clinical decision making, that would depend. Although several series have suggested that wedge excision of the nodule is sufficient, an anatomic lobectomy remains the procedure of choice for a known cancer of the lung. This can often be accomplished by a video-assisted approach. A solitary nodule that turns out to be cancer in early stage and in the absence of metastatic disease and has an up to 80% 5-year survival rate. Unfortunately, the recurrence rate even for stage I tumors or a small nodule is 30% over 5 years. Recurrences are split between local and distant.

WEBSITE

http://www.acssurgery.com

BIBLIOGRAPHY

1. Birim O, Kappetein PA, Stijnen T et al.: Meta-analysis of positron emission tomographic and computed tomographic imaging in detecting mediastinal lymph node metastases in nonsmall cell lung cancer. Ann Thoracic Surgery 79:375-382, 2005.

2. Davies B, Ghosh S, Hopkinson D et al.: Solitary pulmonary nodules: pathological outcome of 150 consecutively resected lesions. Interact Cardiovas Thorac Surg 4:18-20, 2005.

3. Dewey TM, Mack MJ: Lung cancer: surgical approaches and incisions. Chest Surg Clin North Am 10:803-820, 2000.

4. Ginsberg RJ, Rubinstein LV: Randomized trial of lobectomy versus limited resection for T1 N0 non-small cell lung cancer. Lung Cancer Study Group. Ann Thorac Surg 60:615-622, 1995.

5. Khouri NF, Meziane MA, Zerhouni EA et al.: The solitary pulmonary nodule: assessment, diagnosis and management. Chest 91:128-133, 1987.

6. Miller DL, Rowland CM, Deschamps C et al.: Surgical treatment of non-small cell lung cancer 1 cm or less in diameter. Ann Thorac Surg 73:1541-1545, 2002.

7. Nesbitt J, Putnam JB Jr, Walsh GL et al.: Survival in early stage non-small cell lung cancer. Ann Thorac Surg 60:466-472, 1995.

8. Varoli F, Vergani C, Caminiti R et al.: Management of the solitary pulmonary nodule. Eur J Cardiothorac Surg 33: 461-465. 2008.

9. Walsh GL, Pisters KM, Stevens C: Treatment of stage I lung cancer. Chest Surg Clin North Am 10:17-38, 2001.

CHAPTER 81

DISSECTING AORTIC ANEURYSM

Richard-Tien V. Ha, MD

1. **Why is the term *dissecting aortic aneurysm* really incorrect?**
   The correct term should be **dissecting aortic hematoma** because the lesion is not an aneurysm. Blood passes into the media, creating a hematoma that separates the intima from the media or adventitia. It is unclear whether the inciting event is the intimal tear or blood from the media tearing through the intima. Hence, an intimal tear is not a prerequisite because 5% to 13% of patients do not have one.

2. **When should the diagnosis be entertained?**
   Suspicion is the most important factor because no one feature is common to patients presenting with aortic dissections. In any patient who presents with severe knifelike, ripping chest and back pain, the diagnosis of aortic dissection should be considered. Other symptoms include syncope and neurologic symptoms.

3. **After the diagnosis is entertained, how should the patient be managed?**
   Two thirds of patients are hypertensive, so blood pressure must be controlled to a systolic blood pressure (BP) of <100 mm Hg. Pain must also be managed to reduce catecholamine surge. The other diagnosis to be strongly considered is acute myocardial infarction (MI). An electrocardiogram (ECG) often rules out MI, but some aortic dissections tear off a coronary artery; thus, both acute infarction and aortic dissection occur concurrently (this patient group has a higher mortality).

4. **What is the most significant diagnostic clue on physical examination?**
   A new aortic valvular diastolic murmur, indicating aortic valvular regurgitation caused by distortion of the valve structure by the mural hematoma. In addition, the dissecting hematoma can encircle the lumen or actually cleave the takeoff of the subclavian or femoral vessels, resulting in the loss of pulses or systolic variation between arms. Neurologic findings, including paraplegia and hemiplegia, may also be present because of similar flap occlusion of the great vessels.

5. **Which chest radiograph findings are helpful in diagnosis?**
   Widened mediastinum and loss of aortic knob silhouette—a hematoma surrounding the aorta makes the aortic outline blurry—are helpful findings. In 15% to 25% of patients, a left-sided pleural effusion is present.

6. **How is the diagnosis confirmed? What are the best diagnostic studies?**
   The literature reports the high accuracy of transesophageal echocardiography (TEE) and spiral computed tomography angiography (CTA) in the diagnosis of aortic dissections. On the other hand, unlike these modalities, angiography allows for visualization of the coronary arteries or estimation of aortic valvular insufficiency. The decision to use one modality over the other lies in the stability of the patient and the modalities available at a given institution. TEE should be the first modality if available in unstable patients, followed by

CTA. Angiography may be used in stable patients to define the coronary anatomy and valvular architecture, although studies show that in-house mortality is not improved with coronary angiography.

7. What are the types of dissection?

There are two classification schemes: Debakey and Stanford. Debakey type I involves the ascending aorta and propagates to at least the aortic arch. Type II involves only the ascending aorta. Type III involves the descending aorta. The Stanford classification has both therapeutic and prognostic value:

Ascending (type A) involves only the ascending or both the ascending and descending aorta.

Descending (type B) involves only the descending aorta. Ascending dissections are twice as common as descending dissections and often begin at the right lateral wall and involves the aortic arch in 30%.

8. Who cares whether a dissection involves the ascending (type A) or descending (type B) aorta?

Ascending dissections require early surgical correction to avoid extension into the coronary or carotid arteries, rupture into the pericardium (tamponade), or both. Descending dissections do not involve the ascending aorta and may be managed medically or surgically (see Controversies).

9. What is the key to medical management?

The BP should be lowered to 100 mm Hg (systolic) with a combination of sodium nitroprusside and propranolol. Propranolol or labetalol is particularly important because it decreases the contractility of the myocardium (dp/dt), thereby decreasing the shearing force that prevents propagation of the dissection down the aorta. Conceptually, the BP should be lowered as much as possible, but the patient must continue to perfuse the end organs (i.e., make urine). Sodium nitroprusside may be added for further BP control.

10. What are the principles and advantages of surgical management of acute aortic dissection?

Ascending dissection

1. To close off the hematoma by obliterating the most proximal intimal tear.
2. To restore competency of the aortic valve.
3. To restore flow to any branches of the aorta that have been sheared off and receive blood flow from a false lumen.
4. To protect the heart during these maneuvers and to restore coronary blood flow if a coronary artery has been sheared off.
5. To look for tears in the transverse aortic arch.

Technique: Use of deep hypothermia circulatory arrest with or without retrograde cerebral perfusion is in vogue at present. This technique allows the arch to be inspected and the distal anastomosis of the Dacron graft to be sewn accurately to the distal ascending aorta in an open fashion. Whether to replace or repair the aortic valve is controversial.

Descending dissection

1. To close off the hematoma by obliterating the most proximal intimal tear.
2. To restore blood flow to branches of the aorta fed by the false channel.

Technique: Surgery is performed using partial cardiopulmonary bypass, or the "clamp and run" technique, in which the aorta is cross-clamped and the graft is sewn in as fast as possible (see Controversies). Endovascular repair with stents is gaining popularity and in some clinical situations may be the better choice (see Controversies).

KEY POINTS: DISSECTING AORTIC ANEURYSM

1. The correct term should be *dissecting aortic hematoma* because the lesion is not an aneurysm.

2. A new aortic valvular diastolic murmur, indicating aortic valvular regurgitation caused by distortion of the valve structure by the mural hematoma.

3. Ascending dissections require early surgical correction to avoid extension into the coronary or carotid arteries, rupture into the pericardium, or both.

4. Descending dissections may be managed medically; however, even surgical patients should have blood pressure lowered to 100-110 mm Hg with a combination of sodium nitroprusside and propranolol/labetalol.

11. What are the operative complications?
- Hemorrhage (20%): quite common because of the use of heparin and the poor quality of aortic tissue (like wet Kleenex).
- Renal failure (20%).
- Pulmonary insufficiency (30% higher in repair of descending dissections).
- Paraplegia: often presents before operation; as a surgical complication, it usually occurs only with descending dissections (11%).
- Acute MI or low cardiac output (30%).
- Bowel infarction (5%).
- Death (15%): higher for acute than chronic dissections and higher for repair of ascending dissections.

12. What are the long-term results?
Of patients who survive the operation, two thirds die within 7 years because of comorbid cardiac and cerebrovascular disease.

CONTROVERSIES

13. Which is preferred: surgical or medical management of descending dissections?
Initial surgical management
- Approximately 25% of patients initially treated medically need an operation eventually.
- Operative mortality is much lower today (20% to 30%) than in the past.
- Stent graft repair is showing promise as an early and less morbid treatment.

Initial medical management
- Medical management has a lower in-hospital mortality rate (10% to 15%).
- This avoids unnecessary operation and its attendant cost and complication rate.

14. What is the preferred management of aortic insufficiency in ascending dissections?
Replacement of aortic valve
- Easy (valved conduits now available).
- Eliminates aortic insufficiency completely.
- Should be done in patients with Marfan syndrome.

Repair of aortic valve

- With native valve reconstruction, when done correctly, the need to replace the valve at a later time is only 10%.
- Avoids need for anticoagulation, which is necessary when a mechanical valve is used to replace the aortic valve.

15. What is the preferred repair of descending dissections?

1. Partial left atrial-to-femoral artery bypass

For:

- Allows unloading of the heart.
- Allows distal perfusion to avoid visceral ischemia.
- Allows as much time as needed to complete anastomosis.

Against: requires heparinization.

2. Simple aortic cross-clamping

For: Fast.

Against: Placement of the graft has to be done in <30 minutes or the complication rate, particularly paraplegia, increases significantly.

3. Placement of a stent graft across the intimal tear.

For:

- Decreased in-hospital mortality (10%) compared to surgery.
- Decreased hospital stay, faster recovery, and decreased post procedure pain.
- Allows reexpansion of compressed true lumen.
- Decreased risk of paraplegia.

Against:

- May occlude previously normal branch arteries.
- Effectiveness in stable type B dissections under investigation.
- Long-term results are not known at this time.

WEBSITE

www.acssurgery.com

BIBLIOGRAPHY

1. Barron DJ, Livesey SA, Brown IW et al.: Twenty-year follow-up of acute type A dissection: the incidence and extent of distal aortic disease using magnetic resonance imaging. J Card Surg 12:147-159, 1997.

2. Cigarroa JE, Isselbacher EM, DeSanctis RW et al.: Diagnostic imaging in the evaluation of suspected aortic dissection. Old standards and new directions. N Engl J Med 328:35-43, 1993.

3. Glower DD, Fann JI, Speier RH et al.: Comparison of medical and surgical therapy for uncomplicated descending aortic dissection. Circulation 82(suppl IV):39-46, 1990.

4. Khan IA, Nair CK: Clinical, diagnostic, and management perspectives of aortic dissection. Chest 112:311-328, 2002.

5. Nienaber CA, von Kodolitsch Y, Nicolas V et al.: The diagnosis of thoracic aortic dissection by noninvasive imaging procedures. N Engl J Med 328:1-9, 1993.

6. Okita Y, Takamoto S, Ando M et al.: Mortality and cerebral outcome in patients who underwent aortic arch operations using deep hypothermic circulatory arrest with retrograde cerebral perfusion: no relation of early death, stroke, and delirium to the duration of circulatory arrest. J Thorac Cardiovasc Surg 115:129-138, 1998.

7. Safi HJ, Miller CC, Reardon MJ et al.: Operation for acute and chronic aortic dissection: recent outcome with regard to neurologic deficit and early death. Ann Thorac Surg 66:402-411, 1998.

8. Wheat MW Jr, Palmer RF, Bartley TB et al.: Treatment of dissecting aneurysms of the aorta without surgery. J Thorac Cardiovasc Surg 50:364-373, 1995.

9. Hagan PG, Nienaber CA, Isselbacher EM et al.: The International Registry of Acute Aortic Dissection (IRAD): new insights into an old disease. JAMA 283(7):897-903, 2000.

10. Nienaber CA, Eagle KA: Aortic dissection: new frontiers in the diagnosis and management. Part I: etiology to diagnostic strategies. Circulation 108:628-635, 2003.

11. Nienaber CA, Eagle KA: Aortic dissection: new frontiers in the diagnosis and management. Part II: therapeutic management and follow-up. Circulation 108:772-778, 2003.

12. Ince H, Nienaber CA: Diagnosis and management of patients with acute aortic dissection. Heart 93:266-270, 2007.

HYPERTROPHIC PYLORIC STENOSIS

Denis D. Bensard, MD

CHAPTER 82

1. What is hypertrophic pyloric stenosis?

Hypertrophic pyloric stenosis (HPS) is idiopathic thickening and elongation of the pylorus that produces gastric outlet obstruction. HPS is the most common surgical cause of nonbilious vomiting in infants. Offspring of an affected parent have an increased incidence of HPS (10%); the highest rate (20%) occurs in boys born to affected mothers.

2. Describe the typical presentation of HPS.

The typical presentation is a healthy infant who initially fed normally but who presents at age 2 to 6 weeks with a history of "projectile" vomiting. The emesis is nonbilious. After vomiting, the infant appears hungry and will refeed immediately. With time, the infant becomes dehydrated and, if allowed to progress, malnutrition follows.

3. What are the physical findings?

Affected infants suffer some degree of dehydration. The abdomen is nondistended and soft. A palpable pyloric tumor, known as the "olive," confirms the diagnosis. An olive is palpable in 50% of patients. Associated findings are rare, but mild jaundice occurs in 5% of infants because of reduced glucuronyl transferase activity.

4. How is the diagnosis confirmed?

Ultrasonographic criteria include pyloric diameter >1.4 cm, wall width >4 mm, and pyloric channel length >1.6 cm. Alternatively, a barium upper gastrointestinal (UGI) examination may be used to confirm the diagnosis (gastric outlet obstruction, pyloric channel narrowing). Current analyses suggest that UGI is the most cost-effective initial radiologic diagnostic test because, unlike ultrasound (US), alternative causes of nonbilious vomiting (e.g., gastroesophageal reflux [GERD], malrotation, duodenal stenosis) can be identified.

5. Describe the likely electrolyte abnormalities.

Electrolyte levels are often normal, but long-standing vomiting will eventually result in hypokalemic, hypochloremic metabolic alkalosis because of the loss of gastric acid (HCl). Earlier consideration of the diagnosis has led to a significant reduction in this classic electrolyte abnormality at presentation. Dehydration is corrected with either 0.9% sodium chloride (NaCl) or, in less severe cases, 0.5% NaCl with 30 mEq/L potassium chloride (KCl). After dehydration and electrolytes are corrected, pyloromyotomy is performed.

6. What procedure is recommended for the correction of HPS?

The Fredet-Ramstedt pyloromyotomy is recommended. A superficial incision is made longitudinally over the pyloric muscle in an avascular area, and the muscle fibers are fractured to expose the underlying mucosa. At the conclusion of the pyloromyotomy, the gastric mucosa should bulge upward into the cleft, and the pyloric muscle walls should move independently of one another. Air is injected into the stomach via the nasogastric (NG) tube to identify inadvertent mucosal perforation. Pyloromyotomy may be performed either via a transverse incision in the right upper quadrant (i.e., an open procedure) or via three small (3 mm) incisions in the epigastrium (i.e., a laparoscopic procedure). The results of open and laparoscopic pyloromyotomy appear equivalent.

7. What should be done if a perforation is identified?
The mucosa should be closed with several fine sutures and covered with an omental patch. If the mucosal injury is too extensive, the myotomy should be closed with sutures and a second, parallel myotomy should be made at 45 to 180 degrees from the original myotomy.

8. When can postoperative feeding begin?
Small-volume feedings are started after the infant has recovered from anesthesia (2 to 3 hours) and advanced to goal. Small amounts of vomiting are common (20%), but most infants achieve full feeds within 24 hours postoperatively. Incomplete pyloromyotomy is uncommon (<1%) and is not considered unless symptoms of gastric outlet obstruction persist for 7 to 10 days after surgery.

9. Describe several hypotheses about the pathogenesis of HPS.
Recent studies of the abnormal pyloric complex demonstrate improper innervation of pyloric smooth muscle, excessive contraction of circular pyloric smooth muscle (decreased nitric oxide synthase), increased extracellular matrix proteins (collagen), and increased expression or local synthesis of growth hormones (i.e., insulin-like growth factor-1, transforming growth factor β-1, platelet derived growth factor).

BIBLIOGRAPHY

1. Aspelund G, Langer JC: Current management of hypertrophic pyloric stenosis. Semin Pediatr Surg 16:27-33, 2007.
2. Hall NJ, Van Der Zee J, Tan HL et al.: Meta-analysis of laparoscopic versus open pyloromyotomy. Ann Surg 240:774-778, 2004.
3. Leclair MD, Plattner V, Mirallie E et al.: Laparoscopic pyloromyotomy for hypertrophic pyloric stenosis: a prospective, randomized controlled trial. J Pediatr Surg 42:692-698, 2007.
4. Miozzari HH, Tonz M, von Vigier RO et al.: Fluid resuscitation in infantile hypertrophic pyloric stenosis. Acta Paediatr 90:511-514, 2001.
5. Saur D, Vanderwinden JM, Seidler B et al.: Single-nucleotide promoter polymorphism alters transcription of neuronal nitric oxide synthase exon 1c in infantile hypertrophic pyloric stenosis. Proc Natl Acad Sci USA 101:1662-1667, 2004.
6. van der Bilt JD, Kramer WL, van der Zee DC et al.: Early feeding after laparoscopic pyloromyotomy: the pros and cons. Surg Endosc 18:746-748, 2004.

CHAPTER 83

INTESTINAL OBSTRUCTION OF NEONATES AND INFANTS

Richard J. Hendrickson, MD, and Denis D. Bensard, MD

1. What signs or symptoms suggest intestinal obstruction in the neonate?

Signs and symptoms vary according to the level of obstruction. Proximal intestinal obstruction leads to the early onset of bilious emesis, generally with minimal abdominal distention. In contrast, neonates with distal intestinal obstruction present after the first day of life with bilious vomiting and pronounced abdominal distention. Bilious emesis should always be interrogated further in infants and children because contrast study will demonstrate a surgical cause for bilious emesis will be present in approximately one third of infants.

2. What is the differential diagnosis of intestinal obstruction in neonates?

Look for an anal opening, which eliminates the diagnosis of imperforate anus. Next obtain an abdominal radiograph. The extent of gaseous distention of the bowel implicates a proximal or distal bowel obstruction. No attempts should be made to distinguish small from large bowel obstruction.

Proximal (minimal bowel gas)	**Distal** (significant bowel gas)
Duodenal atresia, stenosis	Ileal atresia
Malrotation with midgut volvulus	Meconium ileus or plug
Jejunal atresia	Hirschsprung's disease

3. When are contrast studies of the gastrointestinal tract indicated?

If peritonitis or pneumoperitoneum is present, proceed to exploratory laparotomy without delay. Malrotation with volvulus must be distinguished from the other cause of congenital duodenal obstruction (duodenal atresia). In this setting, upper gastrointestinal (GI) is the study of choice. In volvulus, the upper GI demonstrates distention of the proximal duodenum, corkscrewing of the distal duodenum, and limited or no progression of contrast into the distal bowel. Conversely, duodenal atresia appears as a blind ending pouch in the first or second portion of the duodenum. Contrast enema is generally the preferred study in all other forms of neonatal intestinal obstruction.

Disorder	Barium enema
Ileal atresia	Microcolon; no reflux into terminal ileum
Meconium ileus	Microcolon; reflux into terminal ileum with filling defects
Meconium plug	Normal colon; large filling defect of left colon
Hirschsprung's disease	Narrowed rectosigmoid; dilated proximal colon

4. Describe intestinal atresia.

Atresia can occur anywhere in the GI tract: duodenal (50%), jejunoileal (45%), or colonic (5%). Duodenal atresia arises from a failure of recanalization during the eighth to tenth week of gestation; jejunoileal and colonic atresia are caused by an in utero mesenteric vascular accident.

5. Distinguish duodenal atresia from other forms of intestinal atresia.

Duodenal atresia is characterized by the onset of bilious vomiting (85% of atresia distal to the ampulla of Vater) within the first day of life; significant abdominal distention is absent.

Approximately 25% of affected infants have trisomy 21. The abdominal radiograph demonstrates a "double bubble" caused by the distended stomach and first or second portions of duodenum. Surgical correction is performed by duodenoduodenostomy.

Jejunoileal atresia produces bilious vomiting at 2 to 3 days of life with moderate to severe abdominal distention. The abdominal radiograph shows dilated loops of bowel with air-fluid levels. Barium enema reveals a microcolon and no reflux of contrast into the dilated bowel. Associated anomalies are uncommon. Surgical correction involves end-to-end anastomosis with or without limited intestinal resection.

Colonic atresia, similar to jejunoileal atresia, is associated with the late onset of bilious vomiting, no passage of meconium, and moderate to severe abdominal distention. The abdominal radiograph reveals dilated loops of bowel with air-fluid levels suggesting distal intestinal obstruction. Barium enema demonstrates a microcolon with a cutoff observed in a proximal colonic segment. Twenty percent of affected infants suffer an associated anomaly of the heart, musculoskeletal system, abdominal wall, or GI tract. Surgical management includes limited colonic resection with primary anastomosis.

6. **Describe malrotation with midgut volvulus.**
   During the sixth to twelfth week of gestation, the intestine undergoes evisceration, growth, return to the abdominal cavity, and counterclockwise rotation with fixation. Malrotation is an error in both rotation and fixation. Abnormal fixation and a narrow-based mesentery predispose to twisting of the midgut on its blood supply (superior mesenteric artery), vascular occlusion (strangulation), and obstruction (malrotation with midgut volvulus). Typically, a previously well neonate or child without a history of surgery presents with bilious vomiting, abdominal distention, and variable degrees of shock. If the infant is acutely ill, no further studies are needed and surgical exploration is indicated. If the diagnosis is in question and the infant is stable, an upper GI study, not a barium enema, is performed. Surgical treatment entails four parts: (1) division of abnormal peritoneal bands, (2) correction of malrotation, (3) restoration of a broad-based mesentery, and (4) appendectomy because of the location of the cecum in the right upper quadrant.

7. **Is midgut volvulus a surgical emergency?**
   Yes! The risk of strangulation caused by the rotational anomaly and abnormal peritoneal bands implies a surgical emergency. Delay places the infant at risk of losing the entire midgut and potentially dying.

8. **What is meconium ileus?**
   Meconium ileus (MI) is the obstruction of the terminal ileum by highly viscid, tenacious meconium. MI is a complication of cystic fibrosis (CF). Fifteen percent of neonates with CF present with MI. The combination of hyperviscous mucus secreted by the abnormal intestinal glands and pancreatic insufficiency leads to abnormal meconium and obstructs the lumen of the terminal ileum. Symptoms of feeding intolerance, bilious emesis, and abdominal distention begin in the second to third days of life. Unlike most forms of neonatal intestinal obstruction, surgery is reserved for patients refractory to nonoperative treatment or complex MI (atresia, volvulus, or perforation). Sixty percent of infants with simple MI can be treated successfully with Gastrografin enemas and rectal irrigation. If an operation is indicated, the objective is to remove the obstructing meconium by limited resection or enterostomy with evacuation of the meconium and irrigation of the distal bowel.

9. **What is Hirschsprung's disease?**
   In this disease, the intestine is innervated by cells originating in the neural crest. During the fifth to twelfth week of gestation, neural crest cells migrate in a craniocaudal direction and disperse within the wall of the intestine (intermuscular to Auerbach's plexus; submucosal to Meissner's plexus). Hirschsprung's disease arises from the failure of normal enteric innervation. The bowel remains in a contracted, spastic state and produces a functional rather than a true

mechanical obstruction. Abdominal distention, feeding intolerance, and delayed or absent meconium within the first 48 hours of life are the presenting findings in infants. Older patients suffer chronic constipation, abdominal distention, and failure to thrive. Because the disease always affects the most distal bowel (80% to 85% rectosigmoid) with a variable involvement of proximal bowel, barium enema demonstrates the characteristic radiographic appearance of a spastic, contracted rectum with dilated proximal bowel. Suction rectal biopsy documenting the absence of ganglion cells and presence of nerve hypertrophy confirms the diagnosis. Surgical correction is performed by excision of the aganglionic (distal colorectal) segment and coloanal anastomosis.

10. **What is intussusception? What are the therapeutic options?**
   Intussusception is the invagination of proximal bowel (intussusceptum) into the distal bowel (intussuscipien). Swelling, vascular compromise, and obstruction follow. Nearly two thirds of cases occur in the first 2 years of life. The cause is thought to be a result of lymphoid hyperplasia in the terminal ileum after viral infection. The diagnosis should be suspected in previously well infants, 6 to 9 months of age, with vomiting, crampy abdominal pain, and bloody stools. Barium or air enema is both diagnostic and therapeutic. Injection of contrast demonstrates colonic obstruction with no reflux into the proximal bowel. Controlled hydrostatic reduction with barium or air is successful in 90% of cases. Delay in diagnosis and therefore, delay in attempted reduction is the primary cause failure of hydrostatic reduction and need for operative reduction. If hydrostatic reduction is unsuccessful or in children with peritonitis, operative reduction is indicated. The risk of recurrent intussusception is 5% for either radiographic or surgical reduction.

11. **What examples of neonatal obstruction can escape early detection and present later in life?**
   Although most conditions are identified within the first week to month of life, lesions other than atresia may be identified in children and even adults.
   Duodenal stenosis. Unlike duodenal atresia, stenosis results in narrowing but not complete obstruction of the duodenum. Thus, infants fed formula or pureed foods may not become symptomatic until childhood. Children with intermittent abdominal pain and symptoms of gastric outlet obstruction require an upper GI study, particularly if they have trisomy 21.
   Malrotation. One third of patients with malrotation are identified after the first month of life. Children present with bilious emesis and intermittent abdominal pain, and malrotation is generally identified by an upper GI series. Malrotation with midgut volvulus should be suspected in any ill child with signs of intestinal obstruction and no history of abdominal surgery. Decision analysis suggests that surgical correction of asymptomatic malrotation is beneficial in children up to the second decade of life but beyond is probably not indicated because of the rare occurrence of midgut volvulus in adults.
   Hirschsprung's disease. One third of patients are diagnosed after the first year of life. A long history of constipation refractory to therapy mandates rectal biopsy, particularly in patients with trisomy 21.
   Intussusception. One third of cases occur after age 2 years. A pathologic lead point (i.e., polyp, tumor, hematoma, Meckel's diverticulum) is present in one third of older patients.

BIBLIOGRAPHY

1. Engum SA, Grosfeld JL: Long-term results of treatment of Hirschsprung's disease. Semin Pediatr Surg 13:273-285, 2004.
2. Escobar MA, Grosfeld JL, Burdick JJ et al.: Surgical considerations in cystic fibrosis: a 32-year evaluation of outcomes. Surgery 138:560-571, 2005.
3. Escobar MA, Ladd AP, Grosfeld JL et al.: Duodenal atresia and stenosis: long-term follow-up over 30 years. J Pediatr Surg 39:867-871, 2004.
4. Godbole P, Stringer MD: Bilious emesis in the newborn: how often is it pathologic. J Pediatr Surg 37:909-911, 2002.

5. Jajivassiliou CA: Intestinal obstruction in neonatal/pediatric surgery. Semin Pediatr Surg 12:241-253, 2003.

6. Malek MM, Burd RS: The optimal management of malrotation diagnosed after infancy: a decision analysis. Am J Surg 191:45-51, 2006.

7. Milar AJ, Rode H, Cywes S: Malrotation and volvulus in infancy and childhood. Semin Pediatr Surg 12:229-236, 2003.

8. Somme S, To T, Langer JC: Factors determining the need for operative reduction in children with intussusception: a population-based study. J Pediatr Surg 41:1014-1019, 2006.

CHAPTER 84

IMPERFORATE ANUS

Frederick M. Karrer, MD, and Denis D. Bensard, MD

1. **What is imperforate anus?**
   It is a congenital defect in which the opening of the anus is absent or misplaced, usually fistulizing anteriorly to the perineum or genitourinary (GU) tract. Anorectal malformations range from slight anterior malpositioning of the anus to complex cloacal deformities. Children with anorectal malformations commonly have other congenital anomalies, such as the VACTERL association.

2. **What is the VACTERL association?**
   Vertebral defects
   Anorectal malformations
   Cardiac anomalies
   Tracheoesophageal fistula
   Esophageal atresia
   Renal anomalies
   Limb defects
   The incidence of renal anomalies increases with the severity of the imperforate anus, from 10% with low lesions to 75% with high lesions.

3. **How do you determine the severity of the defect in boys?**
   The key is whether the boy has a high or low lesion. Low lesions are characterized by a fistula to the perineum somewhere along the midline raphe between the anus and the urethral meatus. After 24 hours, most infants with low lesions demonstrate meconium at the fistula. Other signs of a low lesion include white "pearls" along the raphe or a raised loop of skin, the so-called bucket-handle deformity. Boys with high lesions typically have flat buttocks without a good buttocks crease and may have meconium at the urethral meatus or apparent on urinalysis.

4. **How is the lesion assessed in girls?**
   Most affected girls (>90%) have a rectovestibular or rectovaginal fistula, which usually can be determined by careful perineal examination. Girls with cloacal deformities (i.e., one orifice) have a high incidence of GU obstruction such as hydrocolpos or bladder obstruction. In low lesions, the anal opening is displaced anteriorly on the perineum. The normal location of the anus is halfway between the vaginal orifice and the coccyx.

5. **How are infants with anorectal malformations treated?**
   Infants with high lesions should be managed initially with a sigmoid colostomy and later with a pull-through procedure called posterior sagittal anorectoplasty. Infants with low lesions usually can be managed with immediate anoplasty or dilatation and delayed repair.

6. **What is a posterior sagittal anorectoplasty (PSARP)?**
   PSARP is a procedure performed through a longitudinal incision in the midline of the perineum, which permits visualization of the pelvic musculature and sphincters and clear exposure of the rectum and fistula. After closure of the fistula, the rectum is repositioned within the sphincteric muscle complex, and a neoanus is created.

7. **What are the results after surgical reconstruction?**
   Continence, defined as voluntary bowel movements with no soiling, depends on the type of lesion. Continence approaches 100% for low lesions but is rare with the highest lesions such as cloaca deformities in girls or bladder-neck fistulas in boys. Constipation is present in almost 50% of patients but is more frequent with the simpler defects.

KEY POINTS: IMPERFORATE ANUS

1. Imperforate anus is a congenital defect in which the opening of the anus is absent or misplaced, usually fistulizing anteriorly to the perineum or GU tract.

2. Infants with high lesions should be managed initially with a sigmoid colostomy and later with a pull-through procedure called PSARP.

3. Infants with low lesions usually can be managed with immediate anoplasty or dilatation and delayed repair.

BIBLIOGRAPHY

1. Kuo MF, Fsai Y, Hsu WM et al.: Tethered spinal cord and VACTERL association. J Neurosurgery 106:201-204, 2007.

2. Levitt MA, Pena A: Outcomes from the correction of anorectal malformations. Curr Opin Pediatr 17:394-401, 2005.

3. Niedzielski JK: Invertography versus ultrasonography and distal colostography for the determination of bowel-skin distance in children with anorectal malformations. Eur J Pediatr Surg 15:262-267, 2005.

4. Pena A, Levitt MA, Hong A et al.: Surgical management of cloacal malformations: a review of 339 patients. J Pediatr Surg 39:470-479, 2004.

5. Pena A, Hong AR, Midulla P et al.: Reoperative surgery for anorectal anomalies. Semin Pediatr Surg 12:118-123, 2003.

6. Rosen NG, Hong AR, Soffer SZ et al.: Rectovaginal fistula: a common diagnostic error with significant consequences in girls with anorectal malformations. J Pediatr Surg 37:961-965, 2002.

CHAPTER 85

TRACHEOESOPHAGEAL MALFORMATIONS

Denis D. Bensard, MD, and David A. Partrick, MD

1. What are tracheoesophageal fistula (TEF) and esophageal atresia (EA)?

The trachea and esophagus appear as a ventral diverticulum arising from the primitive foregut during the third week of gestation. The trachea and esophagus undergo separation by the ingrowth of ectodermal ridges during the fourth week of gestation. Failure of separation results in anomalous connection of the trachea to the esophagus (i.e., TEF) with or without incomplete formation of the esophagus (i.e., EA).

2. Describe the three most common variants and the relative incidence of each type.

- Proximal EA with distal TEF ("proximal pouch with distal fistula"): 85%
- Isolated EA: 10%
- TEF without EA ("H fistula"): 5%

3. What other anomalies occur with tracheoesophageal malformations?

TEF and EA result from an insult during the critical phase of embryogenesis (3 to 8 weeks' gestation). Up to 70% of infants with tracheoesophageal malformations suffer one or more concomitant anomalies. Cardiovascular anomalies are the most prevalent (35%), followed by anomalies of the gastrointestinal (GI; 24%), genitourinary (GU; 20%), skeletal (13%), and central nervous (10%) systems. Twenty-five percent of infants born with tracheoesophageal malformation have one or more components of the VACTERL association (see question 2 in Chapter 84).

4. Does the presence of other anomalies alter management and outcome?

Healthy infants without concomitant anomalies generally undergo early repair with a nearly 100% survival rate, whereas infants who are severely premature or have life-threatening anomalies typically undergo delayed repair. Infants with lethal anomalies, such as trisomy 18, receive palliative care only.

5. Describe the clinical presentation, diagnosis, and preoperative management of patients with EA with distal TEF.

Early in the newborn period, affected infants demonstrate excessive salivation (i.e., inability to swallow secretions), choking, or regurgitation with feeding (i.e., inability to swallow feeds). Respiratory distress quickly ensues because of aspiration of secretions or feeds from the esophageal pouch and reflux of gastric acid into the airways and lungs via the distal TEF. A nasogastric (NG) tube cannot be advanced into the stomach. The radiograph demonstrates a blind-ending proximal esophageal pouch and an air-filled stomach caused by the anomalous connection of the distal esophagus to the airway. The infant is maintained in a semi-upright position with sump catheter drainage of the proximal esophageal pouch to minimize contamination of the lungs either because of aspiration or reflux.

6. Describe the clinical presentation, diagnosis, and preoperative management of isolated EA.

Isolated EA is associated with excessive salivation, choking, and regurgitation of feeds. The inability to pass an NG tube into the stomach and a gasless abdomen apparent on radiograph suggests the diagnosis. Preoperative management is directed to the identification of associated anomalies and determination of gap length. Sump catheter drainage of the proximal esophageal pouch is maintained to minimize aspiration. Gastrostomy is generally performed within the first 24 hours of life to permit feeding and assessment of the distal esophageal length. Typically, infants with EA undergo delayed repair to permit growth of the distal esophagus and reduction of gap distance.

7. **Describe the clinical presentation, diagnosis, and preoperative management of TEF without EA.**
   These infants demonstrate repeated choking or cyanotic spells with feeding caused by the reflux of feeds from the esophagus to the lungs via the anomalous tracheoesophageal connection. Older infants and children may present with recurrent bouts of pneumonia or unexplained reactive airway disease resulting from the intermittent contamination of the lungs via the fistula. Video esophagography and bronchoscopy are used to demonstrate the fistula.

8. **How are tracheoesophageal malformations corrected surgically?**
   Surgical treatment entails restoration of esophageal continuity and elimination of the pathologic connection of the esophagus to the airway. Correction of EA with or without TEF is generally performed via thoracotomy, with or without ligation of TEF, and end-to-end esophageal anastomosis. In some centers, the repair is now performed thoracoscopically; although feasible, the long-term results of this approach remain unclear. At 5 to 7 days after surgery, an esophagogram is performed; if no leak is visualized, oral feedings are started and the pleural drain is removed.
   TEF without EA is approached via a cervical incision, avoiding thoracotomy. The fistulous tract is divided and healthy tissue is interposed to prevent recurrence.

9. **What are the early and late complications of surgical repair?**
   Early complications

Anastomotic disruption	5%
Recurrent TEF	5%
Anastomotic leak	15%
Tracheomalacia	15%

   Early complications are related to the basic surgical principles of wound healing. Anastomotic disruption generally results from poor blood supply and tension.
   Late complications

Anastomotic stricture	25%
Gastroesophageal reflux (GER)	50%
Esophageal dysmotility	100%

   Most strictures (50%) respond to one to three dilatations performed in the first 6 months of life. Refractory strictures require identification of associated GER, which may worsen stricture formation. The frequency of GER appears related to gap length (i.e., the greater the gap distance, the greater the risk of significant GER).

KEY POINTS: TRACHEOESOPHAGEAL MALFORMATIONS

1. The three most common variants are proximal EA with distal TEF, isolated EA, and TEF without EA.

2. Early in the newborn period, affected infants demonstrate excessive salivation, choking, or regurgitation with feeding.

3. Surgical treatment entails restoration of esophageal continuity and elimination of the pathologic connection of the esophagus to the airway.

BIBLIOGRAPHY

1. Atzori P, Iacobelli BD, Bottero S et al.: Preoperative tracheobronchoscopy in newborns with esophageal atresia: does it matter? J Pediatr Surg 41:1054-1057, 2007.

2. Keckler SJ, St Peter SD, Valuseck PA et al.: VACTERL anomalies in patients with esophageal atresia: an updated delineation of the spectrum and review of the literature. Pediatr Surg Int 23:309-313, 2007.

3. Koivusalo A, Pakarinen MP, Turunen P et al.: Health-related quality of life in adult patients with esophageal atresia - a questionnaire study. J Pediatr Surg 40:307-312, 2005.

4. Konkin DE, O'hali WA, Webber EM et al.: Outcomes in esophageal atresia and tracheoesophageal fistula. J Pediatr Surg 38:1726-1729, 2003.

5. Lopez PJ, Keys C, Pierro A et al.: Oesophageal atresia: improved outcome in high-risk groups? J Pediatr Surg 41:331-334, 2006.

6. Sinha CK, Haider N, Marri RR et al.: Modified prognostic criteria for oesophageal atresia and tracheoesophageal fistula. Eur J Pediatr Surg 17:153-157, 2007.

7. Spitz L: Esophageal atresia: lessons I have learned in a 40 year experience. J Pediatr Surg 41:1635-1640, 2006.

CHAPTER 86

CONGENITAL DIAPHRAGMATIC HERNIA

Denis D. Bensard, MD, and Richard J. Hendrickson, MD

1. **What is the most common type of congenital diaphragmatic hernia?**
   Congenital abnormalities of the diaphragm include a posterolateral defect (Bochdalek hernia), an anteromedial defect (Morgagni hernia), or the eventration (central weakening) of the diaphragm. The Bochdalek hernia is the most common variant and generally occurs on the left (80%). Approximately 20% occur on the right, and <1% are bilateral.

2. **What signs and symptoms suggest CDH?**
   Neonatal respiratory distress is the most common manifestation of CDH caused by associated lung maldevelopment. At birth or shortly thereafter, the infant develops severe dyspnea, retractions, and cyanosis. On physical examination, breath sounds are diminished on the ipsilateral side; heart sounds can be heard more easily in the contralateral chest; and the abdomen is scaphoid because of the herniation of abdominal viscera into the chest. Mediastinal shift may result impairing venous return and cardiac output (CO).

3. **How is the diagnosis confirmed?**
   A chest radiograph demonstrates multiple loops of air-filled intestine in the ipsilateral thorax. If a chest radiograph is obtained before entry of significant amounts of air into the bowel, a confusing pattern of mediastinal shift, cardiac displacement, and opacification of the hemithorax may be observed. Insertion of a nasogastric (NG) tube followed by repeat chest radiograph often demonstrates the tube (i.e., stomach) in the chest and confirms the diagnosis.

4. **Are other anomalies associated with CDH?**
   Fifty percent of infants with CDH have associated anomalies. Fewer than 10% of patients with multiple major concurrent anomalies survive. Excluding intestinal malrotation and pulmonary hypoplasia, cardiac anomalies (63%) are the most frequent, followed by genitourinary (GU; 23%), gastrointestinal (GI; 17%), central nervous system (CNS; 14%), and other pulmonary (5%) anomalies.

5. **What therapeutic measures should be initiated before transport or operation?**
   Perhaps the easiest and most effective palliative intervention is decompression of the stomach with an NG tube, which prevents further distention of the bowel and lung compression. Endotracheal intubation permits adequate ventilation and oxygenation. Protective lung strategies of minimal ventilatory pressures (<30 mm Hg), rapid ventilation(40 to 60 breaths/min), or high frequency oscillatory ventilation are employed to avoid barotrauma to the lungs, which in severe cases are often hypoplastic. Venous access and fluid resuscitation complete preliminary resuscitation.

6. **What is the "honeymoon period"?**
   The honeymoon period describes the interval of time in which a neonate demonstrates adequate oxygenation and ventilation in the absence of maximal medical therapy. Regardless of subsequent deterioration, a honeymoon period suggests that pulmonary function (i.e., lung development) is compatible with survival.

7. **Describe the operative approach.**

CDH results in a physiologic derangement of the lungs that is not reversed by surgical reconstruction of the diaphragm. Thus, repair of CDH is not a surgical emergency. The infant must be stabilized before surgical repair is attempted. A transabdominal (laparotomy) approach allows reduction of the herniated abdominal viscera from the chest; repair of the diaphgramatic defect without obstructed vision or tension; correction of malrotation; and stretching of the abdominal cavity; or creation of a ventral hernia with a prosthetic patch if the reduced viscera are not easily accommodated in the abdomen. In some centers, thoracoscopic or laparoscopic repair has been reported for left-sided CDH but has not become uniformly accepted because of the alterations in physiology imposed by insufflation of CO_2 into the chest (pneumothorax) or abdomen (pneumoperitoneum) of infants who are already critically ill. The approach may be useful in stable infants requiring minimal support or older children with delayed diagnosis of CDH.

8. **What is the most feared complication of diaphragmatic hernia?**

The most feared complication is persistent fetal circulation (PFC). In CDH, one or both lungs are hypoplastic, the pulmonary vascular bed is reduced, and the pulmonary arteries exhibit thickened muscular walls that are hyperreactive. Newborns with CDH are particularly prone to the development of pulmonary hypertension. PFC arises from a sustained increase in pulmonary artery pressure. Blood is shunted away from the lungs, and the unoxygenated blood is diverted to the systemic circulation (right-to-left shunt) through the patent ductus arteriosus and patent foramen ovale. PFC results in hypoxemia, profound acidosis, and shock. PFC is triggered by acidosis, hypercarbia, and hypoxia, all potent vasoconstrictors of the pulmonary circulation.

9. **Is PFC correctable? If so, how?**

Yes. Various strategies are used to prevent or reverse PFC:
 1. **Monitoring:** Oximetry or arterial sampling (preductal in the right upper extremity; postductal in the lower extremity) permits early detection of shunting of unoxygenated blood to the systemic circulation.
 2. **Ventilation:** Hypercarbia is corrected by mechanical ventilation; adequate sedation; and, if necessary, pharmacologic paralysis.
 3. **Oxygenation:** Hypoxemia is corrected by adequate ventilation and high concentrations of inspired oxygen (generally fraction of inspired oxygen [FiO_2] = 100%).
 4. **Resuscitation:** Metabolic acidosis is managed by restoring adequate tissue perfusion (intravenous [IV] fluids or blood, inotropes, and sodium bicarbonate).
 5. **Rescue:** Salvage therapies include administration of pulmonary vasodilators via the ventilatory circuit (nitric oxide) or systemic circulation (priscoline, prostaglandin E2), high-frequency ventilation, and extracorporeal membrane oxygenation (ECMO).

10. **What is the survival rate for patients with CDH?**

The overall survival rate is 60%. The major determinants of survival are the degree of pulmonary hypoplasia and associated major congenital anomalies. Among infants surviving the early newborn period without significant lung dysfunction, the survival rate approaches 100%.

11. **Does in utero intervention have a role in the treatment of patients with CDH?**

To date, fetal surgery for CDH remains experimental. In a prospective trial reported in 1997, the results of intrauterine repair of CDH were compared with conventional postnatal surgery with similar outcome. The investigators concluded that because open fetal surgery with diaphragmatic repair does not improve survival or outcome, prenatally diagnosed CDH should be treated postnatally. Techniques of in-utero endoscopic tracheal occlusion promoting lung growth and development followed by postnatal repair of the diaphragmatic hernia are currently being investigated.

BIBLIOGRAPHY

1. Chiu PP, Sauer C, Mihailovic A et al.: The price of success in the management of congenital diaphragmatic hernia: is improved survival accompanied by an increase in long-term morbidity? J Pediatr Surg 41:888-892, 2006.

2. Clugston RD, Greer JJ: Diaphragm development and congenital diaphragmatic hernia. Semin Pediatr Surg 16:94-100, 2007.

3. Kinsella JP, Ivy DD, Abman SH: Pulmonary vasodilator therapy in congenital diaphragmatic hernia: acute, late, and chronic pulmonary hypertension. Semin Perinatol 29:123-128, 2005.

4. Kitano Y: Prenatal intervention for congenital diaphragmatic hernia. Semin Pediatr Surg 16:101-108, 2007.

5. Lally KP, Lally PA, Lasky RE et al.: Defect size determines survival in infants with congenital diaphragmatic hernia. Pediatrics 120:e651-e657, 2007.

6. Logan JW, Rice HE, Goldberg RN et al.: Congenital diaphragmatic hernia: a systematic review and summary of best-evidence practice strategies. J Perinatol 27:535-549, 2007.

7. Migliazza L, Bellan C, Alberti D et al.: Retrospective study of 111 cases of congenital diaphragmatic hernia treated with early high-frequency oscillatory ventilation and presurgical stabilization. J Pediatr Surg 42: 1526-1532, 2007.

8. Rozmiarek AJ, Qureshi FG, Cassidy L et al.: Factors influencing survival in newborns with congenital diaphragmatic hernia: the relative role of timing of surgery. J Pediatr Surg 39:821-824, 2004.

CHAPTER 87

ABDOMINAL TUMORS

Frederick M. Karrer, MD, and Denis D. Bensard, MD

1. **What are the most common malignant solid abdominal tumors in children?**
   Neuroblastomas, Wilms' tumors, and hepatoblastomas, in that order. Neuroblastomas are
   derived from neural crest tissue; in the abdomen, they originate from the adrenal glands
   and paraspinal sympathetic ganglia. Wilms' tumor (nephroblastoma) derives from the kidney,
   and hepatoblastomas originate in the liver.

2. **Is it tough to differentiate Wilms' tumor from neuroblastomas clinically?**
   Yes. Both tumors present as an asymptomatic abdominal mass. The differences are summarized
   in Table 87-1. In addition, because neuroblastomas produce hormones, affected children
   may exhibit flushing, hypertension (catecholamine release), watery diarrhea, periorbital
   ecchymosis, and abnormal ocular movements.

TABLE 87-1. DIFFERENTIATION BETWEEN WILMS' TUMOR AND NEUROBLASTOMA

	Wilms' Tumor	Neuroblastoma
Age at presentation	3–4 yr	1–2 yr
Extend across midline	Rare	Common
Surface on palpation	Smooth	Knobby
X-ray calcifications	No	Yes

3. **How are Wilms' tumors and neuroblastomas treated?**
   See Table 87-2.

TABLE 87-2. TREATMENT OF WILMS' TUMOR AND NEUROBLASTOMA

	Wilms' Tumor	Neuroblastoma
Primary surgical excision	Important (likely)	Important (less likely)
Chemotherapy	Enormous impact	Less responsive

4. **What are the major prognostic factors in neuroblastomas and Wilms' tumor?**
   In **neuroblastomas,** age at presentation is the major prognostic factor. Children younger
   than 1 year have an overall survival rate >70%, whereas the survival rate for children older than 1 year
   is <35%. Shimada proposed a prognostic classification based on evaluation of histologic
   parameters (tumor differentiation, mitosis-karyorrhexis index [MKI]) and age. Aneuploid tumors,
   tumors with low MKI, and tumors with <10 copies of the n-myc gene also have better outcomes.

Age is also important in children with **Wilms' tumors,** but the prognosis is better because the tumors are more readily excised and much more sensitive to chemotherapy.

5. What are the differences between hepatoblastomas and hepatocellular carcinomas? How are the tumors treated?

Hepatoblastomas usually occur in infants and young children, whereas hepatocellular carcinoma usually occurs in children older than 10 years. Hepatocellular carcinoma usually is associated with cirrhosis and hepatitis B and is histologically identical to the adult form. Surgical resection is the primary therapy for both tumors. Hepatoblastomas often have a good response to adjunctive chemotherapy, whereas hepatocellular carcinoma rarely responds to chemotherapy.

CONTROVERSY

6. Should patients with hepatoblastoma receive preoperative chemotherapy to shrink the tumors?

Preoperative chemotherapy does shrink tumors, resulting in easier hepatic resection and lower surgical morbidity. This benefit must be weighed against the considerable toxicity of chemotherapeutic agents.

KEY POINTS: ABDOMINAL TUMORS

1. The most common malignant solid abdominal tumors in children are neuroblastomas, Wilms' tumor, and hepatoblastomas.

2. In neuroblastomas, age at presentation is the major prognostic factor.

3. Hepatoblastomas usually occur in infants and young children, whereas hepatocellular carcinomas usually occur in children older than 10 years.

BIBLIOGRAPHY

1. Kim S, Chung DH: Pediatric solid malignancies: neuroblastoma and Wilms' tumor. Surg Clin North Am 86:469-487, 2006.

2. La Quaglia MP: Surgical management of neuroblastoma. Semin Pediatr Surg 10:132-139, 2001.

3. Pham TH, Iqbal CW, Grams JM et al.: Outcomes of primary liver cancer in children: an appraisal of experience. J Pediatr Surg 42:834-839, 2007.

4. Pritchard-Jones K: Controversies and advances in the management of Wilms' tumour. Arch Dis Child 87: 241-244, 2002.

5. Ritchey ML, Shamberger RC, Haase G et al.: Surgical complications after primary nephrectomy for Wilms' tumor: report from the National Wilms' Tumor Study Group. J Am Coll Surg 192:63-68, 2001.

6. Shimada M: Tumors of the neuroblastoma group. Pathology 2:43-59, 1993.

7. Tiao GM, Bobey N, Allen S et al.: The current management of hepatoblastoma: a combination of chemotherapy, conventional resection, and liver transplantation. J Pediatr 148:204-211, 2006.

8. von Schweinitz D: Management of liver tumors in childhood. Semin Pediatr Surg 15:17-24, 2006.

9. Wu HY, Snyder HM 3rd, D'Angio GJ: Wilms' tumor management. Curr Opin Urol 15:273-276, 2005.

CHAPTER 88

CONGENITAL CYSTS AND SINUSES OF THE NECK

Frederick M. Karrer, MD, and Denis D. Bensard, MD

1. **What are branchial cleft anomalies?**

   Cysts, sinuses, and fistulas that result from incomplete obliteration of the first, second, or third branchial clefts and are present in early fetal development.

2. **Which anomaly is the most common?**

   Second branchial cleft anomalies are by far the most common, presenting near the mid- to upper border of the sternocleidomastoid (SCM) muscle. First branchial remnants are less common and third clefts are quite rare (see Table 88-1).

3. **How do patients with branchial cleft anomalies present?**

   Those with complete fistulas or sinuses present with intermittent drainage of a mucoid fluid on the neck. Patients with cysts usually present later with a mass (sterile or infected). Complete surgical excision is the treatment of choice.

TABLE 88-1. BRANCHIAL CLEFT ANOMALIES

Branchial Cleft	Internal Opening	Exterior Opening	Frequency
First	External auditory canal	Angle of the jaw	8%
Second	Tonsillar fossa	Anterior border of the SCM	>90%
Third	Piriform sinus	Suprasternal notch	<1%

4. **What are the major operative hazards of branchial cleft remnant excision?**

   The second branchial cleft tracts through the bifurcation of the carotid artery. The facial nerve is in close proximity to the first branchial cleft fistula. The superior laryngeal nerve and the recurrent laryngeal nerve are both at risk in dissection of a third branchial cleft.

5. **What is a thyroglossal duct cyst?**

   A thyroglossal duct cyst is the most common congenital cyst found in the neck. It is caused by failure of normal obliteration of the migration tract of the thyroid gland. Embryologically, the thyroid descends from the base of the tongue (foramen caecum) to its normal location in the low anterior neck.

6. **How do patients with thyroglossal duct cysts present?**

   They present with a paramidline mass in the upper neck; if infected, they may present with fever, tenderness, and erythema.

KEY POINTS: CONGENITAL CYSTS AND SINUSES OF THE NECK

1. The most common branchial cleft anomaly is the second branchial cleft anomaly presenting near the mid- to upper border of the sternocleidomastoid muscle.

2. A thyroglossal duct cyst is the most common congenital cyst found in the neck.

3. A cystic hygroma is a congenital lymphatic malformation that is benign and usually presents as a soft mass in the lateral neck.

7. How are thyroglossal duct cysts treated?
The best treatment is complete excision of the cyst along with the tract. Because embryologically the thyroid descends before formation of the hyoid cartilage, the tract may pass right through the hyoid. Therefore, complete tract removal requires excision of the central portion of the hyoid and dissection up to the base of the tongue (i.e., the Sistrunk procedure).

8. What is a cystic hygroma?
A cystic hygroma is a congenital lymphatic malformation with a predilection for the neck. It is a benign lesion that usually presents as a soft mass in the lateral neck. Excision is often challenging because the lymph cysts do not respect the fascial planes and often intertwine with the neurovascular structures in the neck. Near-total excision is the treatment of choice.

BIBLIOGRAPHY

1. Bloom DC, Perkins JA, Manning SC: Management of lymphatic malformations. Curr Opin Otolaryngol Head Neck Surg 12:500-504, 2004.

2. Foley DS, Fallat ME: Thyroglossal duct and other congenital midline cervical anomalies. Semin Pediatr Surg 15:70-75, 2006.

3. Lieberman M, Kay S, Emil S et al.: Ten years of experience with third and fourth branchial remnants. J Pediatr Surg 37:685-690, 2002.

4. Okazaki T, Iwatani S, Yanai T et al.: Treatment of lymphangioma in children: our experience of 128 cases. J Pediatr Surg 42:386-389, 2007.

5. Ostlie DJ, Burjonrappa SC, Snyder CL et al.: Thyroglossal duct infections and surgical outcomes. J Pediatr Surg 39:396-399, 2004.

6. Schroeder JW Jr, Moyuddin N, Maddalozzo J: Branchial anomalies in the pediatric population. Otolaryngol Head Neck Surg 137:289-295, 2007.

7. Tracy TFJr, Muratore CS: Management of common head and neck masses. Semin Pediatr Surg 16:3-13, 2007.

LIVER TRANSPLANTATION

Jeffrey Campsen, MD, Michael Zimmerman, MD, and Thomas E. Bak, MD

CHAPTER 89

1. **When and where was the first liver transplant performed?**
   Dr. Thomas Starzl performed the first operation on March 1, 1963, at the University of Colorado in Denver. The recipient was a 3-year-old boy with biliary atresia.

2. **Is liver transplantation considered a safe and effective operation?**
   Yes. Although still a major operation with significant risks, patient and graft survival have continuously improved. One-year and 5-year survival should be well over 90% and 70%, respectively, in major centers.

3. **What are the most common indications for liver transplantation in the United States?**
   Noncholestatic cirrhosis characterizes >50% of the recipients. This group includes those with viral hepatitis, alcoholic cirrhosis (Laennec's), and Budd-Chiari syndrome. Cholestatic cirrhosis makes up an additional 15%, with primary sclerosing cholangitis (PSC), primary biliary cirrhosis, and autoimmune hepatitis heading this group. Other indications include biliary atresia, acute hepatic necrosis, malignant neoplasms, and metabolic disease.

4. **Has the most common disease requiring transplantation shifted over the years?**
   Yes. The largest percentage of people now being transplanted have hepatitis C. There are also more retransplants performed because some diseases, such as hepatitis C and PSC, can recur in transplanted livers. Biliary atresia is the main indication for transplant in children.

5. **How is the waiting list run?**
   Changes have been made to the list so that the sickest patients get transplanted first. A new scoring system (Model for End-stage Liver Disease [MELD] score) has been devised to give more weight to objective markers of illness including serum creatinine, bilirubin, and the international normalized ratio (INR); rather than the more subjective medical criteria used in the past. The MELD score provides the best available 3-month mortality estimates for liver disease. This point system has also minimized the importance of time spent on the waiting list. The goal of these changes is to reduce waiting list mortality.

6. **What are some of the recent advances in liver transplant surgery?**
   Operative techniques have improved such that some liver transplant recipients do not require a stay in the intensive care unit (ICU), venovenous bypass, or external biliary drainage, and operative times are shorter (4 to 5 hours). Improved immunosuppression medications have reduced rejection rates and side effects. Live donor transplantation of both right-sided and left-sided liver fragments are also performed.

7. **How long can a liver be kept "on ice"?**
   Optimal cold ischemia should be <12 hours.

8. **What are some common postoperative complications of liver transplantation?**
Postoperative bleeding, infection, and biliary complications are the most common. Primary nonfunction (<5%) and early hepatic artery thrombosis (5%) are less common, but they usually require an urgent retransplant. Long-term recurrence of disease can require retransplantation in the 10% to 20% range.

9. **What is the "piggy-back" technique?**
This is a technique in which the recipient's sick liver is carefully resected off of the vena cava, which is left in situ. The upper donor cava is then sewn to a common cuff of native hepatic veins. The donor's lower cava is ligated. Using this method, it is possible to do the complete transplant with minimal if any vena caval occlusion, resulting in less intraoperative hemodynamic instability.

10. **Is living-donor liver transplantation an option?**
Yes. Initially used in the pediatric population using an adult left lateral segment graft, this procedure has evolved into fairly common practice. The Far East has had a large number of adult-to-adult left lobe graft series. Elsewhere, this has been replaced with a right lobe donor operation. Both the donor and recipient liver lobes quickly regenerate to near normal size. Results in experienced centers mimic those of cadaveric transplant with similar patient survival, albeit at higher complication and retransplant rates. There are reports of both donor and recipient morbidity and mortality.

KEY POINTS: LIVER TRANSPLANTATION

1. The most common indication for liver transplantation in the United States is noncholestatic cirrhosis, usually for viral disease.

2. Optimal cold ischemia time for the liver is <12 hours.

3. TIPS can be used in potential transplant recipients as a bridge to transplantation.

11. **How have transjugular intrahepatic portosystemic shunts (TIPS) improved this field of surgery?**
TIPS can be used in potential transplant recipients as a bridge to transplantation. This procedure is quite effective in controlling portal hypertension without the need for a major abdominal operative shunt. A prior portocaval shunt does complicate a liver transplant, but it is not a contraindication to liver transplantation.

CONTROVERSIES

12. **Should liver transplants be performed in individuals with alcoholic liver disease?**
Transplant centers have strict criteria that alcohol-induced liver transplant recipients must undergo extensive psychological testing and abstain from alcohol before being placed on the waiting list. The recidivism rate (i.e., transplant patients who start drinking again) remains low. Financially, the cost is comparable, if not lower, than continued medical management of end-stage liver disease. We currently do provide care for other self-inflicted medical problems, such as cigarette smokers. The public must realize that people are not being pulled off bar stools and taken to the hospital for their transplant.

13. Should patients with hepatic malignancies have liver transplants?

Patients with hepatocellular carcinoma (single tumor <5 cm or up to three tumors each <3 cm) can be successfully transplanted with good long-term results. Other hepatic malignancies, including cholangiocarcinoma, are generally considered contraindications to transplantation; however, neoadjuvant chemotherapy and brachytherapy coupled with transplant in select cases have shown promising results. Whether scarce donor livers should be allocated to these patients continues to be a complex issue.

14. Should adult-to-adult living donors be used?

The evolving field of adult-to-adult living donor liver transplant (ALDLTx) requires a healthy donor to undergo a major, potentially life-threatening operation. The benefits include a timely, life-saving procedure for a loved one, reducing the recipient's risk of not having a cadaveric liver available in time. The ethics of whether to subject the donor to major liver resective surgery remains debatable. The complication rate in donors is reported to be approximately 30% with biliary complications as the most common type.

15. Should non-heart-beating donors be used for transplant?

Non-heart-beating donors (NHBD) is a relatively new way of obtaining more donor liver grafts. After withdrawal of support by a patient's primary care team, if death occurs rapidly, organ recovery can still proceed in select cases. NHBD experience cardiac arrest before the organs are recovered. Long-term data on these organs is still being gathered, but biliary complication rates and retransplant rates are significantly higher in these grafts. However, with patients dying on the waiting list this technique expands the donor pool and allows for more transplants.

WEBSITE

www.transplantation-soc.org

BIBLIOGRAPHY

1. Bak T, Wachs M, Trotter JF et al.: Adult-to-adult living donor liver transplant using right lobe grafts: results and lessons learned from a single center experience. Liver Transpl 7:680-686, 2001.

2. Busuttil R, Klintmalm, G, editors: *Transplantation of the liver*, 2nd ed., Philadelphia, 2005, Elsevier Saunders.

3. Ghabril M, Dickson RC, Machicao VI et al.: Liver retransplantation of patients with hepatitis C infection is associated with acceptable patient and graft survival. Liver Transpl 13(12):1717-1727, 2007

4. Lok ASF, Villamil FG, McDiarmid SV, editors: Liver transplantation for viral hepatitis [entire volume]. Liver Transpl 8(suppl 1), 2002.

CHAPTER 90

KIDNEY AND PANCREAS TRANSPLANTATION

Jeffrey Campsen, MD, Michael Zimmerman, MD, and Thomas E. Bak, MD

1. **What are the most common indications for kidney transplantation?**
   End-stage renal disease (ESRD) caused by hypertension, diabetes, glomerulonephritis, and polycystic kidney disease.

2. **Why should patients be taken off dialysis and have kidney transplants?**
   Although not a life-saving transplant like liver or heart transplantation, kidney transplantation will improve patients' quality of life. Patient 5-year survival is higher posttransplant when compared with continued dialysis. Finally, there is a cost savings with kidney transplantation compared with long-term dialysis.

3. **How long is kidney graft survival?**
   Cadaveric kidney transplant survival rates have steadily improved over the years. Currently, 1-year graft survival is 90%, with a 10-year graft survival of >50%. Overall 5-year survival for live donor kidney transplants is >75%, which is greater than cadaveric.

4. **How long can kidneys be kept "on ice"?**
   Kidneys can survive and function after longer cold ischemia time than other solid organs. Function can be maintained up to 72 hours, although optimal function is achieved if cold ischemia is kept under 24 hours (most centers transplant before 36 hours). "Pumping" cadaveric kidneys with perfusion machines is a potential way of increasing cold ischemic time and decreasing delayed graft function. Patients on the waiting list frequently continue to work and travel and still have plenty of time to get to the hospital for transplant. Also, United Network of Organ Sharing (UNOS) kidneys are frequently sent via commercial airlines all across the country.

5. **Where is the transplanted kidney placed?**
   Most commonly, the kidney is placed in the right iliac fossa. The peritoneal cavity is reflected superiorly, not entered, and the external iliac vessels are exposed. The renal artery and vein are then anastomosed end-to-side to the iliac vessels and the ureter is anastomosed directly into the bladder.

6. **What are the indications for native nephrectomy?**
   Indications for nephrectomy include chronic infection, symptomatic polycystic kidney disease, intractable hypertension, and heavy proteinurea. The majority of transplant recipients do not need to undergo native nephrectomies.

7. **Are kidney transplants from a living donor recommended?**
   There are definite advantages to receiving a kidney from a living donor. The average survival times of these kidneys are significantly better, 75% at 5-years versus 65% for cadaveric kidneys. Also, the long cadaveric kidney waiting time (usually measured in years) can be avoided. Donors are carefully screened to ensure health and lack of any coercion.

8. **Is donating a kidney a major operation for living donors?**
The standard of care for donor operations has become a laparoscopic donor nephrectomy. This technique has proven to be safe, with no negative effects on the kidney. The benefits of this modification over the open technique are much quicker recovery and shorter return-to-work time. This has generally increased the number of people interested in being living donors. The most common complications are wound infections and hernias.

9. **What are the indications for kidney-pancreas transplantation?**
In general, all type 1 diabetics who have poorly controlled diabetes despite optimal medical management should be considered for kidney-pancreas (K-P) transplantation as long as they are acceptable surgical risks. Unfortunately, many older patients have significant, even prohibitive, comorbidities. A pancreas transplant adds significant morbidity and mortality risks over a kidney-only transplant.

10. **Can a patient undergo pancreas transplantation before or after a kidney transplant?**
Yes. Patients can receive a simultaneous K-P transplant (SKP). This is the most common course, and the operation is done through a midline abdominal incision with the pancreas and kidney placed on opposite iliac vessels. Patients can also receive a pancreas-only transplant (PTA) or pancreas-after-kidney transplant (PAK). The survival for these grafts are at 5 years: SKP is 69% and PAK and PTA are 58%. The SPK has a higher graft survival because transplant physicians can monitor rejection of the pancreas in SPK transplants through the kidney. Some centers are now shifting to portal drainage of the pancreas, with the venous outflow established to the superior mesenteric vein.

KEY POINTS: KIDNEY AND PANCREAS TRANSPLANTATION

1. The most common indication for kidney transplantation is ESRD caused by hypertension, diabetes, glomerulonephritis, and polycystic kidney disease.

2. Cadaveric kidney transplant survival rates have steadily improved over the years, with current 1-year graft survival rates of 90% and a 10-year graft survival rate of >50%.

3. Kidney transplants from live donors have a significantly higher graft survival rate than cadaveric kidneys.

4. In general, all type 1 diabetics with poorly controlled diabetes despite optimal medical management should be considered for K-P transplantation as long as they are acceptable surgical risks. SKP have a higher pancreatic graft survival at 5 years than PTA and PAK. There is significant debate currently whether the risk of PAK is warranted.

11. **How are digestive enzymes drained in a pancreas transplant?**
The donor pancreas is procured with a duodenal cuff still attached, with enzymatic drainage from the graft into this cuff intact. The duodenal cuff is then drained into a piece of recipient's small intestine with an enteric anastomosis. An alternative is to attach the duodenal cuff to the bladder. This allows amylase levels to be followed in the urine, but metabolic and infectious complications frequently require a conversion to enteric drainage.

12. **What are some complications commonly seen with pancreas transplant?**
Leakage from the duodenal cuff, graft venous thrombosis, infection, rejection, and graft pancreatitis are all potential complications. Rejection in PTA is hard to detect early. By the time

there are detectable rises in glucose, amylase, or other markers it is sometimes too late to save the graft. SKP can improve surveillance because serum creatinine is a sensitive indicator of rejection. The incidence of these complications is decreasing as more experience is gained, and pancreas graft survival now approaches kidney graft survival.

CONTROVERSIES

13. Is human leukocyte antigen matching still important?

It is somewhat important. Historically, human leukocyte antigen (HLA) matching was an important consideration when matching cadaver kidneys to recipients. HLA-DR is the most important overall. With today's improved immunosuppressive agents, many transplant surgeons believe that HLA matching is no longer critical. Six antigen match kidneys are still shared nationally and do enjoy some improvement in long-term graft survival. Donor organ quality remains the primary determinant in how well the transplanted organ functions. For example, a poorly matched kidney from a living donor will still usually outlast a well-matched cadaveric kidney. Panel reactive antibody (PRA) detects preformed recipient antibodies using a panel of typing cells and gets a percentage of cells that the serum reacts. This percentage is now also used to help determine management of immunosuppression.

14. Does pancreas transplantation halt the progression of diabetic disease?

This is still unproven. Logically, we would expect it to. Regression of neuropathy and eye dysfunction has been reported. Recently, long-term recipients have exhibited some regression of microscopic nephropathy.

15. Are islet cell transplants the answer in the future?

Probably, although this has been frustratingly slow to achieve. Recent protocols using new immunosuppressive regimens and new islet cell isolation techniques have shown promise, but long-term data are still not widely available. The process requires that isolated islet cells be extracted from a donor pancreas. Most patients need a total islet cell mass that must be prepared from two or more donors to become insulin independent. These cells are then injected into the portal vein, lodge in the liver, and produce insulin. Theoretically, patients achieve the benefit of a pancreas transplant without the surgical risk; however, there are reported complications including hepatic bleeding, hepatic infarct, splenic hemorrhage, portal hypertension, and portal vein thrombosis. Until the logistic and islet cell yield (mass) problems have been solved, pancreas transplantation will remain the most efficient use of most donor organs.

WEBSITE

www.transplantation-soc.org

BIBLIOGRAPHY

1. Bartlett ST: Laparoscopic donor nephrectomy after seven years. Am J Transpl 2:896-897, 2002.
2. Donovitch G: *Handbook of kidney transplantation*, 3rd ed., Philadelphia, 2001, Lippincott Williams & Wilkins.
3. Fiorina P, Secchi A: Pancreatic islet cell transplant for treatment of diabetes. Endocrinol Metab Clin North Am 36(4):999-1013, 2007.
4. Lipshutz GS, Wilkinson AH: Pancreas-kidney and pancreas transplantation for the treatment of diabetes mellitus. Endocrinol Metab Clin North Am 36(4):1015-1038, 2007.

CHAPTER 91

HEART TRANSPLANTATION

Paul R. Crisostomo, MD, Alexandra McMillan, and
Daniel R. Meldrum, MD, FACS

1. **Who performed the first experimental heart-lung transplant?**
   Alexis Carrel, a French-born U.S. surgeon, developed the vascular techniques required for heart-lung transplantation and performed the first experimental heart-lung transplant in 1907. He transplanted the lungs, heart, aorta, and vena cava of a 1-week-old cat into the neck of a large adult cat. For devising the technique of vascular anastomosis and other outstanding accomplishments, Carrel received the Nobel Prize in 1912 (the first Nobel Prize awarded to a scientist working in a U.S. laboratory).

2. **Who performed the first experimental orthotopic heart-lung transplant?**
   Vladimir Demikhov performed the first intrathoracic heart-lung transplant in a dog in 1962.

3. **Who developed the first surgical strategy required for human heart transplantation?**
   Norman Shumway.

4. **Who performed the first human heart transplant? When?**
   Christian Barnard performed the first human heart transplant in December 1967 (in Capetown, South Africa, after visiting Dr. Shumway), although Dr. Shumway set the stage by developing the technique in animals. Shumway and the Stanford group performed the first heart transplant in the United States and accomplished the first successful clinical series.

5. **Who performed the first successful heart-lung transplant? When?**
   Dr. Bruce Reitz at Stanford in 1981 on a 21-year-old woman with pulmonary hypertension secondary to an atrial septal defect.

6. **How many heart transplants are performed annually? Is the number increasing or decreasing?**
   In 1995 approximately 6500 heart transplants were performed worldwide. By 2003, the number had decreased to approximately 5000 and remains relatively stable between 5000 and 5500.

7. **What anastomoses (surgical connections) must be performed for a combined heart and lungs transplant?**
   The operation requires only a right atrial-to-cava (inflow) anastomosis and an aortic (outflow) anastomosis with a connection at the trachea. Heart-lung transplant is less complicated (fewer anastomoses) than heart transplant alone, which may explain why heart-lung transplant was attempted first.

8. **What anastomoses must be performed for a heart transplant?**
   Left atrial, right caval, aortic, and pulmonary arterial.

9. **What is the preferred surgical technique?**
   Orthotopic heart transplant is the standard. The "classical" lower-Shumway technique consisted of a biatrial anastomosis. However, subsequent studies found that the biatrial technique

results in distortion of atrial geometry and abnormal ventricular filling, right ventricular dysfunction, atrioventricular (A-V) valve insufficiency, and sinus node dysfunction. Currently, the bicaval technique (two caval anastomoses are done separately while the left atrial anastomosis is still done as a cuff) is the most common procedure.

10. **Who is an acceptable cardiac donor?**
Acceptable cardiac donors meet the following criteria:
1. Age <55
2. Absence of cardiac disease and few coronary artery disease (CAD) risk factors.
3. Normal electrocardiogram (ECG) and echocardiogram.
4. Normal heart by inspection during organ recovery.
And standard transplant donor criteria:
1. Requirements for brain death.
2. Consent from next of kin.
3. ABO blood group compatibility with recipient.
4. No human immunodeficiency virus (HIV), hepatitis, or untreated acute infections.
5. No systemic malignancy.

11. **Who is an acceptable cardiac recipient?**
Cardiac transplant criteria:
- Deteriorating cardiac function, maximum amount of oxygen per milliliter per kilogram of body weight (VO_2max) <14 ml/kg, ejection fraction (EF) <25%, <1 year prognosis for survival, irremediable New York Heart Association (NYHA) class IV.
- No fixed pulmonary hypertension (pulmonary vascular resistance <6 Wood units).
- Age <70 years.
General transplant criteria:
- No active malignancy, acute infection, HIV, or collagen disorder.
- Normal renal, hepatic, and central nervous system (CNS) function.
- Reasonable physiological status and psychosocial stability.
- No alcohol, tobacco, or drug abuse.

12. **What does UNOS stand for? What is the difference between status I and status II patients?**
UNOS stands for United Network for Organ Sharing. Any available donor hearts would first be offered to status 1A patients on the UNOS list—patients who are critically ill and in the intensive care unit (ICU) requiring advanced life support (ventricular assist device [VAD], intraaortic balloon pump [IABP], ionotropes, etc). Status 1B is the next highest priority; these patients require ionotropic support, but may not need ICU care. Status 2 patients do not require ionotropes and are not hospitalized while they wait.

13. **What are the most common indications for heart transplant in adults and in children?**
In adults, CAD (ischemic cardiomyopathy) and idiopathic cardiomyopathy each account for approximately 45% of transplants.
In children, congenital heart disease and cardiomyopathy are most common, with hypoplastic left-sided heart being the most common congenital malformation requiring heart transplantation, deteriorating cardiac function, and having a prognosis of less than 1 year to live.

14. **What percentage of potential recipients (on the transplant list) die while waiting for a heart transplant?**
Between 15% and 40%.

15. **What are the extended donor criteria? Who would benefit most?**
A persistent shortage of donor hearts has forced the criteria of organ procurement to be extended. High-risk recipients (status 1) who received hearts from older (age >55) donors, hepatitis B (core immunoglobulin M [IgM]-negative) or C positive donors, or donors with mild left ventricular hypertrophy (LVH; wall thickness = 13 mm) demonstrate superior survival to that of patients who were listed but never transplanted.

16. **At what point does donor heart ischemic time influence mortality?**
Donor heart ischemic time >6 hours definitely increases mortality. Ischemic times between 4 and 6 hours stun the donor heart. Most transplant teams try to keep ischemic times (from donor harvest to perfusion in the recipient) to <4 hours.

17. **When is prolonged donor ischemic time appropriate?**
Donor heart ischemia time >4 hours is a significant predictor of adult mortality. However, in the pediatric population, donor heart ischemia times extended as long as 8.5 hours may be safe and have showed no difference in survival.

18. **Who pioneered hypothermic myocardial preservation?**
Henry Swan at the University of Colorado. He submerged anesthetized children in a bathtub of ice water before cardiac procedures.

19. **What are the major causes of death after heart transplantation?**
Non-specific graft failure (ischemia reperfusion injury, reimplantation edema, etc.), days to weeks
Non-cytomegalovirus (CMV) infection, months
Acute rejection, months
Cardiac allograft vasculopathy, years

20. **What is the typical infection pattern for a patient after transplant?**
First postoperative month: conventional bacterial pathogens encountered in surgical patients.
1 to 4 months: opportunistic pathogens, especially CVM.
>4 months: both conventional and opportunistic infections.

21. **How is cardiac allograft rejection prevented?**
Immunosuppression consists of preoperative induction therapy or postoperative maintenance therapy. Induction therapy is primarily either interleukin-2 receptor (CD25) antibodies or antithrombocyte globulin. OKT3 is no longer recommended for induction because of a higher incidence of pulmonary edema, hypotension, and high fevers. Maintenance therapy usually consists of a calcineurin inhibitor (tacrolimus > cyclosporine), an antiproliferative agent (mycophenolate mofetil > rapamycin), and prednisone.

KEY POINTS: CRITERIA FOR ACCEPTABLE HEART DONORS

1. Age <55.

2. Absence of cardiac disease and few CAD risk factors.

3. Normal ECG and echocardiogram.

4. Normal heart by inspection during organ recovery.

22. **Should all transplant patients receive induction therapy?**
    No. Only 50% of patients undergoing heart transplants currently receive induction therapy. Patients with circulating preformed antibodies (multiparous women, reoperative sternotomy, post-transfusions, VAD, etc.) are at risk for early rejection and may benefit. Patients at risk for renal dysfunction may also benefit because induction therapy may allow delayed use of nephrotoxic calcineurin inhibitors.

23. **Does human leukocyte antigen mismatch influence the incidence of rejection after heart transplantation? Is human leukocyte antigen typing routinely performed before heart transplantation?**
    Yes and no. Human leukocyte antigen (HLA) mismatch (2 to 6 versus 0 or 1 antigen matches) is associated with an increased incidence of rejection. However, recent studies reveal that HLA mismatches are no longer significant risk factors for 5-year mortality as they were in previous eras. HLA typing is also not routinely done before heart transplantation; many patients with heart disease have a poor prognosis and require urgent transplant so that they cannot wait for an organ with a high degree of HLA matching to become available.

24. **Is ABO compatibility necessary for cardiac transplantation?**
    No. Hyperacute rejection resulting from ABO incompatibility requires preformed recipient AB and complement activation. Infants have an incompetent complement system, and serum titers of anti-A and anti-B antibodies are usually low until 1 year of age. West and colleagues first described a series of successful ABO incompatible infant heart transplants.

25. **How is cardiac allograft rejection diagnosed?**
    Clinical suspicion is raised by new-onset cardiac arrhythmia, fever, or hypotension. Diagnosis depends on endomyocardial biopsy, which is performed at regular intervals to detect histologic evidence of rejection before signs or symptoms occur. Gene expression profiling of peripheral blood lymphocytes is a novel and increasingly accepted noninvasive tool for diagnosis of rejection. Its negative predictive value is >99%, avoiding the need for biopsy in certain settings.

26. **What is the most serious complication of transvenous endomyocardial biopsy?**
    Cardiac perforation occurs in 0.5% of cases. This can rapidly lead to tamponade and circulatory collapse.

27. **What is the incidence of cardiac allograft vasculopathy? What are the risk factors?**
    Cardiac allograft vasculopathy (VAC; also known as transplant vasculopathy, transplant CAD or accelerated graft arteriosclerosis) occurs in more than 50% of patients by 5 years after transplant and is the main factor limiting long-term survival. Risk factors for CAV include male gender of the donor or recipient, older donor age, donor hypertension, recipient pretransplant CAD, and HLA-DR mismatches.

28. **What is the difference between nontransplant coronary artery disease or atherosclerosis and cardiac allograft vasculopathy?**
    Unlike nontransplant CAD, CAV is a diffuse, concentric process involving large- and medium-sized vessels. Preservation injury, alloimmune responses (cellular and humoral), and possibly chronic CMV infection may contribute to its pathogenesis.

29. **How is CAV diagnosed and treated?**
    CAV is diagnosed predominantly by angiogram and more recently by intravascular ultrasound (IVUS). Statin therapy ± diltiazem decreases the incidence of developing CAV. In patients with established CAV, rapamycin may reduce subsequent cardiac events. Otherwise, treatment

has been disappointing. Retransplantation is no longer recommended in many centers because of only a 55% 1-year survival rate and a 46% incidence of recurrent CAV. Coronary angioplasty ± stenting has been primarily palliative as a result of the diffuse nature of CAV.

30. **Are 3-hydroxy-3-methylglutaryl coenzyme A reductase inhibitors ("statin" drugs) generally recommended for patients post cardiac transplant?**
Yes. Hyperlipidemia is common after cardiac transplantation, and 3-hydroxy-3-methylglutaryl coenzyme A (HMG-CoA) reductase inhibitors reduce the incidence and severity of CAV. In addition, statins have an early effect on mortality, which suggests that these drugs may also have immunosuppressive effects.

31. **What are ventricular assist devices?**
These devices are designed to unload either the right (RVAD) or left (LVAD) ventricle while supporting the pulmonary or systemic circulation. Patients with these VADs may be ambulatory, and the devices may be worn for weeks to months. VADs may be used as a bridge to transplant (when the patient is listed for transplantation) or as destination therapy (when no transplant is planned).

32. **When should a heart transplant be performed after VAD implantation?**
The ideal time to transplant is between 2 weeks to 6 months after VAD implantation. Patients have a 92% 1-year survival rate if transplanted within this time period compared to 75% otherwise.

33. **Is stem cell transplantation for heart failure a reality? What are the mechanisms of its benefit?**
Clinical trials such as TOPCARE-CHF already demonstrate that stem cell transplantation in patients with chronic heart failure is safe. Stem cell transplantation may mediate its effects via regeneration, angiogenesis, and beneficial remodeling of injured cardiac tissue. Stem cell transplantation is an exciting and novel therapeutic modality that may improve myocardial function in heart failure and allow explantation of VADs without the need for heart transplantation.

34. **Is the transplanted heart denervated?**
Initially, yes, but it is believed that partial reinnervation begins within 1 year. Because of this, the heart's anatomically mediated reflexes are blunted (e.g., higher resting heart rate because of decreased or absent vagal tone).

35. **Can one heart be successfully transplanted twice?**
Yes. Meiser and colleagues transplanted the same heart a second time on March 19, 1991, 42 hours after the initial transplantation. Second transplant of the same heart has since been reported by others.

36. **What is "domino heart transplant"?**
The good heart from a heart-lung recipient is transplanted into a patient requiring a heart transplant. Some patients with primary lung dysfunction have secondary irreversible cardiac dysfunction (i.e., Eisenmenger's syndrome); others, however, such as patients with cystic fibrosis, have good cardiac function. Patients with good cardiac function may serve as donors and increase the donor pool.

37. **Is the heart capable of making tumor necrosis factor (TNF)? What does TNF have to do with heart transplantation?**
Tumor necrosis factor (TNF), typically described as a macrophage-derived or monocyte-derived inflammatory cytokine, is also produced in large quantities by the heart. TNF released by the heart after ischemia-reperfusion probably contributes to immediate injury (dysfunction) and possibly to later rejection. Anti-TNF strategies are intuitively promising (but undocumented) therapeutic strategies.

38. **What is the overall 30-day mortality rate after heart transplant? What is the breakdown in mortality between adult and pediatric patients?**

The registry of the International Society for Heart and Lung Transplantation, which has data for approximately 76,000 heart transplants, has recorded a 30-day mortality rate of 10%. The 30-day mortality rate for adult recipients is about 8%; for pediatric recipients, it is slightly higher.

39. **What are the 5- and 10-year actuarial survival rates for heart transplant recipients?**

They are 75% and 50%, respectively (and the quality of life is dramatically improved).

40. **What work remains to be done in heart transplantation?**

The future of heart transplantation is bright. Knowledge gained in experimental myocardial ischemia-reperfusion injury and protection is accelerating. New, exciting ways to manipulate myocardial inflammation (stem cells) and immunology (e.g., signal transduction, gene therapy, chimerism) will improve postoperative myocardial function and graft tolerance. Ultimately, genetic alteration of donor hearts will increase the donor pool.

WEBSITE

www.transplantation-soc.org

BIBLIOGRAPHY

1. Al-khaldi A, Robbins RC: New directions in cardiac transplantation. Annu Rev Med 57:455-471, 2006.

2. Canter CE, Shaddy RE, Bernstein D et al.: Indications for heart transplantation in pediatric heart disease: a scientific statement from the American Heart Association Council on Cardiovascular Disease in the Young; the Councils on Clinical Cardiology, Cardiovascular Nursing, and Cardiovascular Surgery and Anesthesia; and the Quality of Care and Outcomes Research Interdisciplinary Working Group. Circulation 115(5):658-676, 2007.

3. Crisostomo PR, Wang M, Markel TA et al.: Stem cell mechanisms and paracrine effects: potential in cardiac surgery. Shock 28:375-383, 2007.

4. Rahmani M, Cruz RP, Granville DJ et al.: Allograft vasculopathy versus atherosclerosis. Circ Res 99(8):801-815, 2006.

5. Scheule AM, Zimmerman GJ, Johnston JK et al.: Duration of graft cold ischemia does not affect outcomes in pediatric heart transplant recipients. Circulation 106(12 Suppl 1):I163-I167, 2002.

6. Steinman TI, Becker BN, Frost AE et al.: Guidelines for the referral and management of patients eligible for solid organ transplantation. Transplantation 71(9):1189-1204, 2001.

7. Taylor DO, Edwards LB, Boucek MM et al.: Registry of the International Society for Heart and Lung Transplantation: twenty-fourth official adult heart transplant report—2007. J Heart Lung Transplant 26(8):769-781, 2007.

8. Uber PA, Mehra MR. Induction therapy in heart transplantation: is there a role? J Heart Lung Transplant 26(3):205-209, 2007.

9. Wang M, Tsai BM, Crisostomo PR et al.: Tumor necrosis factor receptor 1 signaling resistance in female myocardium during ischemia. Circulation 114(1 Suppl):I282-I289, 2006.

10. West LJ, Pollock-Barziv SM, Dipchand AI et al.: ABO-incompatible heart transplantation in infants. N Engl J Med 344(11):793-800, 2001.

11. Zaroff JG, Rosengard BR, Armstrong WF et al.: Consensus conference report: maximizing use of organs recovered from the cadaver donor: cardiac recommendations, March 28-29, 2001, Crystal City, Va. Circulation 106(7):836-841, 2002.

CHAPTER 92

MECHANICAL CIRCULATORY SUPPORT

T. Brett Reece, MD, Anne Cannon, RN, BSN, and
Joseph C. Cleveland, Jr., MD

1. **What are the indications for ventricular assist device (VAD)?**
   a. Bridge to transplant: Patients are in need of and are eligible for transplant, but their clinical course is such that they will not survive until a donor organ is available. Thus, mechanical circulatory support is required to "bridge" the gap until an organ is available. The ultimate goal for these patients is heart transplantation and must be listed for transplant before VAD placement.
   b. Destination therapy: Patients are those with end-stage heart disease who are not eligible or candidates for heart transplantation. Although they are not candidates for transplantation at the time of device implantation, these patients can evolve into heart transplant candidates in some cases where the ventricular unloading leads to other hemodynamic changes, for instance, improvement in pulmonary hypertension. Goals of destination therapy are to prolong life, reduce hospitalizations, and improve quality of life. Destination therapy is an alternative to medical management for those who have class III to IV heart failure. To qualify for destination therapy, patients should receive optimal medical management (OMM) for at least 60 out of the last 90 days. Destination therapy is also known as "durable long-term support."
   c. Recovery: Patients with acute situations that may improve fall into this category. Most commonly this involves post-infarct cardiogenic shock or failure to separate from cardiopulmonary bypass (CPB). Shorter term devices can allow for recovery or further workup for longer term devices or transplantation. Some recovery devices use the same cannulas as in CPB, facilitating their implantation.

2. **What are contraindications for VAD?**
   a. Lack of social support
   b. Intellectual
   c. Infection
   d. Size (for Heartmate XVE)
   e. Severity of disease

3. **What workup needs to be done prior to VAD placement?**
   a. Cultures need to be sent. Remember that these patients tend to have central lines, Foleys, etc., so infection remain a huge problem for them.
   b. Echocardiogram (ECHO) looking for clot in the ventricles. Thrombus may not exclude the patient alone, but may make stoke more of a risk. ECHO should also evaluate status of valves if repair or replacement is needed and can be done concurrently with VAD placement. If mechanical valve is in place, it should be changed out for bioprosthetic valve at time of implant.
   c. Optimize nutrition because this is a huge indicator of long-term and short-term outcome.
   d. Left ventricular assist device (LVAD): The right ventricle needs to be evaluated closely, because some right ventricular (RV) failure may be secondary to left ventricular (LV) failure. However, the right ventricle may not be able to tolerate the VAD placement either. Unfortunately, predictors of RV failure do not rule out the need for biventricular support.

e. Right ventricular assist device (RVAD): Pulmonary hypertension may be the most important issue to be defined in RV support. If the ventricular issues arise from the pulmonary vasculature, the VAD may not be able to overcome the resistance, or it wears out prematurely.

4. **What is optimal medical management prior to VAD placement?**
Optimizing heart failure management with β-blocker, ace inhibitor, hydralazine, diureses, and possibly digoxin as indicated.

5. **What predicts outcomes with VAD placement?**
Preoperative renal function, nutritional status, mechanical ventilation, redo sternotomy, elevated central venous pressure (CVP), and prothrombin time (PT) and international normalized ratio (INR) have all demonstrated correlation with poor outcomes. Several risk scores have been developed to try to predict outcome that use multiple preoperative factors.

6. **How long do the devices last?**
Durability is device dependent. The short-term devices should probably either be removed are changed to a longer term device within a 1 to 2 weeks because of increased risk of infection and thromboembolism. The long-term devices should last from 1 to 4 years or even more. Short-term devices that are intended for recovery actually can be in for a number of weeks depending on the device. A paracoporeal ventricular assist device (PVAD)—not to be confused with a percutaneous ventricular assist device (pVAD)—can be in for weeks to months (i.e., Thoratec PVAD, Abiomed Ventricle). Extra-corporeal VADs (i.e., CentriMag) are really only approved by the Food and Drug Administration (FDA) for hours but most are left in for days to weeks.

7. **How does the presence of a VAD affect transplantation?**
Despite the complexity of the dissection in the removal of the devices, the transplant outcomes are not compromised. This is thought to be secondary to many of the patients with a VAD being better stabilized than their heart failure counterparts. However, the explanting surgeon must be wary of the outflow tracts, whether they are to the pulmonary artery or aorta.

8. **What are the general classes of devices used today, and what are their advantages and disadvantages?**
   a. Internal
      1. Advantage: the device is protected within the abdomen and thorax.
      2. Disadvantage: devices require sufficient space in the abdomen for the device and the drive line remains an issue for both wound healing and infection. Further, the size of the devices can limit utilization in smaller patients.
   b. External
      1. Advantage: Size of the device does not exclude smaller patients.
      2. Disadvantage: The inflow and outflow of the device traverse the skin, which can be more difficult to prevent infection. Further, the external devices may not allow for the patient to actually leave the hospital.
   c. Axial Flow
      1. Advantage: In general the devices are much smaller.
      2. Disadvantage: Loss of pulsatility creates an abnormal environment for the systemic vascular bed. Also, the medical staff needs further education on how to take and evaluate the vitals of patients with these devices.
   d. Percutaneous
      1. Advantage: They are small, can be placed in the catheter lab through peripheral vessels, and do not need to be placed on CPB for implantation. May be best suited for short-term recovery.

2. Disadvantage: Their durability is still being evaluated. They are not long-term devices. Their implantation may not prevent infection in the long term. These devices do not augment flow as well as the other devices.

9. **What are the perioperative issues that must be observed or addressed?**
   a. Coagulopathy: notorious procedures for postoperative bleeding
   b. Volume status: related to bleeding, but also to preoperative volume status
   c. Afterload: directly affects pump output, most important in axial flow devices
   d. Other ventricle: most difficult to deal with
   e. Thrombosis or embolism

10. **What needs to be done for anticoagulation for these devices?**
   Anticoagulation is device specific. For the most part, all patients with VAD need to be anticoagulated with Coumadin and possible a laundry list of antiplatelet agents. There are devices that do not require anticoagulation beyond aspirin.

11. **What long-term management issues must be addressed?**
   a. Teaching the patient, family, and local medical services how to deal with the VAD
   b. Nutrition
   c. Drive line healing closely related to nutrition
   d. Anticoagulation (which is device specific)
   e. Follow echocardiography: evaluate for ventricular function, valve opening, inflow and outflow orientation, and any indication of device dysfunction including thrombus formation or valve degeneration
   f. Emergency procedures with community education because these issues may not arise near the implantation institution

12. **When to transplant the bridges?**
   The patient needs to recover from the VAD placement. This is an opportunity to address overall body volume issues, improve the patient's nutrition, and improve activity status. Although transplants are done shortly after device placement, the decision to list takes many different factors into account that might improve the transplant outcome. This is not a patient to place a marginal donor organ into because of fear for deterioration. On the other hand, device complications may accelerate the need for transplantation.

13. **What must be evaluated before explantation?**
   Explantation can be a difficult call to make. The heart function can be temporarily lessened by explantation process, so some reserve must be present to tolerate removal in the perioperative period. Pathology can play a significant role, especially if the recovery of the myocardium is possible. ECHO plays a real role as the assist device can be turned down to evaluate the underlying ventricular function. Finally, the decision for assist device explantation must be multidisciplinary including the patient in these discussions.

BIBLIOGRAPHY

1. Birks EJ, Tansley PD, Hardy J et al.: Left ventricular assist device and drug therapy for the reversal of heart failure. N Engl J Med 355:1873, 2006.
2. Lietz K, Long JW, Kfoury AG: Outcomes of left ventricular assist device implantation as destination therapy in the post-REMATCH era: implications for patient selection. Circulation 1165:497-505, 2007.
3. Rao V, Oz MC, Flannery MA et al.: Changing trends in mechanical circulatory assistance. J Card Surg 194: 361-366, 2004.
4. Rose EA, Gelijns AC, Moskowitz AJ et al.: Long-term mechanical left ventricular assistance for end-stage heart failure. N Engl J Med 34520:1435-1443, 2001.

CHAPTER 93

LUNG TRANSPLANTATION

Paul R. Crisostomo, MD, Nadia McMillan, and Daniel R. Meldrum, MD, FACS

1. **Which human organ transplant was performed first, the heart or the lung?**
   Although heart transplantation has progressed more rapidly, the first human lung transplant preceded the first heart transplant.

2. **Who performed the first human lung transplant? When?**
   James Hardy performed the first human lung transplant in 1963; however, more than 20 years passed before lung transplantation was performed routinely in clinical practice (during that 20-year period, only one patient did well enough to leave the hospital). This delay was caused by initial graft failure secondary to inadequate organ preservation, long ischemic times, lack of good immunosuppressive agents, and technical difficulties (primarily with the bronchial—not the vascular—anastomoses).

3. **What are the general types of lung transplants?**
   Single, double (bilateral), and heart-lung.

4. **How many lung transplants are performed annually? Is the number increasing or decreasing?**
   Although first performed in 1963, significant numbers were not performed until the late 1980s (in 1986, 1 lung transplant; in 1989, 132 lung transplants). Since 1994, the number of single lung transplants performed annually has remained stable (around 700). However, bilateral lung transplantations have rapidly increased from approximately 100 in 1994 to more than 1400 in 2005 and continue to increase worldwide.

5. **Why is the number of combined heart-lung transplants performed annually decreasing?**
   Approximately 250 heart-lung transplants were performed in 1990; the number has decreased to approximately 75 in 2005. As the results of single lung and double lung transplants have improved, the need to perform heart-lung transplants in patients with isolated pulmonary disease has been obviated.

6. **Who is a candidate for a lung transplant?**
   Candidates include patients with no other medical or surgical alternative who are likely to die of pulmonary disease within 2 to 3 years, are younger than 65 years, are not ventilator dependent, and do not have a history of malignancy. Psychological stability in the recipient is also important.

7. **What are the most common indications for single lung transplant?**
   Emphysema (50%)
   Idiopathic pulmonary fibrosis (25%)
   α-1 antitrypsin deficiency (7.5%)
   Cystic fibrosis (CF; 2%)
   Sarcoidosis (2%)

8. **What are the most common indications for a double lung transplant?**
   CF (30%)
   Emphysema (25%)
   Idiopathic pulmonary fibrosis (13%)
   α-1 antitrypsin deficiency (8.5%)
   Primary pulmonary hypertension and pulmonary hypertension secondary to correctable congenital heart disease (6%)

9. **What are the most common indications for heart-lung transplant?**
   Primary pulmonary hypertension (25%) and CF (15%) are instances in which bad lungs have ruined a good heart. Conversely, with congenital heart disease (34%), a bad heart has destroyed good lungs.

10. **What is sewn to what during a single lung transplant? A double lung transplant?**
    During a single lung transplant, recipient-to-graft bronchial, pulmonary artery, and pulmonary vein (atrial cuff) anastomoses are required. Anastomoses for double transplant are the same; however, cardiopulmonary bypass (CPB) is required more often during double lung transplant. During implantation of the second lung, diversion of the entire cardiac output (CO) to the freshly ischemic lung often results in reperfusion lung edema and hypoxemia.

11. **Which diagnoses carry the best results for single lung transplants?**
    Patients with emphysema, α-1 antitrypsin deficiency, and CF do significantly better, with 1-year survival rates of approximately 75%. However, patients with CF or idiopathic pulmonary fibrosis may derive more of a survival benefit from lung transplantation than patients with chronic obstructive pulmonary disorder (COPD) because mortality without transplantation is higher.

12. **Are the survival rates different for single lung and double lung transplants?**
    Yes. Although survival rates for single and bilateral transplant recipients are similar for the first year, in subsequent years, bilateral lung transplants (half life = 5.9 years) have significantly improved survival compared to single lung transplants (half life = 4.4 years).

13. **What are the most common complications after lung transplant?**
    Hypertension (85%)
    Renal dysfunction (38%)
    Hyperlipidemia (52%)
    Diabetes (33%)
    Bronchiolitis obliterans (33%)

14. **What are the major causes of death after lung transplantation?**
    Primary graft dysfunction (days)
    Non-cytomegalovirus (CMV) infection (weeks to years)
    Bronchiolitis obliterans (months to years)

15. **What is primary graft dysfunction (PGD)? How is it treated?**
    PGD is a form of acute lung injury resulting from ischemia or reperfusion injury, edema, preservation, surgical technique, and recipient or donor risk factors. It manifests clinically as poor oxygenation, compliance, and edema. Treatment consists of increased ventilatory support, diuretics, pulmonary vasodilation (prostaglandins and inhaled nitric oxide), surfactant replacement (nebulized synthetic), extracorporeal membrane oxygenation, and retransplantation.

16. **What is the most common nonbacterial cause of pneumonia in lung transplant patients?**

    CMV, usually occurring 4 to 8 weeks postoperatively. Primary CMV infection usually results in more serious illness than reactivation disease. CMV-seronegative recipients should receive only blood products that are serologically negative.

17. **In addition to immune suppressive therapy, what other factors put transplanted lungs at risk for infection?**

    Lung denervation, interruption of lymphatic clearance and bronchial circulation, and impaired mucociliary clearance.

18. **What is bronchiolitis obliterans?**

    Bronchiolitis obliterans, a major cause of long-term morbidity after lung transplantation, is a chronic irreversible scarring process that results in progressive obliteration of the small airways of the lung allograft and resultant obstructive lung disease. Clinically, it is characterized by dyspnea and airflow obstruction.

19. **How does bronchiolitis obliterans develop?**

    Lymphocytes infiltrate the bronchiole submucosa, and migrate through the basement membrane to the airway mucosa. Cytotoxic alloreactive injury and epithelial necrosis follow. In response to ulceration, fibropurulent exudent forms within the airway and is accompanied by proliferation of fibroblasts, endothelial cells and lymphocytes. This myxoid tissue partially or completely can occlude the airway.

20. **What are the risk factors for the development of bronchiolitis obliterans after lung transplant?**

    Episodes of acute allograft rejection is undoubtedly the most important risk factor. CMV infection, noncompliance with immunosuppresive medications, and lymphocytic bronchitis are also important risk factors.

21. **How is lung allograft rejection prevented?**

    Immunosuppressive practices for lung transplantation have generally paralleled those for heart transplantation. Less than half receive induction therapy (interleukin-2 receptor [CD25] antibodies > antithrombocyte globulin). Maintenance therapy usually consists of a calcineurin inhibitor (tacrolimus > cyclosporine), an antiproliferative agent (mycophenolate mofetil > rapamycin), and prednisone.

22. **What is the incidence of acute rejection? How is lung transplant rejection diagnosed?**

    Almost 50% of recipients are treated for acute rejection during the first year after transplant. Unlike heart transplants, the diagnosis of rejection in transplanted lungs is imprecise and can be difficult to distinguish from infection. Transbronchial biopsy remains the gold standard, but often requires three or several more "good" biopsies. Bronchoscopy with bronchoalveolar lavage and clinical assessment are also necessary for diagnosis.

23. **What additional tests can help distinguish between acute rejection and infection?**

    Polymerase chain reaction (PCR) assays for CMV, *Aspergillus* and *Pneumocystis jirovecii* pneumonia and multiplex PCR for multiple community-acquired and opportunistic infective agents, can supplement standard transbronchial biopsy staining, and may facilitate discrimination of occult infection from acute rejection.

24. **Describe the phenomenon of chimerism in transplantation.**
Transplant mixed chimerism is a condition in which cells from the recipient engraft into the donor transplant so that the allograft becomes a genetic composite of both the donor and recipient. Chimerism enhances the host's tolerance of the graft because the recipient does not recognize the donor organ as foreign.

25. **Does chimerism develop in the heart and the lungs?**
Yes. The first evidence of heart transplant chimerism was observed in 2002 by Quaini and colleagues in male patients who received hearts from female donors. In 2003, Kleeberger and colleagues also demonstrated evidence of lung transplant chimerism in lung epithelium, type II pneumocytes, and seromucous glands.

26. **Why is chimerism exciting?**
Nature is trying to teach us how to perform transplantation without the use of immunosuppression. Our job is to learn why chimerism is induced in some recipients and not in others. That is, we should dissect the mechanisms of chimerism induction so that we may therapeutically induce chimerism in all recipients.

27. **What are the major types of preservation solutions for heart and lung grafts?**
For nearly two decades, Euro-Collins (EC) solution or University of Wisconsin (UW) were considered the gold standard for lung transplant. Perfadex is increasingly accepted for lung transplant and improves posttransplant lung function and decreases PGD in comparison to other solutions.
The gold standard for heart transplant is crystalloid cardioplegia (arrest) and UW solution (preservation). Celsior is a novel combination arrest and preservation solution for heart transplants that requires further study.

28. **What are the main differences in composition between Euro-Collins and University of Wisconsin solutions and Perfadex and Celsior?**
EC and **UW** are high potassium intracellular preservation solutions originally developed for kidney transplant. In lung transplant, they cause severe vasoconstriction. **Perfadex** is a low potassium extracellular dextran plus glucose solution that demonstrates less vasoconstriction and decreased interstitial edema formation. **Celsior** is also extracellular.

29. **What percentage of pulmonary blood flow goes to the transplanted lung after single lung transplant?**
Predictably, almost all of the pulmonary blood flow passes through the lower resistance circuit of the transplanted lung (depending on the pulmonary vascular resistance of the contralateral native; i.e., sick lung). If a preoperative perfusion scan exists, other factors being equal, the lung with the best perfusion is preserved and the bad lung is replaced.

KEY POINTS: LUNG TRANSPLANTATION

1. The most common indication for single lung transplant is emphysema.

2. The most common indication for double lung transplant is CF.

3. Chimerism is a condition in which cells from the recipient engraft into the donor transplant so that the allograft becomes a genetic composite of both donor and recipient.

4. Bronchiolitis obliterans, a major cause of long-term morbidity after lung transplantation, is a chronic irreversible scarring process that results in progressive obliteration of the small airways of the lung allograft and resultant obstructive lung disease.

30. **Is cardiopulmonary bypass required for lung transplantation?**
No. However, for patients with pulmonary hypertension (primary or secondary), CPB is routinely used before removal of the recipient's lung. CPB is always on standby. This is tricky anesthesia. One lung is transiently excised from a patient who is living (barely) on two bad lungs.

31. **Is living-related lung transplant possible?**
Yes. Living-related lung transplants are an innovative approach to increasing the donor pool. Typically, one lobe from each of two to three donors are used to replace a whole lung in the recipient.

32. **How can stem cells improve pulmonary function before and after lung transplantation?**
Recent studies show that stem cells have acute paracrine effects that result in repair and protection of injured tissue. Specifically, stem cells transplanted to the lung produce antiinflammatory factors, such as IL-10 and TGF-β. These antiinflammatory factors and other angiogenic and antiapoptotic factors may improve pulmonary function after acute lung injury and transplantation.

33. **What is lung volume reduction surgery? How may it be important to patients on the lung transplant waiting list?**
Lung volume reduction surgery offers a therapeutic option for patients who are either not candidates to receive a lung transplant or on a long waiting list. Lung volume reduction surgery removes nonfunctional or destroyed lung. Removal of defunctionalized lung makes more room for airflow in the functional lung, resulting in decreased mortality and increased function.

34. **Who is the best candidate for lung volume reduction surgery?**
The National Emphysema Treatment Trial (NETT) suggests that the best candidates (lowest mortality) are patients with an obvious upper lobe apical target, marked thoracic distention, forced expiratory volume (FEV$_1$) >20%, diffusing capacity of the lung for carbon monoxide (DLCO) >20%, and age <70.

35. **What are the contraindications to lung reduction surgery?**
Pulmonary hypertension (mean pulmonary artery pressure [PAP] >35 mm Hg or systolic PAP >45 mm Hg).
Clinically significant heart disease.
Previous thoracotomy or pleurodesis (visceral and parietal pleural fusion).
Diffuse disease without target.
FEV <20%.
Hypercarbia, partial pressure of carbon dioxide (pCO$_2$) >55.

36. **What are the 1-year, 3-year, and 5-year actuarial survival rates for single lung retransplants?**
Actuarial survival rates are 60%, 50%, and 45%, respectively. Predictably, such patients do significantly worse. These poor results and the donor shortage make retransplantation of the lung an ethical dilemma.

37. **Is a simultaneous lung and pancreas transplant possible?**
Yes. In 2006, the first simultaneous double lung and pancreas transplant was performed in a patient with CF at Methodist Hospital, Indiana.

WEBSITE

www.transplantation-soc.org

BIBLIOGRAPHY

1. Boku N, Tanoue Y, Kajihara N et al.: A comparative study of cardiac preservation with Celsior or University of Wisconsin solution with or without prior administration of cardioplegia. J Heart Lung Transplant 25:219-225, 2006.

2. Crisostomo PR, Markel TA, Wang M et al.: In the adult mesenchymal stem cell population, source gender is a biologically relevant aspect of protective power. Surgery 142(2):215-221, 2007.

3. Crisostomo PR, Meldrum DR: Stem cell delivery to the heart: clarifying methodology and mechanism. Crit Care Med 35(11):2654-2655, 2007.

4. Fishman A, Martinez F, Naunheim K et al.: A randomized trial comparing lung-volume-reduction surgery with medical therapy for severe emphysema. N Engl J Med 348:2059-2073, 2003.

5. Kawut SM, Lederer DJ, Keshavjee S et al.: Outcomes after lung retransplantation in the modern era. Am J Respir Crit Care Med 177:114-120, 2008.

6. Kleeberger W, Versmold A, Rothamel T et al.: Increased chimerism of bronchial and alveolar epithelium in human lung allografts undergoing chronic injury. Am J Pathol 162:1487-1494, 2003.

7. Oto T, Griffiths AP, Rosenfeldt F et al.: Early outcomes comparing Perfadex, Euro-Collins, and Papworth solutions in lung transplantation. Ann Thorac Surg 82:1842-1848, 2006.

8. Quaini F, Urbanek K, Beltrami AP et al.: Chimerism of the transplanted heart. N Engl J Med 346:5-15, 2002.

9. Snell GI, Boehler A, Glanville AR et al.: Eleven years on: a clinical update of key areas of the 1996 lung allograft rejection working formulation. J Heart Lung Transplant 26:423-430, 2007.

10. Trulock EP, Christie JD, Edwards LB et al.: Registry of the International Society for Heart and Lung Transplantation: twenty-fourth official adult lung and heart-lung transplantation report—2007. J Heart Lung Transplant 26:782-795, 2007.

11. Wilkes DS, Egan TM, Reynolds HY: Lung transplantation: opportunities for research and clinical advancement. Am J Respir Crit Care Med 172:944-955, 2005.

THE SURGICAL APPROACH TO INFERTILITY

Randall B. Meacham, MD, and Alex J. Vanni, MD

CHAPTER 94

1. **How common a problem is infertility?**

   Infertility is the inability to establish a pregnancy during 1 year of well-timed intercourse. This affects 15% of all couples in the United States. In 50% of such couples, the woman is responsible; in 30% of couples, a male factor prevents pregnancy; and in 20% of couples, it is a combination of both.

2. **What are the odds that a fertile couple will become pregnant after a single episode of well-timed intercourse?**

   During a given ovulatory cycle, 18% of fertile couples become pregnant after well-timed intercourse.

3. **What is the best timing for intercourse if a couple is trying to conceive?**

   Sperm can survive in the cervical mucus for 48 hours. To achieve pregnancy, therefore, the most effective timing of intercourse is every other day, starting a few days before ovulation.

4. **What environmental factors may play a role in male infertility?**

   Although reproductive function is relatively durable, various toxins have a negative impact on male fertility. Cigarette smoke and alcohol have been implicated as dose-dependent gonadotoxins, as have recreational drugs, including marijuana, cocaine, and heroin. Radiation (in amounts as low as 200 rads) can influence spermatogenesis, as can chemotherapeutic agents. Calcium channel blockers may interfere with the ability of sperm to fertilize eggs.

5. **Can a vasectomy be successfully reversed?**

   Yes, but the success rate is affected by the amount of time since the original vasectomy. Among patients who are less than 3 years from vasectomy, the conception rate after reversal is roughly 75%. This success rate declines to about 50% when the reversal is performed 3 to 8 years after vasectomy and further declines to 30% when 15 or more years have passed.

6. **What is in vitro fertilization (IVF)?**

   With IVF, eggs are harvested from a woman and combined with sperm in a laboratory setting. The resulting embryos are then transferred to the uterine cavity, where they mature into a fetus. In a specialized version of this technology (i.e., intracytoplasmic sperm injection), an individual sperm is injected into each egg, thus facilitating fertilization and allowing pregnancy even in the presence of small numbers of motile sperm.

7. **What is the role of IVF in male infertility?**

   Because use of IVF greatly reduces the number of motile sperm needed to generate a pregnancy, it can be quite helpful in men with poor semen quality. The IVF team needs only as many motile sperm as there are oocytes (eggs) to be fertilized.

8. **Can sperm obtained directly from the testicle be used to generate a pregnancy?**
For the past several years, it has been recognized that incubation of testicular tissue generally yields small numbers of motile sperm. Through the use of IVF, such sperm can generate pregnancies. Even among men suffering from severe testicular failure, it may be possible to retrieve adequate sperm for use in IVF.

9. **What is the role of sperm freezing in the treatment of infertility?**
Sperm can be frozen (cryopreserved) with relative ease. After they are cryopreserved, sperm remain viable for extended periods (years). Cryopreservation can be helpful among men planning to undergo treatment with chemotherapy or radiation therapy.

10. **Does wearing boxer shorts versus tight underwear affect male fertility?**
No.

KEY POINTS: SURGICAL APPROACH TO INFERTILITY

1. Infertility is defined as the inability to establish pregnancy during 1 year of well-timed intercourse.

2. In 50% of infertile couples a female factor prevents pregnancy, in 30% of couples a male factor prevents pregnancy, and in 20% of couples infertility is the result of a combination of both female and male factors.

3. The most common cause of male infertility is varicocele.

11. **Because normal levels of testosterone are necessary for sperm production, is it helpful to give subfertile men additional testosterone?**
Although decreased levels of testosterone can cause impaired male fertility, giving additional testosterone to men with normal testosterone levels can actually cause a dramatic decline in semen quality. Administration of exogenous testosterone causes the patient to cease production of native testosterone within the testes. The resultant decrease in intratesticular testosterone actually results in a decline in sperm production.

12. **What is the most common cause of male infertility?**
Varicocele, a collection of dilated veins above one or both testes. Among men presenting for treatment of infertility, 40% have a varicocele. Correction of varicocele leads to improvement in semen quality in 70% of patients.

13. **If we can clone Dolly (a sheep derived from cloning a fully differentiated mammary cell), can we clone humans?**
Although for a number of critical ethical reasons cloning technology is not currently used in human reproduction, it theoretically allows the cloning of any individual, creating a genetic duplicate. However, cloning probably will not play a role in the treatment of human infertility.

14. **Is in vitro fertilization associated with an increase in genetic abnormalities?**
This issue is controversial, but probably no. At least one recent publication suggested that infants conceived by either intracytoplasmic sperm injection or IVF have twice the risk of major birth defects compared with naturally conceived infants.

15. Will giving supplemental testosterone improve male fertility?

No. Exogenous testosterone induces a profound decrease in spermatogenesis and has been explored as a means of male contraception.

16. What is cloning as it pertains to humans?

Just like Dolly the sheep, human cloning involves nuclear transplantation of the desired clone into an egg devoid of its nucleus. Rather than creating whole human beings, the more controversial ethical dilemma is whether to permit cloning of cells or organs for subsequent transplantation in order to cure human disease.

17. Are undescended testes associated with male infertility?

Yes. Cryptorchidism is associated with male infertility. The decreased fertility correlates with severely reduced total germ cell counts in prepubertal undescended testes. Bilateral testicular maldescent does decrease semen quality. Interestingly, unilateral cryptorchidism may impair semen quality as well. This suggests that both the abnormally descended testis and its normally positioned counterpart are adversely affected. Surgical repositioning of the testis improves semen quality; the earlier it is done, the better.

WEBSITE

www.auanet.org

BIBLIOGRAPHY

1. Cortes D, Thorp JM, Visfeldt J: Cryptorchidism: aspects of fertility and neoplasms. A study of 1,335 consecutive boys who underwent testicular biopsy simultaneously with surgery for cryptorchidism. Horm Res 55:21-27, 2001.

2. Hansen M, Kurinczuk JJ, Bower C et al.: The risk of major birth defects after intracytoplasmic sperm injection and in vitro fertilization. N Engl J Med 346:725-730, 2002.

3. Hargreave T, Ghosh C: Male fertility disorders. Endocrinol Metab Clin North Am 27:765-782, 1998.

4. Ismail MT, Sedor J, Hirsch IH: Are sperm motion parameters influenced by varicocele ligation? Fertil Steril 71:886-890, 1999.

5. Johnson MD: Genetic risks of intracytoplasmic sperm injection in the treatment of male infertility: recommendations for genetic counseling and screening. Fertil Steril 70:397-411, 1998.

6. Kim ED, Winkel E, Orejuela F et al.: Pathological epididymal obstruction unrelated to vasectomy: results with microsurgical reconstruction. J Urol 160(6 pt 1):2078-2080, 1998.

7. Meriggiola MC, Costantino A, Cerpolini S: Recent advances in hormonal male contraception. Contraception 64:269-272, 2002.

8. Naysmith TE, Blake DA, Harvey VJ et al.: Do men undergoing sterilizing cancer treatments have a fertile future? Hum Reprod 13:3250-3255, 1998.

9. Palermo GD, Schlegel PN, Hariprashad JJ et al.: Fertilization and pregnancy outcome with intracytoplasmic sperm injection for azoospermic men. Hum Reprod 14:741-748, 1999.

10. Pellegrino ED, Kilner JF, Fitzgerald KT et al.: Therapeutic cloning. N Engl J Med 347:1619-1622, 2002.

11. Rutkowski SB, Geraghty TJ, Hagen DL et al.: A comprehensive approach to the management of male infertility following spinal cord injury. Spinal Cord 37:508-514, 1999.

12. Scherr D, Goldstein M: Comparison of bilateral versus unilateral varicocelectomy in men with palpable bilateral varicoceles. J Urol 162:85-88, 1999.

13. Wilmut I: Cloning for medicine. Sci Am 279:58-63, 1998.

CHAPTER 95

URINARY CALCULUS DISEASE

Brett B. Abernathy, MD

"I will not cut persons laboring under the stone, but will leave this to be done by men who are practitioners of this work." (Hippocratic Oath)

Hippocrates and the ancient Greeks recognized that cutting for stone was dangerous business. Fortunately, in the era of modern urology, and with the technology that is now available, it is rare to need to actually cut for stone.

1. **How common are stones of the urinary tract?**
   1. In the United States, the prevalence of stone disease has been estimated at 10% to 15%.
   2. One of eight white men will likely experience stone disease by age 70. Although men are more frequently affected than women, the difference appears to be lessening.
   3. Urinary tract stone disease accounts for approximately 600,000 emergency department (ED) visits and more than 177,000 hospitalizations in the United States annually. This represents an enormous financial burden with an expenditure in excess of $2 billion per year.

2. **How are stones in the urinary tract diagnosed?**
   1. Symptomatic stones are commonly associated with pain in the flank area that is colicky. The pain can radiate to the ipsilateral groin.
   2. Patients are usually quite agitated and have difficulty getting in a comfortable position.
   3. Most often (85%) there is microscopic or gross hematuria.
   4. Nausea and vomiting commonly accompany ureteral colic as a result of pressure on the renal capsule.
   5. Asymptomatic, or nonobstructing stones, are commonly diagnosed on computed tomography (CT) scans done for other conditions.

3. **What are the best studies to diagnose stones?**
   1. **Rapid sequence helical CT scan** has become the most common study for diagnosis of stone disease. The advantages of this study include no need for contrast, rapidly performed, and ability to diagnose all common stones of the urinary tract including uric acid and cystine stones that can be radiolucent on standard imaging.
   2. **Intravenous pyelogram (IVP)** and **CT urogram** can also be used and provide additional information about renal function and degree of obstruction. However, these studies do require intravenous (IV) contrast.
   3. **Ultrasonography** can be particularly helpful in pregnant women. However, stones in the mid to distal ureter can be quite difficult to identify with ultrasound (US).

4. **What are the indications for admitting the patient to the hospital with stone disease?**
   1. Any sign of infection (fever, leukocytosis, or bactiuria). Infection behind an obstructing stone may result in urosepsis and death.
   2. Severe pain requiring parenteral analgesics.

3. Intractable vomiting requiring IV fluids.
4. Obstruction in a solitary kidney or bilateral obstructing stones.
5. The degree of hydronephrosis identified on radiologic imaging is not necessarily an indication for admission.

5. What are the common types of urinary tract stones found in the United States?

1. Calcium stones (calcium oxalate, calcium phosphate, or mixed calcium stones): 80%.
2. Struvite or magnesium ammonium phosphate stones, commonly associated with infection: 7%.
3. Uric acid stones: 7%.
4. Cystine stones:1% to 3%.

6. What are the treatment options for renal stones?

1. Expectant management in small, asymptomatic noninfectious stones. Treatment would be indicated for increase in stone burden, or symptoms.
2. Shockwave lithotripsy (SWL) is the least invasive treatment option and is quite successful especially in stones less than 2 cm in size.
3. Ureterorendoscopy with holmium laser lithotripsy is also now an option as a result of the improvement in flexible deflectable ureteroscopes.
4. Percutaneous nephrostolithotomy is especially useful in larger stone burden >2 cm.
5. Combination therapy with percutaneous nephrostolithotomy and SWL. This combination is commonly used with complex stones and large stone burden.
6. One can still cut for stone using laparoscopic or open lithotomy technique. Results are far better than in the days of Hippocrates!

7. What are the treatment options for ureteral stones?

1. Expectant management. Recent meta-analysis studies demonstrate stones <5 mm have a 68% chance of spontaneous passage. Stones between 5 mm and 10 mm have a 47% rate of spontaneous passage. Stones greater than 10-mm are unlikely to pass spontaneously. If the stone is going to pass it is likely to occur within 4 to 6 weeks of diagnosis.
2. Medical expulsive therapy (MET). Treatment with oral α-blocker therapy has been shown to significantly increase the rate of stone passage by 29%. The most commonly studied α-blocker for MET is tamsulosin. The mechanism behind this effect is probably relaxation of ureteral smooth muscle.
3. Ureteroscopy (URS) with laser lithotripsy or stone basket extraction. This technique can be used for stones in the distal, mid, and proximal ureter. If intervention is necessary, URS demonstrates the highest stone free rate for distal and mid ureteral stones. As a result of the advancement in technology of the flexible deflectable ureteroscopes URS now has a similar success rate to SWL in the proximal ureter as well.
4. SWL. SWL can be used for treatment of stones in any portion of the ureter. Localization can be problematic in the mid ureter because of the difficulty identifying stones over the bony pelvis. Although less invasive than URS, success rates in the distal ureter for SWL are not as high as URS. SWL is quite successful (83% stone free) for stones <10 mm in the proximal ureter.
5. Percutaneous antegrade URS can be indicated in selected cases of large stones impacted in the proximal ureter, or when combined with percutaneous nephrostolithotomy and in patients with urinary diversions.
6. Laparoscopic and open stone surgery are rarely indicated, but still useful in selected cases.

8. **What is a stent, and when are they used?**

A stent is a small plastic tube that coils in the renal pelvis, traverses the ureter, and coils in the bladder. They are useful to relieve ureteral obstruction temporarily, and can facilitate stone passage once the stent is removed. Stents often result in some degree of temporary ureteral dilatation. Routine stenting is not recommended as part of SWL in the ureter. Stenting is optional following uncomplicated URS. Stents are also indicated in the treatment of large stone burden, solitary kidneys, and bilateral treatment.

9. **What are the potential complications of treatment for stone disease?**

1. Sepsis. Bactiuria and signs of clinical infection should be treated and cleared if at all possible before definitive treatment of stone disease. Urosepsis should be treated with immediate percutaneous nephrostomy drainage or stenting combined with appropriate antibiotic therapy. Definitive management of the stone can await clearing of the infection.
2. Perinephric hematoma or renal damage following SWL.
3. Disruption of the ureter or ureteral stricture following URS or open surgery.
4. Failure to access or identify the stone or incomplete fragmentation of the stone requiring additional treatment.
5. Steinstrasse (German for stone street) is a pileup of small stone fragments in the ureter resulting in obstruction after lithotripsy.

10. **What is medical management of stone disease?**

Medical management of stone disease involves identifying the type of stone by stone analysis. Serum studies and 24-hour urine collections are then performed to identify the specific causative factors for a patient's stone formation. Based on the specific findings, management can then consist of increase in hydration, dietary changes, and specific drug therapy to try to prevent further stone formation. All stones formers benefit from excellent hydration to provide a urine output of at least 2.0 to 2.5 L daily. Most will also benefit from oral citrate therapy because citrate is an inhibitor of stone formation. Medical management can reduce the risk of recurrent stone disease, and potentially reduce patient morbidity and cost of stone treatment. Identification of primary hyperparathyroidism can also be definitively treated with parathyroidectomy.

11. **Can stones be dissolved?**

1. Uric acid stones can often be dissolved using a combination of alkalinization and hydration.
2. Calcium-based stones cannot be dissolved by medical therapy.

12. **Does a diet high in calcium increase risk of stone disease?**

This is a controversial issue. An adequate dietary intake of calcium is necessary to protect against osteoporosis. In addition, calcium helps to bind oxalate in the intestine that can actually reduce the risk of oxalate absorption and formation of oxalate containing stones. However, there are conditions in which increased absorption of calcium is a contributing factor to calcium stone formation. Currently, the best approach is probably recommending a normal calcium intake or a modest restriction of calcium in the diet and avoiding foods high in oxalate to reduce the risk of calcium oxalate stone formation.

BONUS QUESTION

13. **Who were the "Lithotomists"?**

As noted, removal of stones from the bladder and perineum was banned by Hippocrates. This was probably as a result of poor outcomes. Until the sixteenth century, lithotomy was regarded with disfavor and was usually carried out by itinerant surgeons who specialized in this technique. They were referred to as "Lithotomists." Eventually they developed some unique and fairly barbaric techniques for removing lower urinary tract stones. In one famous case in 1651, a courageous blacksmith named Jan de Doot removed his own stone from the perineum using a kitchen knife. Somehow, cystoscopy under anesthesia with laser lithotripsy seems like progress.

BIBLIOGRAPHY

1. Kraft K, Pattaras JG: Medical management of urolithiasis. AUA Update Series Vol. 27 Lesson 36, 2007.

2. Murphy LJT: *The history of urology*, Springfield, 1972, Charles C. Thomas.

3. Pearle MS, Lotan Y: Urinary litihiasis: etiology, epidemiology, and pathogenesis. In Wein AJ, Kavoussi LR, Novick AC et al., editors: *Campbell-Walsh urology*, 9th ed., Philadelphia, 2007, Saunders Elsevier.

4. Preminger GM, Tiselius H, Assimos DG et al.: 2007 Guideline for the management of ureteral calculi. J Urol 178:2418–2434, 2007.

CHAPTER 96

RENAL CELL CARCINOMA

Fernando J. Kim, MD, FACS, and Mario F. Chammas, Jr., MD

1. **How common is renal cell carcinoma (RCC)?**
   In the United States, approximately 30,000 new cases of renal cell carcinoma are diagnosed each year, about 3% of all adult malignancies.

2. **What is the etiology of RCC?**
   The etiology is unknown, but cigarette smoking is a well-known risk factor. Recurrent RCC is a common manifestation in patients with Von Hippel-Lindau disease.

3. **What are the signs and symptoms of RCC?**
   The most common presenting signs and symptoms are gross or microscopic hematuria. The classic triad of hematuria, flank pain, and an abdominal mass is found in only about 10% to15% of RCC cases. Patients with metastatic disease may present with symptoms of lung or bone metastasis, such as dyspnea, cough, or bone pain.
   About 20% of RCCs are associated with a paraneoplastic syndrome. Many solid renal tumors are detected incidentally by a computed tomography (CT) scan of the abdomen performed for another reason.
   Stauffer's syndrome is diagnosed with elevated liver function tests (LFTs) in the presence of RCC that normalize after nephrectomy and tumor removal; it is thought to be a type of paraneoplastic syndrome.

4. **Are all solid masses in the kidney renal cell carcinoma?**
   No. Other solid masses include angiomyolipomas, oncocytomas, sarcomas, and metastatic lesions. However, all solid masses should be presumed to be RCC until proven otherwise.

5. **What is the unique relationship between renal cell carcinoma and its vasculature?**
   RCC has a tendency to invade its own venous drainage. Tumor thrombus may extend along the renal vein into the inferior vena cava (IVC) and even to the right atrium.

6. **How should suspected involvement of the vena cava be evaluated?**
   Magnetic resonance imaging (MRI) or venacavography.

7. **How is renal cell carcinoma treated?**
   Surgery is the optimal treatment for localized RCC. The standard operation is a radical nephrectomy, including everything within Gerota's fascia. Radical nephrectomy can also be performed laparoscopically or with hand-assisted laparoscopic techniques.

8. **When is nephron-sparing nephrectomy indicated in cases of renal cell carcinoma?**
   Tumors <4 cm in size may be treated with laparoscopic or open Nephron-sparing surgery. Ablative technology (i.e.; cryoablation and radiofrequency ablation) are still under investigation with encouraging results.

9. **How is metastatic renal cell carcinoma treated?**

Chemotherapy has been disappointing. Historically, encouraging results were achieved with cytoreductive radical nephrectomy and interleukin-2 (IL-2) treatment. Currently, targeted therapy with tyrosine kinase inhibitors offers some evidence of definite durable responses. Research is ongoing using different targeted therapy strategies.

KEY POINTS: RENAL CELL CARCINOMA

1. The classic triad is hematuria, flank pain, and an abdominal mass is usually found in advanced cases of RCC.

2. Surgery is the optimal treatment for localized RCC.

3. Stauffer's syndrome is diagnosed with elevated liver function tests (LFTs) in the presence of RCC that normalize after nephrectomy and tumor removal; it is thought to be a type of paraneoplastic syndrome.

WEBSITE

www.transplantjournal.com

BIBLIOGRAPHY

1. Kim FJ, Rha KH, Hernandez F et al.: Laparoscopic radical versus partial nephrectomy: assessment of complications. J Urol 170:408, 2003.

2. Greenlee RT, Hill-Harmon MB, Murray T et al.: Cancer statistics 2001. CA Cancer J Clin 51:15, 2001.

3. Figlin RA: Renal cell carcinoma: management of advanced disease. J Urol 161:391, 1999.

CHAPTER 97

BLADDER CANCER

Fernando J. Kim, MD, FACS, and Mario F. Chammas, Jr., MD

1. **What is the incidence of transitional cell carcinoma (TCC) of the bladder?**
   More than 60,000 new cases of bladder cancer are diagnosed each year in the United States, accounting for approximately 13,000 deaths annually. Recently, the overall incidence of bladder cancer has appeared to be rising maybe as a result of the overall aging of our population and latent effects of tobacco abuse and industrial carcinogens.

2. **What are the risk factors associated with bladder TCC?**
   Age (peak incidence in seventh decade), cigarette smoking, occupational exposure to aniline dyes or aromatic amines, phenacetin abuse, and chemotherapy with cyclophosphamide.

3. **What are the signs and symptoms of bladder TCC?**
   Painless hematuria (gross or microscopic) is the most common finding and is present in up to 90% of patients. Frequency, urgency, and dysuria also may be presenting symptoms, especially for carcinoma in situ (CIS).

4. **What is the most common histologic type of bladder cancer?**
   TCC makes up >90% of bladder cancers. Other histologic types include adenocarcinoma, squamous cell carcinoma, and urachal carcinoma.

5. **How do you evaluate a patient with hematuria and bladder mass?**
   Urine analysis, culture and bladder washings for cytology; bimanual examination (usually performed under anesthesia); upper tract imaging study (rule out concomitant upper tract disease); either cystoscopy with biopsy (if small or atypical lesion) or transurethral resection of bladder tumor (TURBT) of suspicious lesions.

6. **How do you manage bladder TCC?**
   The bladder tumor should be removed with endoscopic transurethral resection and fulguration. Further treatment is determined by the pathologic stage of the disease.

7. **What is the recurrence rate of TCC after initial transurethral resection of bladder tumor?**
   Approximately 45% of patients will have tumor recurrence within 12 months of TURBT alone.

8. **How often do you expect to see a high grade muscle invasive bladder TCC?**
   The vast majority (70% to 75%) of bladder TCC present as superficial (nonmuscle invasive) lesions. Furthermore, the greater part of lesions are categorized as low grade with only 2% to 4% categorized as high grade.

9. **How often should superficial lesions be followed with surveillance cystoscopy and urine cytology?**
   Every 3 months in the first 3 years after initial diagnosis followed by every 6 months for the subsequent 2 to 3 years, and then annually thereafter. Surveillance includes periodic upper tract imaging, especially for high-risk patients.

10. **Is there a chance of concurrent urothelial cancers?**
About 5% of patients with bladder cancer will have urothelial carcinoma outside the bladder (i.e., renal pelvis, ureter, or urethra).

11. **Is CIS a less aggressive type of bladder cancer?**
No. TCC in situ is a flat but poorly differentiated tumor. It can metastasize and should be treated as an aggressive form of bladder cancer.

12. **How do you manage bladder carcinoma in situ?**
Immunotherapy with intravesical bacillus Calmette-Guérin (BCG) is the first-line treatment. Response rates to BCG approach 70%. Other intravesical agents, such as mitomycin C, are generally less effective than BCG.

13. **What are the other indications of intravesical BCG?**
The presence of multifocal or large volume low grade superficial tumors; high grade superficial tumors; or in recurrent superficial tumors.

14. **What are the side effects of BCG?**
Mild symptoms of urinary frequency, urgency, and dysuria are common. Myalgias and low-grade fever (flulike symptoms) also occur. High or persistent fever suggests a more serious problem requiring antituberculous therapy. Rarely, death from BCG has been reported.

15. **When can we start the intravesical BCG treatment?**
Initiation of intravesical BCG therapy is usually delayed for 2 to 3 weeks following TURBT.

16. **What is the most important pathological finding when choosing the treatment?**
The presence of muscle invasion. Nonmuscle invasive cancers can be treated with surveillance and repeated TURBT. The presence of muscle invasive cancer mandates a more aggressive approach (i.e., radical cystectomy [or cystoprostatectomy in men] with some form of urinary diversion).

17. **What types of urinary diversion are used with radical cystectomy?**
Diversion techniques require either a conduit or a continent reservoir. The most common is an ileal conduit. The stoma collection device must be worn with a conduit. Continent reservoirs can be made with either small bowel or with large intestine and must be emptied via the urethra or a continent stoma.

18. **How is metastatic bladder cancer treated?**
Metastatic bladder cancer requires chemotherapy. Most regimens include a platinum-based agent.

19. **In certain countries, TCC is not the predominant form of bladder cancer. What is the predominant histologic type? Why?**
In countries such as Egypt, where schistosomiasis is endemic, squamous cell carcinoma of the bladder is common.

20. **Are there any molecular markers that can be used to help predict the prognosis of bladder TCC?**
The p53 tumor suppressor protein may be helpful in assessing the biologic behavior of the tumor and can assist with treatment option decisions. Monoclonal antibody MIB-1 may also be useful in predicting outcome for stage T2 or grade 2 tumors.

KEY POINTS: BLADDER CANCER

1. Bladder cancer presents as painless hematuria.
2. The most common histologic type of bladder cancer is transitional cell carcinoma.
3. CIS of the bladder is treated with intravesical BCG.

WEBSITE

www.auanet.org/guidelines/bladcan07.cfm

BIBLIOGRAPHY

1. Greenlee RT, Hill-Harmon MB, Murray T et al.: Cancer statistics 2001. CA Cancer J Clin 51:15, 2001.
2. Herr HW, Bajorn DF, Scher HL: Can p53 help select patients with invasive bladder cancer for bladder preservation? J Urol 161:20, 1999.
3. Hendricksen K, Witjes JA: Current strategies for first and second line intravesical therapy for nonmuscle invasive bladder cancer. Curr Opin Urol 17:352, 2007.
4. Soloway MS, Lee CT, Steinberg GD et al.: Difficult decisions in urologic oncology: management of high-grade T1 transitional cell carcinoma of the bladder. Urol Oncol 25:338, 2007.
5. Hall MC, Chang SS, Dalbagni G et al.: Guideline for the management of nonmuscle invasive bladder cancer (stages Ta, T1, and Tis): 2007 update. J Urol 178:2314, 2007.

CHAPTER 98

PROSTATE CANCER

Fernando J. Kim, MD, FACS, and Mario F. Chammas, Jr., MD

1. **What is the prevalence of prostate cancer in the United States?**
   It is the most common malignancy diagnosed in men in the United States; approximately 200,000 new cases are diagnosed every year.

2. **Do most men die with prostate cancer, rather than from it?**
   Yes, but more than 31,500 men will die of prostate cancer annually in the United States. Thus, it should not be treated as a benign disease.

3. **What are the early symptoms of prostate cancer?**
   There are none. By the time significant symptoms develop, the disease is likely to be advanced. This is an argument for screening to detect prostate cancer.

4. **What is the best screening method for prostate cancer?**
   Digital rectal examination (DRE) combined with serum prostate-specific antigen (PSA). Since PSA testing was introduced, there has been a stage migration with less metastatic disease and more local-regional disease being detected.

5. **How is prostate cancer diagnosed?**
   It is diagnosed with prostate biopsy, which is a biopsy using transrectal ultrasound (US) for guidance or incidentally after transurethral resection of the prostate (TURP) for benign prostatic hyperplasia (BPH) is performed.

6. **When is prostate biopsy indicated?**
   When either the PSA or DRE result is abnormal.

7. **Does an elevated PSA level mean a man has prostate cancer?**
   No. PSA can be elevated with BPH, prostatitis, or after prostate trauma. It is prostate specific, not prostate cancer specific.

8. **What is a free PSA?**
   Free PSA is the percentage of PSA that is not bound to a serum protein carrier. The ratio of free to total PSA is helpful in determining when to do a prostate biopsy. "Free" is good because a higher ratio of free to total PSA is less likely to represent prostate cancer.

9. **Are there any known risk factors for prostate cancer?**
   Yes. African American men and men with a family history of prostate cancer are at an increased risk. A high-fat diet may play a role in increasing risk of many cancers, including prostate cancer.

10. **What is Gleason's sum?**
    It is a score that the pathologist gives prostate cancer to estimate its aggressiveness. The two predominant patterns of cancer are scored 1 to 5, and the sum is, therefore, between 2 and 10. Tumors can be well differentiated (2, 3, 4), moderately differentiated (5, 6, 7), or poorly differentiated (8, 9, 10).

11. **How is clinically localized prostate cancer treated?**
    Surgery (radical prostatectomy), radiation therapy by external beam or interstitial seed implant, cryotherapy, high intensity focused ultrasound (HIFU), or watchful waiting.

12. **How is advanced metastatic prostate cancer treated?**
    Hormonal ablation therapy (orchiectomy or luteinizing hormone-releasing hormone agonist drugs) or chemotherapy, but these treatments are palliative and not curative.

13. **What is the best treatment for prostate cancer?**
    This is highly controversial. Patients must weigh factors such as age, overall health, grade and stage of the disease, and risk of side effects versus complications from the various treatment options.

KEY POINTS: PROSTATE CANCER

1. Prostate cancer is the most common malignancy diagnosed in men in the United States.

2. The best screening method is a combination of DRE and serum PSA.

3. Clinically localized prostate cancer is treated with surgery, radiation, cryotherapy, or watchful waiting.

WEBSITES

www.prostatecancerfoundation.org/

www.cancer.gov/cancertopics/types/prostate

BIBLIOGRAPHY

1. Catalona WJ: Clinical utility of free and total prostate specific antigen. Rev Prostate 7(suppl):64, 1996.

2. D'Amico AV, Whittington R, Malkowicz SB et al.: Biochemical outcome after radical prostatectomy, external beam radiation therapy, or interstitial radiation therapy for clinically localized prostate cancer. JAMA 280:969, 1998.

3. Denberg TD, Kim FJ, Flanigan RC et al.: The influence of patient race and social vulnerability on urologist treatment recommendations in localized prostate carcinoma. Med Care 44(12):1137, 2006.

4. Greenlee RT, Hill-Harmon MB, Murray T et al.: Cancer statistics 2001. CA Cancer J Clin 51:15, 2001.

5. Keetch DW, Humphrey PA, Smith DS et al.: Clinical and pathological features of hereditary prostate cancer. J Urol 155:1841, 1996.

6. Polascik TJ, Pound CR, DeWeese TL et al.: Comparison of radical prostatectomy and iodine-125 interstitial radiotherapy for the treatment of clinically localized prostate cancer: a 7-year biochemical (PSA) progression analysis. Urology 51:884, 1998.

URODYNAMICS AND VOIDING DYSFUNCTION

Mario F. Chammas, Jr., MD, and Fernando J. Kim, MD, FACS

CHAPTER 99

1. **What is urodynamics?**

   Urodynamic studies assess the functional aspects of the storage and emptying ability of the lower urinary tract (LUT). The principles of urodynamic studies originated from hydrodynamics. The components of urodynamic studies are cystometrogram, leak point pressures, urethral profile pressures, pressure-flow studies, uroflowmetry, and electromyography. These studies have evolved into videourodynamic with the addition of fluoroscopy (i.e., video).

2. **What is uroflowmetry?**

   Uroflowmetry is the measurement of voided urine (in milliliters) per unit of time (in seconds). The important elements of the test are voided volume (which should be >150 ml), maximum flow rate (Q_{max}), and the curve of the flow (which should be bell shaped). In men a Q_{max} is >15 ml/sec is considered normal, whereas a Q_{max} of less than 10 ml/sec is considered abnormal. Assigning normal values in females is more difficult. In women, uroflowmetry is characterized by the shorter urethra and no resistance, such as that caused by the prostate gland in the male. Normal values are described as a Q_{max} between 20 to 36 ml per second.

3. **What is benign prostatic hyperplasia (BPH)?**

   BPH is benign enlargement of the prostate gland that may lead to bladder outlet obstructive symptoms in men. These symptoms have been termed lower urinary tract symptoms (LUTS).

4. **What is an American Urological Association Symptom Score?**

   It is a self-reported questionnaire developed and popularized by the American Urological Association (AUA) for the assessment of bothersome LUTS in men. This questionnaire has seven questions with a maximum score of 35. The higher the score the more bothersome The AUA Symptom Score has become an index for both the diagnosis and evaluation of treatment outcome in patients with LUTS.

5. **What are the main functions of the LUT?**

   Storage and emptying of urine are the main functions. For practical purposes, all symptoms of LUT dysfunction can be categorized into the malfunction of either storing or emptying ability.

6. **What are the control mechanisms for LUT function?**

   The control mechanisms for LUT function are recognized as central and peripheral. The central control mechanism consists of the cortical portion of the frontal lobe of the brain and pontine micturition center. The peripheral control mechanism includes the thoracic sympathetic and lumbar parasympathetic innervations and neuromuscular apparatus of the LUT organs.

7. **What is the role of the autonomic nervous system in the function of the LUT?**

   Sympathetic fibers, which originate from the T10-L2 portion of the spinal cord, innervate the bladder neck and proximal urethra. These fibers mostly control the contraction of the proximal urethra or bladder neck and relaxation of the bladder, which results in storage of urine. The parasympathetic fibers, which originate primarily from the S2-S4 portion of the spinal cord, innervate the bladder body. The parasympathetic innervation allows contraction of the bladder smooth muscle, leading to bladder emptying.

8. **Is there a better way to memorize this function?**
   Yes. Parasympathetic: Piss; Sympathetic: Storage.

9. **What is the role of the somatic nervous system in the function of the LUT?**
   Voluntary control of the striated muscle of the external urinary sphincter is controlled by the somatic nervous system. Somatic fibers are conveyed to the sphincter by the pudendal nerve.

10. **What is the bulbocavernosal reflex?**
    Bulbocavernous reflex tests the integrity of the peripheral neurological control of the LUT. This reflex is elicited by stimulation of the glans penis in men or clitoris in women, which causes contraction of the external anal sphincter or bulbocarnosus muscle. Alternatively, the reflex may be stimulated by pulling the balloon of a Foley catheter against the bladder neck. This reflex is present in all normal men and in approximately 70% of normal woman. Absent of this reflex in men is strongly suggestive of a sacral neurological lesion.

11. **What is the most common cause of urinary incontinence in the geriatric population?**
    The most common are transient causes, mostly external, that disrupt the fragile balance of LUT function in elderly patients and cause urinary incontinence. These causes can be recalled with the mnemonic **DIAPPERS:**
    Delirium
    Infection
    Athrophic urethritis or vaginitis
    Pharmaceuticals
    Psychological (depression)
    Endocrine (hypercalcemia, hyperglycemia)
    Restricted mobility
    Stool impaction

12. **What is spinal shock? What type of urinary dysfunction does it cause?**
    Spinal shock is the loss of contractility of the smooth muscle below the level of spinal cord injury, leading to difficulty in bladder emptying or urinary retention. This phenomenon may last from hours to several months with a high chance of reversibility if the spinal cord injury is not permanent.

13. **What is autonomic dysreflexia? How is it treated?**
    Autonomic dysreflexia results from systematic outpouring of sympathetic discharge, as in patients with spinal cord lesions above T6 level. This dysreflexia is triggered by distention of the bladder or other stimulus of the bowel or LUT. It is manifested by hypertension, bradycardia, hot flush, sweating, and headache. Initial treatment consists of the removal of the stimulus, such as emptying the bladder and placing the patient in a sitting position. Antihypertensive drugs may be used as either prophylaxis or treatment of severe episodes. This condition may lead to significant cerebrovascular complication if untreated.

14. **What type of bladder dysfunction is frequently seen in patients with diabetes?**
    Patients with diabetes may develop diabetic cystopathy, which is a chronic complication of diabetes with a classic triad of symptoms: decreased bladder sensation, increased bladder capacity, and impaired detrusor contractility. Impaired detrusor contractility may lead to incomplete bladder emptying and subsequently result in voiding difficulty, urinary retention, chronic urinary tract infection (UTI), and upper urinary tract damage.

15. What type of bladder dysfunction is frequently seen in patients with multiple sclerosis (MS)?

Urgency (83%), urge incontinence (75%), detrusor hyperreflexia (62%), and detrussor sphincter dyssynergia (25%) are among the most common LUT symptoms in patients with MS. The worsening of bladder dysfunction correlates with the increasing spinal cord involvement and the neurological symptoms in MS. Variation in symptoms depends on the site of involvement by MS. Involvement of pontine pathways (tegmentum) is associated with a much higher rate of urinary symptoms.

16. Which sacral roots control the micturition physiology?

They are S2-S4.

17. What are the causes of urinary retention after abdominal or pelvic surgery?

They are injuries or disruption of pelvic plexus innervation of the LUT.

18. What is Ogilvie's syndrome?

Acute massive dilatation of the cecum and ascending and transverse colon with no evidence of distal colonic obstruction is known as Ogilvie's syndrome. This syndrome is usually associated with a recent, significant medical illness or surgical procedure. Other common associations are trauma, infection, and cardiac disease, possibly as a result of an imbalance in parasympathetic stimulation of the colon.

KEY POINTS: URODYNAMICS AND VOIDING FUNCTION

1. Uroflowmetry is the measurement of voided urine (in milliliters) per unit of time (in seconds).

2. BPH is benign enlargement of the prostate gland that may lead to bladder outlet obstructive symptoms in men.

3. The sacral roots involved in micturition physiology are S2-S4.

WEBSITE

www.icsoffice.org

BIBLIOGRAPHY

1. Cole EE, Dmochowski RR: Office urodynamics. Urol Clin North Am 32:353, 2005.

2. de Sèze M, Ruffion A, Denys P et al.: The neurogenic bladder in multiple sclerosis: review of the literature and proposal of management guidelines. Mult Scler 13:915, 2007.

3. Gibbs CF, Johnson TM 2nd, Ouslander JG: Office management of geriatric urinary incontinence. Am J Med 120:211, 2007.

4. Hashim H, Abrams P: Overactive bladder: an update. Curr Opin Urol 17:231, 2007.

5. Messelink B, Benson T, Berghmans B et al.: Standardization of terminology of pelvic floor muscle function and dysfunction: report from the pelvic floor clinical assessment group of the International Continence Society. Neurourol Urodyn 24:374, 2005.

CHAPTER 100

PEDIATRIC UROLOGY

Kirstan K. Meldrum, MD, and Mark P. Cain, MD

1. **A healthy 3-year-old girl develops a febrile urinary tract infection. How should she be evaluated?**
   After treatment of the infection, the patient should undergo a urinary tract evaluation with a renal-bladder sonogram and voiding cystourethrogram (VCUG). Approximately 50% of children under the age of 12 presenting with a urinary tract infection (UTI) are found to have abnormalities of the genitourinary (GU) tract. The most common abnormalities identified are vesicoureteral reflux (VUR), obstructive uropathies, and neurogenic bladder. In the absence of anatomic abnormalities, the most common causes of UTI in children are constipation and dysfunctional voiding.

2. **What is vesicoureteral reflux disease?**
   The reflux of urine from the bladder into the upper urinary tract. Primary VUR is caused by an inadequate valvular mechanism at the ureterovesical junction, presumably related to a shortened submucosal ureteral tunnel. One half of children with culture-documented UTIs have VUR.

3. **Is VUR damaging to the kidney?**
   Sterile reflux is unlikely to cause renal damage; however, the reflux of infected urine can lead to pyelonephritis and subsequent renal scarring. Currently, renal scarring is the fourth leading cause for renal transplantation in children. The combination of VUR and elevated bladder storage pressures (e.g., neuropathic bladder or bladder outlet obstruction) is harmful to the kidney, and a concurrent UTI makes this situation particularly dangerous!

4. **What are the indications for surgical correction of VUR?**
   Reflux disappears spontaneously in many children; however, high-grade reflux, especially when bilateral, is unlikely to resolve spontaneously. Children with high-grade reflux or breakthrough UTIs despite antibiotic prophylaxis should be managed surgically. Surgical management is also appropriate in children with reflux persisting into late childhood or adolescence.

5. **What is the most common cause of antenatal hydronephrosis?**
   Ureteropelvic junction (UPJ) obstruction. Hydronephrosis is the most common abnormality detected on prenatal ultrasound (US) and accounts for 50% of all prenatally detected lesions. Fifty percent of prenatal hydronephrosis, in turn, is caused by UPJ obstruction. UPJ obstruction is bilateral in approximately 20% of cases and associated with VUR in 15% of cases.

6. **What is the most common cause of UPJ obstruction?**
   Intrinsic stenosis. Less common causes include a lower pole (renal) crossing vessel, anomalous ureteral insertions (high in the renal pelvis), and peripelvic fibrosis.

7. **Can UPJ obstruction resolve spontaneously? What are the indications for pyeloplasty?**
   Yes. Ultimately, only about 25% of children with evidence of UPJ obstruction require pyeloplasty. The indications for surgical intervention include worsening hydronephrosis, poor or declining renal function, pain, infection, and the presence of a solitary kidney or bilateral hydronephrosis.

8. **What is the Meyer-Weigert law?**
This law refers to the position of the ureteral orifices in patients with complete ureteral duplication. Occasionally, two ureteral buds develop independently from the mesonephric duct. As the ureteral buds are absorbed into the developing bladder, the bud located in a lower position along the duct (draining the lower pole of the kidney) is carried to a more cranial and lateral position. The ureteral bud located in a higher position along the duct (draining the upper pole of the kidney) is carried to a more caudal and medial position within the bladder. Lower pole ureters are more likely to reflux because of their lateral position within the bladder, whereas upper pole ureters are more frequently obstructed and are more often associated with a ureterocele.

9. **What is a ureterocele?**
A ureterocele is a cystic dilatation of the distal portion of the ureter. Ureteroceles are usually associated with the upper pole ureter of a duplicated collecting system; however, they also may develop from single ureters. They are usually ectopic (i.e., some portion of the ureterocele is positioned at the bladder neck or urethra) and frequently cause ureteral obstruction.

10. **What is an ectopic ureter?**
A ureter with an ectopic opening (at or caudal to the level of the bladder neck).

11. **What is the most common presenting symptom in a girl with an ectopic ureter?**
Incontinence. In females, an ectopic ureter will usually drain into the bladder neck, proximal urethra, or vestibule. The orifice may also be located in the vagina (25%) and occasionally the uterus. When the ectopic ureteral orifice is positioned below the external sphincter or within the female genital tract, incontinence can develop. Infection is also a common presenting symptom of an ectopic ureter, occurring as a consequence of ureteral obstruction.

12. **Do boys with ectopic ureters present with incontinence?**
No. The ectopic pathway in boys extends from the bladder neck through the posterior urethra to the mesonephric duct derivatives (i.e., vas deferens, epididymis, and seminal vesicle). Therefore, the ectopic ureteral orifice is always positioned above the continence mechanism.

13. **What percentage of full-term male infants have an undescended testicle?**
Three percent. This number decreases to 0.8% by 1 year of age.

14. **What is the most common location of an undescended testicle?**
The inguinal canal (72% of undescended testicles). The testicle also may be located in the abdomen (8%) or prescrotal area (20%). Twenty percent of undescended testicles are nonpalpable at presentation; of these, 20% are absent completely.

15. **Why should the testicle be brought back into the scrotum?**
Patients with cryptorchidism have a 15-40 fold increased risk of germ cell cancer compared with the normal population. Although positioning of the testicle within the scrotum does not alleviate this risk, it does permit routine, thorough, testicular examination. Patients with cryptorchidism are also at risk for infertility. Histologic studies have demonstrated progressive germ cell loss in the undescended testicle beginning at 18 months of age. Early orchiopexy can minimize the extent of germ cell loss and thereby decrease the chance of future infertility. In general, the higher the testicle (i.e., within the abdomen), the greater the risk of cancer and infertility.

16. **What is the most common cause of bladder outlet obstruction in boys? In girls?**
Posterior urethral valves and ureterocele, respectively.

17. **What are the urinary manifestations of posterior urethral valves?**

    Posterior urethral valves are congenital leaflets of tissue, which extend from the verumontanum to the anterior urethra in boys. They occur at an incidence of 1/8000 live male births. Posterior urethral valves cause bladder outlet obstruction, which in turn, leads to variable degrees of bladder and renal injury. Severe obstruction may result in oligohydramnios, pulmonary hypoplasia, bladder hypertrophy, VUR, hydroureteronephrosis, and renal dysplasia. Fifty percent of affected children have reflux, and 33% progress to end-stage renal disease.

18. **What is a myelomeningocele? What are its urologic consequences?**

    A myelomeningocele is a hernial protrusion of the spinal cord and its meninges through a defect in the vertebral column. The resulting neurologic injury causes, among other problems, bladder dysfunction. Patients with myelomeningocele are usually incontinent because of detrusor hyperactivity, detrusor hypoactivity, poor bladder compliance, inadequate outlet resistance, detrusor-outlet dyssynergy, or a combination of these factors. More importantly, patients with hyperactive, high-pressure bladders may develop upper urinary tract deterioration. Life-long follow-up is necessary for these children because the neurologic lesion can change with time. Treatment goals include maintenance of a low-pressure urinary reservoir, prevention of UTIs, prevention of upper urinary tract deterioration, and the achievement of continence.

19. **What is the most common cause of ambiguous genitalia in the newborn?**

    Congenital adrenal hyperplasia, most commonly as a result of a 21-hydroxylase deficiency.

20. **What diagnostic evaluation should be performed in any male infant presenting with hypospadias and cryptorchidism?**

    The presence of cryptorchidism and hypospadias should alert the physician to the possibility of an androgenized female. A karyotype should always be obtained before surgical intervention.

21. **What is the most common solid renal mass in infancy? In childhood?**

    In **infancy:** congenital mesoblastic nephroma. This is a benign tumor of the kidney that can be managed with surgical excision alone. In **childhood:** Wilm's tumor. Wilm's tumor is associated with Beckwith-Wiedemann syndrome, isolated hemi-hypertrophy, and congenital aniridia. The most important prognostic factors are tumor stage and histology. Treatment is multimodal, consisting of surgery, chemotherapy, and radiation.

BIBLIOGRAPHY

1. Baker LA, Silver RI, Docimo SG: Cryptorchidism. In Gearhart JP, Rink RC, Mouriquand PDE editors: *Pediatric urology* Philadelphia, 2001, WB Saunders.

2. Chang SL, Shortliffe LD: Pediatric urinary tract infections. Pediatr Clin North Am 53:379-400, 2006.

3. Cooper CS, Snyder HM: Ureteral duplication, ectopy, and ureteroceles. In Gearhart JP, Rink RC, Mouriquand PDE editors: *Pediatric urology*, Philadelphia, 2001, WB Saunders.

4. Diamond DA: Sexual differentiation: normal and abnormal. In Wein AJ, Kavoussi LR, Novick AC et al., editors: *Campbell-Walsh urology*, Philadelphia, 2007, Saunders Elsevier.

5. Greenbaum LA, Mesrobian HG: Vesicoureteral reflux. Pediatr Clin North Am 53: 413-427, 2006.

6. Herndon CD: Prenatal hydronpehrosis: differential diagnosis, evaluation, and treatment options. Scientific World Journal, 6:2345-2365, 2006.

7. Hutson JM, Clarke MC: Current management of the undescended testicle. Semin Pediatr Surg 16:64-70, 2007.

8. Shortliff LM: Infection and inflammation of the pediatric genitourinary tract. In Wein AJ, Kavoussi LR, Novick AC et al.: *Campbell-Walsh urology*, Philadelphia, 2007, Saunders Elsevier.

9. Yeung CK, Sihoe JDY, Bauer SB: Voiding dysfunction in children non-neurogenic and neurogenic. In Wein AJ, Kavoussi LR, Novick AC et al., editors: *Campbell-Walsh urology*, Philadelphia, 2007, Saunders Elsevier.

10. Yohannes P, Hanna M: Current trends in the management of posterior urethral valves in the pediatric population. Urology 60:947-953, 2002.

CAN HEALTH CARE BE REFORMED?

Alden H. Harken, MD

CHAPTER 101

1. Is health care reform an oxymoron?
Yes.

2. What is fee for service?
The doctor establishes the price, and the patient agrees to pay it. This traditional system of exchange has great merit if both parties understand the value of the service provided. If either party (usually the patient) cannot estimate the service value, it is possible (even likely) that the doctor will honestly escalate the service value in a fashion unchecked by the patient's perceptions. Thus, in a fee-for-service system, medical prices tend to increase.

3. What is discounted fee for service?
The patient gets together with a group of friends, and they come to the doctor with the following proposition: "Hey, Doc, you can dazzle us with your fancy medical talk, but we still think that your prices are too high. How about my pals and me will pay you 80% of what you charge us?"

4. Is there a difference between hospital costs and hospital charges?
Absolutely. Hospital cost is the sum of the expenses (e.g., sutures, nurses' salaries, electricity, instrumentation sterilization, Band-Aids) that are expended in suturing a laceration, for example. The hospital typically charges about twice the cost (100% markup) for repairing a cut finger. This markup is highly industry specific. Thus, whereas intensely competitive food chains may make a profit of only one penny on a loaf of bread, hospitals and liquor stores usually charge twice the cost.

5. What are fixed costs?
After accounting for light, heat, and staff (nurses, housekeepers, administrators) at a hospital but before seeing a single patient, doctors and the hospital have already spent a huge amount of money. Doctors and hospitals must pay fixed costs whether or not they provide any medical services at all.

6. What are actual costs?
These are the incremental costs of actually providing a service in a hospital (in addition to the fixed costs of light and heat). For example, a patient shows up in the emergency department at midnight complaining of a lump on the tip of his nose. The doctor, with characteristic erudition, says, "Yep, you have a wart on your nose," and sends the patient home with a bill for $500. The actual cost of this encounter is obviously negligible. The patient is really paying for the fixed costs of nurses and emergency resuscitative equipment should he have a cardiac arrest.

7. Is hospital accounting a precisely scientific and objective analysis of financial data?
No.

8. **What is health insurance?**

Traditionally, people can purchase insurance that may pay either all or a portion of their hospital and physician charges if they become ill. Insurance companies make a profit, therefore, only if the patient stays healthy. Insurance companies have elaborate tables to predict who will get sick, and they prefer to sell policies exclusively to young, healthy individuals. This practice is termed "skimming." The insurance company takes all of the risk—and they like to keep it low. Conversely, hospitals must cover fixed costs—and the more expensive (and more frequent) the health care that physicians provide, the better it is for the hospitals.

9. **What are health maintenance organizations?**

Health maintenance organizations (HMOs) are complex systems composed, in their most comprehensive form, of hospitals, doctors plus offices, and an insurance company. HMOs contract with large groups of people (potential patients) to maintain their health. Enrollees pay a monthly fee (just like health insurance) so that all hospital and physician charges are covered if the enrollees become ill. Unlike health insurance, however, in the HMO model, hospitals and physicians get paid whether or not the enrollee gets sick. So, it is better for everyone if enrollees stay healthy—and out of the hospital.

10. **Initially, a lot of physicians did not like HMOs. Why?**

Because physicians are fiercely independent. They did not want a bunch of business managers telling them how to manage patients.

11. **Why are physicians fiercely independent?**

We were probably born that way.

12. **Is that good?**

Probably not. Eventually, everyone will need to work together and not hit each other when they are mad.

13. **Do HMO administrators really dictate how physicians manage their patients?**

Yes and no. Physicians have developed medically effective and optimally efficient strategies—termed clinical pathways—for caring for many common illnesses. Although physicians must treat each patient individually, when we adhere to predetermined treatment guidelines (as encouraged by HMO administrators), patients usually get better faster and cheaper.

14. **Do physicians follow these clinical pathways?**

Traditionally, no.

15. **What do HMO managers do?**

They evaluate each physician's use of expensive resources (within the predetermined clinical pathways) relative to the health of the physician's patients.

16. **Do physicians welcome this kind of scrutiny?**

No.

17. **What is a preferred provider organization (PPO)?**

A PPO is a group of doctors who have elected to remain legally independent of a hospital and insurance company (if they joined together, they would be an HMO) and, most of all, patients. But PPOs maintain their independence as physicians, even though most PPOs require administrators to coordinate programs, keep the books, and keep the doctors from hitting each other. PPOs have the perception of independence, however.

18. Is health care expensive?
Unfortunately, yes. Physicians argue that patients pay a lot but also get a lot. In the United States, patients expect unlimited access to liver transplantation and magnetic resonance imaging (MRI) for every headache. Americans believe that fancy, expensive health care is not just a privilege, it is a right.

19. So what is the problem?
The chief executive officers (CEOs) of big U.S. corporations argue that the obligatory expense of health care is driving up the cost of U.S. products and making U.S. companies less competitive in the global market—there is more health care than steel in a new Chevrolet.

20. Does big business have a solution?
They think so. The CEOs still want unlimited access to the most modern health care for themselves and their families. Without sounding cynical, the CEOs want to save health care dollars spent on their employees and "other people's families." They want to limit access to health care, but they do not want to wield the ax personally. So they developed the idea of capitation.

21. What is capitation?
The CEOs of large businesses come to hospitals, HMOs, or PPOs and say: "Why don't you provide all health care for all my employees at a fixed price, say, $180 per month per head?" (hence, capitation). In this model, physicians make the decisions about who gets how much medical care (satisfying their urge for independence), but they also promise to provide all necessary medical care for a prearranged price. Thus, they take all of the risk. CEOs like this model because they can still offer health care as an employee benefit and budget the cost in advance.

22. Why do physicians not like capitation?
All of a sudden physicians may have acquired a little more independence than they bargained for. Now they are paid in advance so that all costs of patients' health care are subtracted from the money they negotiated up front. Now they must advise against an MRI for every headache and break the news to Granny that she will not think better if they dialyze her blood urea nitrogen (BUN) down to 50. This is the reverse of the good old days when physicians were rewarded if their patients got sick and stayed sick. Physicians could ply them with a smorgasbord of drugs and technologies. Now physicians are trying to control health care costs.

23. Is all this change good?
Absolutely. Medicine has always changed—and the faster, the better. Physicians were initially attracted to medicine as an intellectually stimulating discipline because medicine and surgery evolve rapidly.

24. Can physicians keep up with all this change?
Absolutely.

25. Despite all of the medical Chicken Littles who sonorously declare that the sky is falling, is medicine (and even more clearly, surgery) still the most gratifying, stimulating, and rewarding profession?
Absolutely.

BIBLIOGRAPHY

1. Blumenthal D: Controlling health care expenditures. N Engl J Med 344:766-769, 2001.
2. Dudley RA, Luft HS: Managed care in transition. N Engl J Med 344:1087-1092, 2001.
3. Fuchs VR: What's ahead for health insurance in the United States? N Engl J Med 346:1822-1824, 2002.
4. Iglehart JK: Changing health insurance trends. N Engl J Med 347:956-962, 2002.
5. Schroeder SA: Prospects for expanding health insurance coverage. N Engl J Med 344:847-852, 2001.
6. Wilensky GR: Medicare reform-now is the time. N Engl J Med 345:458-462, 2001.
7. Wood AJ: When increased therapeutic benefit comes at increased cost. N Engl J Med 346:1819-1821, 2002.
8. Wright JG: Hidden barriers to improvement in the quality of health care. N Engl J Med 346:1096, 2002.

CHAPTER 102

ETHICS IN THE SURGICAL INTENSIVE CARE UNIT

Brian P. Callahan, MD, and Kathryn Beauchamp, MD

1. **What are the four principles of medical ethics?**
   1. **Beneficence** describes the active role of doing good by intervention.
   2. **Nonmaleficence** is equivalent to saying, "First do no harm."
   3. **Autonomy** accounts for informed consent, competence, and the patient's right to refuse treatment and to know what's going on.
   4. **Justice** means that all patients should receive fair and equal care but that one patient's care should not squander limited resources for others.

2. **What is a do-not-resuscitate order?**
   A do-not-resuscitate (DNR) order instructs the physician not to intervene if the patient is found pulseless or apneic; however, a DNR order is much more involved and complicated than the acronym would have you believe. DNR is not absolute. A DNR order does not have any implications on any other treatment decision. The Joint Commission for the Accreditation of Healthcare Organizations (JCAHO) mandates that hospitals have written guidelines that promote accountability for DNR orders. All DNR orders must be documented in writing, similar to all other orders, in the appropriate section of the patient's chart. They should specify the treatments to be withheld and treatments that the patient wishes to have implemented. Patients and families must participate in the DNR decision. Moreover, the DNR status should be discussed and reviewed with the other members of the healthcare team. Finally, a DNR order does not mean do not treat. DNR patients should not be medically abandoned.

3. **What is the difference between withdrawing and withholding support?**
   Withdrawing care is when all life-supporting measures are removed, whereas withholding support means no acceleration in care. Both decisions change the treatment goal from maintaining life and restoring health to maintaining comfort during the dying process. There is no moral or ethical distinction between withdrawal and withholding of support. Either of the two allows natural progression of disease without the interface of medical technology. The decision to withdraw or withhold support does not equate with patient death, although the probability of death may be greater. After the decision has been made, appropriate management should focus on the patient's comfort and psychosocial support.

4. **What is an advance directive?**
   An advance directive is a method of delineating a competent patient's wishes for application at a time when he or she is no longer competent. It maximizes the patient's autonomy, assists physicians in decision making, optimizes the use of medical resources, and provides protection from litigation. Medical management or the lack thereof can be based on the patient's wishes rather than a perceived sense of what is best for the patient. Advance directives may be an informal document, such as a living will, or a formal legal document, such as medical durable power of attorney. Advance directive laws vary state to state and are activated when

a patient is in a terminal state, state or permanent unconsciousness, or persistent vegetative state. Despite increased awareness of advance directives, only 25% of adults have them.

5. **What is durable power of attorney?**

A durable power of attorney is a patient-appointed proxy decision maker. The proxy decision maker becomes active as soon as the patient is no longer able to make competent medical decisions. Hence, the durable power of attorney must have been established in advance of the cognitive decline of the patient.

6. **What is a living will?**

A list of instructions made by a competent person about future medical treatment. It produces a preillness guideline for future care givers in accordance with the patient's wishes.

7. **What is included in informed consent?**

Informed consent is a voluntary decision made by the patient or on behalf of the patient by a proxy decision maker. It consists of an explanation of the patient's condition that is to be treated. It explains the proposed treatment in laymen's terms. It details the possible benefits and risks that are reasonably possible. It also includes a discussion of alternative therapies, and their likely outcomes. Importantly, it should also mention the outcome if no treatment is performed. Lastly, all of the patient's or proxy's questions and concerns should be addressed.

8. **What are futile care and medical futility?**

Ultimately, old age and disease will conquer us all. The definition of medically futile or inappropriate treatment is still debated. Nonetheless, there are four main concepts of medical futility:

1. Healthcare professionals are not required to provide **physiologically futile** treatment.
2. **Imminent demise** argues against treatment if the patient has no likelihood of survival to discharge.
3. Under the concept of **lethal condition,** medical care is considered futile if the patient will survive temporarily but ultimately expire as a result of the ongoing disease process.
4. Quality of life or **qualitative futility** argues against treatment if the patient's quality of life is so poor that it would be unreasonable to prolong life.

Care must be taken, however, in making medical decisions based on futility because these decisions may lead to self-fulfilling prophecies.

9. **What are the clinical determinants of brain death?**

Many of the current concepts of brain death are based on the 1968 report from the ad hoc committee at Harvard Medical School, which called for a new neurologic definition of brain death. But it was not until 1981 that James Bemat justified the neurologic criteria of brain death by stressing the need for intact brainstem integrative function for a person to function as a whole. The Uniform Determination of Death Act (UDDA) defines the legal definition of brain death in the United States as determination of death, using neurological criteria, of a patient who has sustained irreversible cessation of all function of the brain, including the brainstem. This determination should be made by accepted medical standards. The accepted medical standards vary state to state and hospital to hospital.

The first step is to document a cause for the permanent loss of brain functions. This is usually done by obtaining a computed tomography (CT) scan. This usually shows massive edema or diffuse ischemia. Reversible causes of decreased neurological function need to be ruled out. This includes metabolic derangements (electrolyte or acid-base) and intoxication. A toxicity screen should be performed on all patients. There should be an absence of all sedative and neuromuscular agents for at least 5 to 7 half-lives of the drug. Hypothermia, hypotension, and hypoxia need to be corrected. The clinical examination includes showing no motor response to noxious stimuli, absence of brain stem reflexes (fixed pupils, no corneal, occulocephalic, occulovestibular, gag, or cough responses), and no breathing drive after a carbon dioxide (CO_2) challenge (apnea test). If the patient has injuries that do not allow complete neurological testing, such as facial trauma or spinal cord injury, confirmatory tests will need to be performed. These include angiography, transcranial Doppler, electroencephalogram (EEG), or radionucleotide scintigraphy. In children, the process is identical except children between 1 and 18 should have repeat testing after 12 hours, and children <1 should have 48 hours of observation with at least one confirmatory test.

10. **What is a persistent vegetative state?**
In a persistent vegetative state, typically seen after improvement of a comatose state, the patient opens their eyes but shows only reflexive behavior. The patient appears to be awake but does not have awareness of his or her surroundings or higher mental activity. Other names for this entity are coma vigil and akinetic mutism.

11. **What is euthanasia?**
Euthanasia requires that the physician play an active role in assisting in the death of the patient. The concepts of physician-assisted suicide and active and passive euthanasia are highly controversial. In 1992, the Society of Critical Care Medicine published the results of a survey of critical care specialists; 87% had withdrawn life-prolonging support from patients. In addition, the most recent U.S. law pertaining to assisted suicide was passed in Oregon in 1994. This law makes it legal for a physician to prescribe medication to terminally ill patients for the purpose of committing suicide.

12. **Who should approach patients' families about organ donation?**
The organ procurement organization should be the first to approach the family. This is called the decoupling principle, and it eliminates any conflict of interest. Some claim that the physician who has established good rapport with the patient's family should raise the issue of organ donation. The best approach is probably a combined one. After the organ procurement organization has approached the patient, the physicians should be available if the family wishes to speak to them.

13. **What should patients' families be told when organ donation is feasible?**
The surgeon should stress that the patient has died despite an actively beating heart and that they are not suffering or feeling any pain. The family should be questioned about the patient's wishes regarding organ donation. All topics should be based on the concepts of informed consent. The family should be informed of the likelihood that several patients will benefit from the donated organs. The family needs to understand that there is no guarantee that the organs will be suitable for donation. They should be assured that they are not responsible for the cost of care provided after brain death is determined and that they may refuse organ donation without fear of prejudice.

14. **What is organ donation after cardiac death?**
This is the process in which organs are procured on a patient that has not been declared brain dead. Most of these patients have suffered catastrophic brain or spinal cord injuries but have not met the clinical definition of brain death. The same informed consent procedure is performed as with brain dead patients. The patient is taken to the operating room (OR) and care is withdrawn. A doctor, who is not involved in the procurement of the organs or in the transplantation of the organs, is present and declares death. After cardiac death is pronounced, the procurement team enters the OR and proceeds.

15. **What is the role of the hospital ethics committee?**
The hospital ethics committee educates hospital staff members and provides a source of consultation.

The function of education is accomplished through grand rounds, seminars, special lectures, and journal clubs. The hospital ethics committee should be viewed as an intrinsic part of the hospital community. Developed policies should be reviewed by other committees and divisions of the hospital to foster a better sense of cohesiveness when ethical and moral dilemmas arise.

The hospital ethics committee is made up of physicians and ancillary staff with special training in medical ethics. They can and should provide an arena for collaboration and general ethical education within the hospital.

BIBLIOGRAPHY

1. Ad Hoc Committee of the Harvard School to Examine the Definition of Brain Death: A definition of irreversible coma. JAMA 205:337-340, 1968.
2. Bernat JL: How can we achieve uniformity in brain death determinations? Neurology J70(4):284-289, 2008.
3. Harken AH: Enough is enough. Arch Surg 10:1061-1063, 1999.
4. Laureys S, Boly M: What is it like to be vegetative or minimally conscious? Curr Opin Neurol 20(6):609-613, 2007.
5. Luce JM, White DB: The pressure to withhold or withdraw life-sustaining therapy from critically ill patients in the United States. Am J Respir Crit Care Med 177(1):1104-1108, 2008.
6. Mirarchi FL: Does a living will equal a DNR? Are living wills compromising patient safety? J Emerg Med 33(3):299-305, 2007.
7. Nishimura A, Mueller PS, Evenson LK et al.: Patients who complete advance directives and what they prefer. Mayo Clin Proc 82(12):1480-1486, 2007.
8. Steinbrook R: Organ donation after cardiac death. New Engl J Med 357(3):209-213, 2007.
9. Wijdicks EF: 10 questions about the clinical determination of brain death. Neurologist 13(6):380-381, 2007.

CHAPTER 103

PROFESSIONALISM

U. Mini B. Swift, MD, David Altman, MD, MBA, and Alden H. Harken, MD

1. What is a profession?

The professions are the means by which the complex services needed by society are organized. A profession has been defined by the American College of Surgeons as:

> an occupation whose core element is work that is based upon the mastery of a complex body of knowledge and skills. It is a vocation in which knowledge of some department of science or learning, or the practice of an art founded upon it, is used in the service of others. Its members are governed by codes of ethics and profess a commitment to competence, integrity and morality, altruism and to the promotion of the public good within their domain. These commitments form the basis of a social contract between a profession and society, which, in turn, grants the profession a monopoly over the use of its knowledge base, the right to considerable autonomy in practice and the privilege of self-regulation. Professions and their members are accountable to those served and to society.

2. What are the core elements of a profession?

All professions are characterized by four core elements: (1) a monopoly over the use of specialized knowledge; (2) in return for that monopoly that we enjoy, relative autonomy in practice and the responsibility of self-regulation; (3) altruistic service to individuals and society; and (4) responsibility for maintaining and expanding professional knowledge and skills.

3. What is professionalism?

Professionalism describes the cognitive, moral, and collegial attributes of a professional. Ultimately, it is all the reasons that your mother is proud to say that you are a doctor and a surgeon.

4. Why do physicians need a code of professional conduct?

Trust is integral to the practice of surgery. The Code of Professional Conduct clarifies the relationship between the surgical profession and the society it serves. This is often referred to as a social contract. For patients the code of professional conduct crystallizes the commitment of the surgical community toward individual patients and their communities. Trust is built brick by brick.

5. What is the American College of Surgeons Code of Professional Conduct?

The Code of Professional Conduct takes the general principles of professionalism and applies them to surgical practice. The code is the foundation on which we earn our professional privileges and the trust of patients and the public. It is our job description.

6. What are the responsibilities of professionalism described in the American College of Surgeons Code of Professional Conduct?

During the continuum of the preoperative, intraoperative, and postoperative care surgeons have the responsibility to:

1. Serve as effective advocates for our patients' needs.
2. Disclose therapeutic options including their risks and benefits.
3. Disclose and resolve any conflict of interest that might influence the decisions of care.
4. Be sensitive and respectful of patients, understanding their vulnerability during the perioperative period.

5. Fully disclose adverse events and medical errors.
6. Acknowledge patients' psychological, social, cultural and spiritual needs.
7. Encompass within our surgical care the special needs of terminally ill patients.
8. Acknowledge and support the needs of patients' families and
9. Respect the knowledge, dignity, and perspective of other healthcare professionals.

7. **Do other professional societies have a code of professional conduct?**
Yes. Several groups have created professional codes and the American College of Surgeons supports their declarations.

8. **Why do surgeons need their own code of professionalism?**
A surgical procedure is an extreme experience. We impact our patients physiologically, psychologically, and socially. When patients submit themselves to a surgical experience, they must trust that the surgeon will put their welfare above all other considerations. The written code helps to reinforce these values.

9. **What are the fundamental principles of the Code of Professional Conduct and the codes of other professional societies?**
   1. The primacy of patient welfare.
   2. Patient autonomy.
   3. Social justice.

10. **What is the "primacy of patient welfare"?**
This means that the patient's interests always come first. Altruism is central to this concept, and it is the surgeon's altruism that fosters trust in the physician-patient relationship.

11. **What is the "principle of patient autonomy"?**
Patients must understand and make their own informed decisions about their treatment. This is tricky. As physicians we must be honest with our patients so that they make educated decisions. At the same time, we must make sure that their decisions are consistent with ethical practices and do not lead to demands for inappropriate care.

12. **What is the "principle of social justice"?**
As physicians we must advocate for our individual patients while at the same time promoting the health of the healthcare system as a whole. We must balance our patient's needs (autonomy) and not misdirect scarce resources that benefit society (social justice).

13. **How can I apply these lofty ideas to my everyday existence on the medical-surgical unit?**
The American College of Surgeons Code of Professional Conduct lists the responsibilities of being a surgeon specifically. For all other situations, use the guiding principles to dictate your actions. A few examples include:
Pursuit of the *"just and equitable distribution of finite resources"* could mean that you do not order unnecessary tests or even give 20 units of blood to a Child's C cirrhotic.
"Commitment to improving quality of care" is honored by submitting ideas to improve work flow on the wards to your chief resident, program director, or even department chair.
As a student you have a unique opportunity to spend a little extra time with a frightened patient (they are all frightened) and to help explain the nature of the disease and what the plans are to do something. Use little words—not doctor words. Patients and families will love you for doing this. And this understanding promotes patient autonomy.

BIBLIOGRAPHY

1. ABIM Foundation, ACP-ASIM Foundation, European Federation of Internal Medicine: Medical professionalism in the new millennium: a physician charter. Ann Intern Med 136(3):243-246, 2002.

2. Cruess SR, Johnston S, Cruess RL: Professionalism for medicine: opportunities and obligations. Med J Aust 177:208-211, p. 208, 2002.

3. American College of Surgeons Task Force on Professionalism: Code of Professional Conduct. J Am Coll Surg 197:603-604, 2003.

4. American College of Surgeons Task Force on Professionalism: Code of Professional Conduct. J Am Coll Surg 199:734-735, 2004.

5. Kopp M, Bonatti H, Haller C et al.: Life satisfaction and active coping style are important predictors of recovery from surgery. J Psychosom Res 55(4):371-377, 2003.

6. Rosenberger PH, Joki P, Ickovics J: Psychosocial factors and surgical outcomes: an evidence-based literature review. J Am Acad Orthop Surg 14(7):397-405, 2006.

7. Roth RS, Lowery JC, Davis J et al.: Psychological factors predict patient satisfaction with postmastectomy breast reconstruction. Plast Reconstr Surg 119(7):2008-2015; discussion 2016-2017, 2007.

INDEX

Page numbers followed by *t* indicate tables; *f,* figures. Page numbers in **boldface** type indicate complete chapters.